DIETARY FIBER

Basic and Clinical Aspects

DIETARY FIBER

Basic and Clinical Aspects

Edited by

George V. Vahouny

The George Washington University Medical Center
Washington, D.C.

and

David Kritchevsky

The Wistar Institute
Philadelphia, Pennsylvania

PLENUM PRESS • NEW YORK AND LONDON

Library of Congress Cataloging in Publication Data

Washington Symposium on Dietary Fiber (2nd: 1984: Washington, D.C.)
  Dietary fiber.

  "Proceedings of the second Washington Symposium on Dietary Fiber, held
April 25–28, 1984, in Washington, D.C."—T.p. verso.
  Includes bibliographies and index.
  1. High-fiber diet—Congresses. 2. Fiber deficiency diseases—Congresses.
I. Vahouny, George V., 1932–   . II. Kritchevsky, David, 1920–   . III. Title.
[DNLM: 1. Dietary Fiber—congresses. W3 WA33 2nd 1984d/WB 427 W319
1984d]
RM237.6.W36   1984   613.2′8   85-19159
ISBN-13:978-1-4612-9249-4   e-ISBN-13:978-1-4613-2111-8
DOI: 10.1007/978-1-4613-2111-8

Proceedings of the Second Washington Symposium on Dietary Fiber,
held April 25–28, 1984, in Washington, D.C.

© 1986 Plenum Press, New York
Softcover reprint of the hardcover 1st edition 1986

A Division of Plenum Publishing Corporation
233 Spring Street, New York, N.Y. 10013

Contributors

MARGARET J. ALBRINK • Department of Medicine, West Virginia University School of Medicine, Morgantown, West Virginia

R. ALI • Nutritional Research and Development, Bristol-Meyers International Division, New York, New York

JAMES W. ANDERSON • Medical Service, Veterans Administration Medical Center, and Department of Medicine, University of Kentucky College of Medicine, Lexington, Kentucky

ARNOLD BERSTAD • Department of Medicine, Lovisenberg Hospital, Oslo, Norway

SHEILA A. BINGHAM • University of Cambridge and MRC Dunn Clinical Nutrition Centre, Cambridge, United Kingdom

CHARLES T. BONFIELD • Farma Food, Washington, D.C.

CYNTHIA L. BOULANGER • Department of Nutrition and Food Science, and The Statistics Center, Massachusetts Institute of Technology, Cambridge, Massachusetts

WILLIAM J. BRANCH • MRC Dunn Clinical Nutrition Centre, Cambridge, United Kingdom

W. GORDON BRYDON • Wolfson Gastrointestinal Laboratories, Department of Medicine, Western General Hospital, Edinburgh, United Kingdom

ARTHUR W. BULL, Jr. • Department of Surgery, Wayne State University School of Medicine, Detroit, Michigan

DENIS P. BURKITT • The Old House, Stroud, Gloscestershire, United Kingdom

RITVA R. BUTRUM • National Cancer Institute, Bethesda, Maryland

F. ANN CARR • Department of Nutrition and Food Sciences, and The Statistics Center, Massachusetts Institute of Technology, Cambridge, Massachusetts

K. K. CARROLL • Department of Biochemistry, University of Western Ontario, London, Ontario, Canada

MARIE M. CASSIDY • Department of Physiology, George Washington University School of Medicine and Health Sciences, Washington, D. C.

W. J. L. CHEN • Medical Service, Veterans Administration Medical Center, and Department of Medicine, University of Kentucky College of Medicine, Lexington, Kentucky

BERTRAM I. COHEN • Departments of Surgery, Beth Israel Medical Center and Mount Sinai School of Medicine of the City University of New York, New York, New York

BARBARA H. CONNER • Department of Nutrition and Food Science, and The Statistics Center, Massachusetts Institute of Technology, Cambridge, Massachusetts

JOHN H. CUMMINGS • MRC Dunn Clinical Nutrition Centre, Cambridge, United Kingdom

WILLIAM D. DEWYS • National Cancer Institute, Bethesda, Maryland

WILLIAM H. DUMOUCHEL • Department of Nutrition and Food Science, and The Statistics Center, Massachusetts Institute of Technology, Cambridge, Massachusetts

MARTIN A. EASTWOOD • Wolfson Gastrointestinal Laboratories, Department of Medicine, Western General Hospital, Edinburgh, United Kingdom

HANS N. ENGLYST • MRC Dunn Clinical Nutrition Centre, Cambridge, United Kingdom

KATHLEEN FADDEN • PHLS Centre of Applied Microbiology and Research, Bacterial Metabolism Research Laboratory, Salisbury, Wiltshire, United Kingdom

LEO R. FITZPATRICK • Department of Physiology, George Washington University School of Medicine and Health Sciences, Washington, D. C.

THOMAS FRANCIS • Department of Nutritional Sciences, Faculty of Medicine, University of Toronto, Toronto, Canada

PETER GREENWALD • National Cancer Institute, Bethesda, Maryland

ERIK GREGERSEN • Department of Gynecology and Obstetrics, Sct. Maria Hospital, Vejle, Denmark

K. W. HEATON • Department of Medicine, University of Bristol, and Bristol Royal Infirmary, Bristol, United Kingdom

MICHAEL J. HILL • PHLS Centre for Applied Microbiology and Research, Salisbury, Wiltshire, United Kingdom

KATSUMI IMAIZUMI • Laboratory of Nutrition Chemistry, Kyushu University School of Agriculture, Fukuoka, Japan

LUCIEN R. JACOBS • Department of Internal Medicine, Division of Gastroenterology, School of Medicine, University of California, Davis, California

ALEXANDRA L. JENKINS • Department of Nutritional Sciences, Faculty of Medicine, and Division of Endocrinology and Metabolism, St. Michael's Hospital, University of Toronto, Toronto, Canada

DAVID J. A. JENKINS • Department of Nutritional Sciences, Faculty of Medicine, and Division of Endocrinology and Metabolism, St. Michael's Hospital, University of Toronto, Toronto, Canada

PATRICIA A. JUDD • Department of Nutrition, Queen Elizabeth College, University of London, London, United Kingdom

JUNE L. KELSAY • Carbohydrate Nutrition Laboratory, U. S. Department of Agriculture Agricultural Research Service, Beltsville, Maryland

DAVID M. KLURFELD • The Wistar Institute of Anatomy and Biology, Philadelphia, Pennsylvania

DAVID KRITCHEVSKY • The Wistar Institute of Anatomy and Biology, Philadelphia, Pennsylvania

SOON Y. LEE • Department of Nutrition and Food Science, and The Statistics Center, Massachusetts Institute of Technology, Cambridge, Massachusetts

ANTHONY R. LEEDS • Department of Nutrition, Queen Elizabeth College, University of London, and Department of General Medicine and Endocrinology, Central Middlesex Hospital, London, United Kingdom

MICHAEL LEFEVRE • Department of Nutrition, University of California, Davis, California

LINDA F. MCKAY • Wolfson Gastrointestinal Laboratories, Department of Medicine, Western General Hospital, Edinburgh, United Kingdom

ERWIN H. MOSBACH • Departments of Surgery, Beth Israel Medical Center and Mount Sinai School of Medicine of the City University of New York, New York, New York

NORMAN D. NIGRO • Department of Surgery, Wayne State University School of Medicine, Detroit, Michigan

M. I. ODENDAAL • Department of Physiology, University of Potchefstroom, Potchefstroom, South Africa

G. M. OWEN • Nutritional Research and Development, Bristol-Meyers International Division, New York, New York

LEON PROSKY • Experimental Nutrition Branch, Division of Nutrition, Bureau of Foods, Food and Drug Administration, Washington, D. C.

A. VENKETESHWER RAO • Department of Nutritional Sciences, Faculty of Medicine, University of Toronto, Toronto, Canada

N. W. READ • Clinical Research Unit, Royal Hallamshire Hospital, Sheffield, United Kingdom

BANDARU S. REDDY • Naylor Dana Institute for Disease Prevention, American Health Foundation, Valhalla, New York

ADRIANNE E. ROGERS • Department of Pathology, Boston University School of Medicine, Boston, Massachusetts

ANDREAS RYDNING • Department of Medicine, Lovisenberg Hospital, Oslo, Norway

ABIGAIL A. SALYERS • Department of Microbiology, University of Illinois, Urbana, Illinois

L. M. SCHANBACHER • Nutritional Research and Development, Bristol-Meyers International Division, New York, New York

BARBARA OLDS SCHNEEMAN • Department of Nutrition, University of California, Davis, California

I. SEGAL • Department of Gastoenterology, Baragwanath Hospital, Johannesburg, South Africa

DAVID A. T. SOUTHGATE • AFRC Food Research Institute, Norwich, United Kingdom

JON A. STORY • Department of Foods and Nutrition, Purdue University, West Lafayette, Indiana

MICHIHIRO SUGANO • Laboratory of Nutrition Chemistry, Kyushu University School of Agriculture, Fukuoka, Japan

RODNEY H. TAYLOR • Department of Gastroenterology and Nutrition, Central Middlesex Hospital, University of London, London, United Kingdom

LILIAN U. THOMPSON • Department of Nutritional Sciences, Faculty of Medicine, University of Toronto, Toronto, Canada

IRMA H. ULLRICH • Department of Medicine, West Virginia University School of Medicine, Morgantown, West Virginia

GEORGE V. VAHOUNY • Department of Biochemistry, George Washington University School of Medicine and Health Sciences, Washington, D. C.

JOHN E. VANDERVEEN • Food and Drug Administration, Division of Nutrition, Washington, D. C.

A. R. P. WALKER • School of Pathology, South African Institute of Medical Research, and University of the Witwatersrand, Johannesburg, South Africa

MAXINE M. WEBER • The Wistar Institute of Anatomy and Biology, Philadelphia, Pennsylvania

THOMAS M. S. WOLEVER • Department of Nutritional Sciences, Faculty of Medicine, and Division of Endocrinology and Metabolism, St. Michael's Hospital, University of Toronto, Toronto, Canada

Foreword

Only 15 years ago a conference on dietary fiber, let alone an international conference, would have been considered an extremely unlikely, and in fact an unthinkable, event. Yet in recent years a number of such conferences have taken place at the international level and in different parts of the world; the conference of which the present volume is an outgrowth is the second to have been held in Washington, D.C.

This extraordinary development of interest in a hitherto largely neglected component of diet has been reflected by a veritable explosion of scientific literature, with published articles increasing 40-fold, from around ten to over 400 per year, within the decade 1968–1978.

Not only has the growth of interest in and knowledge of fiber made it perhaps the most rapidly developing aspect of nutritional science in recent history if not in all time, but epidemiologic studies relating fiber intake to disease patterns, subsequently broadened to include other food components, have been largely responsible for the current concept of diseases characteristic of modern Western culture and lifestyle. The potential importance of this realization is forcefully underlined by the considered judgment of Thomas MacKeown, epidemiologist and medical historian of Birmingham University, England. He has asserted that just as the recognition that infective disease was related to factors in the environment that could be controlled was the greatest single medical advance in the 19th century, the recognition that the chronic noninfective diseases characteristic of modern Western culture are likewise due to factors in the environment that can be controlled may prove to be the greatest medical advance of the 20th century.

When fiber is seen in this light there is no need to emphasize the significance of what might appear to the uninitiated to be just another conference on fiber. With work and knowledge expanding at its present rate, the potential benefits of bringing together authorities on the increasingly expanding and varied aspects of the subject for an interchange of ideas and discussion of problems could scarcely be exaggerated.

It might be appropriate here to consider fiber's *curriculum vitae,* and the incredibly slow and ignominious progress of its early life, before it took root and began its rapid growth to its present stature.

In the fourth century B.C. Hippocrates commented, "To the human body it makes a great difference whether the bread be made of fine flour or coarse, whether of the wheat with the bran or the wheat without the bran."

Thirteen centuries later a Persian physician, Hakim, wrote: "Wheat is a beneficial cereal. Chuppatis are made from wheat flour. Chuppatis containing more bran come out of the digestive tract quicker. Those containing little bran take a long time to be excreted."

In Shakespeare's play *Coriolanus,* the gut proclaims its unselfish nature. All the nourishment that is put into it is given out again to the various parts of the body. But the gut then says, "Though all at once cannot see what I deliver out to each, yet I can make my audit up, that all from me do back receive the flour of all, and leave me but the bran" (*Coriolanus,* Act 1, Scene 1).

In the 19th century Graham in the U. S. endeavored to draw attention to roughage, as did Allinson in the U. K. The latter had his name erased from the medical register for the unethical practice of selling whole meal (whole wheat) bread, and henceforth the name plate outside his London consulting rooms announced him as "Ex. L.R.C.P."! His name is perpetuated in the U. K. in "Allinson's Bread."

Other lone voices cried largely in the wilderness prior to World War II. Sir Albuthnot Lane, the English society surgeon whose name is still linked to anatomic anomalies and surgical instruments, believed that many ailments were related to stagnation of colonic contents. It is stated, whether apocryphally or factually is open to question, that he treated this condition by excising the colon, before he recognized that the administration of Miller's bran was an equally effective and less drastic remedy.

Sir Robert McCarrison attributed the health of the tribesmen of northern India among whom he worked to their largely vegetarian diet and their consumption of minimally processed foods.

The brothers John and William Kellogg extolled the virtues of bran. Unfortunately, when one of them began to make commercial products, they quarreled to the extent of instituting litigation against one another. Their name is of course perpetuated in breakfast cereal products that continue to make fiber-rich foods available.

The outstanding British protagonist of fiber, then considered as cellulose, in the 1920s, was the British surgeon Arthur Rendle-Short. He was the first doctor to argue convincingly with abundant epidemiological and other evidence that cellulose-depleted diets played a dominant role in the causation of appendicitis.

At about the same time Cowgill and Anderson (1932) were extolling the laxative virtues of wheat bran in the U. S. A few years later, Ted Dimmock, who subsequently worked as a family physician both in Britain and abroad, demonstrated the role of fiber in treating constipation and piles.

It was after World War II that three of the pioneers most responsible for the early development of the fiber hypothesis emerged. T. L. Cleave, a physician in the Royal Navy, acquired a reputation, not always complimentary, for successfully treating constipation in sailors at sea by using Miller's bran. Subsequently he put his ideas in a popular book, *The Saccharine Disease*, published in the mid-1960s. He was among the first to draw attention to the relationship between certain characteristically Western diseases and diets, with emphasis on the danger of sugar, but at the same time recognizing the benefits of fiber. It was not until a few years before his death in 1983 that his work was in any way adequately recognized by the conferral of two prestigious medals.

While Cleave was thinking his revolutionary ideas in England, Dr. Hugh Trowell was thinking along similar lines in East Africa, where he worked as a physician for 35 years. He was the first to list in a medical textbook diseases common in the West but rare in Africa. Although he did not specifically incriminate refined carbohydrate foods in the way Cleave had done, he suspected that the bulky stools passed by Africans were somehow protective against some of these diseases. It was he who first coined the term "dietary fiber." He was one of the first, if not the first, to suggest that fiber could confer protection against diabetes, obesity, and ischemic heart disease.

A third name that must be linked with those of Cleave and Trowell is Walker of South Africa. During the war years he began to recognize a relationship between fiber intake, large stools, and a low incidence of certain gastrointestinal diseases, and he has been making significant contributions to this subject ever since.

My interest in this field was first stimulated by Cleave, whose observations opened my eyes to the enormous possibility of massive disease prevention. However, I had an advantage denied to Cleave, because of my previous work in another field. I was accorded credibility and consequently given the hearing that had been denied to others. Moreover, the information collection network that I had built up in much of the Third World for gathering information on cancer distribution was tailor-made for confirming or refuting Cleave's hypothesis. Although this information might in the initial stages have been considered anecdotal, massive and consistent information of this nature has to be and was taken seriously. Only a few others, notably Southgate and Eastwood, entered the field before the end of the 1960s.

Until recently, those actively involved in the study of dietary fiber and related aspects of diet and disease were a small enough group to be for the most part known to one another personally, with the immense benefits that such relationships bring to cooperative studies. Now that the number has grown, gatherings such as the one that led to the present volume are immensely valuable not only, and not even primarily, to learn the progress of one another's work, but more importantly to renew old and make new friendships, to replace mere names by recognizable faces, and to forge those links of friendship between workers in different fields and in different countries that have so often been the starting point of invaluable new ventures in scientific exploration. It is these meetings among individuals with complementary interests and abilities that are likely to bear much fruit in years to come.

We must all be grateful to those who conceive and organize such conferences, so that workers in this field can enjoy the opportunities of friendly scientific exchange that were denied to its pioneers.

Denis Burkitt

Dedication

SURGEON-CAPTAIN T. L. CLEAVE, MRCS, FRCP
August 8, 1906–September 15, 1983

The son of a Royal Navy Captain and engineer, Peter Cleave (as he was always known) was born in Exeter and educated in Bristol. He finished his training at St. Mary's Hospital and went straight into the Royal Navy. There he was Medical Specialist in various hospitals, ending up as Surgeon-Captain and Director of Medical Research until he retired in 1962.

In the 1970s Cleave received international acclaim as the father of the dietary fiber hypothesis, but for 20 years before that he had been an obscure and ridiculed writer. As a boy he had become convinced of the importance of diet to health. At medical school he was taught by Rendle-Short, who propounded that appendicitis is caused by a lack of cellulose in the diet. At this time he was also profoundly influenced by the writings of Charles Darwin and henceforth he built all his theories on the rock of the adaptation of species to their environment. His great vision was the realization that the human body must be maladapted to the artificial foods of civilization, of which the most artificial were the refined carbohydrates, chiefly sugar and white flour. He reasoned that if man avoided unnatural foods he would surely avoid unnatural diseases, that is, diseases absent in wild animals or primitive communities. He spent his life gathering evidence and developing arguments to support this view, which culminated in his grand hypothesis of a range of diseases caused by maladaptation to the foods and drinks containing refined carbohydrate. These diseases included obesity, diabetes, coronary heart disease, peptic ulcer, dental caries, constipation, appendicitis, and varicose veins. Since they all had a common cause he viewed them as a single master disease, "the Saccharine Disease." His book of this name, published in 1974, sold many thousands of copies. Previously, he had written books on varicose veins and peptic ulcer.

Cleave was slow to achieve recognition for several reasons. At a time when others were learning to trust only randomized trials and probability values, he trusted in the lessons of nature and logical argument. He was recording differences in disease patterns over time and space long before the epidemiology of chronic disease was a recognized discipline. He looked for big differences and had no use for statistical analysis. He painted with broad strokes on the biggest possible canvas when others were focusing on ever more minute areas of investigation. At his own expense, he published his lofty ideas and findings in books, while ordinary mortals submitted humbly to peer review and the rule of editors.

Cleave's most effective advocate was Denis Burkitt, F. R. S., already famous in another field, and the meeting of the two men in 1967 was the turning point in the fortunes of Cleave's hypothesis. Burkitt's connections with 150 Third World hospitals enabled him to confirm many of Cleave's epidemiologic observations and even to add to his list of Western diseases explicable in terms of refined carbohydrate.

The idea of fiber-depletion is inherent in Cleave's concept, but he preferred to emphasize the dangers of sugar, the fiber-depleted extract of sugar cane and sugar beet. However, in 1941 he had been one of the first to advocate raw bran in medical practice. While serving on the battleship *King George V* he had sacks of bran brought on board to combat the constipation that was prevalent in sailors deprived of fresh fruit and vegetables. Bran was so effective that Cleave became known throughout the navy as "the bran man."

In 1979, Cleave was awarded the Harben Gold Medal of the Royal Institute of Public Health and Hygiene (previously awarded to Pasteur, Lister, and Fleming) and the Gilbert Blane Medal for naval medicine, which is awarded jointly by the Royal Colleges of Physicians and Surgeons, but had never before been given to a retired man. A few months later, the Royal College of Physicians published its report *Medical Aspects of Dietary Fibre* which largely vindicated Cleave's theory and summarized the large body of research that it had stimulated. However, the full story is yet to be told. In particular, the full implications of overnutrition and the role of fiber-depleted foods in causing it have not received the emphasis that Cleave believed they deserved. His last work, published in 1977, was an article entitled, "Overnutrition, now the most dangerous cause of disease in westernised countries."

Cleave was certainly one of the most original medical thinkers of the 20th century. His rare combination of panoramic vision, piercing logic, and bulldog tenacity deserves the title of genius. He was a true pioneer, who started a major revolution in scientific thought.

Preface

The first Spring Symposium on Dietary Fiber in Health and Disease was held in Washington, D.C. in 1981 and was an outgrowth of belief that informal discussion among peers was the most effective way to organize our current knowledge and direct our thinking. The Symposium and its published proceedings were considered singularly successful in achieving these goals. It resulted in a free exchange of ideas and established collaborations based on mutual interest and friendship.

The success of this concept is reflected in the composition and quality of the participants of the Second Washington Symposium on Dietary Fibers, which was held in the nation's capital in the spring of 1984. This conference, like its predecessor, was conducted with informality and openness, and was further enriched by the participation of Denis Burkitt and A. R. P. Walker. The conference was honored to have Denis Burkitt as its keynote speaker, and the expression of his historical perspective is included as the Foreword to this volume. Unfortunately, two of the other "founding fathers" of the modern fiber field, Hugh Trowell and T. L. Cleave, were not in attendance. Professor Trowell was unable to attend because of personal reasons, but his influence was felt. Captain Cleave, whose pioneering work is alluded to in the Foreword, had died in the preceding year. We felt it fitting to include a tribute to him in this volume.

This volume presents a current, thorough, and integrative overview of all aspects of the field. It opens with discussions of fiber analyses, progress in relating fiber chemistry and function, and certain socioeconomic and regulatory aspects of dietary fibers in foods and as food supplements.

Chapters on the effects of fiber on gastrointestinal physiology and function are followed by discussions of the application of fiber in specific human disorders. These include disorders of lipid metabolism, overweight and obesity, diabetes, constipation, ulcers, and gallstones. The closing chapters are devoted to various aspects of dietary fiber and cancer, which were organized as a separate satellite with the support of the National Cancer Institute. The scope and depth of the contributions to this volume include material on both basic background and future directions, and provide a valuable resource to others interested in dietary fiber in health and disease.

We are grateful to all of the conferees for their valuable suggestions on the organization of the Symposium and on the inclusion of additional participants. In particular, we wish to acknowledge the invaluable effort of Karen Ries, Pamela Bonfield, and Charlotte Robinson in ensuring the success and efficiency of all aspects of the conference, and of S. Satchithanandam and R. Chanderbhan in audiotaping and slide projection. We also wish to acknowledge Fran Nigro for assistance in the preparation of the index.

The organizers are also indebted to George Washington University and to Farma Food for their interest and generous support for the conference as well as other areas of research and communication involving human health and disease. We also greatly appreciate the supportive role of Drs. W. DeWys and R. Butrum of the National Cancer Institute, U. S. Public Health Service, in developing the satellite on Future Directions in Research on Dietary Fiber and Cancer.

George V. Vahouny

Contents

Analysis of Total Dietary Fiber: The Collaborative Study

LEON PROSKY

1. INTRODUCTION

In the fall of 1979 the Association of Official Analytical Chemists (AOAC) set out to develop and test suitable methods for dietary fiber analysis through collaborative studies. The need for such methods was stimulated by the publications of Burkitt *et al.* (1972), Trowell (1972), and Burkitt (1973), who represented dietary fiber as food ingredients that would cure a number of chronic degenerative diseases. During the past few years the AOAC associate referee for dietary fiber sought (1) to define dietary fiber in terms of chemical components, (2) to perform and/or evaluate intralaboratory methods for quantitatively measuring these components, and (3) to subject the most promising procedures to collaborative study. To help arrive at a definition and method of choice for dietary fiber we contacted more than 100 scientists who were actively engaged in determining dietary fiber. Included in this group were many of the persons who contributed to a joint meeting of the European Economic Community's Committee on Medical Research and the World Health Organization's International Agency for Research on Cancer held in Lyon, France in 1977. In 1981 a volume entitled *The Analysis of Dietary Fiber in Foods* (James and Theander, 1981) appeared, which described the work at that meeting, including the methods then being employed and developed for the analysis of dietary fiber in foods.

LEON PROSKY • Experimental Nutrition Branch, Division of Nutrition, Bureau of Foods, Food and Drug Administration, Washington, D. C. 20204.

The following year *Dietary Fiber in Health and Disease* (Vahouny and Kritchevsky, 1982) was published and stimulated much discussion on the definition and terminology of dietary fiber. The methods of detection employed either were based on direct carbohydrate determinations or were gravimetric procedures. For a complete discussion of the advantages and disadvantages of these methods the reader is referred to these volumes.

In the spring of 1981 at an AOAC workshop in Ottawa, Canada, Asp, Baker, Heckman, Southgate, and Van Soest reported on the advances they had made in their dietary fiber research (Prosky, 1981). The scientists present at the workshop concluded from these reports that two methods for the determination of total dietary fiber (TDF) should be developed: (1) a rapid enzymic gravimetric method based on a modification of methods developed by Hellendoorn *et al.* (1975), Asp *et al.* (1983), Furda *et al.* (1979), and Schweizer and Würsch (1979); and (2) a more comprehensive method, such as a modification of the methods of Southgate (1969a,b) or Theander and Åman (1982), to determine the individual dietary fiber components. In the first method the sum of the soluble and insoluble polysaccharides and lignin would be defined and measured as a unit, while in the second method each of the specific components of TDF would be identified and measured separately (Prosky and Harland, 1981). It was envisioned that the second method would act as a methodology check on the more rapid first method. There was recognition that this chemical method would satisfy the needs of some individuals, e.g., analytical chemists, but not others, e.g., physiologists, who were primarily interested in identifying the fiber fractions that most consistently elicit a physiological response. The gravimetric method may be suitable for the measurement of TDF in food, but not for the same measurement in nutritional balance studies. Van Soest (unpublished, 1983) has recently developed a detergent method which measures soluble and insoluble fiber in foods. This method will certainly warrant further consideration when it appears in the literature.

In this chapter it is my intention to describe the collaborative study of a method for TDF conducted under the auspices of the AOAC. Some of the data have already been published (Prosky and Harland, 1985; Prosky *et al.*, 1984).

2. DEVELOPMENT OF THE METHOD

Enzymatic methods were first employed by Williams and Olmsted (1935). Removal of starch and protein by pancreatin was followed by acid hydrolysis and subsequent identification and measurement of the sugar fractions. Hellendoorn *et al.* (1975) used pepsin for the hydrolysis of protein and pancreatin for subsequent starch hydrolysis. Furda (1977) assessed existing analytical methods and suggested new methodology based on the use of appropriate enzymes and inclusion of the soluble fiber fraction. Asp *et al.* (1983) and Asp (1977) evaluated some of the more widely used methods for the determination of dietary fiber and proposed enzymic modifications using pepsin, pancreatin, and Termamyl, a heat-stable α-amylase. Theander and Åman (1979) introduced the use of the Termamyl enzyme for combined gelatinization and starch degradation in dietary fiber analysis. At the 93rd AOAC Annual Meeting, Furda *et al.* (1979) reported that the use of mammalian as well as bacterial enzymes gave similar values for TDF when these enzymes were free of the activity of the dietary fiber-splitting enzymes cellulase, hemicellulase, and pectinase. In addition, they sought to measure the soluble fractions of dietary fiber.

Heckman and Lane (1981) analyzed several foods by various dietary fiber methods: the acid detergent fiber (ADF) method of Goering and Van Soest (1970); the neutral detergent fiber (NDF) method by the Schaller (1976) modification employing hog pancreas amylase; Robertson and Van Soest's (1977) enzyme-modified NDF method employing *Bacillus subtilis* amylase; the method of Furda *et al.* (1979) for soluble and insoluble dietary fiber using physiological enzymes; the method of Hellendoorn *et al.* (1975) for "indigestible residue"; and the method of Southgate (1969a,b) for TDF. Results showed that enzyme-modified NDF was lower than NDF and was dependent principally upon the starch content of the foods examined. The Furda method, with its capability for measuring soluble dietary fiber and its additional features of simplicity and rapidity, seemed the most promising. Later Englyst *et al.* (1982) measured the nonstarch polysaccharides (the major components of "dietary fiber") of plant foods. They removed starch from samples by adding hog pancreatic α-amylase together with pullulanase and amyloglucosidase, and analyzed the starch-free material after acid hydrolysis by gas chromatography.

A broad collaborative study testing various gravimetric, colorimetric, and gas chromatographic methods on nine food samples was conducted in 1978 and reported by James and Theander (1981). Results varied greatly among different methods, and Southgate's colorimetric method proved difficult to reproduce in different laboratories (Southgate and White, 1981). An enzymatic gravimetric method apparently was the most practical and simplest way to meet the challenge, i.e., the practical approach with the major components identified as total dietary fiber.

The method studied and reported here is based on several methods (Asp, Englyst, Furda, Schweizer, Southgate, Theander, Van Soest) and was developed at General Mills Co., Minneapolis, Minnesota by DeVries and Furda; at Kemicentrum, University of Lund, Sweden by Asp; and at the Nestlé Research Department, La Tour-de-Peilz, Switzerland by Schweizer.

3. PRINCIPLE OF THE METHOD

Duplicate samples of dried foods, fat-extracted if containing >5% fat, are gelatinized with Termamyl (heat-stable α-amylase), and then enzymatically digested with protease and amyloglucosidase to remove the protein and starch. Ethanol is added to precipitate the soluble dietary fiber. The total residue is filtered and then washed with ethanol and acetone. The residues are dried and then weighed. One of the duplicates is analyzed for protein, and the other is incinerated at 525°C and the ash determined. The TDF is the weight of the residue less the weight of the protein and ash.

3.1 Apparatus and Reagents

1. Balance. Analytical, capable of weighing to 0.1 mg.
2. Fritted crucible. Porosity 2, Pyrex 32940, coarse ASTM 40- to 60-μm fritted crucible, available from Scientific Products Co., Columbia, Maryland C-8525-1; V.W.R. Scientific Co., Baltimore, Maryland 23863-040; Fisher Scientific Co., Pittsburgh, Pennsylvania 08237-1A; or Sargent Welch Co., Skokie, Illinois F-243-90-B or F-243-90-C, depending on size needed. Clean the crucible thoroughly, ash at 525°C, soak in water, and rinse in water. Add ~0.5 g Celite 545 to crucibles before drying to obtain constant weight. Dry them at 130°C for 1 h, cool them, and store them in a desiccator until used. The crucibles indicated in the procedure may not be available in Europe. Porosity 2 signifies pores 40–90 μm in Europe and 40–60 μm in the U.S. Several analysts have reported breakage of crucibles when the temperature was increased to 525°C and have recommended Corning no. 36060 Buchner, fritted disk, Pyrex, 60 ml ASTM 40–60 μm, which seemed to break less often and gave the same results.
3. Vacuum source. A vacuum pump or aspirator equipped with an in-line double vacuum flask.
4. Vacuum oven. Seventy degrees centigrade and desiccator. Alternatively, an air oven capable of operating at 105°C can be used.
5. Constant-temperature water bath. Adjustable to 60°C, and equipped to provide constant agitation of digestion flasks during enzymatic hydrolysis. A multistation shaker or multistation magnetic stirrer will suffice for this requirement.
6. Beakers. Tall form, 400 ml.
7. Ethanol. Ninety-five percent, technical grade.
8. Ethanol. Seventy-four percent. Place 250 ml water in a 1-liter volumetric flask. Dilute to volume with 95% ethanol. Mix and dilute to volume again with 95% ethanol if necessary. Mix.

9. Phosphate buffer, pH 6.0. Dissolve 1.5 g sodium phosphate dibasic and 10.0 g sodium phosphate monobasic monohydrate in ~700 ml water. Dilute to 1 liter with water and adjust pH to 6.0 by adding drops of dilute monobasic or dibasic sodium phosphate, if necessary.

10. Termamyl (heat-stable α-amylase) solution, 120L (Novo Laboratories, Wilton, Connecticut). Store enzyme solution in refrigerator after each use.

11. Protease P-5380. Subtilopeptidase A, type VIII (Sigma Chemical Co., St. Louis, Missouri). One unit will hydrolyze casein to produce color equivalent to 100 μm tyrosine (181 μg)/min at pH 7.5 at 37° C. Refrigerate the dry enzyme after each use.

12. Amyloglucosidase A-9268. E.C. 3.2.1.3 (Sigma Chemical Co.). One unit will liberate 1.0 mg glucose from starch in 3 min at pH 4.5 and 55° C. Keep the reagent refrigerated when not in use.

13. NaOH solution, 0.285 N. Dissolve 11.4 g NaOH in ~700 ml water in a 1-liter volumetric flask. Dilute the mixture to volume with water.

14. Phosphoric acid solution, 0.329 M. Dissolve 37.9 g phosphoric acid (85%) in water in a 1-liter volumetric flask. Dilute the mixture to volume with water.

15. Celite 545. Acid-washed (Fisher Scientific Co., Fair Lawn, New Jersey).

3.2. Sample Preparation

For this study, no sample preparation was required other than drying overnight at 70° C in a vacuum oven and cooling in a desiccator before weighing. However, if the fat content is >5%, the sample is defatted with petroleum ether (decant with three 25-ml portions/g sample) before milling. Record the loss of weight due to fat removal and make the appropriate correction to the final percent TDF. Store the dry, milled sample in a capped jar in a desiccator until the analysis is carried out. When sample preparation is necessary, homogenize the sample and dry it overnight as described above; then dry-mill a portion to pass through a 0.3- to 0.5-mm mesh sieve. If the sample cannot be heated, freeze-dry it before milling.

When dealing with unknowns, fat-extract all samples. For fat extraction, place ~10 g of sample in a 250-ml beaker and add 25 ml petroleum ether. Stir the mixture for 15 min, using a magnetic stirrer. Let it stand 1 min; then decant petroleum ether. Repeat this procedure with two 25-ml portions of petroleum ether. Place the beaker in a 70° C oven and dry overnight. If apparatus is unavailable for milling samples to pass through a 0.3- or 0.5-mm mesh sieve, grind in a mortar.

3.3. Determination of Total Dietary Fiber

1. Run a blank through the entire procedure along with samples to measure any contribution from reagents to the final weight of the residue.
2. Weigh, in duplicate, a 1-g sample accurate to 0.1 mg (sample weights should not differ by more than 20 mg) into 400-ml tallform beakers. Add 50 ml of pH 6.0 phosphate buffer to each beaker.
3. Add 100 μl Termamyl solution.
4. Cover beakers with aluminum foil and place in a boiling water bath for 15 min. Gently shake the beakers every 5 min. Increase the incubation time when the number of beakers placed in the boiling water bath makes it difficult for the beaker contents to reach an internal temperature of 100° C; 30 min should be sufficient.
5. Cool the beakers. Adjust to pH 7.5 ± 0.1 by adding 10 ml of 0.285 N NaOH solution.
6. Add 5 mg protease. Since the protease adheres to a spatula, it may be preferable to make an enzyme solution just prior to use with a small amount (about 100 μl) of phosphate buffer and pipet the required amount.
7. Cover the beakers with aluminum foil. Incubate them at 60° C for 30 min with continuous agitation.
8. Cool the beakers. Add 10 ml of 0.329 M phosphoric acid solution to adjust the pH to 4.5 ± 0.2.
9. Add 0.3 ml amyloglucosidase solution.
10. Cover beakers with aluminum foil. Incubate them at 60° C for 30 min with continuous agitation.
11. Add 280 ml of 95% ethanol preheated to 60° C. Mix.
12. Let precipitate form at room temperature for 60 min.
13. Weigh crucible containing Celite to the nearest 0.1 mg. After weighing, redistribute the bed of Celite in the crucible, using a stream of 74% ethanol from a wash bottle. Apply suction to the crucible to draw Celite onto the fritted glass as an even mat. When fiber is filtered in the following step, Celite effectively separates the fiber from the fritted glass of the crucible, allowing for easy removal of the crucible contents.
14. Filter the enzyme digest from step 12 through the crucible.
15. Wash the residue successively with three 20-ml portions of 74% ethanol, two 10-ml portions of 95% ethanol, and two 10-ml portions of acetone. With some materials, gum is formed, trapping liquid. If the surface film that develops after adding the suspension to Celite is broken with a spatula, filtration is improved. Time for filtration and washing will vary from 0.1 to 6 h, averaging 0.5 h/sample.

Long filtration times can be avoided by careful intermittent suction throughout the filtration. Normal suction can be applied at washing. Backbubbling of air is another way of speeding up filtrations, if available.

16. Dry the crucible containing the residue overnight in a 70° C vacuum oven or in a 105° C air oven.

17. Cool in a desiccator and weigh the crucible, Celite, and residue to nearest 0.1 mg.

18. Analyze the residue from one sample of a set of duplicates for protein. Protein is probably most easily analyzed by carefully scraping the Celite and the fiber mat onto filter paper, which can then be folded and digested. A similar piece of filter paper should be analyzed as a blank. Use Kjeldahl analysis as specified in Association of Official Analytical Chemists (1980), Sections 47.021−47.023. Use 6.25 for the protein factor in all cases for which the nature of the protein is unknown. The appropriate protein factor for a particular protein (if known) should be used. For example, the factor for plant protein may be 5.7.

19. Incinerate a second sample of the duplicate set for 5 h at 525° C.

20. Cool the crucible in a desiccator. Weigh the crucible containing the Celite and the ash to the nearest 0.1 mg.

3.4. Calculation of Total Dietary Fiber

The total dietary fiber is calculated as follows:

$$TDF(\%) = \frac{mg\ residue - [(\%\ protein\ in\ residue + \%\ ash\ in\ residue)/100 \times mg\ residue] - blank \times 100}{mg\ sample\ (wt)}$$

3.5 Food Samples Analyzed

Portions of 13 foods were sent to each of the 42 analysts to be analyzed for TDF. The foods, unknown to the analysts, were:

1. Corn bran, donated by A. E. Staley Manufacturing Co., Decatur, Illinois, and used as provided.

2. Iceberg lettuce, mixed with 50 ml deionized water for every 350 g lettuce, and blended in a Waring blender for 2 min until homogeneous, with the slurry then freeze-dried for 48 h and stored in tightly sealed plastic bags at room temperature until shipped.

3. Oats, quick-cooking, donated by the Quaker Oats Co., Barrington, Illinois, blended in a Waring blender for 3 min and stored in plastic bags at room temperature until used.

4. Potatoes, instant, from Giant Foods, Washington, D. C., used directly.

5. Raisins, seedless, from Giant Foods, blended with enough water to make a thick paste, freeze-dried for 48 h, removed from the pan with a spatula, and placed in sample vials.

6. Rice, enriched, long grain, from Giant Foods, ground 5 min in a Straub (Philadelphia, Pennsylvania) model 4E electric mixer to a uniform powder. There was visible separation of the outer coating, leading to a lack of uniformity of particles.

7. Rye bread (Deli-Rye), from Giant Foods, broken into pieces, placed in an aluminum loaf pan, and dried 4 h at 80° C, with the dried pieces then blended in a Waring blender for 2 min.

8. Soy isolate, donated by Ralston-Purina Co., St. Louis, Missouri, used as received.

9. Wheat bran, AACC Certified Food Grade, purchased from the American Association of Cereal Chemists, St. Paul, Minnesota, and used as received.

10. Whole wheat flour (called whole wheat meal in Britain), high extraction, donated by General Mills, Minneapolis, Minnesota, and used as received.

11. White wheat flour, low extraction, donated by General Mills, used as received.

12. A nonvegetarian mixed diet.

13. A lacto-ovo vegetarian mixed diet. The foods comprising items 12 and 13 were those reported by Oberleas and Harland (1981). Casseroles and baked goods were either purchased ready-to-eat or prepared in the Food and Drug Administration laboratory. After all foods listed in the diets were purchased or prepared, homogenates were prepared by adding foods one at a time and blending without adding water until the homogenate was uniform. The homogenates were freeze-dried for 48 h, and the powder was again blended in a Waring blender for 2 min before being placed in sample vials.

Because the proposed method recommended fat extraction if samples contained >5% fat, we calculated the fat content of each item. Samples 1–11 did not require fat extraction. Calculations showed that diet composites 12 and 13 contained >5% fat, so fat extraction was recommended for these samples.

All samples were placed in 25-ml scintillation vials with screw caps and the sample number was taped to each vial.

4. RESULTS AND DISCUSSION

Foods used to test the method under collaborative study were chosen so that they differed in the amounts of dietary fiber and in the distribution of the components of dietary fiber in a variety of cellular matrices. Many dietary fiber methods work well on individual products, but fail when applied to a variety of products. In this study each laboratory took two separate aliquots from each sample. Starch and the bulk of the protein were digested by enzymes. Residual protein was determined on one sample and ash weight on the other. The results from these two separate determinations were used to calculate the percent TDF from the formula given in Section 3.4. This was repeated to arrive at a duplicate value for percent TDF.

Thirty-two of the 42 laboratories submitted results. The remaining ten laboratories either used other procedures or did not send in any analytical results. Some laboratories did only one determination, while others repeated the determination several times. Individual values are reported elsewhere (Prosky *et al.*, 1984). Seven analytical results were not used because they were Cochran outliers (Youden and Steiner, 1982) (the range of replicates was wider than could be accounted for by chance alone). After looking at the results in some detail, it became apparent that one analyst had been unable to perform the procedure. This analyst had some difficulty with step 15; most filtrations took as long as or longer than the maximum. He helped identify the time required at this stage as a major cause of problems with replication; blank, and by inference, sample, precipitation increases extensively during prolonged filtration or standing. He found that high blanks and ash residues were found in replicates that filtered slowly or were left overnight in an attempt to reduce the filtration time. To achieve good replication, this stage must be controlled. At least seven samples gave poor replicates in this analyst's laboratory. Another analyst also had poor replicates in six cases, but the mean results fell in a reasonable range. Since the majority of laboratories provided good replicates, it can be assumed that the problems of these two analysts were not due to the method or to the lack of specific directions.

Statistical evaluation of the results is given in Table I. Of the approximately 834 analyses performed, only five were omitted because they were Grubbs outliers (Youden and Steiner, 1982) (extreme variance). Although there were no apparent statistical correlations between the coefficients of variation (CV) and dietary fiber levels, the foods containing the highest levels of dietary fiber, 89.02%, 42.25%, 23.31%, and 12.92%, had the lower CVs, i.e., 2.95%, 5.29%, 11.79%, and 11.04%, respectively. Conversely, foods containing the lowest amounts of dietary fiber, 3.07%, 3.67%, 4.43%, and 5.90%, had the larger CVs, i.e., 32.95%, 64.15%, 23.12%, and 24.41%. These findings would be of importance because the physiological significance of

TABLE I. Measures of Precision for Determining Dietary Fiber

Sample	Number of laboratories[a]	Average % dietary fiber	Reproducibility (CV), %
1 Corn bran	30	89.02	2.95
2 Lettuce, freeze-dried	32	23.31	11.79
3 Oats, quick-cooking	32	12.47	25.64
4 Potatoes, instant	32	7.22	13.24[b]
5 Raisins, seedless	31	4.43	23.12[b]
6 Rice, powdered	30	3.67	64.15
7 Rye bread, dried	30	5.90	24.41
8 Soy isolate	32	7.51	100.93
9 Wheat bran	31	42.25	5.29
10 Whole wheat flour	30	12.92	11.04[b]
11 White wheat flour	32	3.07	32.95[b]
12 Nonvegetarian mixed diet	32	7.19	26.39
13 Lacto-ovovegetarian mixed diet	32	8.59	22.07[b]

[a] When fewer than 32 results are reported, the laboratory in question did not submit any results for the particular sample.
[b] A Grubbs-outlier laboratory was omitted prior to computing these measures of precision. An outlier rejection level of 0.05 was used in the one-tailed test (Youden and Steiner, 1982, p. 89).

dietary fiber increases as the level in the diet increases, making greater variations in low-fiber values of little importance, particularly with regard to label declaration and claims. On the other hand, foods with a low fiber content (potato or even whole wheat flour, for example) are often eaten in large amounts and may contribute significantly to fiber intake. This would require accurate analyses of low-fiber foods.

Player and Wood (1980) carried out a collaborative study of methods of analysis for crude fiber in flours and found that the CVs were between 9% and 133%, but the largest proportion of values was between 10% and 20%. Although our CVs were within those reported by Player and Wood, the values of dietary fiber for samples 6 (rice; 64% CV) and 8 (soy isolate; 101% CV) were not acceptable in this study. Both samples presented special problems to the analysts.

Rice had the highest amount of starch of any of the foods analyzed, 77%, as determined by method B (Olof Theander, Swedish University of Agricultural Sciences, Uppsala, Sweden, personal communication, 1983). Lack of homogeneity of the sample was suspect because of a noticeable separation of the outer coating after milling. However, the major concern was the ability of the enzyme to digest completely the starch from the food. These steps were accomplished with the use of an active amylase and amyloglucosidase enzyme preparation along with an incubation period sufficient to allow total hydrolysis of the starch. Shipping these enzymes by mail to various parts of this country and to other countries may have been responsible for partial reduction or inactivation of the enzyme activity. In the final analysis, the large CV for TDF in rice was probably due to insufficient milling, making amylase penetration into the hard rice particles difficult and incomplete. This is supported by the fact that one of the analysts, who pulverized the sample in a mortar before analysis, obtained a very low value (1.26%) for dietary fiber. Also other samples with very high starch content (4, potato and 11, white wheat flour) gave no problems with starch removal. If the high starch content or inactive enzyme was the problem, samples 4 and 11 should have presented the same problem.

The other food that had a high CV was sample 8, soy isolate. This food had the highest protein content, 90%, of any of the foods analyzed and therefore would have very little dietary fiber. All analysts were instructed to multiply the nitrogen content by 6.25 to convert to percent protein. While the average factor 6.25 is applied to food in general, specific factors may be used in the case of products for which the protein and nitrogen relations are definitely known. We found that the analysts performed protein analysis by a variety of methods, which may lead to inaccurate protein values and hence to questionable dietary fiber results. The instructions in our next collaborative study have been changed to state that the nitrogen determination must be performed by the Kjeldahl method (Association of Official Analytical Chemists, 1980) and 6.25 is to be used as the protein conversion factor in all cases. If the higher fiber values (higher than 3%) for sample 8 are discarded, the average TDF is 1.38% ± 0.29 (17 laboratory results ranged from 0.12% to 2.78%). The CV was 88%, but the quantity of fiber was so small that this large CV_x becomes almost meaningless under physiological conditions.

Other sources of problems in the determination of TDF may be the products of the Maillard reaction. The effect of various kinds of heat treatment on the determination of TDF appears to be important. When food is heated, the contribution of the noncarbohydrate dietary fiber residue increases because of the formation of modified proteins and new carbohydrate polymers that are different from those in the plant food material (James and Theander, 1981). Products of the Maillard reaction are present in significant amounts in many food products, but presumably in significant amounts only in samples 12 and 13 in this study.

Because there are no known mixtures of dietary fiber nor known true percentages of dietary fiber in foods, it was impossible to do a recovery study. However, for some products we were able to obtain dietary fiber values from the company producing the food. These were:

a. Sample 1. Staley refined corn bran, 88–92% dietary fiber by the method of Goering and Van Soest (1970) and Hart and Fisher (1971).

    b. Sample 9. AACC wheat bran, 40.2% dietary fiber by the method of Van Soest and Wine (1967) modified to use hog pancreatic amylase.

    c. Sample 10. General Mills whole wheat flour, 8–9% dietary fiber by the AOAC method for TDF (Association of Official Analytical Chemists, Sections 7.069–7.071).

    d. Sample 11. General Mills white wheat flour, 0.6–1.0% dietary fiber by the NDF method (American Association of Cereal Chemists, 1978).

The methods used above were suitable for the products analyzed; however, they would not necessarily be suitable for determining fiber in other foods.

Two investigators (Theander and Åman, 1979; Englyst et al., 1982) used their own methods for the determination of dietary fiber to analyze the samples sent out in this study. Their values were not included in the statistical evaluation of the results. Two other investigators (Asp et al., 1983; Schweizer and Würsch, 1979) provided results using both the AOAC method and their own published methods. The values they obtained for TDF by the proposed method were included in the final statistics; however, the values for TDF that they obtained by their own methods were not included in the statistical evaluation of results. The results of the comparison are shown in Figs. 1 and 2. The data showed that the Englyst method gave comparable results with the AOAC procedure; however, the values for dietary fiber were lower in all cases than those obtained by the AOAC method. In using the Englyst method, the analysis of dietary fiber is limited to the determination of nonstarch polysaccharides and does not involve lignin and is therefore not comparable with any accepted definition of TDF. Further, it is not a rapid or robust method and is more complicated to carry out than the proposed AOAC procedure. The food industry certainly and regulatory agencies probably will be reluctant to accept such a procedure. The Englyst procedure does not isolate dietary fiber residues that may serve as the starting material for "research application" of physiologically active fractions. Our procedure gives a TDF fraction from which the TDF components are capable of being isolated and identified. Finally, the additional information on monosaccharide ratios provided by the Englyst method has only limited scientific value because it does not describe the type or character of polysaccharide from which the sugars originated. The AOAC procedure includes enzymatically unhydrolyzable starch as part of the TDF fraction. This may or may not be a major problem, since many nutritionists consider unhydrolyzable starch as part of the dietary fiber fraction. The other three methods were in very good agreement, with the exception of sample 8, soy isolate, a problem that was previously discussed. The fact that these more complicated methods agree with the present rapid and simple procedure demonstrates the suitability of the latter for routine measurements.

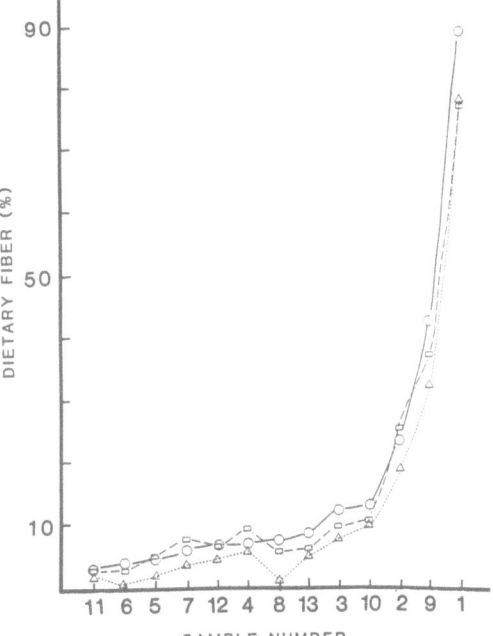

FIGURE 1. Comparison of percent dietary fiber by (O) the proposed method, (Δ) the method of Englyst *et al.* (1982), and (□) the method of Theander and Åman (1982). Data are from Prosky *et al.* (1984).

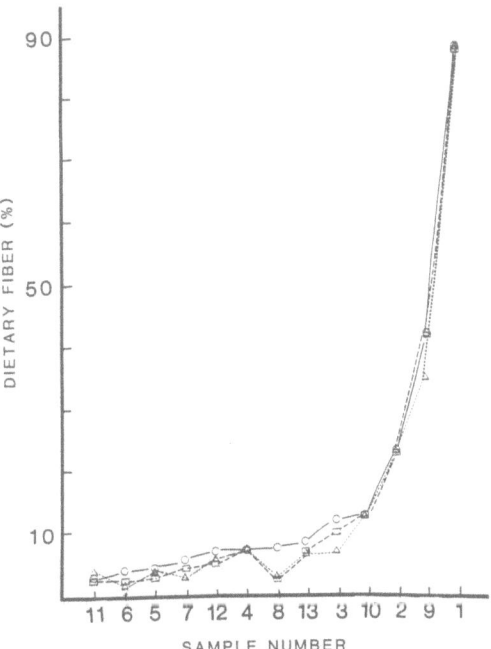

FIGURE 2. Comparison of percent dietary fiber by (O) the proposed method, (Δ) the method of Schweizer and Würsch (1979), and (□) the method of Asp *et al.* (1983). Data are from Prosky *et al.* (1984).

A second collaborative study has been completed. Several changes have been introduced into the procedure, mainly in buffer and ethanol concentrations and some explanatory points. The method has been accepted as Official First Action by the AOAC and will be published in the March, 1985 issue of the AOAC journal.

ACKNOWLEDGMENTS. The work reported here has been a major collaborative effort of the author and Dr. Nils-Georg Asp, Department of Food Chemistry, University of Lund, Lund, Sweden; Drs. Ivan Furda and Jonathan DeVries, General Mills, Minneapolis, Minnesota; Dr. Thomas F. Schweizer, Nestlé Research Department, La Tour-de-Peilz, Switzerland; and Dr. Barbara F. Harland, Food and Drug Administration, Washington, D.C.

The author acknowledges the collaborators in this study: E. L. Anderson, Kellogg Co., Battle Creek, Michigan; N.-G. Asp, University of Lund, Lund, Sweden; K. E. Bach-Knudsen, Carlsberg Research Center, Valby, Denmark; M. Bergstrom-Nielsen and A. Sørensen, National Food Institute, Søborg, Denmark; J. H. Cummings and H. Englyst, Addenbrookes Hospital, Cambridge, England; C. E. Daugherty, Campbell Institute for Research and Technology, Camden, New Jersey; J. DeVries, General Mills, Minneapolis, Minnesota; S. A. Elayda, Quaker Oats Co., Barrington, Illinois; J. G. Faugere, Laboratoire Municipale, Bordeaux, France; F. Fidanza, Institute of Nutrition, Perugia, Italy; M. Fisher, Department of Scientific and Industrial Research, Palmerston, New Zealand; W. Frølich, Norsk Cerealinstitutt Ved, Oslo, Norway; B. Garping, Wasabrod AB Laboratory, Filipstad, Sweden; D. Gordon and D. O. Holst, University of Missouri, Columbia, Missouri; G. Hill and C. Gjersvick, ITT, Continental Baking Co., Rye, New York; T. Howes and T. Pattison, Shaklee Corp., Hayward, California; M. Katan, Agricultural University, Wageningen, The Netherlands; P. Koivistoinen and P. Varo, University of Helsinki, Helsinki, Finland; B. A. Lewis and A. Bucher, Cornell University, Ithaca, New York; C. Lintas, Instituto Nazionale della Nutrizione, Italy; F. Lubin, Chaim Sheba Medical Center, Tel Hashomer, Israel; A. Menger, Federal Research Center of Grain and Potato Processing, Detmold, Germany; R. Mongeau, Health and Welfare Canada, Ottawa, Canada; J. K. Palmer and R. Antenucci, Virginia Polytechnic Institute, Blacksburg, Virginia; G. S. Ranhotra, American Institute of Baking, Manhattan, Kansas; V. E. Rasper, University of Guelph, Guelph, Canada; R. M. Saunders, U. S. Department of Agriculture, Berkeley, California; B. O. Schneeman and S. Hovde, University of California, Davis, California; T. F. Schweizer, Nestlé Research Department, La Tour-de-Peilz, Switzerland; D. A. T. Southgate, Food Research Institute, Norwich, England; G. Testolin, Universita di Milano, Milano, Italy; O. Theander and E. Westerlund, Swedish University of Agricultural Sciences, Uppsala, Sweden; N.

Troisler, Faculty of Nutrition, Rehovoth, Israel; P. J. Van Soest and J. Robertson, Cornell University, Ithaca, New York; P. Venetz, Nestlé Products, LaTour-de-Peilz, Switzerland; J. Zyren and S. Berman, National Food Processors Association, Washington, D.C.

I would like also to acknowledge the invaluable contributions of Dr. Richard Albert, statistician, Clarisse Jones, technician, and Donna Waldrop, typist, in the preparation of this chapter.

REFERENCES

American Association of Cereal Chemists, 1978, *Approved Methods of the AACC, Revisions: Method 32-20,* American Association of Cereal Chemists, St. Paul, Minnesota.

Asp, N.-G., 1977, *Dietary Fibre: Current Developments of Importance to Health,* Food and Nutrition Press, Westport, Connecticut, pp. 21-26.

Asp, N.-G., Johansson, C.-G., Hallmer, H., and Siljeström, M., 1983, Rapid enzymatic assay of insoluble and soluble dietary fiber, *J. Agric. Food Chem.* **31**:476–482.

Association of Official Analytical Chemists, 1980, *Official Methods of Analysis,* 3rd ed., Association of Official Analytical Chemists, Arlington, Virginia.

Burkitt, D. P., 1973, Some diseases characteristic of modern Western civilization, *Br. Med. J.* **1**: 274–278.

Burkitt, D. P., Walker, A. R. P., and Painter, N. S., 1972, Effect of dietary fibre on stools and transit-times, and its role in the causation of disease, *Lancet* **2**:1408–1412.

Englyst, H., Wiggins, H. S., and Cummings, J. H., 1982, Determination of the non-starch polysaccharides in plant foods by gas-liquid chromatography of constituent sugars as alditol acetates, *Analyst* **107**:307–318.

Furda, I., 1977, Fractionation and examination of biopolymers from dietary fibre, *Cereal Foods World* **22**:252–254.

Furda, I., Gengler, S. C., Johnson, R. R., Magnuson, J. S., and Smith, D. E., 1979, *Complete Carbohydrate Analysis—Sugars, Starch and Total Dietary Fiber in Plant Residues and Food Products,* 93rd Annual Meeting of the Association of Official Analytical Chemists, Washington, D.C.

Goering, H. K., and Van Soest, P. J., 1970, *Forage Fiber Analysis,* USDA Agriculture Handbook no. 379, U.S. Department of Agriculture, Washington, D.C.

Hart, F. L., and Fisher, H. J., 1971, *Modern Food Analysis Methods,* Springer, New York.

Heckman, M. M., and Lane, S., 1981, Comparison of dietary fiber methods for foods, *J. Assoc. Off. Anal. Chem.* **64**:1339–1343.

Hellendoorn, E. W., Noordhoff, M. G., and Slagman, J., 1975, Enzymatic determination of the indigestible residue (dietary fibre) content of human food, *J. Sci. Food Agric.* **26**:1461–1468.

James, W. P. T., and Theander, O., 1981, *The Analysis of Dietary Fiber in Food,* Marcel Dekker, New York.

Oberleas, D., and Harland, B. F., 1981, Phytate content of foods: Effect on dietary zinc bioavailability, *J. Am. Diet. Assoc.* **79**:433–436.

Player, R. B., and Wood, R., 1980, Collaborative studies on methods of analysis, Part I: Determinations of crude fibre in flours, *J. Assoc. Public Anal.* **18**:29–40.

Prosky, L., 1981, Panel Discussion on Dietary Fiber, 6th Annual Association of Official Analytical Chemists Spring Workshop, Ottawa, Canada.

Prosky, L., and Harland, B. F., 1981, Definition and Method for Dietary Fiber, 95th Annual Meeting, Association of Official Analytical Chemists, Washington, D.C.

Prosky, L., and Harland, B. F., 1985, Dietary fibre methodology, in: *Dietary Fibre, Fiber-Depleted Foods, and Diseases* (H. C. Trowell, D. P. Burkitt, and K. W. Heaton, eds.), Academic, London, pp. 57–76.

Prosky, L., Asp, N.-G., Furda, I., DeVries, J., Schweizer, T. F., and Harland, B. F., 1984, Determination of total dietary fiber in foods, food products, and total diets: Interlaboratory study, *J. Assoc. Off. Anal. Chem.* **67**:1044–1052.

Robertson, J. B., and Van Soest, P. J., 1977, Dietary fiber estimation in concentrated feedstuff, *J. Anim. Sci.* **45**(Suppl. 1):254.

Schaller, D. R., 1976, *Analysis of Cereal Products and Ingredients*, American Association of Cereal Chemists, New Orleans, Louisiana; also AACC Method 32-20, First Approval 10/26/77, *Methods of the AACC*, Minneapolis, Minnesota.

Schweizer, T. F., and Würsch, P., 1979, Analysis of dietary fibre, *J. Sci. Food Agric.* **30**:613–619.

Southgate, D. A. T., 1969a, Determination of carbohydrates in foods. I. Available carbohydrates, *J. Sci. Food Agric.* **20**:326–330.

Southgate, D. A. T., 1969b, Determination of carbohydrates in foods. II. Unavailable carbohydrates, *J. Sci. Food Agric.* **20**:331–335.

Southgate, D. A. T., and White, M. A., 1981, Commentary on results obtained by the different laboratories using the Southgate method, in: *The Analysis of Dietary Fiber in Food* (W. P. T. James and O. Theander, eds.), Marcel Dekker, New York, pp. 37–50.

Theander, O., and Åman, P. 1979, Studies on dietary fibres. 1. Analysis and chemical characterization of water-soluble and water-insoluble dietary fibres, *Swed. J. Agric. Res.* **9**:97–106.

Theander, O., and Åman, P., 1982, Studies on dietary fibre. A method for the analysis and chemical characterisation of total dietary fibre, *J. Sci. Food Agric.* **33**:340–344.

Trowell, H. C., 1972, Ischemic heart disease and dietary fiber, *Am. J. Clin. Nutr.* **25**:926–932.

Vahouny, G. V., and Kritchevsky, D., 1982 (eds.), *Dietary Fiber in Health and Disease*, Plenum, New York.

Van Soest, P. J., and Wine, R. H., 1967, Use of detergents in the analysis of fibrous feeds. IV. Determination of plant cell-wall constituents, *J. Assoc. Off. Anal. Chem.* **50**:50–55.

Williams, R. D., and Olmsted, W. D., 1935, A biochemical method for determining indigestible residue (crude fiber) in feces: Lignin, cellulose, and non-water-soluble hemicelluloses, *J. Biol. Chem.* **108**:653–656.

Youden, W. J., and Steiner, E. H., 1982, *Statistical Manual of the Association of Official Analytical Chemists*, Association of Official Analytical Chemists, Arlington, Virginia.

2

Measurement of Dietary Fiber as Nonstarch Polysaccharides

HANS N. ENGLYST and JOHN H. CUMMINGS

1. INTRODUCTION

In 1972 Trowell defined dietary fiber as "the skeletal remains of plant cells that are resistant to digestion by enzymes of man." This definition was modified in 1976 to "the plant polysaccharides and lignin which are resistant to hydrolysis by the digestive enzymes of man" (Trowell *et al.*, 1976).

The only plant polysaccharide known to be hydrolyzed by the digestive enzymes of man is starch. Trowell's 1976 definition of fiber is therefore equivalent to defining it as dietary polysaccharides other than starch, or as nonstarch polysaccharides (NSP) and lignin. Much confusion has arisen, however, because the Trowell definition has been interpreted as meaning the "polysaccharides and lignin resisting or escaping hydrolysis by the digestive enzymes of man." This interpretation of Trowell's definition is a physiological one and cannot be defended on the basis of what is known about carbohydrate breakdown in the gut; furthermore, it is inexact and inappropriate as the objective for an analytical procedure. For example, the fate of dietary polysaccharides in the human small bowel is largely unknown, although it is widely believed that starch is totally digested and nonstarch polysaccharides not at all. However, recently there has been speculation that this simple view may not be valid (Anderson *et al.*, 1981; Holloway *et al.*, 1978).

HANS N. ENGLYST and JOHN H. CUMMINGS • MRC Dunn Clinical Nutrition Centre, Cambridge CB2 1QL, United Kingdom.

Starch may resist hydrolysis with α-amylase in the small intestine and in *in vitro* incubations for a variety of reasons. Starch granules from potato, banana, high-amylose corn (Fuwa, 1980), and legumes (Fleming and Vose, 1979) and also the small granules in wheat (Palmer, 1972) show considerable resistance to hydrolysis with α-amylase *in vitro*. Nevertheless, neither these nor starch retrograded during food processing (Englyst *et al.*, 1982) are strictly resistant. They can all eventually be degraded by α-amylase after suitable treatment (Englyst and Cummings, 1984), showing that they are truly starch and not nonstarch polysaccharides, and are therefore not included in Trowell's definition of dietary fiber.

Starch may also escape digestion in the small intestine because of the presence of α-amylase inhibitors from foods (Shainkin and Birk, 1970) or additives (Wolever *et al.*, 1983) or due to complexes formed with other food components, such as fat (Holm *et al.*, 1983) or protein (Anderson *et al.*, 1981), or simply due to excess intake of starch in a less available form, as in unmilled seeds and grains (Snow and O'Dea, 1981). It is of considerable interest for the study of metabolism to know the amount of starch that, for these various reasons, may resist or escape digestion in the small intestine. However, this is a separate problem from the measurement of dietary fiber.

Lignin is included in the definition of dietary fiber by Trowell *et al.* (1976), but with the exception of bran, most plants for human consumption are harvested and eaten before much lignification takes place. Lignin is therefore absent or only a very minor component in human foods, although animal foods may contain substantial amounts (Theander and Åman, 1980).

Lignin may have specific physiological properties (Chang and Johnson, 1980) affecting digestive physiology. For example, the degree of lignification of a tissue may alter a plant's susceptibility to bacterial degradation. Information about the lignin content of plant foods could therefore be useful, but will only be obtained if lignin is measured and given as a value separate from NSP. Unfortunately there is no easy and reliable method available for measurement of lignin at the present time and the values reported are often due to artefacts (Hartley, 1978). Lignin is not a carbohydrate, but a phenylpropane polymer and has properties very different from NSP. No information whatsoever is obtained by including an unspecified amount for lignin in a value for total dietary fiber. Inclusion of uncertain values for lignin may even invalidate a more reliable measurement of NSP. Values for NSP and lignin should therefore be measured and reported separately. In the first place it is most important to get a reliable value for NSP. When an accurate method becomes available it may be of interest to obtain values for lignin and also tannins, cutins, and other cell-wall related components.

In the light of this we have developed a method for the measurement of dietary NSP, a chemically definable group of plant polysaccharides. The method is in accord with the definition of Trowell *et al.* (1976), who defined dietary fiber as polysaccharides *resistant* to the digestive enzymes of man, since only starch (and glycogen) are known to be degraded by human α-amylase. The method does not attempt to measure polysaccharides that pass through the human small bowel undigested, since this is an unpredictable event depending on the source of food, processing, other dietary components, and the digestive action of the individual person. Lignin is not included, because there is no reliable and straightforward method for its measurement at present and for the other reasons already discussed.

2. MEASUREMENT OF DIETARY FIBER AS NSP

The aim of the procedure we have developed is to measure chemically definable cell-wall polysaccharides in plant foods. Plant carbohydrates can be separated into free sugars and polysaccharides (Fig. 1). The polysaccharides may then be subdivided into starch and nonstarch polysaccharides (NSP). NSP can further be separated into cellulose and noncellulosic polysaccharides (NCP) and the constituent sugars measured.

An important objective in setting up any method for the measurement of NSP is to identify and completely recover it without contamination by starch or other carbohydrates. Our overall analysis is based on three main steps:

1. Complete removal of starch and free sugars without loss of NSP.
2. Hydrolysis of NSP.
3. Measurement of constituent sugars released from NSP.

3. STARCH REMOVAL

A major problem in all methods for the measurement of dietary fiber is the removal of starch. The present method depends on the identification of component sugars after acid hydrolysis of NSP. Starch must therefore be removed completely so that any glucose left can be considered as deriving from NSP. Contamination with 2 to 3% of the starch in starch-rich products such as potato and rice will lead to substantial overestimation of NSP.

3.1. Selective Removal of Starch

To avoid loss of NSP, starch must be removed selectively. This is best achieved using enzymes specific for the hydrolysis of the 1,4 and 1,6 glucosidic links in starch. A number of starch-degrading enzyme preparations have been tested and several found to be contaminated with β-glucanase,

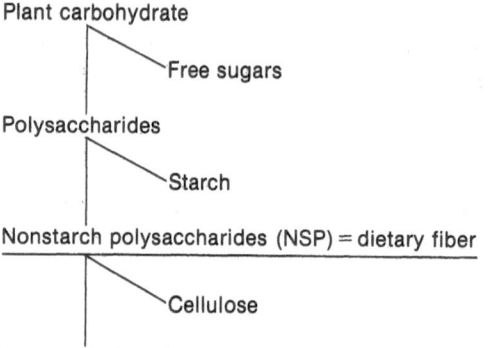

Plant carbohydrate

Free sugars

Polysaccharides

Starch

Nonstarch polysaccharides (NSP) = dietary fiber

Cellulose

Noncellulosic polysaccharides (arabinose, xylose, mannose, galactose, glucose, uronic
acids)

FIGURE 1. Separation of plant carbohydrate.

which limits the number available for selective hydrolysis of starch. For
example, incubation with a number of bacterial amylases leads to significant
losses of β-glucan, and 3 amyloglucosidases also result in loss of β-glucan
and/or other NSP components. β-glucans are important plant cell-wall
polysaccharides found widely in cereal foods such as wheat, rye, barley, and
oats. There is evidence to suggest that they are important in the control of
cholesterol metabolism (Judd and Truswell, 1981). Of the enzymes tested,
only the combination of mammalian α-amylase and pullulanase gave complete removal of starch and full recovery of β-glucan and other NSP components (Englyst et al., 1982).

3.2. Enzymatic Removal of Starch from Unprocessed Foods

Starch granules are hydrolyzed at a much slower rate than dispersed
starch (Walker and Hope, 1963), and so starch granules in some plants such
as potato and banana are highly resistant to hydrolysis with α-amylase. To
achieve complete hydrolysis of starch it is therefore necessary to disperse
starch granules before incubation with enzymes.

A series of experiments (Englyst et al., 1982) showed that treatment for
1 h with 0.1 M acetate buffer at 100°C is sufficient for complete enzymatic
removal of starch from unprocessed foods. The remaining glucose measured
in white flour and potato after removal of starch corresponds well with
detailed structural analyses of wheat endosperm and potato cell-wall material
(Bacic and Stone, 1980; Ring and Selvendran, 1978). No further reduction in
glucose was observed for white flour, potatoes, or a number of other unprocessed starchy foods by doubling the recommended amount of enzyme.

Furthermore, a test for residual starch with potassium iodide failed to reveal any blue color. These findings indicate that starch is completely removed and that the residual glucose can be regarded as true NSP glucose, originating principally from cellulose, although some is present in noncellulosic polysaccharides (e.g., β-glucans).

3.3. Enzymatic Removal of Starch from Processed Foods

During processing, part of the gelatinized starch, especially the amylose fraction, may retrograde to material resistant to hydrolysis with α-amylase. If not redispersed, this starch will result in falsely elevated values for NSP glucose.

Table I shows the effect of various treatments on the production of α-amylase-resistant starch (RS). If potato is analyzed raw, the correct values for NCP glucose and cellulose are obtained and no RS is measured. Boiled potatoes rapidly frozen in methanol–solid CO_2 mixture give similar values, indicating that no resistant starch has been produced. However, boiled potatoes stored for 2 h at $0°$ C prior to rapid freezing or direct analysis show substantial increases in the apparent values for NCP and cellulose. All the difference between the values for the raw and the cooked and stored potatoes can be explained by the production of RS. A number of other treatments used in food processing have effects on starch and may lead to substantial increases in apparent values for NCP glucose and cellulose.

RS may be dispersed with potassium hydroxide and then enzymatically hydrolyzed to glucose. The values obtained can then be subtracted from the apparent NSP glucose to obtain a correct value for NSP (Englyst et al., 1982). Although this technique gives correct values for NSP, it may be regarded as rather complex. A simpler and more direct approach is to

TABLE I. Food Processing and Resistant Starch

Treatment given to raw potato before analysis	Glucose in fraction,[a] g/100 g dry matter			
	NCP	Cellulose	NSP	RS
None (control)	0.07	1.51	1.58	0
Boiled $(CO_2 \rightarrow -25°C)$[b]	0.12	1.52	1.64	0.06
Boiled 2 h at $0°C$	1.93	2.96	4.89	3.31
Boiled, ethanol-extracted	0.70	2.23	2.93	1.35
Boiled, freeze-dried	2.61	3.13	5.74	4.16
Boiled, frozen	1.79	2.25	4.04	2.46

[a] NCP, noncellulosic polysaccharides; NSP, nonstarch polysaccharides; RS, resistant starch.
[b] Frozen in methanol–solid CO_2 mixture, then stored at $-25°C$.

remove all starch, including RS, in one step so that any glucose left, regardless of processing, can be considered as true NCP glucose.

As a result of a number of experiments with various agents known to disrupt hydrogen bonds, it was found that heating the food sample with dimethylsulfoxide for 1 h at 100 ° C dispersed all starch, including RS, without causing any loss of NSP. This technique has been incorporated into a simplified procedure for direct measurement of NSP (Englyst and Cummings, 1984).

4. HYDROLYSIS OF NSP

Experiments with cell wall material have shown that the highest yields of neutral sugars and uronic acids are obtained after treatment for 1 h with 12 M H_2SO_4 at 35°C followed by dilution to 1 M H_2SO_4 and hydrolysis for a further 2 h at 100°C (Englyst et al., 1982). This treatment is used for the measurement of total NSP.

5. MEASUREMENT OF CONSTITUENT SUGARS RELEASED FROM NSP

The sugar composition of NSP can be measured by gas liquid chromatography (GLC) of the constituent sugars as alditol acetates prepared as previously described (Englyst et al., 1982). This procedure is accurate, but rather time-consuming, and an alternative technique using N-methylimidazole to catalyze acetylation has been developed (Connors and Pandit, 1978; Wachowiak and Connors, 1979; Bittner et al., 1980; Blakeney et al., 1983). We have recently described a modification to our earlier procedure, which allows much quicker preparation of alditol acetates (Englyst and Cummings, 1984). In this procedure the hydrolysate is neutralized with NH_3OH, and the sugars are reduced for 1 h and within 10 min acetylated to alditol acetates using N-methylimidazole as catalyst.

6. PROCEDURES FOR MEASUREMENT OF TOTAL NSP AND ITS MAIN COMPONENTS

The technique described allows measurement of total NSP in one simple procedure. If values for cellulose and NCP or soluble and insoluble NSP are required, these can be obtained by simple modification to the procedure A* for total NSP (Fig. 2).

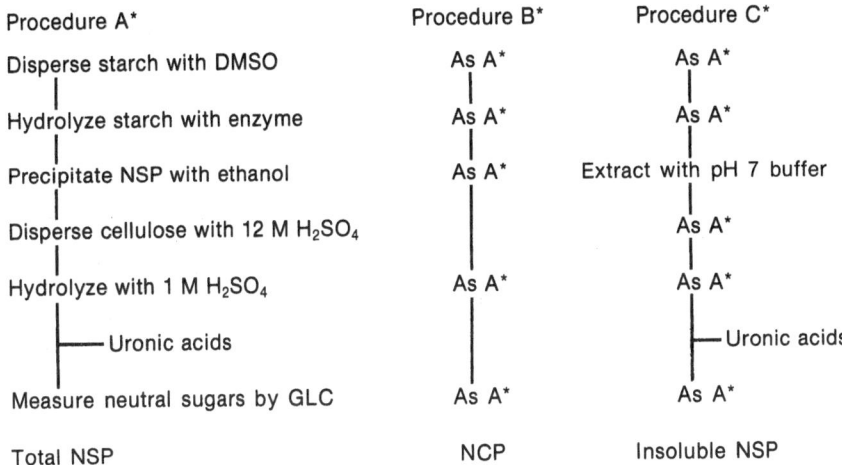

Procedure A*	Procedure B*	Procedure C*
Disperse starch with DMSO	As A*	As A*
Hydrolyze starch with enzyme	As A*	As A*
Precipitate NSP with ethanol	As A*	Extract with pH 7 buffer
Disperse cellulose with 12 M H₂SO₄		As A*
Hydrolyze with 1 M H₂SO₄	As A*	As A*
——Uronic acids		——Uronic acids
Measure neutral sugars by GLC	As A*	As A*
Total NSP	NCP	Insoluble NSP

Calculation of NSP:

Total NSP	= sum of sugars, procedure A*
Cellulose	= glucose, procedure A* − glucose, procedure B*
NCP	= total NSP − cellulose
Insoluble NSP	= sum of sugars, procedure C*
Soluble NSP	= sum of sugars, procedure A* − sum of sugars, procedure C*

FIGURE 2. Analysis for nonstarch polysaccharides (NSP). [From Englyst and Cummings (1984).]

6.1. Determination of Total NSP

Starch is dispersed with DMSO and hydrolyzed with α-amylase and pullulanase, and NSP is precipitated with ethanol. The starch-free residue is then dispersed with 12 M H_2SO_4 and hydrolyzed with 1 M H_2SO_4. Total NSP is calculated as the sum of released neutral sugars measured as alditol acetates by GLC and uronic acids measured colorimetrically.

6.2. Separation of Total NSP into Cellulose and NCP

If dispersion with 12 M H_2SO_4 is omitted in the procedure for total NSP, only NCP is hydrolyzed when treated with 1 M H_2SO_4. A value for cellulose can then be obtained as the difference between total NSP glucose and NCP glucose in the two procedures.

6.3. Separation into Soluble and Insoluble NSP

If the precipitation with ethanol in the procedure for total NSP is replaced by a 1-h extraction with buffer at pH 7, a value is obtained for insoluble NSP. A value for soluble NSP is then calculated as the difference between total NSP and insoluble NSP (Englyst and Cummings, 1984).

6.4. Measurement of RS

RS is not a part of NSP or dietary fiber, but if required, RS can be measured after dispersion with potassium hydroxide as previously described (Englyst *et al.*, 1982) or it can be measured as the difference in glucose between the procedure in which starch is dispersed with DMSO and that in which it is dispersed by acetate buffer (Englyst and Cummings, 1984).

7. RESULTS FOR SOME FOODS

Table II gives detailed values for NSP and the constituent sugars in various foods. White flour has a higher proportion of soluble NSP when compared to whole meal (whole wheat) products and bran. This may lead to more rapid and complete fermentation in the gut of NSP from white flour than that found in whole meal products. Arabinose–xylose-containing poly-saccharides and cellulose are the main components of NSP from wheat products. Cornflakes contain very little NSP, but significant amounts of RS (2.9%). The high content of β-glucan in oats and barley is identified by the high values for soluble NCP glucose in these products. Whole rye flour contains considerably more NSP than whole wheat flour.

Raw and cooked potatoes contain the same NSP, but in addition 2.08% resistant starch is found in the cooked and cooled potatoes. Cabbage is characterized by its high content of uronic acid polymers (péctin) and cellulose.

The main polysaccharide fractions in a number of cereal products are shown in Table III.

8. COMPARISON WITH OTHER METHODS

The values obtained by the crude fiber method (Analytical Methods Committee, 1943) and the neutral detergent fiber method of Goering and Van Soest (1970) are generally lower than those obtained by the present procedure, with the exception of rice and cornflakes. All the hemicellulose

TABLE II. Nonstarch Polysaccharides in Some Foods[a]

Food		Total	Rhamnose	Fucose	Arabinose	Xylose	Mannose	Galactose	Glucose	Uronic acid
								Constituent Sugar		
White flour	Cellulose	0.19	—	—	—	—	—	—	0.19	—
	Soluble NCP	1.96	—	—	0.68	0.89	t	0.18	0.21	—
	Insoluble NCP	1.05	—	—	0.23	0.49	0.07	t	0.26	—
	Total NSP	3.20	—	—	0.91	1.38	0.07	0.18	0.66	—
Whole wheat flour	Cellulose	1.64	—	—	—	—	—	—	1.64	—
	Soluble NCP	2.55	—	—	0.83	1.23	0.06	0.16	0.19	0.08
	Insoluble NCP	6.08	—	—	1.84	3.09	0.09	0.13	0.73	0.20
	Total NSP	10.27	—	—	2.67	4.32	0.15	0.29	2.56	0.28
Whole wheat bread	Cellulose	1.61	—	—	—	—	—	—	1.61	—
	Soluble NCP	2.67	—	—	0.88	1.27	0.05	0.14	0.28	0.05
	Insoluble NCP	5.63	ﾠt	—	1.74	2.90	0.16	0.16	0.47	0.20
	Total NSP	9.91	—	—	2.62	4.17	0.21	0.30	2.36	0.25
	Resistant starch	0.84	—	—	—	—	—	—	0.84	—
All-Bran	Cellulose	4.67	—	—	—	—	—	—	4.67	—
	Soluble NCP	3.94	t	—	1.05	1.80	0.03	0.19	0.76	0.11
	Insoluble NCP	15.22	t	—	4.82	7.88	0.22	0.31	1.36	0.63
	Total NSP	23.83	t	—	5.87	9.68	0.25	0.50	6.79	0.74
	Resistant starch	t	—	—	—	—	—	—	t	—
Cornflakes	Cellulose	0.24	—	—	—	—	—	—	0.24	—
	Soluble NCP	0.18	—	—	0.02	0.02	—	—	0.11	0.03
	Insoluble NCP	0.23	—	—	0.09	0.12	—	—	0.00	0.02
	Total NSP	0.65	—	—	0.11	0.14	—	—	0.35	0.05
	Resistant starch	2.92	—	—	—	—	—	—	2.92	—
Porridge oats	Cellulose	0.41	—	—	—	—	—	—	0.41	—
	Soluble NCP	4.51	t	—	0.35	0.24	t	0.14	3.70	0.08
	Insoluble NCP	2.15	t	—	0.56	0.90	0.09	t	0.45	0.15
	Total NSP	7.07	t	—	0.91	1.14	0.09	0.14	4.56	0.23

(continued)

TABLE II. (Continued)

Food		Total	Rhamnose	Fucose	Arabinose	Xylose	Mannose	Galactose	Glucose	Uronic acid
						Constituent Sugar				
Pearl barley	Cellulose	0.36	—	—	—	—	—	—	0.36	—
	Soluble NCP	4.77	—	—	0.48	0.52	0.13	0.07	3.53	0.04
	Insoluble NCP	2.66	—	—	0.70	1.10	0.21	t	0.63	0.02
	Total NSP	7.79	—	—	1.18	1.62	0.34	0.07	4.52	0.06
Rye flour	Cellulose	1.49	—	—	—	—	—	—	1.49	—
	Soluble NCP	4.61	—	—	1.41	2.14	0.15	0.10	0.73	0.08
	Insoluble NCP	7.80	—	—	2.22	3.62	0.18	0.21	1.45	0.12
	Total NSP	13.90	—	—	3.63	5.76	0.33	0.31	3.67	0.20
Haricot beans (dry)	Cellulose	4.20	—	—	—	—	—	—	4.20	—
	Soluble NCP	7.20	0.10	0.28	4.24	0.73	0.22	0.51	0.22	0.90
	Insoluble NCP	5.38	t	t	1.87	1.05	0.31	0.22	0.18	1.75
	Total NSP	16.78	0.10	0.28	6.11	1.78	0.53	0.73	4.60	2.65
Raw potato	Cellulose	1.77	—	—	—	—	—	—	1.77	—
	Soluble NCP	2.76	0.13	—	0.26	0.01	t	1.25	0.09	1.02
	Insoluble NCP	0.61	t	—	0.08	0.09	0.06	0.35	—	0.03
	Total NSP	5.14	0.13	—	0.34	0.10	0.06	1.60	1.86	1.05
Cooked potato	Cellulose	1.63	—	—	—	—	—	—	1.63	—
	Soluble NCP	2.64	0.12	—	0.23	0.01	0.03	1.19	0.19	0.87
	Insoluble NCP	0.57	t	—	0.08	0.08	0.06	0.32	0.00	0.03
	Total NSP	4.84	0.12	—	0.31	0.09	0.09	1.51	1.82	0.90
	Resistant starch	2.08	—	—	—	—	—	—	2.08	—
Raw cabbage	Cellulose	9.86	—	—	—	—	—	—	9.86	—
	Soluble NCP	13.53	0.85	0.10	3.14	0.19	0.05	1.26	0.38	7.56
	Insoluble NCP	4.21	0.05	0.07	0.84	1.33	0.64	0.76	0.00	0.52
	Total NSP	27.60	0.90	0.17	3.98	1.52	0.69	2.02	10.24	8.08

[a]From Englyst et al. (1982). Values are g/100 g dry matter; t, trace. NCP, noncellulosic polysaccharides; NSP, nonstarch polysaccharides.

TABLE III. Polysaccharide Content of Some Cereal Products[a]

Food	Percent dry matter	Starch	Resistant starch	Cellulose	Noncellulosic polysaccharides		Total NSP
					Soluble	Insoluble	
White bread[b]	60.7	77.5	1.15	0.13	1.91	0.59	2.63
White flour	88.0	79.6	0.19	0.16	1.58	0.86	2.60
White bread crust	76.4	72.4	0.52	0.14	1.81	0.61	2.56
White bread crumb	55.2	75.0	0.98	0.18	1.73	0.67	2.58
Brown bread[b]	58.7	67.7	0.91	1.06	2.33	3.85	7.25
Brown flour	88.0	68.0	0.13	1.29	2.19	4.53	8.01
Brown bread crust	76.6	63.0	0.58	1.03	2.90	3.49	7.42
Brown bread crumb	54.5	63.6	1.00	1.23	2.69	3.78	7.70
Whole meal bread[c]	60.4	64.6	0.80	1.52	2.57	5.48	9.58
Whole meal flour	88.0	64.9	0.12	1.57	2.55	6.03	10.15
Whole meal crust	75.2	60.3	0.42	1.35	3.07	5.00	9.42
Whole meal crumb	54.6	62.0	0.92	1.65	2.86	5.49	10.00
Wheat bran, Arjuna	87.6	16.4	—	8.17	4.25	28.60	41.06
Wheat bran, Allinson's Broad Bran	89.4	14.6	—	7.98	3.22	30.37	41.57
All-Bran (Kellogg's)	94.9	29.1	0.15	4.38	3.94	15.36	23.68
Weetabix	93.8	62.3	0.26	1.59	3.28	5.54	10.41
Shredded Wheat	91.6	64.4	0.88	1.70	2.33	6.70	10.73
Cornflakes	94.9	78.9	3.11	0.26	0.18	0.24	0.68

(*continued*)

TABLE III. (Continued)

Food	Percent dry matter	Starch	Resistant starch	Cellulose	Noncellulosic polysaccharides		Total NSP
					Soluble	Insoluble	
Rice Krispies	95.2	73.9	0.24	0.40	0.20	0.29	0.89
Oatmeal, medium ground	90.4	64.0	t	0.40	3.93	2.96	7.29
Scott's Porage Oats	90.0	65.1	—	0.28	3.98	2.96	7.22
Rye grain	86.0	66.7	0.17	1.52	4.47	7.24	13.23
Rye flour	86.6	62.2	0.21	1.40	4.61	7.68	13.69
Barley grain	87.1	72.1	—	1.44	3.89	6.50	11.83
White rice, round grain	86.5	92.4	t	0.16	0.16	0.35	0.67
Brown rice	86.0	85.8	—	0.70	0.14	1.18	2.02
White rice, long grain	87.4	88.7	—	0.21	0.13	0.24	0.58
Sago	86.5	101.3	0.72	0.35	0.26	—	0.61
Digestive Wheatmeal biscuits	97.1	46.4	0.13	0.33	1.38	1.26	2.97
Rich Tea biscuits	96.8	52.3	0.19	0.14	1.58	0.50	2.22
Semolina	86.5	75.8	0.49	0.31	1.22	1.06	2.59
Macaroni	88.0	76.7	0.22	0.28	1.59	1.11	2.98
Spaghetti	90.1	75.5	0.18	0.20	1.85	0.97	3.02
Spaghetti, whole wheat	90.1	62.9	0.21	1.78	2.42	5.75	9.95
Tapioca	87.0	102.1	—	0.08	0.13	0.23	0.44
Arrowroot	86.5	101.7	—	0.01	0.03	0.02	0.06

[a] From Englyst et al. (1983). Polysaccharide content given as g/100 g dry matter; t, trace; —, none detected.
[b] Average of four samples.

(NCP) is extracted and removed in the crude fiber method. In the neutral detergent procedure the water-soluble polysaccharides are extracted and lost.

Values obtained by Southgate's method (Southgate, 1969, 1976; Sivell and Wenlock, 1983) are normally higher than those found by the present procedure due to the incomplete removal of starch. Differences may also arise because of the less specific colorimetric method for the measurement of sugars.

Table IV compares the mean values obtained by the method tested in the collaborative dietary fiber trial organized by the Association of Official Analytical Chemists (AOAC) (Prosky *et al.*, 1984) with values obtained by the present method, which was used in collaborative studies organized by the Ministry of Agriculture, Fisheries and Food in the U. K. (Cummings *et al.*, 1985). For corn bran, which has a high content of NSP and low content of starch and protein, there is good agreement between the two methods when lignin is taken into account. For products with a high content of starch and/or protein considerable differences are seen between the results obtained by the two methods. Table V shows the values for total NSP in the 13 AOAC trial samples separated into soluble NCP, insoluble NCP, cellulose, and the constituent sugars. Resistant starch values are also given in Table IV. For these largely unprocessed foods the difference in values between the two methods cannot be explained on the basis of resistant starch.

TABLE IV. Percent Dietary Fiber in the 13 AOAC Trial Samples

	AOAC procedure[a]	MAFF procedure[b]	AOAC/MAFF
1 Corn bran	89.02	78.48	1.13
2 Iceberg lettu	23.31	19.24	1.21
3 Oats	12.47	7.59	1.64
4 Instant potato	7.22	4.74	1.52
5 Raisins	4.43	1.89	2.34
6 Rice	3.67	0.62	5.91
7 Rye bread	5.90	3.17	1.86
8 Soy isolate	7.51	0.97	7.74
9 Wheat bran	42.25	32.21	1.31
10 Whole wheat flour	12.92	9.79	1.31
11 White wheat flour	3.07	1.83	1.67
12 Mixed diet, nonvegetarian	7.19	4.11	1.74
13 Mixed diet, vegetarian	8.59	4.96	1.73

[a] Procedure of Prosky *et al.* (1984).
[b] Procedure of Englyst and Cummings (1984).

TABLE V. Nonstarch Polysaccharides (NSP) and Resistant Starch (RS) in the 13 AOAC Trial Samples Analyzed by the Present Procedure[a]

Sample	Total	Constituent Sugar						
		Rhamnose	Arabinose	Xylose	Mannose	Galactose	Glucose	Uronic acid
Corn bran								
Cellulose	16.70	—	—	—	—	—	16.70	—
Soluble NCP	6.57	0.25	2.50	3.00	0.08	0.45	—	0.29
Insoluble NCP	55.21	—	15.60	29.40	0.29	3.59	2.80	3.53
Total NSP	78.48	0.25	18.10	32.40	0.37	4.04	19.50	3.82
Iceberg lettuce								
Cellulose	7.17	—	—	—	—	—	7.17	—
Soluble NCP	9.35	0.55	0.65	0.16	0.04	0.67	0.12	7.16
Insoluble NCP	2.72	—	0.23	0.99	0.40	0.37	0.26	0.47
Total NSP	19.24	0.55	0.88	1.15	0.44	1.04	7.55	7.63
Oats								
Cellulose	0.48	—	—	—	—	—	0.48	—
Soluble NCP	4.86	—	0.26	0.16	0.04	0.09	4.20	0.11
Insoluble NCP	2.25	—	0.59	1.05	0.05	0.04	0.35	0.17
Total NSP	7.59	—	0.85	1.21	0.09	0.13	5.03	0.28
Resistant starch	0.06	—	—	—	—	—	0.06	—
Instant potato								
Cellulose	1.61	—	—	—	—	—	1.61	—
Soluble NCP	2.89	—	0.25	0.05	—	1.35	0.30	0.94
Insoluble NCP	0.24	—	—	—	—	0.20	—	0.04
Total NSP	4.74	—	0.25	0.05	—	1.55	1.91	0.98
Resistant starch	1.33	—	—	—	—	—	1.33	—
Raisins								
Cellulose	0.58	—	—	—	—	—	0.58	—
Soluble NCP	1.12	—	0.13	0.01	0.01	0.12	0.05	0.80
Insoluble NCP	0.19	—	0.02	0.08	0.03	—	0.04	0.02
Total NSP	1.89	—	0.15	0.09	0.04	0.12	0.67	0.82

Rice								
Cellulose	0.26	—	—	—	—	—	0.26	—
Soluble NCP	0.32	—	0.15	0.12	—	—	—	0.05
Insoluble NCP	0.04	—	—	—	—	—	—	0.04
Total NSP	0.62	—	0.15	0.12	—	—	0.26	0.09
Rye bread								
Cellulose	0.39	—	—	—	—	—	0.39	—
Soluble NCP	1.76	—	0.60	0.74	0.04	0.12	0.26	—
Insoluble NCP	1.00	—	0.27	0.42	0.20	0.02	0.06	0.03
Total NSP	3.15	—	0.87	1.16	0.24	0.14	0.71	0.03
Resistant starch	0.74	—	—	—	—	—	0.74	—
Soy isolate								
Cellulose	—	—	—	—	—	—	—	—
Soluble NCP	0.35	—	—	0.07	0.20	0.03	—	0.05
Insoluble NCP	0.62	—	0.06	0.03	0.42	0.06	—	0.05
Total NSP	0.97	—	0.06	0.10	0.62	0.09	—	0.10
Wheat bran								
Cellulose	5.89	—	—	—	—	—	5.89	—
Soluble NCP	3.51	—	1.10	1.7	—	0.08	0.17	0.46
Insoluble NCP	22.81	—	6.92	12.1	0.15	0.28	2.64	0.72
Total NSP	32.21	—	8.02	13.8	0.15	0.36	8.70	1.18
Resistant starch	0.08	—	—	—	—	—	0.08	—
Whole wheat flour								
Cellulose	1.77	—	—	—	—	—	1.77	—
Soluble NCP	1.83	—	0.64	0.88	—	0.12	0.12	0.07
Insoluble NCP	6.19	—	1.93	3.17	0.10	0.08	0.69	0.22
Total NSP	9.79	—	2.57	4.05	0.10	0.20	2.58	0.29
Resistant starch	0.19	—	—	—	—	—	0.19	—
White wheat flour								
Cellulose	0.24	—	—	—	—	—	0.24	—
Soluble NCP	0.94	—	0.40	0.50	—	—	0.02	—
Insoluble NCP	0.65	—	0.14	0.29	0.06	—	0.16	0.02
Total NSP	1.83	—	0.54	0.79	0.06	—	0.42	0.02

(continued)

TABLE V. (Continued)

Sample		Total	Constituent Sugar						
			Rhamnose	Arabinose	Xylose	Mannose	Galactose	Glucose	Uronic acid
Mixed diet, nonvegetarian	Cellulose	1.15	—	—	—	—	—	1.15	—
	Soluble NCP	1.72	—	0.51	0.30	0.07	0.18	0.16	0.50
	Insoluble NCP	1.24	—	0.32	0.45	0.17	0.06	0.05	0.19
	Total NSP	4.11	—	0.83	0.75	0.24	0.24	1.36	0.69
	Resistant starch	0.54	—	—	—	—	—	0.54	—
Mixed diet, vegetarian	Cellulose	1.50	—	—	—	—	—	1.50	—
	Soluble NCP	2.01	—	0.54	0.21	0.03	0.23	0.20	0.80
	Insoluble NCP	1.45	—	0.42	0.55	0.12	0.10	0.07	0.19
	Total NSP	4.96	—	0.96	0.76	0.15	0.33	1.77	0.99
	Resistant starch	0.55	—	—	—	—	—	0.55	—

[a] Values are g/100 g as received. NCP, noncellulosic polysaccharides.

ACKNOWLEDGMENTS. This work has been supported by grants from the National Association of British and Irish Millers and by the Danish Medical, Technical, Agricultural and Veterinary Research Councils.

REFERENCES

Analytical Methods Committee, 1943, *Analyst* **68**:276.

Anderson, I. H., Levine, A. S., and Levitt, M. D., 1981, Incomplete absorption of the carbohydrate in all-purpose wheat flour, *N. Engl. J. Med.* **304**:891.

Bacic, A., and Stone, B., 1980, A (1→3) (1→4) linked β-D-glucan in the endosperm cell-walls of wheat, *Carbohydrate Res.* **82**:372.

Bittner, A. S., Harris, L. E., and Campbell, W. F., 1980, Rapid *N*-methyl imidazole-catalyzed acetylation of plant cell wall sugars, *J. Agric. Food Chem.* **28**:1242.

Blakeney, A. B., Harris, P. J., Henry, R. J., and Stone, B. A., 1983, A simple and rapid preparation of alditol acetates for monosaccharide analysis, *Carbohydr. Res.* **113**:291.

Chang, M. L. W., and Johnson, M. A., 1980, Effect of lignin versus cellulose on the absorption of taurocholate and lipid metabolism in rats fed cholesterol diet, *Nutr. Rep. Int.* **21**:513.

Connors, K. A., and Pandit, N. K., 1978, *N*-Methylimidazole as a catalyst for analytical acetylations of hydroxy compounds, *Anal. Chem.* **50**:1542.

Cummings, J. H., Englyst, H. N., and Wood, R., 1985, Analysis of dietary fibre: Report of collaborative studies. Parts (a) and (b) (in press).

Englyst, H. N., and Cummings, J. H., 1984, Simplified method for the measurement of total non-starch polysaccharides by gas-liquid chromatography of constituent sugars as alditol acetates, *Analyst* **109**:937.

Englyst, H., Wiggins, H. S., and Cummings, J. H., 1982, Determination of the non-starch polysaccharides in plant foods by gas-liquid chromatography of constituent sugars as alditol acetates, *Analyst* **107**:307.

Englyst, H. N., Anderson, V., and Cummings, J. H., 1983, Starch and non-starch polysaccharides in some cereal foods, *J. Sci. Food Agric.* **34**:1434.

Fleming, S. E., and Vose, J. R., 1979, Digestibility of raw and cooked starches from legume seeds using the laboratory rat, *J. Nutr.* **109**:2067.

Fuwa, H., Takaya, T., and Sugimoto, Y., 1980, Degradation of various starch granules by amylases, in: *Mechanisms of Saccharide Polymerization and Depolymerization* (J. J. Marshall, ed.), Academic, New York, p. 73.

Goering, H. K., and Van Soest, P. J., 1970, *Forage Fiber Analysis,* USDA Agricultural Handbook no. 379, U. S. Department of Agriculture, Washington, D.C.

Hartley, R. D., 1978, The lignin fraction of plant cell walls, *Am. J. Clin. Nutr.* **31**:S90.

Holloway, W. D., Tasman-Jones, C., and Lee, S. P., 1978, Digestion of certain fractions of dietary fiber in humans, *Am. J. Clin. Nutr.* **31**:927.

Holm, J., Bjorck, I., Ostrowska, S., Eliasson, A.-C., Asp, N.-G., Larsson, K., and Lundquist, I., 1983, Digestibility of amylose–lipid complexes *in-vitro* and *in-vivo, Starke* **35**:294.

Judd, P. A., and Truswell, A. S., 1981, The effect of rolled oats on blood lipids and fecal steroid excretion in man, *J. Clin. Nutr.* **34**:2061.

Palmer, G. H., 1972, Morphology of starch granules in cereal grains and malts, *J. Inst. Brew. London* **78**:326.

Prosky, L., Asp, N. G., Furda, I., Devries, J. W., Schweizer, T. F., and Harland, B. F., 1984, Determination of total dietary fiber in foods, food products and total diets: Interlaboratory study, *J. Assoc. Anal. Chem.* **67**:1044.

Ring, S. G., and Selvendran, R. R., 1978, Purification and methylation analysis of cell wall material from *Solanum tuberosum, Biochemistry* **17**:745.

Shainkin, R., and Birk, Y., 1970, α-Amylase inhibitors from wheat isolation and characterization, *Biochim. Biophys. Acta* **221**:502.

Sivell, L. M., and Wenlock, R. W., 1983, The nutritional composition of British bread: London area study, *Hum. Nutr. Appl. Nutr.* **37A**:459.

Snow, P., and O'Dea, K., 1981, Factors affecting the rate of hydrolysis of starch in food, *Am. J. Clin. Nutr.* **34**:2721.

Southgate, D. A. T., 1969, Determination of carbohydrates in foods. II. Unavailable carbohydrates, *J. Sci. Food Agric.* **20**:331.

Southgate, D. A. T., 1976, The analysis of fiber, in: *Fiber in Human Nutrition* (G. A. Spiller and R. J. Amen, eds.), Plenum, New York, p. 31.

Theander, O., and Åman, P., 1980, Chemical composition of some forages and various residues from feeding value determinations, *J. Sci. Food Agric.* **31**:31.

Trowell, H., 1972, Crude fiber, dietary fiber and atherosclerosis, *Atherosclerosis* **16**:138.

Trowell, H., Southgate, D. A. T., Wolever, T. M. S., Leeds, A. R., Gassull, M. A., and Jenkins, D. J. A., 1976, Dietary fiber redefined, *Lancet* **1**:967.

Wachowiak, R., and Connors, K. A., 1979, *N*-Methylimidazole-catalyzed acelylation of hydroxy compounds prior to gas chromatographic separation and determination, *Anal. Chem.* **51**:27.

Walker, G. J., and Hope, P. M., 1963, The action of some α-amylases on starch granules, *Biochem. J.* **86**:452.

Wolever, T. M. S., Chan, C., Law, C., Bird, L., Ramdath, D., Moran, J. J., and Jenkins, D. J. A., 1983, The *in vitro* and *in vivo* anti-amylase activity of starch blockers, *J. Plant Foods* **5**:23.

3

The Relation between Composition and Properties of Dietary Fiber and Physiological Effects

DAVID A. T. SOUTHGATE

1. INTRODUCTION

In this chapter I review progress toward an understanding of the relation between the composition and properties of dietary fiber and the physiological effects that are associated with its ingestion. In this context I will use the term dietary fiber for the mixture of complex polysaccharides (Southgate, 1982) and lignin in the diet derived principally from plant cell-wall structures in foods. The complex polysaccharides making up dietary fiber (Table I) are distinguished by the fact that they do not contain α-linked glucosidic polymers and are therefore not susceptible to hydrolysis by the endogenous secretions of the mammalian digestive tract.

This chapter focuses on developments in our knowledge of the chemistry of the plant cell wall, developments in the analysis and characterization of dietary fiber in foods, and, finally, the links between the composition and properties of dietary fiber and its physiological effects.

2. THE CHEMISTRY OF THE PLANT CELL WALL

The major source of dietary fiber is the plant cell wall, and studies of the fundamental chemistry and structure of the plant cell wall form the basis for

DAVID A. T. SOUTHGATE • AFRC Food Research Institute, Norwich NR4 7UA, United Kingdom.

TABLE I. Components of Dietary Fiber

Components of plant cell wall		Isolated polysaccharides natural or added
Lignin	Cellulose,	Modified celluloses
	Noncellulosic	Pectin
	polysaccharides	Gums
	Pectic	Mucilages
	hemicelluloses	Algal polysaccharides

Non-α-glucan polysaccharides
Nonstarch polysaccharides

understanding the behavior of dietary fiber in foods and when consumed in the diet. Major efforts to study the plant cell wall in foodstuffs have led to substantial progress, and recent comprehensive reviews of the extensive information that has accumulated are available (Selvendran, 1983, 1984). Some general conclusions from this work need to be kept in mind in discussing the physiological effects of dietary fiber.

First, the plant cell wall is a complex physical structure, with a detailed molecular architecture (Albersheim, 1977) in which the major elements are polysaccharides, but where the protein and phenolic constituents, ranging from simple acids (Hartly et al., 1976; Hartley and Jones, 1977; Selvendran and O'Neill, 1982) to complex polymeric lignin, play important roles.

Second, the biochemical, chemical, and physical dissection of this structure and the fractionation of the mixture of polysaccharides are delicate and time-consuming operations. Techniques developed for one type of cell wall are rarely applicable in detail to other cell walls (Siegel, 1968).

Fractionation using the mildest techniques produces a range of polymers from most cell walls and these have been characterized in relatively few foods (Selvendran, 1984). A typical diet, with its mixture of foods and therefore types of plant organs, tissues, and cell types, provides the organism with a wide variety of polymeric types bound up, for the most part, within the physical structure of the cell walls themselves. It is therefore difficult to draw conclusions in detail about the role of specific polysaccharides from studies where mixed diets and therefore mixtures of cell walls have been fed. Conversely, the results of studies with isolated polysaccharides where specific isolated polysaccharides are fed at high levels of intake are difficult to relate to the behavior of the polysaccharide when consumed at usual levels of intake and as part of the cell wall.

Selvendran (1983) draws attention to differences due to the type of plant tissue that is the origin of the cell wall material, and their compositional implications. Table II illustrates the compositional differences between mature and immature cell walls from different plant tissues.

The fundamental studies of plant cell-wall chemistry provide the basis for the design and development of analytical methods for dietary fiber measurement (Southgate 1976a), and the results of cell wall analysis from fractionation studies that form part of the elucidation of the molecular architecture of the plant cell wall provide the reference against which analytical methods for dietary fiber must be assessed.

3. PROGRESS IN THE ANALYSIS AND CHARACTERIZATION OF DIETARY FIBER IN FOODS

The definition of dietary fiber as the sum of the polysaccharides and lignin that are not digested by the endogenous secretions of the human digestive tract (Trowell et al., 1976) has been largely accepted as the basis for analytical measurement. The physiological boundary between polysaccharides that are digested and absorbed as carbohydrate and those that resist hydrolysis in the small intestine and may or may not be fermented in the large intestine has been translated in analytical terms as resistance to hydrolysis by amylolytic enzymes (Southgate, 1976b; Southgate et al., 1978; Englyst et al., 1982.

TABLE II. Influence of Source on the Composition of Dietary Fiber[a]

Major food group	Type of tissue present	Major polymers present
Cereals	Parenchymatous endosperm; seed coats, partially lignified	Noncellulosic polysaccharides, arabinoxylans, β-D-glucans, glucurono arabinoxylans; cellulose, phenolic esters, lignin
Vegetables and fruits	Parenchymatous flesh; partially lignified vascular tissues; cutinized epidermal tissues	Noncellulosic polysaccharides, pectic substances, xyloglucans, glucuronoxylans; cellulose, lignin, cutin, and waxes
Seeds other than cereals, e.g., seed legumes	Parenchymatous cotyledons; thickened endospermal walls	Noncellulosic polysaccharides, pectic substances, xyloglucans, galactomannans; cellulose
Polysaccharide food additives	Amorphous, soluble, or dispersible	Gums; algal polysaccharides, alginates, sulfated galactans; cellulose esters and ethers; modified starches

[a] Based on Selvendran (1984).

The boundary is *de facto* defined empirically by the choice of enzyme(s) and the conditions used for the enzymatic hydrolysis (Southgate, 1974). It is important to emphasize the critical nature of this boundary in the analysis. Incomplete hydrolysis of starch results in inflated values for the dietary fiber polysaccharides, and over-rigorous hydrolytic conditions may lead to solubilization of dietary fiber compounds and underestimation. Of these, the former is most often seen and also involves problematic issues relating to the presence of "resistant starch," i.e., starch that resists *in vitro* enzymatic hydrolysis (Englyst *et al.*, 1982, and is formed in many starchy foods during thermal processing and storage.

In procedures for "unavailable carbohydrate" (Southgate, 1969; Southgate *et al.*, 1978), enzymes derived from fungal sources were used to remove and measure starch, but several workers have suggested that mammalian α-amylases would be more appropriate. Hellendoorn *et al.* (1975) used pancreatin, and much recent work uses a combination of mammalian and fungal enzymes.

The analysis of dietary fiber has recently been reviewed (Selvendran and Du Pont, 1984) and it is not necessary to deal at length with the large volume of work in this field. At the risk of oversimplification, one can state that two analytical approaches have been subjected to collaborative trial and give the indication that analysis has reached the stage where agreed methods are likely within a year or so. The approach developed by Asp *et al.* (1983) from the principles originally proposed by Williams and Olmsted (1935) and developed by Hellendoorn *et al.* (1975) has already been reviewed by Prosky (this volume, Chapter 1), and it is sufficient to summarize its principles as shown in Fig. 1; this method is designed to give a value for total dietary fiber. In the U. K. it was felt that a more detailed method that characterized the dietary fiber polysaccharides (Englyst *et al.*, 1982) was desirable for statutory food labeling purposes. The principles are shown in Fig. 2; the method is

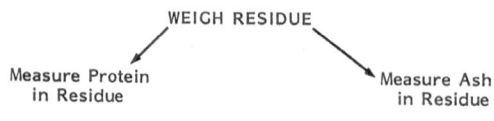

ANALYSIS AFTER STARCH REMOVAL
GRAVIMETRIC APPROACH

FOOD SAMPLE

Gelatinised with Thermamyl, Proteoylic enzyme
Amyloglucosidase

WEIGH RESIDUE

Measure Protein   Measure Ash
in Residue   in Residue

RESIDUE minus protein + ash ≡ TOTAL DIETARY FIBRE

FIGURE 1. Analysis after starch removal by the gravimetric approach.

MEASUREMENT OF NONSTARCH POLYSACCHARIDES

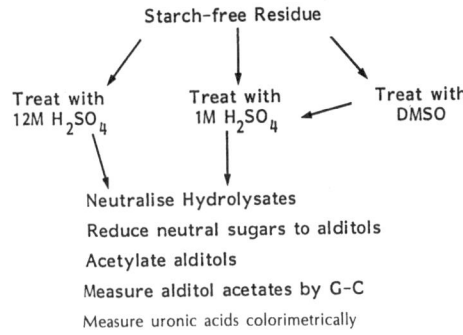

FIGURE 2. Measurement of non-starch polysaccharides. GLC, gas-liquid chromatography.

designed to measure the nonstarch polysaccharides and provides an estimate of resistant starch.

In collaborative trials both these methods performed quite reasonably, but the gravimetric procedures do show a poorer precision at dietary fiber concentrations of less than 10 g/100 g. Both methods are probably a little more time-consuming than is desirable for quality control purposes.

However, it is important to emphasize that a range of methods giving comparable results now exists to measure the sum of the nonstarch polysaccharides, so that confusion resulting from authors comparing different values for "total dietary fiber" (e.g., as unavailable carbohydrates plus lignin, and detergent fiber or crude fiber) and using the discrepancies to raise doubts concerning the significance of "so-called dietary fiber" is no longer justified.

The principles for the analysis of dietary fiber, especially the polysaccharide components, are clear (Selvendran and Du Pont, 1984); technical problems will arise as the methods are applied more widely, but these will not involve matters of principle. It is worth reemphasizing that dietary fiber is a complex mixture, and as with all natural materials (especially carbohydrates), its analysis requires intelligent application of the principles (Southgate, 1976b).

4. RELATION BETWEEN COMPOSITION AND PHYSIOLOGICAL EFFECTS

In this section I review progress toward our understanding of the link between the composition of ingested dietary fiber and physiological effects. It is clear that the physical properties of ingested dietary fiber are also important determinants of physiological effects, and it is better to consider composition and properties together.

The level of dietary fiber in diets that are composed of actual foods, in contrast to formulated semisynthethic meals, has a profound effect on the diet as a whole. High levels of fiber intake (30–40 g/day) can only be achieved if the diet contains a high proportion of plant foods and in particular, high-extraction cereals. The ratio of dietary fiber to energy content in foods imposes finite practical limits on dietary composition (Southgate and Penson, 1983), and very high intakes (>50 g) can only be achieved with low-fat diets, where the bulk of the energy intake is derived from complex polysaccharides, as in the typical diet eaten by the rural African (Bingham and Cummings, 1980), or where specially processed sources of dietary fiber or isolated polysaccharides are used.

Diets rich in dietary fiber have characteristic physical properties and the cell wall structure in themselves impart special properties to the food. As yet no system has been devised for quantifying these structural properties except in crude terms, such as particle size; however, cell wall thickness, proportion of intact cell wall structures, surface area of cell walls, etc., are likely to be important.

The perceived textural properties of these diets also is characteristic and affects the degree of mastication required and almost certainly dietary acceptance (Heaton, 1973). The nutritional significance of these properties has yet to be explored.

The direct effects of the physical structure of a food on satiety (Haber *et al.*, 1977) have not been related to specific properties or dietary composition. These effects are probably related to the "structure" of the diet and are not due to the specific contribution of dietary fiber.

4.1. Gastrointestinal Motility

Effects of changes in dietary fiber intake, usually produced by changes in the foods making up the diet, are associated with changes in motility (McCance *et al.*, 1953; Grimes and Goddard, 1977). As with effects on ingestion, these do not appear to be related to dietary fiber *per se,* but to changes in the structure of the diet and components associated with the dietary fiber. Changes in the viscosity or water binding and bulking of gastric contents can be produced by starches or complex nonstarch polysaccharides, proteins, or synthetic polymers; however, it is likely that quantitative starch is a major dietary factor in relation to gastric motility, and the rate of solubilization of starch in a meal is a factor that may or may not be associated with dietary fiber content and has an influence on gastric emptying (Grimes and Goddard, 1977).

The feedback control of gastric emptying, which is apparently dependent on the delivery of energy-yielding nutrients (Hunt and Stubbs, 1975), may be indirectly related to dietary fiber content if this affects starch hydrolysis by steric or direct effects on enzymatic activity.

4.2. Intestinal Absorption

The effect of complex nonstarch polysaccharides on the rate of absorption of glucose is clearly established and is dependent on the complex nonstarch polysaccharide being intimately associated with the test meal (Jenkins, 1980). The effect is not seen with cell wall preparations from foods such as wheat bran (Jenkins *et al.*, 1979) and is only associated with water-soluble or dispersible polysaccharides such as guar gum or pectin and possibly with foods containing complex nonstarch polysaccharides with similar physical properties. The effect is seen with neutral galactomannans such as guar and with acidic galacturonans such as pectin and is not attributable to chemical properties *per se* but to the capacity of these materials to produce viscous solutions or dispersions (Johnson and Gee, 1981; Gee *et al.*, 1983). Materials such as guar gum increase the viscosity of the contents of the stomach and small intestine *in vivo,* and *in vitro* studies show that there is an effect on glucose transport that is related to viscosity and is independent of the type of polysaccharide. The effect on transport can be seen *in vivo* in animals (Blackburn and Johnson, 1981) and in man (Blackburn *et al.*, 1984): the mechanism of action appears to be due to an increase in the physiologically unstirred layer at the mucosal surface. At the present time it is not possible to exclude the possibility that an increase in viscosity also slows the bulk movement of the intestinal contents and consequently the delivery of digesta to intestinal sites of absorption.

4.3. Bile Salt Binding

There is reasonably clear evidence for the binding of bile salts by cell wall preparation *in vitro* (Story *et al.*, 1979), but it is not possible to identify any clear association between chemical structure and binding. The physical properties of the cell wall preparations, including their large surface area and cellular structure, may be involved. Evidence that associated materials such as saponins are involved (Potter *et al.*, 1979; Topping *et al.*, 1980) is somewhat equivocal, but intuitively one would expect any surface-active component to elicit some effects, and that with complex cell wall preparations ascribing effects to defined fractions without considering associated components (Eastwood and Girdwood, 1968) is naive.

4.4. Binding of Inorganic Constituents

The position here is also unclear; some structural elements, such as uronic acid residues of pectin, clearly bind divalent ions *in vitro* (James *et al.*

1978); however, binding by cell wall preparations is not interpretable on a simple structural basis.

The major obstacle to establishing the structural basis for any binding effects is the need to use defined materials. Virtually all procedures for preparing cell wall preparations involve treatments that have effects on detailed polysaccharide structures. Thus, cellulose preparations from cell walls invariably involve some oxidative removal of lignin, and the preparation of detergent fiber preparations, while milder, involve treatments that modify the ionic state of carboxyl groups. The use of enzymatically prepared fractions seems to offer the most promise and it has been argued that the gravimetric procedures for measuring dietary fiber offer the possibility of making studies of binding effects after measurement of total dietary fiber (Asp *et al.*, 1983).

A major difficulty in establishing the structural features involved in binding is the presence of associated materials (Oberleas and Harland, 1977). Phytic acid, which is associated with many cereal cell walls and starch polysaccharide fractions from legumes such as soya, confounds many studies of cell wall preparations on the absorption of divalent ions. In the cell wall phytates are integral with the wall structures and are difficult to remove without chemical modification. Studies with preparations where the fiber–phytate ratios have been modified either by the addition of phytate or by enzymatic dephylinization suggest that the effects of phytate on iron absorption may be much more important than that of fiber, but that effects of phytate on zinc absorption are significant (Fairweather-Tait, 1982; Caprez and Fairweather-Tait, 1982).

Studies with isolated polysaccharides and binding of ions *in vitro* have demonstrated clear evidence of binding (Branch *et al.*, 1978), but extrapolation of these effects *in vivo* (Cummings *et al.*, 1979) has not shown effects of physiological importance, and extrapolation to effects of analogous polysaccharides within intact cell walls is difficult.

4.5 Large Intestine Effects

Much of the effort in dietary fiber research has been directed toward relating effects in the large intestine to the composition of the ingested dietary fiber. Substantial progress has been made in relation to these direct effects of dietary fiber.

4.5.1 Fecal Bulking

A detailed discussion of the mechanism of the effects of dietary fiber on fecal bulking is given in Chapter 7 and is summarized here. First, it is clear that the source and therefore composition of the dietary fiber have important effects. Thus it is not possible to generalize about the relationship between total dietary fiber intake and fecal bulking. Both composition and physical state, especially particle size, are important.

A relationship between fecal bulking and dietary fiber with regard to the intake of pentose-containing polysaccharides (Cummings et al., 1978), but it is not clear whether pentose polysaccharides merely provide an index of the fermentability of cell wall material (Bacon, 1979). Stephen and Cummings (1980a) have postulated that the degree of fermentability of a dietary fiber preparation is a major factor in its effect on fecal bulk. Selvendran (1984) has pointed out that the pentose effect may be due to structural features of the cereal cell wall, which in many of the fiber-rich diet studies provided a major proportion of the pentose polysaccharide intake. The greater effects of cereal cell walls on fecal bulking may thus be related to structural features that inhibit bacterial degradation and thus permit more of the cereal cell-wall polysaccharides to survive in the large intestine and contribute to fecal bulk.

Water binding of ingested fiber does not appear to be correlated with fecal bulk (Stephen and Cummings, 1979), but it may be postulated that polysaccharides with water-binding properties (McConnell et al., 1974) that are resistant to bacterial degradation would have the more important fecal bulking effects.

4.5.2 Bacterial Degradation in the Large Intestine

Considerable interest has been reawakened in the degradation of dietary fiber in the large intestine. It has been clear for many years (McCance and Laurence, 1929; Mangold, 1934) that considerable degradation of the polysaccharides in dietary fiber occurs in the large intestine. The extent of degradation appears to vary among individuals and is dependent on the source and composition of the dietary fiber (Table III). Individual variation in the extent of degradation is partially dependent on transit time, of which residence time in the large intestine is a major component (Southgate and Penson, 1983).

The effects of the composition of dietary fiber on degradation appear somewhat confused, primarily because of analytical problems. The choice of analytical method is of great importance, but the difficulties of precisely controlling human studies, and especially of marking fecal collections, produce some element of uncertainty.

Bacterial degradation is dependent on the physical state of the dietary fiber. Soluble polysaccharides are readily accessible to the microflora, whereas cell wall preparations are degraded by surface activity (Bacon, 1979), so

TABLE III. Influence of Source on the Degradation of Cellulosic Material

Source	Intake, g/day	Apparent digestibility, %	Degradation rate, g/day	Reference
Wheat bran	6.8	31.6	2.1	Williams and Olmsted (1935)
		24.0	1.7	
		33.0	2.2	
Cabbage	9.1	61.3	5.6	—
		43.5	4.0	
		59.2	5.4	
Carrot	8.7	72.5	6.3	—
		62.3	5.4	
		65.6	5.7	
Mixed diet	2.6	14.3	0.3	Southgate and Durnin (1970)
	8.0[a]	15.5	1.2	
Purified cellulose	6.0–8.5	57.0	3.4	Milton-Thompson and Lewis (1971)
		(85.0–13)		
Mixed diets	10.5	74.5	7.8	Farrell et al. (1978)
	18.8[a]	62.6	11.8	

[a] In both these studies dietary fiber from wheat accounted for much of the increase.

that thin cell walls are readily degraded, and particle size and the extent of exposure of cell wall surfaces will influence the extent of degradation.

One interesting feature that has emerged in these studies concerns bacterial growth (Stephen and Cummings, 1980b) on high-fiber diets, where the evidence suggests that the amounts of dietary fiber degraded are inadequate to account for this growth. This implies that other polysaccharide substates such as starch are available. This raises important issues relating to the inclusion or exclusion of enzymatically resistant starch within dietary fiber (Englyst et al., 1982, 1983).

The complex bacterial flora in the large intestine is capable of degrading the whole range of natural polysaccharides present in dietary fiber, and while structural features may have slight effects on the proportions of short-chain fatty acids produced (Cummings, 1981; McNeil et al., 1978), the physical state and cell wall architecture are most important (Van Soest, 1973).

5. SUMMARY

The physiological effects of dietary fiber ingestion are only weakly dependent on structural composition per se. Effects on dietary ingestion and satiety are dependent on higher levels of structure in the diet and on the integrity of the plant tissues in the diet. Effects in the small intestine are mediated by the physical effects of soluble or dispersible components on the viscosity of the intestinal contents. Binding effects may be structurally dependent, but remain to be clearly established. Effects in the large intestine on fecal bulking are apparently dependent on polysaccharide composition,

TABLE IV. Relation between Physiological Effect and Dietary Fiber

Physiological effect	Property or feature involved	Major determinant	Specific effects of dietary fiber
Food intake satiety	Dietary structure	State of foodstuffs ingested	Cell wall integrity
Gastric effects	Water-holding capacity of diet	Presence of hydratable components	Complex polysaccharides, starch, gums, mucilages, hydrocolloid additives
Absorption in small intestine	Presence of nonhydrolyzable hydrocolloid	Viscosity of intestinal contents	Soluble or dispersible polysaccharides forming gels or viscous solutions
Binding of bile salts; binding of inorganic ions		Surface activity?; functional groups on polysaccharides or lignin	Components associated with plant cell walls; uronic acid groups; lignin; associated components
Fecal bulking	Presence of nonabsorbable components	Nonstarch polysaccharides; balance between fermentable and nonfermentable components	Solubility; particle size; pentosans; associated components, e.g., lignin, determining fermentability

but these effects may be due to cell wall architecture and the presence of associated constituents in the cell wall.

Bacterial degradation is primarily dependent on solubility and the physical state of the dietary fiber ingested.

Much still remains to be done to establish the actual nature of effects in the small intestine and the long-term effects of dietary fiber ingestion on mucosal structure and function, in order to relate these effects to polysaccharide composition and properties.

In the large intestine detailed studies are required to establish the role of cell wall architecture in susceptibility to bacterial degradation. The relation between polysaccharide composition and the bacterial flora and metabolism is clearly of considerable importance in understanding whether, and in what directions, polysaccharide composition can influence the pattern of metabolites produced.

ACKNOWLEDGMENTS. I would like to acknowledge the role that discussions with my colleagues at the Food Research Institute, especially Dr. I. T. Johnson and Dr. R. R. Selvendran, played in developing the themes in this chapter.

REFERENCES

Albersheim, P., 1977, The primary cell wall, In: *Plant Biochemistry* (J. Bonner and J. E. Varner, eds.), Academic, New York, pp. 226–227.

Asp, N.-G., Johansson, C.-G., Hallmer, H., and Siljestrom, M., 1983, Rapid enzymatic assay of insoluble and soluble dietary fibre, *J. Agric. Food Chem.* **31**: 476–482.

Bacon, J. S. D., 1979, Plant cell wall digestibility and chemical structure, *Rep. Rowett Res. Inst.* **35**:99–108.

Bingham, S., and Cummings, J. H., 1980, Sources and intakes of dietary fibre in man, in: *Medical Aspects of Dietary Fibre* (G. A. Spiller and R. McPherson Kay, eds.), Plenum, New York, pp. 261–284.

Blackburn, N. A., and Johnson, I. T., 1981, The effect of guar gum on the viscosity of the intestinal contents and on glucose uptake from the perfused jejunum in the rat, *Br. J. Nutr.* **46**:239–246.

Blackburn, N. A., Redfern, J. S., Jarjis, H., Holgate, A. M., Hanning, I., Scarpello, J. H. B., Johnson, I. T., and Read, N. W., 1984, The mechanism of action of guar gum in improving glucose tolerance in man, *Clin. Sci.* **66**:329–336.

Caprez, A., and Fairweather-Tait, S. J., 1982, Effect of heat treatment and particle size of bran on mineral absorption in rats, *Br. J. Nutr.* **48**:467–475.

Cummings, J. H., 1981, Short chain fatty acids in the human colon, *Gut* **22**:763–779.

Cummings, J. H., Southgate, D. A. T., Branch, W., Houston, H., Jenkins, D. J. A., and James, W. P. T., 1978, Colonic response to dietary fibre from carrot, cabbage, apple, bran and guar gum, *Lancet* **i**:5–9.

Cummings, J. H., Southgate, D. A. T., Branch, W., Wiggins, H. S., Houston, H., Jenkins, D. J. A., Jibraj, T., and Hill, M. W., 1979, The digestion of dietary pectin in the human gut,

Eastwood, M. A., and Girdwood, R. H., 1968, Lignin: A bile salt sequestering agent, *Lancet* **ii**:1170–1172.

and its effect on calcium absorption and large bowel function, *Br. J. Nutr.* **41**:477–485.

Englyst, H. N., Anderson, V., and Cummings, J. H., 1983, Starch and non-starch polysaccharides in some cereal foods, *J. Sci. Agric.* **34**:1434–1440.

Englyst, H. N., Wiggins, H. S., and Cummings, J. H., 1982, Determination of the non-starch polysaccharides in plant foods by gas-liquid chromatography of constituent sugars as alditol acetates, *Analyst* **107**:307–318.

Farrell, D. J., Girle, L., and Arthur, J., 1978, Effects of dietary fibre on the apparent digestibility of major food components in men, *Aust. J. Exp. Biol. Med. Sci.* **56**:469–479.

Fairweather-Tait, S. J., 1982, The effects of different levels of wheat bran on iron absorption in rats from breads containing similar amounts of phytate, *Br. J. Nutr.* **47**:243–249.

Gee, J. M., Blackburn, N. A., and Johnson, I. T., 1983, The influence of guar gum intestinal cholesterol transport in the rat, *Br. J. Nutr.* **50**:215–224.

Grimes, D. S., and Goddard, J., 1977, Gastric emptying of wholemeal and white bread, *Gut* **18**:725–729.

Haber, G. B., Heaton, K. W., Murphy, D., and Burroughs, L. F., 1977, Depletion and disruption of dietary fibre, effects on satiety, plasma glucose and serum insulin, *Lancet* **ii**:679–682.

Hartley, R. D., and Jones, E. C., 1977, Phenolic components and degradability of cell walls of grass and legume species, *Phytochemistry* **16**:1531–1534.

Hartley, R. D., Jones, E. C., and Wood, T. M., 1976, Carbohydrates and carbohydrate esters of ferulic acid released from cell walls of *Lolium multiflorum* by treatment with cellulolytic enzymes, *Phytochemistry* **15**:305–307.

Heaton, K. W., 1973, Food fibre as an obstacle to energy intake, *Lancet* **ii**:1418–1421.

Hellendoorn, E. W., Noordhoff, M. G., and Slagman, J., 1975, Enzymatic determination of the indigestible residue (dietary fibre) content of human foods, *J. Sci. Food Agric.* **26**: 1461–1468.

Hunt, J. N., and Stubbs, D. F., 1975, The volume and energy content of meals as determinants of gastric emptying, *J. Physiol.* **245**:209–225.

James, W. P. T., Branch, W. J., and Southgate, D. A. T., 1978, Calcium binding by dietary fibre, *Lancet* **1**:636–639.

Jenkins, D. J. A., 1980, Dietary fibre and carbohydrate metabolism, in: *Medical aspects of dietary fibre* (G. A. Spiller and R. Macpherson-Kay, eds.), Plenum, New York, pp. 175–192.

Jenkins, D. J. A., Reynolds, D., Leeds, A. R., Waller, A. L., and Cummings, J. H., 1979, Hypocholesterdemic action of dietary fibre unrelated to faecal bulking effect, *Am. J. Clin. Nutr.* **32**:2430–2435.

Johnson, I. T., and Gee, J. M., 1981, Effect of gel-forming gums on the intestinal unstirred layer and sugar transport *in vitro*, *Gut* **22**:398–403.

Jenkins, D. J. A., Reynolds, D., Leeds, A. R., Waller, A. L., and Cummings, J. H., 1979, Hypocholesterolemic action of dietary fibre unrelated to faecal bulking effect, *Am. J. Clin. Nutr.* **32**:2430–2435.

Johnson, I. T., and Gee, J. M., 1981, Effect of gel-forming gums on the intestinal unstirred layer and sugar transport *in vitro*, *Gut* **22**:398–403.

Mangold, D. E., 1934, The digestion and utilisation of crude fibre, *Nut. Abs. Rev.,* **3**, 647–656.

McCance, R. A., and Lawrence, R. D., 1929, The Carbohydrate Content of Foods, Special Report Series, Medical Research Council, no. 135 Her Majesty's Stationery Office, London.

McCance, R. A., Prior, K. M., and Widdowson, E. M., 1953, A radiological study of the rate of passage of brown and white bread through the digestive tract of man, *Br. J. Nutr.* **7**:98–104.

McConnell, A. A., Eastwood, M. A., and Mitchell, W. D., 1974, Physical characteristics of vegetable foodstuffs that could influence bowel function, *J. Sci. Food Agric.* **25**:1457–1464.

McNeill, N. I., Cummings, J. H., and James, W. P. T., 1978, Short chain fatty acid absorption by the human large intestine, *Gut* **19**:819.

Milton-Thompson, G. J., and Lewis, B., 1971, The breakdown of dietary cellulose in man, *Gut* **12**:853–854.

Oberleas, D., and Harland, B. F., 1977, Nutritional agents which affect metabolic zinc status in zinc metabolism, in: *Current Aspects in Health and Disease*, A. R. Liss, New York, pp. 11–24.

Potter, J. D., Topping, D. L., and Oakenfull, D., 1979, Soya, saponins and plasma cholesterol, *Lancet* i:223.

Selvendran, R. R., 1983, The chemistry of plant cell walls, in: *Dietary Fibre* (G. G. Birch and K. J. Parker, eds.), Applied Science, London, pp. 95–147.

Selvendran, R. R., 1984, The plant cell wall as a source of dietary fibre: chemistry and structure, *Am. J. Clin. Nutr.* **39**:320–337.

Selvendran, R. R., and Du Pont, M. S., 1984, The analysis of dietary fibre, in: *Food Analysis Techniques*, Volume 3 (R. D. King, ed.), Applied Science, London, pp. 1–68.

Selvendran, R. R., and O'Neill, M. A., 1982, Plant glycoproteins, in: *Plant Carbohydrates I* (F. A. Loewus and W. Tanner, eds.), Springer, Berlin, pp. 515–583.

Siegel, S. M., 1968, The biochemistry of the plant cell wall, in: *Comprehensive Biochemistry*, Volume 26A (M. Florkin and E. H. Stotz, eds.), Elsevier, Amsterdam, pp. 1–51.

Southgate, D. A. T., 1969, Determination of carbohydrates in foods II Unavailable carbohydrate, *J. Sci. Food Agric.* **20**:331–335.

Southgate, D. A. T., 1974, Problems in the analysis of polysaccharides in food-stuff, *J. Assoc. Pub. Anal.* **12**:114–118.

Southgate, D. A. T., 1976a, The analysis of dietary fibre, in: *Fibre in Human Nutrition* (G. A. Spiller and R. J. Amen, eds.), Plenum, New York, pp. 73–107.

Southgate, D. A. T., 1976b, *Determination of Food Carbohydrates*, Applied Science, London.

Southgate, D. A. T., 1982, Definition and terminology of dietary fibre, in: *Dietary Fibre in Health and Disease* (G. A. Vahouny and D. Kritchevsky, eds.), Plenum, New York, pp. 1–7.

Southgate, D. A. T., and Durnin, J. V. G. A., 1970, Calorie conversion factors; An experimental re-assessment of the factors used in the calculation of the energy value of human diets, *Br. J. Nutr.* **24**:517–535.

Southgate, D. A. T., and Penson, J. M., 1983, Testing the dietary fibre hypothesis, in: *Dietary Fibre* (C. G. Birch and K. J. Parker, eds.), Applied Science, London, pp. 1–19.

Southgate, D. A. T., Hudson, G. J., and Englyst, H., 1978, The analysis of dietary fibre, the choices for the analyst, *J. Sci. Food Agric.* **29**:979–998.

Stephen, A. M., and Cummings, J. H., 1979, Water-holding by dietary fibre *in vitro* and its relationship to faecal out-put in man, *Gut* **20**:722–729.

Stephen, A. M., and Cummings, J. H., 1980, Mechanism of action of dietary fibre in human colon, *Nature* **284**:283–284.

Stephen, A. M., and Cummings, J. H., 1980b, The microbial contribution to human faecal mass, *J. Med. Microbiol.* **13**:45–56.

Story, J. A., Kritchevsky, D., and Eastwood, M. A., 1979, Dietary fibre and bile acid interactions, in: *Dietary Fibres, Chemistry and Nutrition* (G. E. Inglett and S. I. Falkenhag, eds.), Academic, New York, pp. 49–55.

Topping, D. L., Storer, G. B., Calvert, C. D., Illman, R. J., Oakenfull, D. G., and Weller, R. A., 1980, Effects of dietary saponins on faecal bile acids and neutral sterols, plasma lipids and hypo-protein turnover in the pig, *Am. J. Clin. Nutr.* **33**:783–786.

Trowell, H., Southgate, D. A. T., Wolever, T. M. S., Leeds, A. R., Gassull, M. A., Jenkins, D. A., 1976, Dietary fibre redefined (letter), *Lancet* **1**:967.

Van Soest, P. J., 1973, The uniformity and nutritive availability of cellulose, *Fed. Proc.* **32**:1804–1808.

Williams, R. D., and Olmsted, W. H., 1935, A biochemical method for determining indigestible residue (crude fibre) in faeces lignin, cellulose and non-water soluble hemicelluloses, *J. Biol. Chem.* **108**:653–666.

4

Federal Regulations

JOHN E. VANDERVEEN

Health claims for fiber-containing foods have been made for more than a century. Although not described as fiber, removal of fiber-containing portions of wheat from flour was the subject of much debate in the 19th century (Deutsch, 1977). The effects of wheat bran on promoting increased bowel evacuation were also recognized. In the early 1900s health claims for wheat bran were common in breakfast cereal advertisements. In one advertisement, the statements "Put a handful of health in the bread!" and "Doctors are stressing the importance of more bran or 'bulk' in the diet" were used to draw attention to bran cereals. This same advertisement included a guarantee that, if eaten according to directions and did not relieve constipation safely, the purchase price would be refunded (McCall's Magazine, 1927). Identical claims made directly on the package were largely unregulated until after the Federal Food, Drug and Cosmetic Act of June 25, 1938.

On October 31, 1940 the Food and Drug Administration held a hearing on dietary properties of food purporting to be or represented for special dietary uses. On November 22, 1941 the agency published findings of fact and regulations, which included labeling requirements for "non digestable carbohydrates" (FDA, 1941; Federal Register, 1941). Although the hearing record is no longer available, it is apparent from the findings of fact that the valued properties of foods having a high-fiber content were primarily attributed to the lowering of the caloric content of foods. These findings are as follows:

> Some carbohydrate substances are not digested or assimilated by the human organism and supply no food energy. Only the carbohydrates which may be digested and assimilated are available to the metabolic processes of the organism.

JOHN E. VANDERVEEN • Food and Drug Administration, Division of Nutrition, Washington, D.C. 20204.

Carbohydrates which are nonavailable to the metabolic processes have a theoretical caloric value but supply no calories to the human organism.

The value of a food for special dietary use may depend on the presence therein of a constituent which is not utilized in normal metabolism and which consequently has no nutritive value.

Its use may be for the reduction of caloric intake, as in the case of mineral oil; for the promotion of laxation, as in the case of fibrous plant matter; or for the satisfaction of taste desires without increasing food value, as in the case of saccharin.

Information necessary to inform the purchaser of the value of a food for special dietary use by reason of its content of such a constituent includes a statement of the percent by weight of the constituent in the food, preceded or followed by the word "nonnutritive," except as hereinafter noted in finding 98 with respect to saccharin.

If such constituent is fibrous plant matter it is commonly determined as and expressed as crude fiber.

The regulation that resulted from these findings of fact read as follows:

Label statements relating to nonnutritive constituents. If a food purports to be or is represented for special dietary use by man by reason of the presence of any constituent which is not utilized in normal metabolism, the label shall bear a statement of the percent by weight of such constituent, and in juxtaposition with the name of such constituent, the word "nonnutritive." If such constituent is fibrous plant matter, it shall be considered to be crude fiber and its percent expressed as such.

This regulation remained in effect for over 38 years. In 1979 this regulation was withdrawn from the published regulations, along with other parts of regulations concerning special dietary foods, because of a successful court suit brought against the agency regarding vitamin and mineral supplements (Federal Register, 1979a,b).

For some time the agency has recognized the need for revision of the labeling of fiber to include other fractions of carbohydrates that are not digested by human enzymes; however, the scientific base for such rule-making has not yet been established. For example, on December 21, 1979 the agency made the following statement (Federal Register, 1979c):

Fiber is an essential dietary component for normal bowel function. Some advocates of higher fiber diets have theorized that the incidence of bowel cancer and other intestinal diseases may be related to the decreased amount of fiber in western diets, and these theories have gained a measure of public currency. Some segments of the food industry, especially cereal manufacturers, have increased the use of fiber declaration on product labels in response to the increased public interest. The question here is whether to increase information food labels provide about fiber content.

Until recently, scientists and consumers had only a limited interest in the fiber content of foods. The biomedical aspects of fiber in its various forms are unsettled and the subject still generates considerable controversy. There is no scientific consensus on a definition of "fiber." Both the government and industry are still conducting research to solve the methodological problems related to the several types of dietary fiber. The only official method of analysis currently available is for "crude fiber," which is just a fraction of total dietary fiber.

Finally, the relationship of dietary fiber to health remains controversial. FDA regulations [21 CFR 105.3(d)]* now require that any disclosure of fiber content must be expressed as "crude fiber" and declared as a percent by weight.

Despite the lack of regulations on fiber content, the agency has permitted declaration of fiber on breakfast cereals and other products provided such information has been truthful and not misleading.

Current regulatory initiatives continue to focus on the caloric aspects of dietary fiber. On September 22, 1978 the FDA published a final regulation on label statements relating to usefulness in reducing or maintaining caloric intake or body weight (21 CFR 105.66) (Federal Register, 1978a). In this regulation the use of nonnutritive ingredients is addressed as follows:

> Any food ... that achieves its special dietary usefulness by use of a nonnutritive ingredient (i.e., one not utilized in normal metabolism) shall bear on its label a statement that it contains a nonnutritive ingredient and the percentage by weight of the nonnutritive ingredient.

A proposal was published in conjunction with the final order, which, had it been finalized, would have permitted reduced calorie claims for breads that achieved only a one-fourth reduction in lieu of the one-third reduction required under §21 CFR 105.66 (Federal Register, 1978b). The rationale for proposing a lower requirement for bread was that inclusion of fiber at levels necessary to achieve a one-third reduction in digestable calories as measured by crude fiber measurements resulted in an organoleptically unacceptable product. After due consideration of the fact that significant levels of undigestable carbohydrates were not measured by the crude fiber method, which would have achieved the difference between a one-fourth and a one-third reduction in calories, it was decided to withdraw the proposal and propose methods for measuring dietary fiber and calculating available calories. This withdrawal of the bread exemption and the proposal for a method for measuring dietary fiber was published on August 13, 1984 (Federal Register, 1984a). Together with a correction published on September 17, 1984 (Federal Register, 1984b), the regulations for nutrition labeling of food would be amended as follows:

> Caloric content will be determined by the Atwater method as described in A. L. Merrill and B. K. Watt, "Energy Value of Foods-Basis and Derivation," USDA Handbook 74 (1955), except that the nondigestible dietary fiber may be subtracted from the total carbohydrate content before calculation of the calories

*As noted earlier, this provision in 21 CFR 105.3(d) was deleted.

contributed by the carbohydrate portion of the food. The nondigestible dietary fiber will be determined by the method entitled, "Total Dietary Fiber, AOAC Collaborative Study, January, 1984." Both methods are incorporated by reference.

Dietary fiber has also had consideration in federal regulations relative to its laxative effects. On March 21, 1975 the agency published an advanced notice of public rule-making (monograph) that addresses the properties of bran and other foods that were noted for laxative effects (Federal Register, 1975). The scientific information relating to this subject is as follows:

> Wheat bran consists largely of hemicellulose, cellulose and "crude fiber" of uncertain chemical composition. When fed to animals and man as bran, these components escape digestion and result in decreased intestinal transit time and increased stool bulk, weight and water content.
>
> Bran's laxative action seems related to its hydrophilic properties and to the direct action on the colon of undefined substances produced by the bacterial action on the bran.
>
> Dietary fiber seems to play the major role in the action of bran. The role of fiber in the gut is not precisely understood because of the incomplete knowledge of its composition and the inadequate techniques for measuring each component.
>
> Bran-rich breakfast cereals and wholewheat bread are convenient sources of crude fiber: 100 grams of bran flakes (various brands) contain between 2.7 to 6.5 grams of crude fiber and one slice of wholewheat bread contains 1–2 grams. As with other bulk laxatives, intestinal obstruction may occur if bran is given for constipation in patients with partial obstruction of the digestive tract.
>
> Bran tablets, as opposed to dietary bran, are classified in category III (insufficient evidence that this form is an effective laxative).

Comments made to this notice of advanced rule-making are on file and available for review. The agency is expecting to publish a proposed rule on laxatives in which the policy relative to labeling claims for the laxative effects of foods will likely be addressed. Two aspects are probable: (1) claims for laxative effects of foods or food-derived substances will be regarded as drug claims; and (2) such claims will have to be substantiated through analysis of clinical data.

SUMMARY

The statement made in notice of advanced rule-making published on December 21, 1979 (Federal Register, 1979c), that the biomedical aspects of fiber in its various forms are unsettled and the subject still generates considerable controversary, remains valid today. Consequently, it is impossible for the FDA or other regulatory agencies to promulgate regulations pertaining to claims for the usefulness of these substances in human diets except in reducing available calories or promoting laxation. It is evident from data reported in the scientific literature that the various forms of fiber have vastly different properties in binding undesirable dietary lipid component, bile acids, and other substances suspected of contributing to the incidence of such degenerative diseases as atherosclerosis and cancer. It appears also that the beneficial effects of individual fiber components on promoting a more desirable rate of absorption of simple carbohydrates in diabetic individuals also vary greatly. Consequently, it is premature to permit claims other than those already permitted by regulation.

In the future as more scientific data become available it seems probable that the inclusion of information on levels of specific nondigestible plant material in food labeling information may be permitted by regulation. However, the inclusion of such information could only be justified on the basis of evidence that such nondigestible plant materials provided discrete biomedical benefits to significant numbers of individuals in segments of the population or the entire population. To permit claims for specific dietary fiber components in the absence of such scientific evidence would be misleading to the public.

In the case where a specific component(s) of dietary fiber were shown to be beneficial in the dietary management of a specific disease(s) for very small numbers of population segments, specific claims for such substances may be warranted as either a medicinal food and/or a drug. Again, the criteria for proposing regulations to allow such claims should be based on carefully designed clinical studies that provide evidence of efficacy.

In summary, inclusion of truthful information on dietary fiber content that is not misleading is now being permitted on food labels and required in association with calorie claims made on the basis of the presence of dietary fiber in such foods. In addition, claims for certain fibrous plant materials may also be made for preparations sold as over-the-counter drugs. More scientific evidence is needed before claims for dietary fiber or components of dietary fiber can be made for other biomedical conditions.

REFERENCES

Advertisement for "All Bran," *McCall's* **1927**(March), 78.

Deutsch, R. M., 1977, *The New Nuts among the Berries,* Bull, San Alto, California.

FDA, 1941, Regulations Promulgated on Food for Special Dietary Uses, Press release, U. S. Food and Drug Administration, Washington, D.C.

Federal Register, 1941, Label statements concerning dietary properties of foods purporting to be or represented for special dietary uses, *Fed. Regis.* **6**:5921.

Federal Register, 1975, Over-the-counter drugs; Proposal to establish monographs for OTC laxative; Antidiarrheal, emetic, and antiemetic products, *Fed. Regis.* **40**(56):12902.

Federal Register, 1978a, Foods for special dietary use, *Fed. Regis.* **43**(185):43248.

Federal Register, 1978b, Special dietary foods label statements; Misleading statement, calorie labeling for bread, *Fed. Regis.* **43**(185):48261.

Federal Register, 1979a, Vitamin and mineral products: Revocation of regulation, *Fed. Regis.* **44**(53):16005.

Federal Register, 1979b, Foods for special dietary use, vitamin and mineral products: Revocation of regulation, *Fed. Regis.* **44**(166):49665.

Federal Register, 1979c, Food labeling: Tentative position of agencies (DHEW, FDA; USDA; FSPS; FTC; BCP), *Fed Regis.* **44**(247):75991.

Federal Register, 1984a, Food labeling; Nutrition labeling of food; Calorie content, *Fed. Regis.* **49**(157):32216.

Federal Register, 1984b, Nutrition labeling of food; Calorie content; Correction, *Fed. Regis.* **49**(181):36405.

5

Socioeconomic Aspects of a Fiber-Deficient Public Diet

CHARLES T. BONFIELD

1. INTRODUCTION

Increasing evidence in the world literature is confirming the relationship between diets deficient in dietary fiber and the prevalence of certain gastro-intestinal, cardiovascular, metabolic, and, perhaps, oncologic diseases. Pioneering ideas and observations in this area of human nutrition are presented in reviews by Cleave et al. (1966), (1974) and Burkitt and Trowell (1975). More recently, two rather extensive literature reviews with regard to the value of dietary fiber in health and disease have been undertaken and reported by the Federation of American Societies for Experimental Biology under grants provided by the Bureau of Food of the U. S. Food and Drug Administration (Kimura, 1977; Talbot, 1980). Some evidence for the association between fiber deficiency and consequent disease has been demonstrated in well-controlled animal and human investigations. Other data have been extracted from epidemiologic information and from inference.

Dietary fiber research is currently in its renaissance. Laboratory methods intended to be used for the chemical analysis and classification of dietary fiber are being developed and improved in a number of scientific centers around the world (Prosky et al., 1984; Englyst and Cummings, 1984; Theander and Åman, 1982; Asp, et al., 1983). Techniques that can be used to measure the physiological effects and the clinical benefits of dietary fiber are also being developed by Albrink, Anderson, Bingham, Cummings, Eastwood, Heaton, Hill, Jenkins, Kelsay, Kritchevsky, Leeds, Read, Salyers, Schneeman, Southgate, Story, Vahouny, Walker, and others (Vahouny and Kri-

CHARLES T. BONFIELD • Farma Food, Washington, D.C. 20007.

tchevsky, 1982). Since this is a relatively new and rapidly growing field, there is considerable controversy among research workers with respect to the validity of various scientific methods and the reliability and reproducibility of the results of current research activities. Consequently, it has not been possible to obtain a reasonable consensus among international experts toward establishing a recommended dietary guideline for dietary fiber in human nutrition. Indeed, expert opinion varies widely with respect to the quantities of dietary fiber required to promote and sustain public health. It is even more difficult to establish agreement about the approximate balance that should be provided from various sources of dietary fiber derived from grains, vegetables, fruits, and other foods. This ambiguous environment has inhibited the development of a public policy with regard to recommended levels of dietary fiber in the public diet.

This situation should and must be changed. The accumulated knowledge about human requirements for dietary fiber, even though controversial, is surely adequate to formulate some broad public dietary guideline for this essential macronutrient. A more educated and better informed public is seeking and should be given recommended guidelines for average daily intake of dietary fiber.

While it does not seem likely that, even in the near future, current dietary fiber research will provide the hard scientific evidence that most scientists would find necessary as the basis for establishing a dietary fiber guideline, we cannot in good conscience further delay this decision. Continued procrastination in setting guidelines will perpetuate public diets deficient in dietary fiber and thereby result in a continued high prevalence of associated deficiency diseases. It is essential that a compromise be made and that a guideline be established as soon as possible, even if it is a temporary one. Thereafter, adjustments in the recommended quantities and types of dietary fiber required for normal human nutrition can be made, when substantial evidence is presented from current and future research. Surely, a range of approximately 30–40 g of dietary fiber per day from mixed food sources is a reasonable compromise for a public guideline and can be substantiated with current scientific knowledge. Such a guideline has all the potential to do some good, and certainly cannot do any harm.

2. SOCIOECONOMIC ASPECTS

Clearly, the social, medical, and economic costs of perpetuating a public diet deficient in dietary fiber outweigh the risk that our recommendations may be slightly inaccurate. The human suffering and the socioeconomic costs that result from dietary fiber deficiency diseases are enormous. The list of diseases associated with this macronutrient deficiency is extensive, but can be grouped for the purposes of this discussion into three general categories: (1) systemic/metabolic diseases, (2) digestive diseases, and (3) cancer. The health literature in the U. S. contains considerable information about the prevalence and the associated costs of diseases in these three categories.

3. SYSTEMIC/METABOLIC DISEASES

The socioeconomic costs of systemic/metabolic diseases, including hypertension, diabetes, coronary heart disease, obesity–overweight, gallstones, varicose veins, and other conditions that may result from fiber-deficient diets, cannot realistically be estimated. It is obvious, however, that the cost of human suffering, medical care, time lost from work, and other factors associated with these diseases represents a large share of our annual health care expenditure and loss of productivity. Reducing this medical and socioeconomic burden to any reasonable degree would make a significant contribution to the welfare and well-being of mankind. The problem, of course, is how to get started. Many of these disease conditions and syndromes do not have a single, simple etiology. Indeed, most systemic/metabolic problems are complex and are associated with a number of interrelated and complicated etiologic factors, not the least of which are age, sex, and certain inherited or genetic predispositions to various health problems. Even so, current well-controlled animal and human clinical research studies highlight the importance and significance of human nutrition in preventing, controlling, and/or ameliorating many of these disease conditions. For example, while certain individuals are sensitive to sodium, their hypertension can be sufficiently well-controlled with low-sodium diets. Also, most individuals bothered by bouts of simple constipation can be quite effectively treated and relieved with the addition of wheat bran or other sources of dietary fiber to their diet.

The nutritional factors that come into play in hypertension, diabetes, obesity, and other systemic/metabolic diseases are also interrelated and complex. However, there is firm clinical evidence that overweight–obese individuals are more prone to earlier mortality (Dublin, 1953; Society of Actuaries, 1979), hypertension (Ashley and Kannel, 1974; Larsson *et al.*, 1981; Rimm *et al.*, 1975; Reisin, *et al.*, 1978; Jung *et al.*, 1979; Tuck *et al.*, 1981), diabetes (Bray *et al.*, 1979; Westlund and Nicolayson, 1972; Ashley and Kannel, 1974; Keen, 1975; Rimm *et al.*, 1975), hypercholesterolemia (Ashley and Kannel, 1974; Olefsky *et al.*, 1975; Leelarthaepin *et al.*, 1974; Alexander, 1975), coronary heart disease (Garrow, 1974; Bray, 1979; Lew and Garfinkel, 1979; Cook, 1978; Rabkin *et al.*, 1977; Ashley and Kannel, 1974), gallbladder disease (Mabee *et al.*, 1976; Rimm *et al.*, 1975; Bray *et al.*, 1979; Heaton, 1975), and other serious health problems. There is also firm evidence that this complex of diseases can be ameliorated or controlled by reducing the amount of fat and by increasing the amount of dietary fiber in the diet. The reduction of fats—particularly saturated fats—in the American diet is most probably the single most important nutritional factor contributing to the rapidly falling incidence of strokes and other cardiovascular disease in the U. S. population during the past 20 years. An increase in the levels of dietary fiber would follow as a second order of priorities in nutritional mangement of these diseases.

Foods high in dietary fiber are normally low in fats. It is therefore difficult to compare epidemiologic information with regard to disease incidence obtained from populations consuming a diet high in dietary fiber to information from populations with dietary fiber deficiencies. The former tend to consume less dietary fat, while the low-fiber eaters tend to consume higher quantities of fat. The relative importance of reducing levels of dietary fats versus increasing levels of dietary fiber and the potential impact of these actions on reducing hypertension, coronary heart disease, diabetes, overweight, and other serious diseases cannot be determined at this time. Certainly, reducing the level of dietary fat appears to be the most important factor; however, clinical evidence would indicate that increasing levels of dietary fiber is also important. What, then, are the potential socioeconomic consequences of reducing dietary fats and increasing dietary fiber in the public diet?

3.1 High Blood Pressure

Approximately 60 million Americans have elevated blood pressures (above 140/90 mm Hg) and are at increased risk for illness and death. Of these people, 35 million—15% of the U. S. population—have blood pressures at or above 160/95 mm Hg, which puts them at substantial risk from heart attack, heart failure, stroke, and kidney failure (U. S. Department of Health and Human Services, 1980). It is also estimated that 30% of all employed Americans—30 million people—have elevated blood pressures or are on antihypertensive medicines. Also, 125,000 employed Americans die each year due to cardiovascular disease associated with high blood pressure and 29 million workdays, representing over $2 billion in earnings are lost each year due to problems related to high blood pressure (U. S. Department of Health and Human Services, 1983). The total health care costs of high blood pressure and its related health problems are obviously very large. In 1980, the U. S. Department of Health and Human Services established 10-year goals to reduce two primary risk factors for high blood pressure. These goals propose that by 1990 the average daily sodium ingestion for adults should be reduced to at least the 3- to 6-g range and the prevalence of significant overweight (120% or more of "desired weight") among the U. S. population should be decreased to 10% of men and 17% of women without nutritional impairment (U. S. Department of Health and Human Services, 1980). Some progress is being made toward lowering dietary sodium intake; however, a major portion of the population continues to be overweight or obese.

3.2 Diabetes

Diabetes also contributes substantially to the U. S. health care expenditure. Total costs are estimated to run $9.7 billion per year. The indirect costs alone (loss of life, disability, lost time from work, etc.) are estimated to be $4.9 billion per year, whereas direct costs of medical care are estimated to be $4.8 billion per year. A breakdown of the medical costs are estimated to be: hospital costs, $2.2 billion; nursing home care, $1.2 billion; physician care, $840 million; drugs, $380 million; and other health costs, $140 million (American Diabetes Association, 1983). Health statistics in the U. S. show that diabetics have twice as many heart attacks and more than twice as many strokes as do nondiabetics. Also, the risk of death from cardiovascular disease is more than twice as great in diabetic men as in nondiabetic men. For diabetic women the risk is five times greater than for other women. Diabetics who are overweight are at a substantially higher risk for cardiovascular disease, especially in combination with hypertension and elevated plasma cholesterol levels (U. S. Department of Health and Human Services, 1981).

3.3 Overweight

Overweight (110%–120% of ideal body weight) and obesity (greater than 120% of ideal body weight) are two of the most underrated and underestimated health care problems in the U. S. Overweight *per se* is not usually regarded to be a significant health care problem. It is therefore difficult to attract the interest of the scientific and medical community to the importance of the medical consequences of overweight, which in fact is one of the severest forms of malnutrition in industrialized communities. Health statistics in the U. S. show that 14% of American men and 24% of American women between the ages of 20 and 74 are obese (U. S. Department of Health and Human Services, 1980). It is also clear that overweight–obese individuals are at a greater risk for complications from hypertension and diabetes than the rest of the population. It is not possible, therefore, to estimate the overall socioeconomic costs of overweight and obesity in our population. However, it is substantial.

Clinical studies have demonstrated that certain types of dietary fiber have satiating properties, presumably due to the absorption of water, thereby swelling and producing a feeling of fullness in the stomach (McCance *et al.*, 1953; Heaton, 1973, 1978, 1980; Evans and Miller, 1975; Haber *et al.*, 1977; Grimes and Gordon, 1978; Mickelsen *et al.*, 1979). Several investigators have shown that some types of dietary fiber also delay stomach emptying (Holt *et al.*, 1979; Wilmshurs ˙ Crawley, 1980; Leeds *et al.* 1981). This property tends to prolong the   ation of satiety. Other workers have shown that certain types of dietary fiber interfere with, delay, or spread nutrient (calorie) absorption over a longer period of time in the small intestine. This in turn prevents rapid skyrocketing raises in serum glucose levels, improves insulin sensitivity, and thereby avoids the deposition of fat caused by glucose–insulin imbalances. Excellent reviews on the effects of dietary fiber on nutrient metabolism and absorption have been prepared by Leeds (1982), Kritchevsky (1982), Ali *et al.* (1982), and Anderson (1982). At the present time there is circumstantial evidence that dietary fiber—not metabolized by human digestive enzymes—may entrap some nutrients (calories), thereby carrying them into the large intestine, where the food is either utilized by colonic bacteria or excreted as unmetabolized nutrients. This evidence has been reviewed by Southgate (1982). Several recent clinical studies in this area of research, comparing a fiber tablet supplement to placebo in subjects on reduced-calorie diets, have shown significantly greater weight losses in the fiber subjects than in the placebo subjects (Solum, 1983; Ryttig, *et al.*, 1984). Since all subjects were consuming the same reduced-calorie diet, the increased weight loss in the fiber subjects is clearly due to reduced availability or increased loss of energy (calories).

All of these actions provide natural methods of long-term weight control, thereby reducing the propensity for hypertension, diabetes, hypercholesterolemia, and other serious health problems.

Efforts to modify the public diet by reducing the amount of dietary fat and increasing the amount of dietary fiber would be one of the most significant and effective actions that could be taken to reduce the human suffering and the socioeconomic burden of this group of widespread and interrelated diseases. It is important, therefore, that we begin to take first steps toward making progress in this area. Public guidelines for dietary fiber must be established and the importance of increasing fiber in the diet must be communicated to the public.

4. DIGESTIVE DISEASE

The group of digestive diseases that includes hiatus hernia, irritable bowel syndrome, constipation, diverticulosis, hemorrhoids, and related problems has long been associated with fiber-deficient diets. A recent consumer survey conducted by Louis Harris and Associates in consultation with the National Digestive Diseases Advisory Board showed that Americans know less about the nature and symptoms of digestive diseases than they know about cancer, heart disease, and a number of other major disease conditions (Harris and Associates, 1983). In view of this limited understanding of digestive diseases and digestive disease origins, it is not surprising to find that Americans do not consider digestive diseases to be very serious health problems. This, however, is not the case. Digestive diseases are quite a considerable socioeconomic burden. In point of fact, up to 100 million Americans suffer from intermittent forms of digestive diseases and the estimated total cost in lost work, lost wages, and medical costs is $50 billion per year. It is also estimated that 200,000 workers miss work every day due to digestive problems. Health statistics also show that more Americans are hospitalized due to diseases of the digestive tract than for any other group of disorders. The direct medical costs of these diseases is estimated to be $17 billion per year (National Digestive Diseases Advisory Board, 1983). Annual sales of prescription and over-the-counter drug products used for digestive diseases is $1.2 billion per year and is growing at a steady 10% rate (Consumer Expenditure Study, 1983). The breakdown is as follows:

Laxatives	$450,000,000
Antacids	$600,000,000
Antihemorrhoidals	$115,000,000
Antidiarrheals	$50,000,000

These diseases, therefore, are a significant public health problem and contribute substantially to our overall health care costs. Increasing the level of dietary fiber in the public diet would reduce the incidence of these diseases and their consequent health costs.

5. CANCER

Doll and Peto (1981) have conducted an extensive review of the epidemiologic, clinical, and scientific literature and have been able to prepare a list of the most important factors contributing to the incidence of cancer in the U. S. These authors have estimated that by changing dietary patterns of Americans it may be possible to reduce the cancer death rate by as much as 35%. It has been determined from this and other research that the most important factors contributing to the incidence of cancer in the U. S. are as follows (Office of Cancer Communications, 1984):

Diet	35%
Tobacco	30%
Viruses	5%

Occupation	4%
Alcohol	3%
Excess sunshine	3%
Environmental pollution	2%
Medicine and medical procedures	1%
Food additives	$\leq 1\%$

The National Cancer Institute has now incorporated these findings into a major public information program, and in March 1984 launched an education and awareness campaign to inform the American public of dietary and environmental factors that may reduce the risk of cancer. The major recommendations of this campaign are:

1. Do not smoke or use tobacco in any form.
2. Make changes in your diet to increase your intake of fiber and reduce the fat you eat.
3. If you drink alcoholic beverages, do so only in moderation—one or two drinks a day.

The National Cancer Institute estimates that as many as 20,000 lives per year can be saved through a healthier diet, which includes more fiber and less fat (Office of Cancer Communications, 1984). The human and socioeconomic impact of this program could obviously be substantial.

Thus, substantial progress could be made toward promoting health and preventing disease if the dietary fiber content of the public diet could be increased to healthier levels. This can and should be accomplished by formulating a public guideline and by launching a substantial and continuing promotional and public awareness campaign.

6. PUBLIC GUIDELINES

There are a number of public guidelines available in the U. S. that provide recommendations with regard to dietary fiber. The most familiar documents are as follows:

Dietary Guidelines for Americans (U. S. Department of Agriculture and U. S. Department of Health and Human Services, 1980).

Promoting Health/Preventing Disease-Objectives for the Nation (U. S. Department of Health and Human Services, 1980).

Recommended Dietary Allowances (National Research Council, 1980).

Diet, Nutrition and Cancer (National Research Council, 1982).

Cancer Prevention Awareness Campaign (Office of Cancer Communications, 1984).

Diet Guidelines (American Cancer Society, 1984).

All of these documents acknowledge that the average American's diet is deficient in dietary fiber and in every case the guidelines recommend that the level of dietary fiber be increased by most Americans.

In addition to these public interest documents, the shelves of book stores are replete with books and pamphlets written by clinicians, scientists, nutritionists, and other individuals who have developed some concept, scheme, or idea about adding dietary fiber to the daily diet. Most of these books promote the use of specialized fiber diets for use as an adjunct in treating body overweight, digestive diseases, diabetes, and other conditions. The concepts in some of these books are rational, reasonable, and supported by scientific evidence. Some are not.

One would think that with this abundant evidence in both the public and the private literature we should be making substantial progress toward increasing fiber in the average American diet. But we are not. There is some indication that literate, well-educated, affluent Americans have become knowledgeable about dietary fiber and have adopted a healthier, higher fiber diet; however, very little progress has been made in educating the average American citizen. The following results of a recent study conducted in Washington, D. C. emphasize our problems at the grass roots level.

7. A CASE STUDY

The American Health Foundation, a nonprofit public interest group, is conducting a study of 1500 elementary school children in nine Washington, D. C. public schools under a grant sponsored by the National Heart, Lung and Blood Institute of the National Institutes of Health. The program is called the "Know Your Body Evaluation Project" and is basically a survey and health project (American Health Foundation, 1984). The current study is just beginning; however, a pilot program was conducted in one school in Washington, D. C. in November 1982. The results of this study are alarming.

The pilot study included 205 children in grades 1-6 at the K. C. Lewis School in Northwest Washington. Physicians from the Howard and Georgetown University Schools of Medicine conducted miniscreens of these children to include: height, weight, blood pressure, skinfold thickness, exercise test, and blood cholesterol levels. The results of this pilot program have raised some substantial questions about health risk in these young citizens and in the general public.

1. Nearly three out of four children screened as part of this innovative health education program at this Washington, D. C. *elementary* school were *already* at risk of developing chronic illnesses, such as cancer and heart disease, or of becoming susceptible to strokes later in life.

2. Of the 205 students in grades 1–6 (6– 12 years of age) tested at the
    K. C. Lewis School, 43% had blood cholesterol levels of 180
    mg/100 ml or greater, and 24% of these had levels of more than 200
    mg/100 ml. This compared with current average cholesterol levels
    in American children of 160–180 mg/100 ml, although the optimum
    level for children is considered to be 140 mg/100 ml.
3. Nearly 17% (of the 205 students in grades 1–6 tested at the K. C.
    Lewis School) were considered overweight or 20% above the mean
    weight established for their age and sex.
4. Nearly 9% of the 205 students (in grades 1–6 tested at the K. C.
    Lewis School) had a systolic blood pressure of 120 mm Hg or
    above and 22% had a diastolic pressure of 80 mm Hg or above,
    which is in the upper ranges for the norms established for elemen-
    tary school children.

These findings are obviously not all related to fiber-deficient diets nor to
any one factor. Nor could an increase in dietary fiber improve all of these
parameters. However, in combination with a reduction in saturated fat it
could certainly help. Clearly, unless the dietary patterns of these children
and similar groups of children around the world are changed, the health
risks and socioeconomic burden of these health risks are predetermined.

8. CONCLUSION

The association between diets deficient in dietary fiber and certain
human diseases has been established in well-controlled animal and human
research programs and in epidemiologic studies. The human suffering and
socioeconomic costs of these fiber deficiency diseases is enormous. It is
therefore appropriate at this time to formulate a public guideline to advise
the average citizen about the daily quantities of dietary fiber required to
promote general health and to help in the prevention of disease. There
should also be an advocacy on the part of research workers and educators in
this field to not only encourage the formulation of a public guideline, but
also to advise about the necessity to launch extensive and continuing public
relations and public awareness campaigns to promote the increase of dietary
fiber in the public diet.

REFERENCES

Alexander, J. K., 1975, Interactions of hyperlipidaemia, hypertension and obesity as coronary
    risk factors, *Triangle* 14:1.
Ali, R., Staub, H., Leveille, G. A., and Boyle, P. C., 1982, Dietary fiber and obesity: A review,

in: *Dietary Fiber in Health and Disease* (G. V. Vahouny and D. Kritchevsky, eds.), Plenum, New York, pp. 139–149.

American Cancer Society, 1984, Diet Guidelines, American Cancer Society, New York.

American Diabetes Association, 1983, National Diabetes Data Group, April 4, 1983, New York.

American Health Foundation, 1984, Know Your Body Evaluation Project, supported by National Heart, Lung and Blood Institute, NIH Grant 1 R 18 HL 30610.

Anderson, J., 1982, Dietary fiber and diabetes, in: *Dietary Fiber in Health and Disease* (G. V. Vahouny and D. Kritchevsky, eds.), Plenum, New York, pp. 151–167.

Ashley, F. W., Jr., and Kannel, W. B., 1974, Relation of weight changes to changes in atherogenic traits. The Framingham study, *J. Chronic Dis.* **27**:103.

Asp, N.-G., Johansson, C.-G., Hallmer, H., and Siljestrom, M., 1983, *J. Agric. Food Chem.* **31**:476–482.

Bray, G. A. (ed.), 1979, *Obesity in America*, Proceedings of the 2nd Fogarty International Centre Conference on Obesity, U. S. Department of Health, Education and Welfare, Washington, D. C.

Burkitt, D. F., and Trowell, H. C. (eds.), 1975, *Refined Carbohydrate Foods and Disease*, Academic Press, London,

Cleave, T. L., 1974, *The Saccharine Disease*, Wright, Bristol, England.

Cleave, T. L., Campbell, G. D., and Painter, N. S., 1966, *Diabetes, Coronary Thrombosis, and the Saccharine Disease*, Wright, Bristol, England.

Consumer Expenditure Survey, 1983, Product Marketing/Cosmetic and Fragrances Retailing Magazine, August 1983, pp. 12–15.

Cook, L., 1978, Relationship of blood pressure, serum cholesterol, smoking habit, relative weight and E. C. S. abnormalities to incidence of major cornary events: Final report of the Pooling Project. The Pooling Project Research Group, *J. Chronic Dis.* **31**:201.

Doll, R., and Peto, R., 1981, The causes of cancer: Quantitative estimates of avoidable risks of cancer in the United States today, *J. Natl. Cancer Inst.* **66**:1191–1308.

Dublin, L. I., 1953, Relation of obesity to longevity, *N. Engl. J. Med.* **248**:971.

Englyst, H. N., and Cummings, J. H., 1984, Simplified method for measurement of total non-starch polysaccharides by gas-liquid chromotography of constituent sugars as alditol acetates, *Analyst* **109**:937–942.

Evans, E., and Miller, D. S., 1975, Bulking agents in the treatment of obesity, *Nutr. Metab.* **18**:199–203.

Garrow, J. S., 1974, *Energy Balance and Obesity in Man*, North-Holland, Amsterdam.

Grimes, D. S., and Gordon, C., 1978, Satiety value of wholemeal and white bread, *Lancet* **2**:106.

Haber, G. B., Heaton, K. W., Murphy, D., and Burroughs, L., 1977, Depletion and disruption of dietary fibre. Effects on satiety, plasma-glucose and serum-insulin, *Lancet* **2**:679–682.

Harris, L., and Associates, 1983, *Public Perceptions of Digestive Diseases*, Prepared for the National Institute of Arthritis, Diabetes, Digestive and Kidney Diseases of the National Institutes of Health, Bethesda, Maryland.

Heaton, K. W., 1973, Food fibre as an obstacle to energy intake. *Lancet* **2**:1418–1421.

Heaton, K. W., 1975, Bile salts and fibre, in: *Fiber Deficiency and Colonic Disorders* (R. W. Reilly and J. P. Kirsner, eds.), Plenum, New York), p. 27.

Heaton, K. W., 1978, Fibre, satiety and insulin—A new approach to overnutrition and obesity, in: *Dietary Fibre, Current Developments of Importance to Health* (K. W. Heaton, ed.), Newman, London, pp. 141–149.

Heaton, K. W., 1980, Food intake regulation and fiber, in: *Medical Aspects of Dietary Fiber* (G. A. Spiller and R. M. Kay, eds.), Plenum, New York, pp. 223–238.

Holt, S., Heading, R. C., Carter, D. C., Prescott, L. F., and Tothill, P., 1979, Effect of gel fibre on gastric emptying and absorption of glucose and paracetamol, *Lancet* **1**:636–639.

Jung, R. T., Shetty, P. S., James, W. P. T., Barrand, M., and Callingham, B. A., 1979, Reduced thermogenesis in obesity, *Nature* **279**:322.

Keen, H., 1975, The incomplete story of obesity and diabetes, in: *Recent Advances in Obesity Research I* (A. Howard, ed.), Newman, London, pp. 116–127.

Kimura, K. K., 1977, *The Nutritional Significance of Dietary Fiber,* Prepared for Food and Drug Administration, Washington, D. C., by Life Sciences Research Office, Federation of American Societies for Experimental Biology, Bethesda, Maryland; available from National Technical Information Service, Springfield, Virginia.

Kritchevsky, D., 1982, Fiber, obesity and diabetes, in: *Dietary Fiber in Health and Disease* (G. V. Vahouny and D. Kritchevsky, eds.), Plenum, New York, pp. 133–137.

Larsson, B., Bjorntorp, P., and Tibblin, G., 1981, The health consequences of moderate obesity, *Int. J. Obesity* **5**:97.

Leeds, A. R., 1982, Modification of intestinal absorption by dietary fiber and fiber components, in: *Dietary Fiber in Health and Disease* (G. V. Vahouny and D. Kritchevsky, eds.), Plenum, New York, pp. 53–71.

Leeds, A. R., Ralphs, D. N. L., Ebied, F., Metz, G., and Dilawri, J. B., 1981, Pectin in the dumping syndrome: Reduction of symptoms and plasma volume changes, *Lancet* **1**: 1075–1078.

Leelarthaepin, B., Woodhill, J. M., Palmer, A. J. and Blackett, R. B., 1974, Obesity, diet and type II hyperlipidaemia, *Lancet* **2**:1217.

Lew, E. A., and Garfinkel, L., 1979, Variations in mortality by weight among 750,000 men and women, *J. Chronic Dis.* **32**:563.

Mabee, T. M., Meyer, P., Den Besten, L., and Mason, E. E., 1976, The mechanisms of increased gallstone formation in obese human subjects, *Surgery* **79**:460.

McCance, R. A., Prior, K. M., and Widdowson, E. M., 1953, A radiological study of the rate of passage of brown and white bread through the digestive tract, *Br. J. Nutr.* **7**:98–104.

Mickelsen, O., Makdani, D. D., Cotton, R. H., Titcomb, S. T., Colmey, J. C., and Gatty, R., 1979, Effects of a high fiber diet on weight loss in college age males, *Am. J. Clin. Nutr.* **32**:1703–1709.

National Digestive Diseases Advisory Board, 1983, *Annual Report to the National Institute of Arthritis, Diabetes, Digestive and Kidney Diseases,* National Institutes of Health; Document no. NIH 83-2482, available from National Digestive Diseases Education Information Clearinghouse, Bethesda, Maryland.

National Research Council, 1980, *Recommended Dietary Allowances,* National Research Council, National Academy of Sciences, Washington, D. C.

National Research Council, 1982, *Diet, Nutrition and Cancer,* National Research Council, National Academy of Sciences, Washington, D. C.

Office of Cancer Communications, 1984, Cancer Prevention: A Program to Inform the Public about Cancer Risk and Cancer Prevention, National Cancer Institute, Bethesda, Maryland, January, 1984.

Olefsky, J., Crapo, P. A., Ginsberg, H., and Reaven, G. M., 1975, Metabolic effects of increased caloric intake in man, *Metabolism* **24**:495.

Prosky, L., Asp, N.-G., Furda, I., DeVries, J. W., Schweizer, T. F., and Harland, B. F., Determination of total dietary fiber in foods, food products and ingredients: Collaborative study, *J. Assoc. Off. Anal. Chem.* (in press).

Rabkin, S. W., Mathewson, F. A. L., and Hsu, P. H., 1977, Relation of body weight to development of ischaemic heart disease in a cohort of young North American men after a 26-year observation period: The Manitoba study, *Am. J. Cardiol.* **39**:452.

Reisin, E., Abel, R., Modan, M., Silverburg, D. S., Eliahou, H. E., and Modan, B., 1978, Effect of weight loss without salt restriction on the reduction of blood pressure in overweight hypertensive patients, *New Engl. J. Med.* **298**:1.

Rimm, A. A., Werner, L. H., Van Yserloo, B., and Bernstein, R. A., 1975, Relationship of obesity and disease in 73,532 weight-conscious women, *Public Health Rep.* **90**:44.

Ryttig, K., Larsen, S., and Haegh, L., 1984, Treatment of slightly to moderately overweight persons, *J. Norw. Med. Assoc.* **104**(14):989–991.

Society of Actuaries, 1979, *Build Study 1979,* Association of Life Insurance Medical Directors of America.

Solum, T., 1983, Fiber tablets, Dumo Vital, as a means to achieve weight reduction, *J. Norw. Med. Assoc.* **103**(24):1707–1708.

Southgate, D. A. T., 1982, Digestion and absorption of nutrients, in: *Dietary Fiber in Health and Disease* (G. V. Vahouny and D. Kritchevsky, eds.), Plenum, New York, pp. 45–52.

Talbot, J. M., The Role of Dietary Fiber in Diverticular Disease and Colon Cancer, Prepared for Food and Drug Administration, Washington, D.C., by Life Sciences Research Office, Federation of American Societies for Experimental Biology, Bethesda, Maryland; available from National Technical Information Service, Springfield, Virginia.

Theander, O., and Amen, P., 1982, Studies on dietary fiber. A method for the analysis and chemical characterization of total dietary fiber, *J. Sci. Food Agric.* **33**:340–344.

Tuck, M. L., Sowers, J., and Dornfeld, L., *et al.*, 1981, Effect of Weight Loss in Reducing Blood Pressure in Hypertensive Obese Patients, *New Eng. J. Med.* **304**:930.

U. S. Department of Agriculture and U. S. Department of Health and Human Services, 1980, *Dietary Guidelines for Americans,* Home and Garden Bulletin no. 232; available through U. S. Government Printing Office, Washington, D. C.

U. S. Department of Health and Human Services, 1980, Promoting Health/Preventing Disease—Objectives for the Nation, U. S. Government Printing Office, Washington, D. C.

U. S. Department of Health and Human Services, 1981, *Cardiovascular Primer for the Workplace,* National Institutes of Health, Bethesda, Maryland.

U. S. Department of Health and Human Services, 1983, *Statement of High Blood Pressure in the Workplace,* National Institutes of Health, Bethesda, Maryland.

Vahouny, G. V., and Kritchevsky, D. (eds.), 1982, *Dietary Fiber in Health and Disease,* Plenum, New York.

Westlund, K., and Nicolayson, R., 1972, A ten-year mortality and morbidity related to serum cholesterol. A follow-up of 3,751 men aged 40–49, *Scand. J. Clin. Lab. Invest.* **30**(Suppl. 127):1.

Wilmshurst, P., and Crawley, J. C. W., 1980, The measurement of gastric transit time in obese subjects using 24Na and the effects of energy content and guar gum on gastric emptying and satiety, *Br. J. Nutr.* **44**:1–6.

6

Dietary Fiber, Gastrointestinal, Endocrine, and Metabolic Effects: Lente Carbohydrate

DAVID J. A. JENKINS,
THOMAS M. S. WOLEVER,
ALEXANDRA L. JENKINS, and
RODNEY H. TAYLOR

1. INTRODUCTION

Considerable use has been made of purified fiber as a model to explore the possible mechanisms of action of fiber in foods within the gut. It is possible that direct extrapolation to the whole food of all the results obtained with purified fiber may be inappropriate. Nevertheless, these studies have aided in defining specific aspects of the physiology of the gut in relation to nutrient absorption and subsequent metabolic effects. In addition, the findings have suggested possible new approaches to the management of a range of disorders, such as diabetes, the dumping syndrome, hyperlipidemia, and obesity. It is the aim of this chapter to review these effects of fiber in relation to carbohydrate metabolism.

DAVID J. A. JENKINS, THOMAS M. S. WOLEVER, and ALEXANDRA L. JENKINS • Department of Nutritional Sciences, Faculty of Medicine, and Division of Endocrinology and Metabolism, St. Michael's Hospital, University of Toronto, Toronto M5S 1A8, Canada
RODNEY H. TAYLOR • Department of Gastroentrology and Nutrition, Central Middlesex Hospital, University of London, London NW10, United Kingdom.

2. EXTENSION OF THE DIETARY FIBER HYPOTHESIS

Initially the dietary fiber hypothesis focused on the fact that fiber within the lumen of the bowel may delay the absorption of nutrients (Trowell and Burkitt, 1975; Southgate, 1973). Thus, nutrients, for example, carbohydrate in fiber-rich foods, would be released from the stomach in more energy-dilute form and travel along the length of the small intestine releasing their products of digestion more slowly (Fig. 1A) (Jenkins, 1982). On the other hand, energy-dense foods would leave the stomach and be rapidly absorbed high up in the small intestine (Fig. 1B). Reasons for this may be: changes in the rate of gastric emptying or nutrient delivery to the small intestine; alterations in small intestinal motility with possible increases in thickness of the unstirred water layer; and overall impedance of diffusion of nutrients from the lumen to the absorptive surface of the enterocyte. All these would contribute to the altered metabolite and endocrine responses seen (Fig. 2). Thus, in the case of the high-fiber food, a more undulant blood glucose response would be observed (Fig. 2A), while in the fiber-depleted food, high rises, with possibly an undershoot in blood glucose, would be the reflection of the absorption profile (Fig. 2B). The former characteristics would be desirable in the food for the treatment of diabetes and other disorders where low blood glucose responses were required. The importance of being able to select useful carbohydrate foods has been emphasized by the recent guidelines issued internationally by the various Diabetes Associations (Committee of the American Diabetes Association on Food and Nutrition, 1979; Special Report Committee of the Canadian Diabetes Association, 1981; Nutrition Sub-Committee of the British Diabetic Association's Medical Advisory Committee, 1982) recommending that carbohydrate intakes should be increased. For some years now we have been used to thinking in terms of rapid- and slow-acting insulins. One of the features of the dietary fiber hypothesis has been the evolution of these concepts in terms of foods.

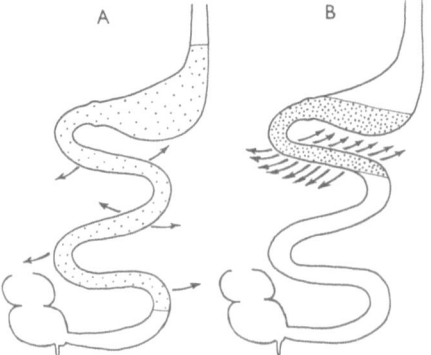

FIGURE 1. Stomach and small intestine, showing (A) slow absorption of energy-dilute nutrient in a fiber-rich "primitive" diet, and (B) rapid absorption of energy-dense nutrient from low-fiber, modern Western foods.

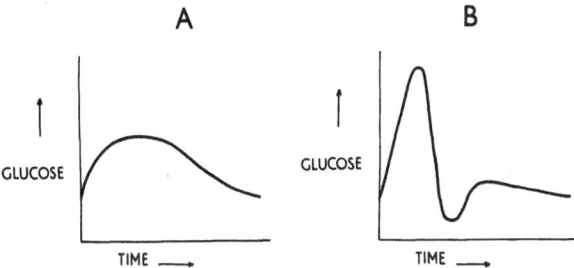

FIGURE 2. Postprandial glycemia following (A) slow absorption from starchy, fiber-rich meals, and (B) rapid absorption with undershoot due to excessive insulin release following refined, fiber-depleted carbohydrate foods.

3. EFFECT OF FIBER ON ABSORPTION AND GLYCEMIC RESPONSE

Early studies using viscous fibers (e.g. guar) demonstrated that they could impede the diffusion of glucose from fiber-glucose solutions in dialysis bags (Jenkins *et al.*, 1977b; Jenkins, 1983). There are now many studies indicating that such fibers added to glucose tolerance tests result in flattened glycemic responses and also flattened insulin and gastric inhibitory polypeptide (GIP) responses (Jenkins *et al.*, 1978a, 1976; Holt *et al.*, 1979; Morgan *et al.*, 1979; Levitt *et al.*, 1980; Gold *et al.*, 1980). In comparative studies the most viscous fibers seem to be the most effective in this respect (Jenkins *et al.*, 1978a). Bran has little effect, while guar and tragacanth, the most viscous, produce the largest response (Jenkins *et al.*, 1978a). The results in normal volunteers (Jenkins *et al.*, 1978a; Holt *et al.*, 1979) have also been confirmed in diabetics (Jenkins *et al.*, 1976; Morgan *et al.*, 1979; Levitt *et al.*, 1980; Gold *et al.*, 1980). Although the results do not appear to be related to increased insulin secretion, the question remains as to whether fiber has induced carbohydrate malabsorption.

4. POTENTIAL CARBOHYDRATE MALABSORPTION WITH DIETARY FIBER

A number of studies have been undertaken to explore the possible effects of dietary fiber in inducing carbohydrate malabsorption. Xylose has been added to dietary fiber test meals and complete urine collections made over the folowing 8 h to determine the xylose losses in the urine (Jenkins *et al.*, 1978a). Despite considerable flattening in the glycemic response induced by guar in the test meal, no difference in total urinary xylose excretion was seen to suggest carbohydrate malabsorption (Jenkins *et al.*, 1978a). Nevertheless, looking at the 2-h aliquots, it was found that the absorption profile with guar was shifted to the right, indicating delayed carbohydrate absorption (Fig. 3) (Jenkins *et al.*, 1978a). Similar results have been obtained with guar-containing meals using paracetamol as a marker of absorption (Holt *et al.*, 1979). Furthermore, studies where breath hydrogen measurement was made after guar–glucose mixtures were consumed have revealed that no hydrogen was evolved (Jenkins *et al.*, 1977b). This provides additional evidence that carbohydrate is not malabsorbed, since when the nonabsorbable carbohydrate sugar lactulose was added to guar test meals, hydrogen was evolved as predicted over the same time course (Jenkins *et al.*, 1977b). Thus, although there may be some increased losses of available carbohydrate from whole foods or from purified fiber preparations that employ starch as the test carbohydrate rather than glucose, carbohydrate malabsorption does not provide the explanation for the flattening of glycemic response discussed here in relation to glucose and purified fiber.

5. LENTE CARBOHYDRATE: METABOLIC EFFECTS

Studies using fiber-free glucose solutions have also helped in defining the possible mechanisms of action of dietary fiber. In a study involving a maturity-onset diabetic patient, 240 g of glucose was given either as three discrete boluses over a 12-h period or by continuous sipping (Fig. 4) (Jenkins *et al.*, 1983). Each bolus resulted in a high rise in blood glucose followed by an undershoot. Continuous ingestion, on the other hand, resulted only in a relatively small rise in blood glucose, which fell to the same low level as seen after the third bolus by the end of the experimental period (Jenkins *et al.*, 1983). Correspondingly, the insulin results for the boluses showed high rises,

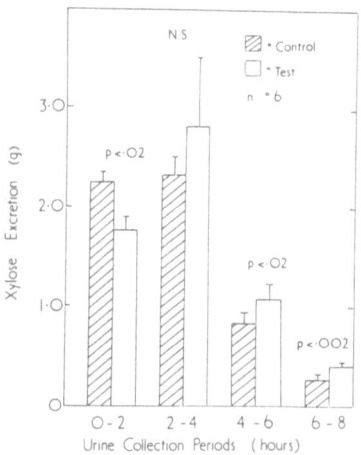

FIGURE 3. Effect of 14.5 g guar on urinary xylose excretion (g/2 h) over the first 8 h postprandial collected in 2-h aliquots, compared with the control meal. (From Jenkins *et al.*, 1978a.)

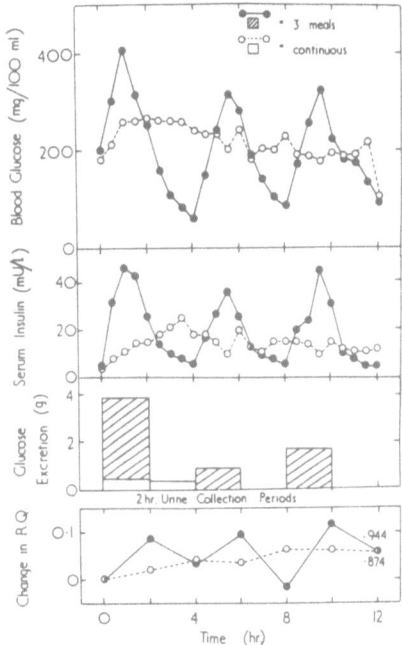

FIGURE 4. Blood glucose, insulin, 2-h urinary glucose losses, and respiratory quotient (RQ) measured over 12 h shown in a diabetic controlled on diet. On one occasion 80-g glucose drinks were taken at 0, 4, and 8 h and on another 5 g glucose in solution was taken every 15 min by continuous sipping. (From Jenkins *et al.*, 1983.)

while on continuous sipping the total insulin area was reduced by more than 20%. Most dramatically, the urinary glucose losses were reduced to virtually zero on the glucose sipping test. As a reflection of the overall metabolic events, with continuous sipping, the respiratory quotient (RQ) rose through the experimental period, whereas when the glucose was taken as boluses the RQ assumed a sawtooth appearance, with the peak RQ corresponding to each bolus (Jenkins *et al.*, 1983). Such results illustrate the possible benefit that slow release or sustained absorption of carbohydrate may confer, irrespective of the presence of fiber.

The theoretical importance of this concept is further highlighted by the studies of Radzuic *et al.* (1978). They demonstrated (Fig. 5) that after a 40-g glucose load the peripheral blood glucose level had returned to normal at a time when glucose absorption from the gut was still proceeding at a near maximal rate. In other words, this suggested that toward the end of a glucose tolerance test the absorption of glucose from the gut into the circulation is matched by its removal by the tissues and reflects a progressive fall in resistance to glucose uptake with time. Theoretically this would mean that if one could prolong the time over which absorption took place, then carbohydrate uptake by tissues would be more effective in the latter part of the glucose tolerance test and the total area above the fasting blood glucose

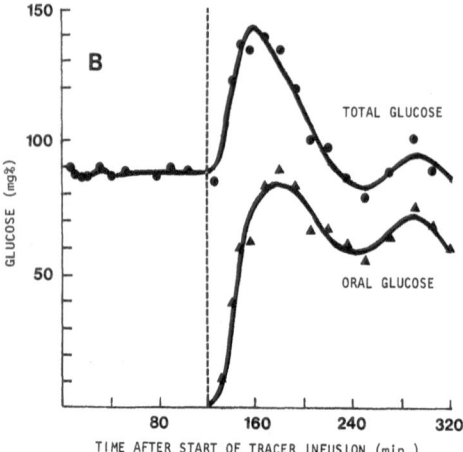

FIGURE 5. Experiment showing the relative time courses of the rise and fall in blood glucose concentration at a time when absorption of glucose from the gut continues at a high level. Forty-five grams of glucose labeled with [1-14C]glucose infusion was also started at zero time. Total glucose = blood glucose concentration, i.e., endogenous glucose and glucose absorbed from the gut; oral glucose = concentration of glucose absorbed from the gut. (From Radzuik et al., 1978.)

response curve would be reduced. The same principles may apply to the absorption of carbohydrate from foods. This then may be one of the advantages of dietary fiber.

Such a possibility has been further explored using dietary fiber to delay the absorption of glucose and then studying the blood glucose response to a second, fiber-free glucose load (Jenkins et al., 1980c). The results indicated that when fiber had been given in the preceding meal, the fiber-free test meal that followed 4 h later showed a considerable flattening in the blood glucose response compared with that taken 4 h after a fiber-free meal (Fig. 6) (Jenkins et al., 1980c). Changes in free fatty acids and ketone bodies appeared to provide part of the explanation for this phenomenon. Peripheral blood levels of these metabolites were low 4 h after the slowly absorbed fiber-containing meal, but were considerably elevated 4 h after the fiber-free meal (Jenkins et al., 1980c). Thus, after the fiber-containing meal, the second glucose load was taken against a background of low free fatty acid and ketone body levels. This was associated with lower blood glucose and insulin responses than when the second glucose load was taken 4 h after the fiber-free meal, when free fatty acid and ketone body levels were elevated (Jenkins et al., 1980c).

Free fatty acids and ketone bodies have been implicated in impairing glucose uptake and utilization by peripheral tissues (Randle et al., 1963). Through their prolonged suppression by slow-release carbohydrates, however this is achieved, glucose tolerance for the subsequent meal may be improved. Thus, fiber, although it remains within the gut, through its effects in changing the rate of nutrient delivery and endocrine responses may produce secondary metabolic effects in peripheral tissues. These events in turn will influence the handling of further substrates from the gut.

6. MECHANISM BY WHICH FIBER MAY CREATE LENTE CARBOHYDRATE

There has been considerable debate as to whether the effects of dietary fiber lie primarily through its ability to delay gastric emptying, a property only shared by some fiber preparations, or its ability to prolong carbohydrate absorption from the small intestine. Early studies focused attention on the effects of the viscous fibers in delaying gastric emptying (Leeds *et al.*, 1978a). This property of fiber was illustrated by gamma camera studies, which illustrated the ability of guar to slow the emptying of labeled indium in man (Leeds *et al.*, 1981). These findings were supported by gastric emptying and small intestinal studies using the rat as a model (Leeds *et al.*, 1978a). However, it was never possible to show a direct relationship between the flattening of glycemic response and the rate of gastric emptying in a given group of individuals (Leeds *et al.*, 1978b).

This has made the second hypothesis of delayed absorption (Jenkins *et al.*, 1978a) as a small intestinal event more acceptable as originally implicated by the dialysis model. Recently a number of studies have confirmed that delayed small intestinal absorption is likely to be of major importance. The elegant studies of Read *et al.* using direct small intestinal intubation in man showed that glucose was absorbed less rapidly when guar was added to

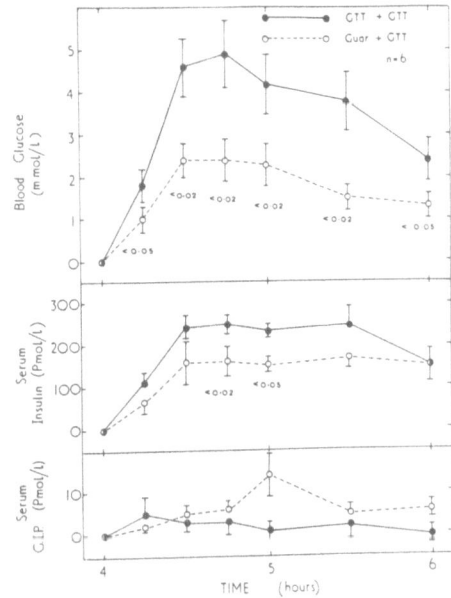

FIGURE 6. Mean rises in blood glucose, serum insulin, and gastric inhibitory polypeptide (GIP) levels in six subjects after the second of two 80-g glucose drinks with or without 22.3 g guar added to the first drink (guar control). (From Jenkins *et al.*, 1980c.)

glucose solutions (Read, this volume, Chapter 7). Similar conclusions have been reached using isolated loops of pig small intestine *in vivo* (Rainbird *et al.*, 1982) and by studying the intake of both glucose and amino acids by segments of rat intestine *in vitro* (Elsenhaus *et al.*, 1980).

Studies that have indicated that fiber has little effect in reducing post-prandial glycemia in diabetic patients with autonomic neuropathy and gastroparesis (Levitt *et al.*, 1980) might now be explained by the fact that such patients, due to reduced small intestinal motility, already have a slow rate of small intestinal absorption. In this respect it is of interest that such patients tended to have flatter blood glucose responses than patients without marked autonomic neuropathy and with more normal gastrointestinal function (Levitt *et al.*, 1980).

7. DIABETES

As already mentioned, when added to test meals, viscous fibers have been shown to flatten the glycemic response in both normal and diabetic individuals. Viscous fiber, notably guar (Jenkins *et al.*, 1977d; 1978b), has been shown to reduce urinary glucose losses by half in 5-day metabolic trials and at the same time reduce urinary ketone body losses (Jenkins *et al.*, 1979). The effects have been maintained on intermediate (Aro *et al.*, 1981) and long-term (Jenkins *et al.*, 1980b) administration. Incorporation of guar into the meal plan also reduced insulin requirements in patients on the artificial pancreas (Christiansen *et al.*, 1980). Of considerable interest are the studies using cellulose (Miranda and Horwitz, 1978) or high-wheat-bran diets (Bo-sello *et al.*, 1980). In these studies, too, improvement in diabetic control has been noted, although no ready explanation or mechanism of action is agreed upon. One study in patients with diverticular disease, however, indicated that there were long-term effects of wheat bran supplementation, which re-sulted in improved glucose tolerance (Brodribb and Humphreys, 1976). The apparent beneficial effect of nonviscous fiber may therefore manifest itself in long-term alterations perhaps in gastrointestinal physiology or morphology.

8. DUMPING SYNDROME

Because of the purported beneficial effect of dietary fiber in reducing the rate of gastric emptying, early studies focused on the effect of viscous fiber in the treatment of the dumping syndrome. It was shown that the addi-tion of pectin to glucose test meals abolished hypoglycemic symptoms, re-sulted in a flatter glucose, insulin, and GIP responses, and even minimized carbohydrate malabsorption (Jenkins *et al.*, 1977a; 1980a). The lessening of carbohydrate malabsorption was evidenced by reduced breath hydrogen levels after pectin administration (Jenkins *et al.*, 1977a). Further studies, which confirmed the overall reduced rate of gastric emptying when pectin was added to glucose solutions, also showed that there was a reduced effective osmotic action of glucose as manifest by a smaller degree of hemoconcentration after glucose plus pectin (Leeds *et al.*, 1981). These results further indicated the profound changes in gastrointestinal physiology that may accompany addition of unabsorbed materials to nutrient loads. In longer term studies the effect of addition of pectin to the diet of patients with the dumping syndrome was shown to reduce the severity and frequency of attacks (Jenkins *et al.*, 1977a).

However, although in both diabetes and the dumping syndrome possible therapeutic gains may be made by the use of fiber, the lack of commercially available sources in palatable form does not allow the immediate application of these findings to the clinical situation.

9. LONG-TERM EFFECTS

The long-term effects of fiber supplementation may include an alteration of small intestinal morphology and gastrointestinal motor function. In this respect it is of interest that in rat studies, diets supplemented with pectin resulted in flattening of the villus structure and a reduction in the concentrations of brush border enzymes (Tasman-Jones *et al.*, 1982; Thompson and Tasman-Jones, 1982; Cassidy *et al.*, 1981). No such change was seen with cellulose supplementation, which had little effect on carbohydrate absorption (Tasman-Jones *et al.*, 1982).

In studies in man, long-term administration of pectin resulted in a reduced rate of gastric emptying (Schwartz *et al.*, 1982). This was seen even when no pectin was present in the test meal. Nevertheless, in normal volunteers, chronic high doses of pectin (30 g/day for 6 weeks) had no long-term effect on glucose tolerance or insulin response (Jenkins *et al.*, 1977c). The relevance of possible long-term adaptive responses therefore remains to be defined (Cassidy *et al.*, 1981).

10. CONCLUSION

Studies with purified fiber have proved useful in indicating possible mechanisms of action of fiber and fiber-rich food within the gastrointestinal tract. Obvious differences between fiber mixed with a food, and fiber actually present in the cell wall structure of the food are acknowledged. Nevertheless, using viscous fiber, which can to some extent coat the different food forms and food particles, it has been possible to demonstrate alterations in nutrient absorption, endocrine responses, and their metabolic consequences. Attention has been focused on the importance of the rate of release of nutrients and their absorption from the gastrointestinal tract. Prolongation of the rate of absorption of carbohydrate, for example, may result in more effective uptake by peripheral tissues. This phenomenon may have advantages in the treatment of disorders of carbohydrate metabolism such as diabetes and possibly hypertriglyceridemia. Further studies have illustrated the possible importance of fiber in reducing the effective osmotic load delivered to the small intestine. Together with the effect of fiber in delaying gastric emptying, these actions may result in fiber being of benefit to patients with the dumping syndrome. Such properties should be looked for in fiber in whole foods. It is also possible that pharmacological development of purified forms of fiber and the other plant materials with similar actions may allow new pharmacological approaches to the therapy of disorders of carbohydrate metabolism.

ACKNOWLEDGMENTS. Work by the authors was supported by funds from the Natural Sciences and Engineering Research Council.

REFERENCES

Aro, A., Uusitupa, M., Vontilainen, E., Hersio, K., Korhonen, T., and Siitonen, O., 1981, Improved diabetic control and hypocholesterolemic effect induced by long-term dietary supplementation with guar gum in type 2 (insulin-dependent) diabetes, *Diabetologia* 21: 29–33.

Bosello, O., Ostuzzi, R., Armellini, F., Micciolo, R. M., and Ludovico, A. S., 1980, Glucose tolerance and blood lipids in bran fed patients with impaired glucose tolerance, *Diabetes Care* 3:46–49.

Brodribb, A. J. M., and Humphreys, D. M., 1976, Diverticular disease: Three studies. Part III—Metabolic effect of bran in patients with diverticular disease, *Br. Med. J.* 1:428–430.

Cassidy, M. M., Lightfoot, F. G., Gray, L. E., Story, J. A., Kritchevsky, D., and Vahouny, G. V., 1981, Effect of chronic intake of dietary fibers on the ultrastructural topography of rat jejunum and colon: A scanning electron microscopy study, *Am. J. Clin. Nutr.* 34:218–228.

Christiansen, J. S., Bonnevie-Nielsen, V., Svendsen, P. A., Rubin, P., Ronn, B., and Nerup, J., 1980, Effect of guar gum on 24-hour insulin requirements of insulin-dependent diabetic subjects as assessed by an artificial pancreas, *Diabetes Care* 3:659–662.

Committee of the American Diabetes Association on Food and Nutrition, 1979, Special report: Principles of nutrition and dietary recommendations for individuals with diabetes mellitus, *Diabetes Care* 2:520–523.

Elsenhaus, B., Sufke, U., Blume, R., and Caspary, W. F., 1980, The influence of carbohydrate gelling agents on rat intestinal transport of monosaccharides and neutral amino acids *in vitro*, *Clin. Sci.* 59:373–380.

Gold, L. A., McCourt, J. P., and Merimee, T. J., 1980, Pectin: An examination in normal subjects, *Diabetes Care* 3:50–52.

Holt, S., Heading, R. C., Carter, D. C., Prescott, L. F., and Tothill, P., 1979, Effect of gel fibre on gastric emptying and absorption of glucose and paracetomol, *Lancet* 1:636–639.

Jenkins, D. J. A., 1982, Lente carbohydrate: A newer approach to the dietary management of diabetes, *Diabetes Care* **5**:634–641.

Jenkins, D. J. A., 1983, Fiber and delayed carbohydrate absorption in man: Lente carbohydrate, in: *Delaying Absorption As a Therapeutic Principle in Metabolic Disease* (W. Creutzfeldt and U. R. Folsch, eds.), Thieme-Stratton, New York, pp. 45–56.

Jenkins, D. J. A., Leeds, A. R., Gassull, M. A., Wolever, T. M. S., Goff, D. V., Alberti, K. G. M. M., and Hockaday, T. D. R., 1976, Unabsorbable carbohydrates and diabetes: Decreased post-prandial hyperglycaemia, *Lancet* **2**:172–174.

Jenkins, D. J. A., Gassull, M. A., Leeds, A. R., Metz, G., Dilawari, J. B., Slavin, B., and Blendis, L. M., 1977a, Effect of dietary fiber on complications of gastric surgery: Prevention of postprandial hypoglycemia by pectin, *Gastroenterology* **72**:215–217.

Jenkins, D. J. A., Leeds, A. R., Gassull, M. A., Cochet, B., and Alberti, K. G. M. M., 1977b, Decrease in postprandial insulin and glucose concentrations by guar and pectin, *Ann. Intern. Med.* **86**:20–23.

Jenkins, D. J. A., Leeds, A. R., Houston, H., Hinks, L., Alberti, K. G. M. M., and Cummings, J. H., 1977c, Carbohydrate tolerance in man after six weeks of pectin administration, *Proc. Nutr. Soc.* **36**:60A.

Jenkins, D. J. A., Wolever, T. M. S., Hockaday, T. D. R., Leeds, A. R., Haworth, R., Bacon, S., Apling, E. C., and Dilawari, J., 1977d, Treatment of diabetes with guar gum, *Lancet* **2**:779–780.

Jenkins, D. J. A., Wolever, T. M. S., Leeds, A. R., Gassull, M. A., Dilawari, J. B., Goff, D. V., Metz, G. L., Alberti, K. G. M. M., 1978a, Dietary fibres, fibre analogues and glucose tolerance: Importance of viscosity, *Br. Med. J.* **1**:1392–1394.

Jenkins, D. J. A., Wolever, T. M. S., Nineham, R., Taylor, R. H., Metz, G. L., Bacon, S., and Hockaday, T. D. R., 1978b, Guar crispbread in the diabetic diet, *Br. Med. J.* **2**:1744–1746.

Jenkins, D. J. A., Wolever, T. M. S., Nineham, R., Goff, D. V., Haisman, P., Charnock, P., Taylor, R. H., and Hockaday, T. D. R., 1979, Dietary fibre and ketone bodies: Reduced urinary 3-hydroxybutyrate excretion in diabetics on guar, *Br. Med. J.* **2**:1555–1556.

Jenkins, D. J. A., Leeds, A. R., Bloom, S. R., Sarson, D. L., Albuquerque, R. H., Metz, G. L., and Alberti, K. G. M. M., 1980a, Pectin and post-gastric surgery complications of gastric complications: Normalisation of postprandial glucose and endocrine responses, *Gut* **21**:574–579.

Jenkins, D. J. A., Wolever, T. M. S., Taylor, R. H., Reynolds, D., Nineham, R., and Hockaday, T. D. R., 1980b, Diabetic glucose control, lipids, and trace elements on long term guar, *Br. Med. J.* **1**:1353–1354.

Jenkins, D. J. A., Wolever, T. M. S., Nineham, R., Sarson, D. L., Bloom, S. R., Ahern, J., Alberti, K. G. M. M., and Hockaday, T. D. R., 1980c, Improved glucose tolerance four hours after taking guar with glucose, *Diabetologia* **19**:21–24.

Jenkins, D. J. A., Wolever, T. M. S., Taylor, R. H., Kannan, W., Sarson, D., and Bloom, S. R., 1983, Reply to letter by Abraira and Lawrence, *Am. J. Clin. Nutr.* **37**:153–154.

Leeds, A. R., Bolster, N. R., Andrews, R., and Truswell, A. S., 1978a, Meal viscosity, gastric emptying and glucose absorption in the rat, *Proc. Nutr. Soc.* **36**:44A.

Leeds, A. R., Ralphs, D. N., Boulos, P., Ebied, F., Metz, G. L., Dilawari, J., Elliott, A., and Jenkins, D. J. A., 1978b, Pectin and gastric emptying in the dumping syndrome, *Proc, Nutr. Soc.* **37**:23A.

Leeds, A. R., Ralphs, D. N. L., Ebied, F., Metz, G., and Dilawari, J. B., 1981, Pectin in the dumping syndrome: Reduction of symptoms and plasma volume changes, *Lancet* **1**:1075–1078.

Levitt, N. S., Vinik, A. I., Sive, A. A., Child, P. T., and Jackson, W. P. U., 1980, The effect of dietary fiber on glucose and hormone responses to a mixed meal in normal subjects and in diabetic subjects with and without autonomic neuropathy, *Diabetes Care* **3**:515–519.

Miranda, P. M., and Horwitz, D. L., 1978, High fiber diets in the treatment of diabetes mellitus, *Ann. Intern. Med.* **88**:482–486.

Morgan, L. M., Goulder, T. J., Tsiolakis, D., Marks, V., and Alberti, K. G. M. M., 1979, The effects of unabsorbable carbohydrate on gut hormones: Modification of postprandial GIP secretion by guar, *Diabetologia* **17**:85–89.

Nutrition Sub-Committee of the British Diabetic Association's Medical Advisory Committee, 1982, Dietary Recommendations for Diabetics for the 1980s—A policy statement by the British Diabetic Association, *Hum. Nutr. Appl. Nutr.* **36A**:378–394.

Radzuik, J., McDonald, T. J., Rubenstein, D., and Dupre, J., 1978, Initial splanchnic extraction of ingested glucose in normal man, *Metabolism* **27**:657–669.

Rainbird, A. L., Low, A. G., and Zebrowska, T., 1982, Effect of guar gum on glucose absorption from isolated loops of jejunum in conscious growing pigs, *Proc. Nutr. Soc.* **39**:48A.

Randle, P. J., Garland, P. B., Hales, C. N., and Newsholme, E. A., 1963, The glucose–fatty acid cycle: Its role in insulin sensitivity and the metabolic disturbances of diabetes mellitus, *Lancet* **1**:785–789.

Schwartz, S. E., Levine, R. A., Singh, A., Scheidecker, J. R., and Track, N. S., 1982, Sustained pectin ingestion delays gastric emptying, *Gastroenterology* **83**:12–17.

Southgate, D. A. T., 1973, Fibre and the other unavailable carbohydrates and their effects on the energy value of the diet, *Proc. Nutr. Soc.* **32**:131.

Special Report Committee, 1981, Guidelines for the nutritional management of diabetes mellitus: A special report from the Canadian Diabetes Association, *J. Can. Diet. Assoc.* **42**:110–118.

Tasman-Jones, C., Owen, R. L., and Jones, A. L., 1982, Semi-purified dietary fiber and small bowel morphology in rats, *Dig. Dis. Sci.* **27**:519–524.

Thompson, L. L., and Tasman-Jones, C., 1982, Dissaccharidase levels of the rat jejunum are altered by dietary fibre, *Digestion* **23**:253.

Trowell, H. C., and Burkitt, D. P., 1975, Concluding considerations, in: *Refined carbohydrate Foods and Disease* (D. P. Burkitt and H. C. Trowell, eds.), Academic, London, pp. 333–345.

7

Dietary Fiber and Bowel Transit

N. W. READ

1. FUNCTIONAL ROLES OF THE SMALL INTESTINE AND COLON

It normally takes between 1 and 4 days for the residues of a solid meal to pass through the gastrointestinal tract. Most of this time is spent in the colon; passage of food through the stomach and small intestine only takes a few hours (Read *et al.*, 1980).

The small intestine and colon are best considered separately, because they have fundamentally different actions with regard to the digestion and absorption of food. The small intestine is adapted for rapid absorption of large amounts of food; between 80 and 90% of ingested food and digestive secretions are absorbed during a journey that lasts on average between 4 and 6 h.

In contrast, the colon is adapted for the bacterial fermentation of food material that has escaped absorption in the small intestine and for the extraction of salt and water against high transepithelial osmotic and concentration gradients. Both of these functions require relative stasis of colonic contents. The proliferation of the enormous colonic populations of anaerobic bacteria necessary for adequate fermentation requires stagnant hypoxic conditions. Extraction of salt and water in the colon against large gradients is much slower than absorption in the small intestine, and prolonged colonic residence is necessary for it to proceed to completion.

These fundamental differences in function mean that the action of

N. W. READ • Clinical Research Unit, Royal Hallamshire Hospital, Sheffield S10 2JF, United Kingdom.

dietary fiber is different in the two sites and that different types of dietary fiber are effective at each site. For example, viscous polysaccharides, such as guar, delay absorption and slow transit in the small intestine, but are rapidly degraded by colonic bacteria and have a relatively minor influence on colonic function. In contrast, cellulose and bran have little action on the small intestine, but they both accelerate colonic transit and increase stool weight.

2. SMALL BOWEL TRANSIT

2.1 Measurement

Small bowel transit time is the time taken for food to pass from the stomach to the colon. While the passage of a single unabsorbable pellet or marker from stomach to cecum is easy to measure, no single transit time describes the passage of a meal through the small intestine. Food particles leave the stomach at different times and the residues enter the cecum at different times, so there is a range of possible transit times, and an accurate value for mean or median transit time can only be obtained by complex mathematical methods, such as deconvolution. Another problem is that it is only possible to measure the transit time of the unabsorbable components of food and these may not necessarily bear any direct relationship with the transit time of the absorbable components. In practice, this may not be important consideration, since we have found that the profile describing the output of an unabsorbable marker from a terminal ileostomy is virtually identical to the output of protein, fat, or carbohydrate (Holgate and Read, 1983).

A value for small bowel transit time in humans is conveniently obtained by feeding a meal containing a source of unabsorbable carbohydrate, such as lactulose or baked beans (stachyose and raffinose), and measuring the rise in breath hydrogen concentration that occurs when the carbohydrate reaches the cecum and is fermented by colonic bacteria (Bond and Levitt, 1974; Read et al., 1980). It takes less than 5 min for cecal bacteria to generate a detectable increase in breath hydrogen when exposed to carbohydrate. This technique, although convenient, can only be used to measure the transit time of the head of a meal through the small intestine.

A more informative method of measuring small bowel transit in intact human subjects is to measure the gastric emptying and colonic filling of a radiolabeled meal by means of a gamma camera (Read et al., 1983). This has the advantage of recording the whole profile of colonic filling or gastric emptying. The disadvantage with this method is the problem of how to measure the entry of the radioactive label into the colon when there are loops of small intestine overlapping the cecum.

In animals, detailed information can be gained about the patterns of movement of food down the small intestine by administering a radiolabeled meal and then killing the animal and measuring the amount of marker in each region of the small intestine.

2.2. The Importance of Small Bowel Transit

The movement of a meal down the small intestine resembles a non-steady-state perfusion system, in which the transit time provides an approximate measure of the time that food is in contact with the absorptive epithelium: the contact time or residence.

Absorption of food depends on the rate at which nutrients can be taken up from the lumen and the length of time nutrients are in contact with the absorptive epithelium. The degree to which transit time or contact time normally limits absorption is not established. Borgstrom et al. (1957) showed that over 90% of the components of a liquid meal were absorbed by the distal jejunum in normal subjects. Nevertheless, direct measurements of the composition of effluent from ileostomies constructed from the terminal ileum have shown that appreciable amounts of absorbable nutrients may escape absorption in the human small intestine (Holgate and Read, 1983; Nuguid et al., 1961; Kramer et al., 1962). These amounts were increased when transit was accelerated by lactulose, magnesium sulfate, or metoclopramide (Holgate and Read, 1983) (Table I). Absorption of fat was more influenced by changes in transit time than absorption of carbohydrate or protein. However, lactulose, which accelerates transit by increasing the volume and flow of intestinal contents, had a greater influence on absorption than metoclopromide, which has a direct action on smooth muscle, although both had a similar effect on transit. Clearly, absorption of nutrients in these experiments was influenced by other factors, such as the dilution of chyme or the path length from bulk phase to mucosa.

To find out whether transit time could influence small intestinal absorption in intact human subjects, the residues of a radiolabeled liquid carbohydrate meal were aspirated from the ileum (Read, 1984). The results showed that carbohydrate absorption was markedly reduced when transit was accelerated by metoclopramide, and increased when transit was delayed by infusion of lipid into the ileum (Fig. 1) (Read 1984).

Although these experiments suggest that contact time may play a role in limiting absorption in the small intestine, the importance of this factor in the nutrition of normal healthy people is uncertain. This is because food usually remains in the small intestine for enough time to absorb all but about 10% of nutrients and much of this residue may be metabolized by bacteria and salvaged in the colon. In fact, the colon can adapt to absorb 4–5 liters of fluid per day (Debongnie and Phillips, 1978) and up to 50 g carbohydrate per

TABLE I. The Effect of Lactulose, Magnesium Sulfate, and Metoclopramide on Gastric and Small Bowel Transit Times and the Delivery of the Components of the Test Meal in the Ileal Effluent[a]

	Control (n = 14)	Lactulose (n = 7)	MgSO₄ (n = 6)	Metoclopramide (n = 9)
Transit measurements				
Gastric emptying ($t^{1}/_{2}$ - hr)	1.3±0.1	1.3±0.3	1.5±0.3*	1.0±0.2
Small bowel transit time (hr) ($t^{1}/_{2}$ ileal emptying)	6.0±0.6	4.3±0.6*	5.0±1.0*	4.9±0.5*
Composition of ileal effluent				
Wet weight, g	250±24	1191±53**	387±42**	319±41*
Dry weight, g	22.40±1.02	32.81±2.80*	28.83±1.53**	22.94±0.93**
Fat, g	1.25±0.16	3.55±0.27*	2.35±0.27*	1.66±0.13**
Absorbable carbohydrate, g	1.03±0.09	2.13±0.26*	2.10±0.23*	0.90±0.24
Protein, g	5.28±0.32	8.03±0.55**	7.49±0.67*	4.39±0.53
Na⁺, g	0.50±0.06	1.50±0.21**	0.63±0.10*	0.73±0.09**

[a]Results are expressed as means±SEM. Superscripts refer to degree of significance compared with paired controls: * $p < 0.05$; ** $p < 0.01$.

day (Saunders and Wiggins, 1981). It is perhaps because of the prodigious capacity of the colon to adapt to an increased fluid and nutrient load that rapid small bowel transit is not by itself a recognized cause of diarrhea. Nevertheless, it is notable that patients with irritable bowel syndrome and who present with diarrhea have a more rapid small bowel transit than people who present with constipation or with abdominal pain and distension (Cann et al., 1983).

Excessively slow small bowel transit, on the other hand, is a recognized cause of diarrhea. This is because the relative stasis encourages overgrowth of bacteria in the small intestine. Among other actions, the bacteria degrade bile acids, impairing their absorption; the bile acids then pass into the colon, where they stimulate secretion and propulsion (Binder, 1980; Snape et al., 1980).

2.2.1. Transit through the Ileum

The ileum differs from the jejunum in that, although transport of nutrients across the epithelium occurs more slowly, food material remains there longer. This slowing down is partly related to the reduction in luminal volume and partly related to the motor pattern in the ileum; solutes delivered at the same flow rates exhibit a slower rate of transit in the ileum than in the jejunum (Morris and Turnberg, 1980). This increased residence of food in the ileum may mean that under normal circumstances more food is absorbed in the ileum than the jejunum. This possibility has never really been tested. In their classic experiments, Borgstrom *et al.* (1951) showed that approximately 90% of a liquid test meal was absorbed by a point 200 cm from the mouth (distal jejunum); their meal, however, contained nutrients in a simple, well-dispersed form, which required little digestion. It seems unlikely that the same results would be obtained using a normal semisolid meal.

Resection of the ileum results in considerably greater nutritional impairment than resection of the same length of jejunum (Booth *et al.*, 1961; Kalser *et al.*, 1960; Nygaard, 1966). This must be partly related to the depletion of bile acids and impairment of fat absorption that occurs after ileal resection. However, the fact that small bowel transit is also much more rapid after ileal resection than after jejunal resection (Nygaard, 1967) suggests that the reduction in small bowel contact time may also play an important role.

2.3. Control of Small Bowel Transit Time

The rate of passage of food through the small intestine must depend upon its rate of entry from the stomach, the propulsion through the small intestine, and the rate at which it is expelled from the ileum.

2.3.1. Ileal Expulsion

Logically, the rate of ileal expulsion should have the predominant influence on small bowel transit, not only because it is the last part of the system, but also because contact time is longer in the ileum than the jejunum.

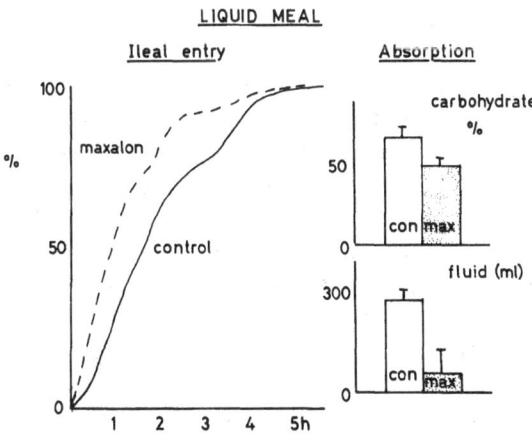

FIGURE 1. The cumulative delivery of a liquid carbohydrate meal and the degree of absorption of carbohydrate and fluid after administration of (---) metoclopramide (Maxalon) or (—) placebo.

It is, however, the factor we know least about, because nobody has studied ileal emptying under standardized conditions. Studies using the gamma camera have shown that the ileum empties at a remarkably constant rate after a meal (Read *et al.*, 1984b) and that the rate increases upon ingestion of a subsequent meal.

2.3.2. Gastric Emptying

Small bowel transit time may be considerably accelerated in patients who have undergone partial or total gastrectomy and may be delayed in patients with diabetic gastroparesis, although the delay in that condition may be related to direct involvement of the extrinsic and intrinsic nerve supply to the intestine by the diabetic process. In normal subjects, however, there is no correlation between the half-time for gastric emptying of a solid meal and small bowel transit time of the head or 50% of the meal (Read *et al.*, 1982). Furthermore, factors such as diet, exercise, and drugs that influence gastric emptying do not necessarily affect small bowel transit time (Read *et al.*, 1982; Cammack *et al.*, 1982; Cann *et al.*, 1984a,b).

2.3.3. Small Intestinal Motor Activity

The manner in which small bowel motor activity influences intestinal transit has been little investigated. It seems logical that the rate at which small intestinal contents are propelled downstream depends not only on the frequency of contractions in the segment under investigation, but also on the extent to which these contractions are propagated distally and the length of bowel over which they are propagated. Contractions that are static or only propagated over a short distance may obstruct the flow of contents, while those that are propagated over a long distance will move contents rapidly downstream. Summers and Dusdieker (1981) recently showed that in the canine duodenum, bursts of myoelectrical spiking activity, which normally generate contractions, behave as if they are always propagated downstream, but vary according to the distance of propagation. If this observation applies to other species, including man, then the frequency of contractions should be directly related to the degree of propagation. In a recent study we found that the half-time taken for food residues to enter the colon was inversely related to the contraction frequency in the upper small bowel, but not in the ileum (Read *et al.*, 1984b).

The passage of food to the colon was also affected by the return of the fasting motor pattern. The entry of food residues to the ileum was much more complete in subjects in whom an activity front (phase III of the interdigestive migrating motor complex) had travelled all the way to the distal ileum (Read *et al.*, 1984b).

2.3.4. The Ileal Brake

Infusion of fat emulsions or a protein hydrolysate into the ileum slows the transit through the small intestine of a bolus of lactulose infused at the ligament of Treitz (Read *et al.*, 1984a). This effect is not observed when fats or protein are infused into the jejunum or the colon. Ileal infusion of fat also slows the passage of a meal through the stomach and small intestine (Read *et al.*, 1984a). (Fig. 2) and increases the degree of absorption (Holgate and Read, 1985). This "ileal brake" may be an important feedback mechanism for regulating absorption in the small intestine. Studies in which the passage of labeled meals has been monitored have shown that the head of the meal often travels rapidly to the distal or pelvic small intestine, while the rest of the meal travels through the upper small intestine in a much more gradual manner (Poulakos and Kent, 1973; Jian *et al.*, 1979). It is possible that the more sedate progress is induced by activation of the ileal brake by nutrients in the head of the meal, and this may serve to optimise absorption.

The observation that transit is very much faster and absorption much reduced after ileal resection compared with resection of an equivalent length of jejunum (Nygaard, 1967) is compatible with a physiological role for the "ileal brake."

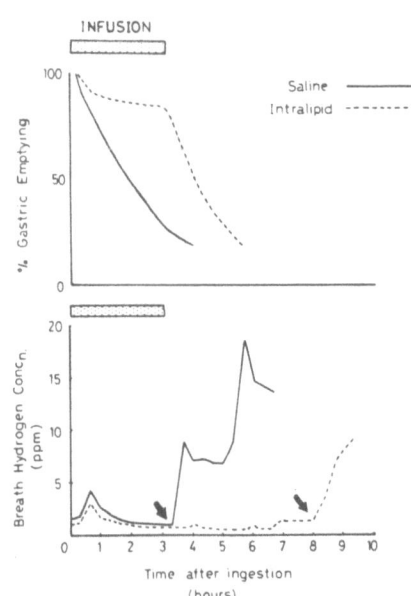

FIGURE 2. The effect of infusion of intralipid (dotted line) on the profiles of gastric emptying and the breath hydrogen following ingestion of a solid meal. The arrows indicate small bowel transit time of the head of the meal. (From Read *et al.*, 1984a.)

2.4. Action of Dietary Fiber on Small Bowel Transit

Jenkins (1978) used the breath hydrogen technique to investigate the action of a variety of different dietary fibers or fiber analogues on the small bowel transit time of the head of a 400-ml drink containing glucose, xylose, and lactulose. Addition of 14.5 g of either guar, tragacanth, or pectin or 12 g of cholestyramine delayed transit. Methylcellulose had no effect, while a much larger amount of bran (41.5 g) accelerated transit. In general, the delaying action of fibers on small bowel transit time was directly proportional to the viscosity of the solution. Other workers have confirmed the action of viscous polysaccharides on small bowel transit.

Although no allowance was made for the rate of gastric emptying in these studies, viscous polysaccharides can slow small bowel transit without having any significant action on gastric emptying (Fig. 3). Moreover, Caspary *et al.* have found that guar slows small bowel transit time even in patients who have had a partial gastrectomy (personal communication).

If a delay in gastric emptying cannot always explain a reduction in glucose absorption, it is possible that viscous polysaccharides may confine the nutrients to a smaller area of small intestine, reducing the number of available absorptive sites. In a recent study utilizing the gamma camera (Blackburn *et al.*, 1984b) we have shown that over the time when guar reduces blood glucose levels there is no difference in the distribution of a radiolabeled glucose drink in the upper small intestine. Thus, it seems likely that viscous polysaccharides have a more pronounced action on the distal intestine, especially since the viscosity would be greater in the distal small intestine as more fluid is absorbed. Leeds (1982) has reported that addition of guar gum to meals slows their transit through the middle third, but not the proximal third of the rat small intestine.

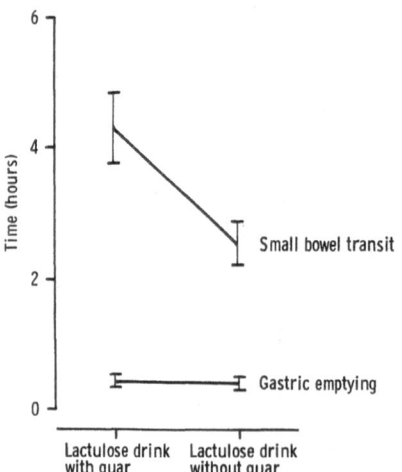

FIGURE 3. Action of 9 g guar gum on the half-time for gastric emptying and the small bowel transit time of the head of a drink of lactulose.

2.4.1. The Effect of Fiber on Patterns of Contractions

Only one study has attempted to investigate patterns of motor activity in the small intestine in relation to small bowel transit. Bueno *et al.* (1981) used strain gauges to record small intestinal motor activity in dogs after feeding meals containing 30 g of either guar gum, bran, or cellulose. All three agents delayed the transit time through the jejunum, measured by dye dilution techniques, although cellulose and guar were more effective than bran. The normal postprandial pattern of duodeno–jejunal motor activity in dogs contained bursts of 4–10 rhythmic contractions separated by periods of 1–2 min. Bran and cellulose enhanced the bursting pattern of small intestinal motor activity, causing an increase in the number of contractions per burst. Since this pattern of activity can be induced by luminal distension (Summers *et al.*, 1983) or obstruction, and may be acting to propel luminal contents rapidly downstream (Fleckenstein *et al.*, 1982), it may represent a response to the increased luminal bulk. Guar induced a different pattern of activity: regular small-amplitude contractions. This may have been related to the considerable increase in luminal volume caused by guar compared with the other two agents. The reason cellulose was so effective in delaying transit in this study, but not in Jenkins' study (Jenkins *et al.*, 1978), may be related to the very large quantities used, the difficulties in measuring flow rate and transit by marker dilution techniques in the presence of viscous agents, and the difference in species. The observation that bran delayed transit through the jejunum but accelerated transit through the whole small intestine (Jenkins *et al.*, 1978) may indicate that the dominant action of bran in the small intestine is to accelerate ileal transit.

2.4.2. Mechanism of Action

It seems likely that the action of viscous substances on the small intestine is to reduce convection induced by smooth muscle contractions (Blackburn *et al.*, 1984a). Not only would this impair the action of propulsive contractions, slowing transit, but it would also reduce the degree of mixing, preventing the access of nutrients in the luminal bulk phase to the absorptive epithelium. The reduction of mixing is thought to reduce the rate of absorption, allowing more food material to travel further down the gut before absorption takes place (Jenkins, 1983). Thus the presence of extra nutrients in the ileum may trigger the ileal brake (see above), which would contribute to the slowing of small bowel transit by viscous polysaccharide. Ileal nutrients also slow the delivery of food from the stomach (Read *et al.*, 1984a), which could in turn reduce food intake (Fig. 4).

If the delay in transit did not take place, then administration of viscous polysaccharides would probably cause significant malabsorption of nutrients. As it is, the question of whether viscous polysaccharides cause malabsorp-

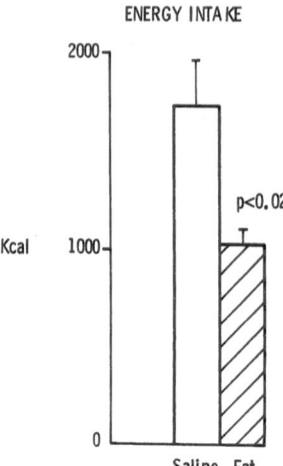

ENERGY INTAKE

FIGURE 4. The effect of ileal infusion of intralipid on intake of calories from an excessively large test meal.

tion of nutrients has not been satisfactorily answered. That bran increases fecal nitrogen and fat is well known (Burrows *et al.*, 1982; Cummings *et al.*, 1976a; Walters *et al.*, 1975), although much of this increase could come from an increase in excretion of bacterial cells. In the study of Jenkins *et al.* (1978), urinary excretion of ingested xylose was delayed by guar gum, but it was not actually reduced. Administration of bran to patients with ileostomies increased the total wet weight and dry weight of effluent, but did not influence the delivery of protein and available carbohydrate (Sundberg *et al.*, 1981). To my knowledge, nobody has investigated the action of guar gum on the composition of ileal effluent in man.

3. COLONIC TRANSIT

3.1. Measurement

Colonic transit time is defined as the time taken from entry of food residues through the ileocecal valve to expulsion at the anus. It is about ten times as long as mouth to cecum transit time, and is the dominant component of transit through the gut. To obtain accurate values, colonic transit should either be measured independently of mouth to cecum transit time or the latter should be deducted from values of whole-gut transit time. This is rarely done.

Whole-gut transit time is commonly measured by administering a marker by mouth and measuring the time taken for this to appear at the anus. Although a number of substances have been used as markers—polyethylene glycol (PEG), radiolabeled bran, chromium salts, carmine red—the most convenient is undoubtedly small radio-opaque plastic shapes. In our laboratory, we regularly use small (0.4×0.2 cm) segments of radio-opaque tubing. In the most frequently used method (Hinton *et al.*, 1969) the markers are ingested with a meal and the results of every bowel action over the next few days are collected and X-rayed and the number of markers determined. The time taken to pass a standard percentage of these markers (50%, 80%) is the whole-gut transit time. Measurement of transit time using radio-opaque markers bears a close relationship with measurements using PEG, carmine red, or chromium mordanted onto particles of bran (Wrick *et al.*, 1983; Read *et al.*, 1980).

This method of measurement is impaired by the considerable daily variations in whole-gut transit. To avoid this, a mean value for transit time can be obtained by administering a small number of markers three times a day over a period of weeks and measuring the daily delivery of markers in the stool. From these data, the amount of marker retained in the gut at any time may be calculated and from this the turnover or mean transit time (MTT) (Cummings *et al.*, 1976b). Changes caused by irregularities in bowel habit can be overcome by taking a 5-day moving average of the daily MTT values.

The number of markers present in the gut can also be measured on an abdominal X-ray. This has the added advantage of providing a measure of the transit time through each part of the colon. The importance of segmental transit measurements relates to the difference in function of different areas of the colon; the proximal colon is the region where most fermentation of carbohydrate takes place, whereas the transverse and distal colonic segments are perhaps concerned more with extraction of salt and water from colonic contents. Transit time through the right colon is much shorter than through the left colon (Wiggins and Cummings, 1976).

3.2. The Importance of Colonic Transit

3.2.1. Stool Weight

Colonic transit time is inversely related to stool weight (Burkitt *et al.*, 1973; Read *et al.*, 1980). Rapid transit is associated with large stool weights and diarrhea, while slow transit times are associated with low stool weight and constipation.

This association can occur because of a primary effect of transit time on colonic absorption or because of the effect of an increase in bulk of colonic contents on propulsion.

The colon extracts salt and water against high transepithelial concentration and osmotic gradients. This process requires material to remain in the colonic lumen for very long periods of time. If transit is too rapid, there may be insufficient contact with the epithelium for adequate absorption of salt and water, and the subject will experience diarrhea (Read, 1982). Adequate colonic residence is also necessary for the salvage of unabsorbed carbohydrate by bacterial conversion to short-chain fatty acids, which are rapidly absorbed (McNeil et al., 1978; Ruppin et al., 1980). Rapid transit may well lead to retention of sugars in the colonic lumen, which could further impair salt and water absorption by their osmotic activity. In addition, the increase in flow of colonic contents could impair colonic salvage of carbohydrate by flushing out the bacterial flora.

If transit time is prolonged, then more fluid may be extracted from the colonic contents, converting them into hard masses that are difficult to pass. This situation may lead to high colonic pressure and diverticular disease (Burkitt et al., 1972).

It would be incorrect to assume that the change in transit is always the primary action. Increases in luminal volume can reduce transit time by directly increasing flow rate and possibly also by inducing propulsive colonic contractions.

3.2.2. Metabolic Activity of Colonic Bacteria

The colonic bacteria carry out an enormous variety of metabolic processes besides converting carbohydrates to short-chain fatty acids, and the formation of metabolic products may be increased if the colonic residence is increased and *vice versa*. Relationships have been demonstrated between mean transit time and fecal ammonia levels (Cummings et al., 1978), neutral steroid conversion products (coprostanol and coprostanone) (Davignon et al., 1968), urinary phenol (Cummings et al., 1979b), and the digestibility of cellulose (Cummings et al., 1979a). Of critical importance is the possible formation of carcinogens. Both ammonia and secondary bile acids have been implicated in the pathogenesis of colonic cancer (Hill et al., 1975; Topping and Visek, 1976), which is more prevalent in people who have slow colonic transit (Burkitt et al., 1972).

3.3. Factors That Influence Colonic Transit

Colonic transit can be affected by the load of material arriving at the cecum, the motor patterns in the colon itself, and the expulsion of fecal matter from the anus.

3.3.1. Ileal Emptying

Few studies have attempted to relate cecal input with stool output in man under controlled physiological conditions. Nevertheless, it is known that the colon is able to absorb 4–5 liters of isotonic saline infused at a steady rate throughout the day (Debongnie and Phillips, 1978), although infusion of 500 ml over 1 h results in diarrhea. It seems likely that rapid perfusion of large volumes of fluid into the colon induces a propagative motor pattern that propels fluid rapidly to the anus (Chauve et al., 1976).

3.2.2. Motor Patterns

For most of the time, the motor activity of the colon consists of ringlike or haustral contractions that are either stationary or are propagated in an anal or aboral direction. The sigmoid colon exhibits a particularly high degree of phasic and tonic contractile activity and may function as a sphincter, holding material back in the more proximal colon (Baker and Mann, 1981), creating the stagnant conditions appropriate for fermentation. This pattern may be thought of as an obstructive or holding pattern. Then, from time to time, particularly after meals, the colon adopts another pattern of activity. This consists of contractions that appear to occupy a longer length of intestine and propel food rapidly downstream (mass movements). Studies in animals and man suggest that rapid transit is associated with a reduction in haustral contractions and/or an increase in propagated contractions, while slow transit is associated with an increase in haustral contractions (Read, 1983).

Certain factors may alter the pattern of motor activity and influence transit. Exercise and eating are thought to increase the number of mass movements (Holdstock et al., 1970). Bile acids may have the same effect (Snape et al., 1980).

3.4. Action of Dietary Fiber on Colonic Transit

Some fibers such as bran, ispaghula, or cellulose, accelerate colonic transit and produce a larger, softer stool that contains more water and is easier to pass. These are useful in treating constipation. Other forms of dietary fiber, such as guar, pectin, or cabbage, have comparatively little influence on colonic transit or stool weight, although they, too, can increase the water content, making the stool softer and easier to pass (Wrick et al., 1983). The reason for this distinction is not clear. However, guar, pectin, and cabbage are rapidly metabolized by colonic bacteria to volatile fatty acids, which are absorbed by the colon, whereas bran and other fibers are less easily digested by colonic bacteria.

The mechanism by which certain fibers reduce colonic transit time and increase stool bulk is unclear. It is not known, for example, whether the increase in the bulk of colonic contents stimulates colonic peristalsis or whether the fiber has a primary action on colonic motor activity. The following mechanisms may contribute to the laxative action of fiber on the colon:

1. Retention of fluid in the fiber matrix.
2. Carriage of bile acid into the colon.
3. Fermentation to poorly absorbed short-chain fatty acids.
4. Inhibition of salt and water absorption by low pH.
5. Increase in bacterial cell mass.
6. Increase in mucus production.
7. Distension due to gas production.

3.4.1. Retention of Fluid

The lack of correlation between the water-holding properties of different fibers *in vitro* and their action on transit time and stool bulk (Stephen and Cummings, 1979) does not necessarily imply that fibers do not exert their action on colonic function by retaining water; viscous polysaccharides such as guar have enormous capacities for hydration, but are rapidly degraded by colonic bacteria and so lose these properties. The positive correlation between stool weight and ingestion of pentose-containing polysaccharides (Cummings *et al.*, 1978) may be related in part to the greater water-holding capacity of pentoses and the fact that they are less well-fermented compared with polysaccharides containing a greater proportion of hexose (Prynn and Southgate, 1979). The effect of different fibers on stool weight is also related to their lignin content. This suggests that lignin in the cell wall may confer protection from fermentation. Nevertheless, chemical delignification of bran did not affect the fecal recovery of dietary fiber from bran (Bertrand *et al.*, 1981). The properties of bran that appear to be related to its action on colonic transit and stool bulk are that it should have a sufficiently large particle size to ensure an intact cell wall structure and sufficient lignification to resist extensive fermentation. Coarse bran loses both its water-holding properties and some of its laxative effect when it is finely ground (Brodribb and Groves, 1978; Heller *et al.*, 1980; Smith, 1982).

3.4.2. Increase In Bacterial Cell Mass

Fibers that are easily broken down, such as guar and cabbage, are a rich substrate for colonic bacteria, and increase bacterial cell mass (Stephen and Cummings, 1980). Since bacteria contain a large percentage of water, ingestion of such substances softens the stool by increasing water content and may be useful in promoting laxation (Wrick *et al.*, 1983). However, the stools of subjects on diets rich in easily fermented fiber substances are not always bulky and the transit time is not necessarily accelerated. In other words, such substances may enhance laxation without increasing the bulk or transit time of colonic contents (Wrick *et al.*, 1983), although their laxative properties are less than those of bran.

3.4.3. Binding of Bile Acids

Certain fibers, particularly bran, are known to bind bile acids. It is possible that bran may act as a vehicle for the transport of increased amounts of bile acid into the colon. Although direct measurement of the amounts of bile acid leaving the terminal ileum have not been carried out, the increase in deconjugation of bile acid that occurs in people given bran (Pomare and Heaton, 1973) suggests that it may be so. An increased load of bile acids could enhance laxation by increasing colonic secretion and propulsive motor activity (Binder, 1980; Snape *et al.*, 1980; Kirwan *et al.*, 1975). This hypothesis needs to be tested, although the observation that fecal excretion of bile acid is not necessarily increased in subjects on a diet rich in bran (Kay and Truswell, 1980; Pomare and Heaton, 1973) may argue against it.

3.4.4. Production of Short-Chain Fatty Acids

Colonic bacteria ferment carbohydrate to short-chain fatty acids. Since most of these are so rapidly absorbed, and they stimulate salt and water absorption (Ruppin *et al.*, 1980; McNeil *et al.*, 1978), it seems that this action would decrease the bulk of the stool rather than increasing it. However, if fermentation reduces the pH of the colonic contents, this will inhibit salt and water absorption directly (Rousseau and Sladen, 1971) and encourage the production of lactic acid (Cummings, 1981). The latter is poorly absorbed by the colon and its osmotic activity may contribute to the laxative action of certain polysaccharides.

3.5. Is the Action of Bran on Colonic Transit Useful?

The production of a softer, bulkier stool certainly helps some patients with mild constipation, but has little action in patients with severe constipation, except to make them feel bloated and uncomfortable. The action of bran in the irritable bowel syndrome is also controversial. Some studies have found it helpful (Soltoft *et al.*, 1976; Manning *et al.*, 1977). Others have found that it may improve constipation but does not help other symptoms, such as abdominal pain (Cann *et al.*, 1984a). At least one group has suggested that bran regularizes transit, slowing it in patients with diarrhea and accelerating it in those with constipation (Payler *et al.*, 1975; Harvey *et al.*, 1973). Other workers have failed to confirm any action on diarrhea, except to increase the percentage of unformed stools (Cann *et al.*, 1984a) (Table II). Many patients with irritable bowel syndrome cannot tolerate bran; their

TABLE II. Response of Whole-Gut Transit Time and Stool Weight, Frequency, and Consistency to Bran Treatment in Patients with Irritable Bowel Syndrome Who Had Constipation at Presentation and Those Who Had Diarrhea[a]

	Constipation (n = 17)		Diarrhea (n = 18)	
	Baseline	Bran	Baseline	Bran
Percent patients with improvement in symptom	—	71	—	28
Percent patients with deterioration in symptom	—	12	—	17
Daily stool frequency	1.1±0.2	1.2±0.1	2.2±0.3	2.2±0.3
Whole-gut transit time (50% markers), h	74±8	52±8	39±6	41±6
Stool weight, g/24 hr	76±24	135±19[b]	168±22	170±19
Percent unformed stools (median)	39	69[b]	69	94[b]

[a]Values are mean±SEM.
[b]Significant difference from baseline ($p < 0.05$).

bowels are as irritable to bran as they are to other factors (Cann *et al.*, 1984a).

Finally, epidemiologic data suggest that high-fiber diets may protect against colonic cancer (Burkitt *et al.*, 1972; IARC, Intestinal Microecology Group, 1977). If this is a cause and effect relationship, it is possible that other factors may be involved, such as binding of carcinogens or promoters or their dilution in the increased stool bulk.

REFERENCES

Baker, W. N. W., and Mann, C. V., 1981, The rectosigmoid junction zone: Another sphincter?, in: *Alimentary Sphincters and Their Disorders,* (P. A. Thomas, and C. V. Mann, eds.), MacMillan, London, pp. 201–211.

Bertrand, D., Brillouet, J. M., Rasper, V. F., Bouchet, B., and Mercier, C., 1981, *Cereal Chem.* **58**:468.

Binder, H. J., 1980, Pathophysiology of bile acid and fatty acid induced diarrhoea, in: *Secretory Diarrhea* (M. Field, J. S. Fordtran, and S. G. Schultz, eds.), American Physiological Society, Baltimore, pp. 159–178.

Blackburn, N. A., Redfern, J. S., Jarjis, M., Holgate, A. M., Hanning, I., Scarpello, J. H. B., Johnson, I. T., and Read, N. W., 1984a, The mechanism of action of guar gum in improving glucose tolerance in man, *Clin. Sci.* **66**:329–336.

Blackburn, N. A., Holgate, A. M., and Read, N. W., 1984b, Small intestinal contact area— another mechanism by which guar reduces postprandial hyperglycaemia in man, *Br. J. Nutr.* **52**:197–204.

Bond, J. H., and Levitt, M. D., 1974, Investigation of small bowel transit time in man utilising pulmonary H_2 measurements, *J. Lab. Clin. Med.* **85**:546–559.

Booth, C. C., Alldis, D., and Read, A. E., 1961, Studies on the site of fat absorption. 2. Fat balances after resection of varying amounts of small intestine in man, *Gut* **2**:168–174.

Borgstrom, B., Dahlquist, A., Lundh, G., and Sjovall, J., 1951, Studies of intestinal digestion and absorption in human, *J. Clin. Invest.* **36**:1521–1536.

Brodribb, A. J. M., and Groves, C., 1978, Effect of bran particle size in stool weight, *Gut* **19**:60-63.

Bueno, L., Praddaude, F., Fioramonti, J., and Ruckebusch, Y., 1981, Effect of dietary fiber on gastrointestinal motility and jejunal transit time, *Gastroenterology* **80**:701-707.

Burkitt, D. P., Walker, A. R. P., and Painter, N. S., 1972, Effect of dietary fibre on stools and transit times, and its role in the causation of disease, *Lancet* **2**:1408-1412.

Burrows, C. F., Kronfield, D. S., Banta, C. A., and Merritt, A. M., 1982, Effects of fiber on digestibility and transit time in dogs, *J. Nutr.* **112**:1726-1732.

Cammack, J., Read, N. W., Cann, P. A., Greenwood, B., and Holgate, A. M., 1982, Effect of prolonged exercise on the passage of a solid meal through the stomach and small intestine, *Gut* **23**:957-961.

Cann, P. A., Read, N. W., Brown, C., Hobson, N., and Holdsworth, C. D., 1983, The irritable bowel syndrome (IBS) Relationship of disorders in the transit of a single solid meal to symptom patterns, *Gut* **24**:405-411.

Cann, P. A., Read, N. W., and Holdsworth, C. D., 1984a, What is the benefit of coarse wheat bran in patients with the irritable bowel syndrome, *Gut* **25**:168-173.

Cann, P. A., Read, N. W., Holdsworth, C. D., and Barends, D., 1984b, Role of loperamide and placebo in the management of the irritable bowel syndrome (I.B.S.), *Dig. Dis. Sci.* **29**: 239-247.

Chauve, A., Devroede, G., and Bastin, E., 1976, Intraluminal pressures during perfusion of the human colon *in situ, Gastroenterology* **70**:336-340.

Cummings, J. H., Hill, M. J., Jenkins, D. J. A., Pearson, J. R., and Wiggins, H. S., 1976a, Changes in faecal composition and colonic function due to cereal fibre, *J. Clin. Nutr.* **29**:1468-1473.

Cummings, J. H., Jenkins, J. D. A., and Wiggins, H. S., 1976b, Measurement of the mean transit time of dietary residue through the human gut, *Gut* **17**:210-217.

Cummings, J. H., Southgate, D. A. T., Branch, W., Houston, H., Jenkins, D. J. A., and James, W. P. T., 1978, The colonic response to dietary fibre from carrot, cabbage, apple, bran and guar gum, *Lancet* **i**:5-9.

Cummings, J. H., Southgate, D. A. T., Branch, W., Wiggins, H. S., Houston, H., Jenkins, D. J. A., Jibraj, T., and Hill, M. W., 1979a, The digestion of dietary pectin in the human gut and its effect on calcium absorption and large bowel function, *Br. J. Nutr.* **41**:488-485.

Cummings, J. H., Hill, M. J., Jirraj, T., Houston, H., Branch, W. J., and Jenkins, D. J. A., 1979b, The effect of meat protein and dietary fiber on colonic function and metabolism, *Am. J. Clin. Nutr.* **32**:2086-2093.

Cummings, J. H., 1981, Short chain fatty acids in the human colon, *Gut* **22**:763-769.

Davignon, J., Simmonds, W. J., and Alunen, E. H., 1968, Usefulness of chromic oxide as an internal standard for balance studies in formula fed patients and for assessment of colonic function, *J. Clin. Invest.* **47**:127-138.

Debongnie, J. C., and Phillips, S. F., 1978, Capacity of the human colon to absorb fluid, *Gastroenterology* **74**:698-703.

Fleckenstein, P., Bueno, L., Fioramonti, J., and Ruchebusch, Y., 1982, Minute rhythm of electrical spike bursts of the small intestine of different species, *Am. J. Physiol.* **242**: G654-G659.

Harvey, R. F., Pomare, E. W., and Heaton, K. W., 1973, Effects of increased dietary fibre on intestinal transit, *Lancet* **i**:1278-1280.

Heller, S. N., Mackler, L. R., Rivers, J. M., Van Soest, P. J., Roe, D. A., Lewis, B. A., and Robertson, J., 1980, Dietary fibre: The effect of particle size of wheat bran on colonic function in young adult men, *Am. J. Clin. Nutr.* **33**:1734-1744.

Hill, M. J., Drasar, B. S., Williams, R. E. O., Meade, T. W., Cox, A. G., Simpson, D. E. P., and

Morson, B. C., 1975, Faecal bile acids and clostridia in patients with cancer of the large bowel, *Lancet* i:535-538.

Hinton, J. M., Lennard-Jones, J. E., and Young, A. C., 1969, A new method for studying gut transit times using radio-opaque markers, *Gut* **10**:842-847.

Holdstock, D. S., Misiewicz, J. J., Smith, T., and Rowlands, E. N., 1970, Propulsion (mass movements) in the human colon and its relationship to meals and somatic activity, *Gut* **11**:91-99.

Holgate, A. M., and Read, N. W., 1983, The relationship between small bowel transit time and absorption of a solid meal: Influence of metoclopramide, magnesium sulfate and lactulose, *Dig. Dis. Sci.* **28**:812-819.

Holgate, A. M., and Read, N. W., 1985, Effect of ileal infusion of intralipid on gastrointestinal transit—Ileal flow rate and carbohydrate absorption in humans after a liquid meal, *Gastroenterology,* **88**:1005-1011.

IARC (International Agency for Research on Cancer), Intestinal Microecology Group, 1977, Dietary fibre, transit time, fecal bacteria steroids and colon cancer in two Scandinavian populations, *Lancet* **2**:207-211.

Jenkins, D. J. A., 1983, Fiber and delayed carbohydrate absorption in man: Lente carbohydrate, in: *Delaying Absorption As a Therapeutic Principle in Metabolic Diseases* (W. Creutzfeldt and U. R. Folsch, eds.), Thieme Stuttgart, pp. 45-56.

Jenkins, D. J. A., Wolever, T. M. S., Leeds, A. R., Gassull, M. A., Haisman, P., Dilawari, J., Goff, D. V., Metz, G. L., and Alberti, K. G. M. M., 1978, Dietary fibres, fibre analogues and glucose tolerance: Importance of viscosity, *Br. Med. J.* i:1392-1394.

Jian, R., Pecking, A., Najean, Y., and Bernier, J. J., 1979, Etude de la progression d'un repas dans l'intestine grele de l'homme par une methode scintigraphique, *Gastroenterol. Clin.* **3**:755-762.

Kalser, M. M., Rother, J. L. A., Tumen, M., and Johnson, T. A., 1960, Relation of small bowel resection to nutrition in man, *Gastroenterology* **38**:458-468.

Kay, R. M., and Truswell, A. S., 1980, Dietary fibre: Effects on plasma and biliary lipids in man, in: *Medical Aspects of Dietary Fibre* (G. A. Spiller and R. M. Kauf, eds.), Plenum, New York, pp. 153-173.

Kirwan, W. O., Smith, A. N., Mitchell, W. D., Falconer, J. D., and Eastwood, M. A., 1975, Bile acids and colonic motility in the rabbit and the human, *Gut* **16**:894-900.

Kramer, P., Kearney, M. M., and Ingelfinger, F. Z., 1962, The effect of specific foods and water loading on the ileal excreta of ileostomised human subjects, *Gastroenterology* **42**:535-546.

Leeds, A. L., 1982, Modification of intestinal absorption by dietary fiber and fiber components, in: *Dietary Fiber in Health and Disease* (G. V. Vahouny and D. Kritchevsky, eds.), Plenum, New York, pp. 53-72.

Manning, A. P., Heaton, K. W., Harvey, R. F., and Uglass, P., 1977, Wheat fibre and irritable bowel syndrome, *Lancet* **2**:417-418.

McNeil, N. I., Cummings, J. A., and James, W. P. T., 1978, Short chain fatty acid absorption by the human large intestine, *Gut* **19**:819-822.

Morris, A. I., and Turnberg, L. A., 1980, The influence of a parasympathetic agonist and antagonist on human intestinal transport *in vivo, Gastroenterology* **79**:861-866.

Nuguid, T. P., Bacon, H. E., and Bantwell, J., 1961, An investigation of the volume of output and chemical content of ileal discharges following total colectomy and ileostomy, *Surg. Gynecol. Obstet.* **113**:733-742.

Nygaard, K., 1966, Resection of the small intestine in rats. I. Nutritional status and adaptation of fat and protein absorption, *Acta Clin. Scand.* **132**:731-742.

Nygaard, K., 1967, Resection of the small intestine in rats. IV: Adaptation of gastrointestinal motility, *Acta Clin. Scand.* **133**:407-416.

Payler, D. U., Pomare, E. W., Heaton, K. W., and Harvey, R. F., 1975, The effect of wheat bran on intestinal transit, *Gut* **16**:209-213.

Pomare, E. W., and Heaton, K. W., 1973, Alteration of bile salt metabolism by dietary fibre (bran), *Br. Med. J.* **4**:262–264.

Poulakos, L., and Kent, T. H., 1973, Gastric emptying and small intestinal propulsion in fed and fasted rats, *Gastroenterology* **64**:962–967.

Prynn, C. J., and Southgate, D. A. T., 1979, The effects of a supplement of dietary fibre on faecal excretion by human subjects, *Br. J. Nutr.* **41**:495–503.

Read, N. W., 1982, Diarrhoea: The failure of colonic salvage, *Lancet* **ii**:481–483.

Read, N. W., 1983, Speculations on the role of motility in the pathogenesis and treatment of diarrhoea, *Scand. J. Gastroenterol.* **18**(Suppl. 84):45–63.

Read, N. W., 1984, The control of gastrointestinal transit by luminal nutrients, in: *Intestinal Absorption and Secretion* (K. H. Soegel, ed.), MTP, Lancaster, England, pp. 153–160.

Read, N. W., Miles, C. A., Fisher, D., Holgate, A. M., Kime, N. D., Mitchell, M. A., Reeve, A. M., Roche, T. B., and Walker, M., 1980, Transit of a meal through the stomach, small intestine, and colon in normal subjects and its role in the pathogenesis of diarrhea, *Gastroenterology* **79**:1276–1282.

Read, N. W., Cammack, J., Edwards, C., Holgate, A. M., Cann, P. A., and Brown, C., 1982, Is the transit time of a meal through the small intestine related to the rate at which it leaves the stomach? *Gut* **23**:824–828.

Read, N. W., Al Janabi, M. N., Bates, T. E., Barber, D. C., 1983, The effect of gastrointestinal intubation on the passage of a solid meal through the stomach and small intestine in humans, *Gastroenterology* **84**:1568–1572.

Read, N. W., MacFarlane, A., Kinsman, R., Bates, T., Blackhall, N. W., Farrar, G. B. J., Hall, J. C., Moss, G., Morris, A. P., O'Neill, B., and Welch, I., 1984a, Effect of infusion of nutrient solutions into the ileum on gastrointestinal transit and plasma levels of neurotensin and enteroglucagon in man, *Gastroenterology* **86**:274–280.

Read, N. W., Al-Janabi, M. N., Barber, D. C., and Edwards, C. A., 1984b, The relationship between post-prandial motor activity in the human small intestine and the gastrointestinal transit of food, *Gastroenterology* **86**:721–727.

Rousseau, B., and Sladen, G. C., 1971, Effect of luminal pH on the absorption of water, sodium and chloride by the rat intestine *in vivo*, *Biochim. Biophys. Acta* **233**:591–593.

Ruppin, H., Bar-Meir, S., Soergel, K. H., Wood, C. M., and Schmitt, M. G., 1980, Absorption of short chain fatty acids by the colon, *Gastroenterology* **78**:1500–1507.

Saunders, D. R., and Wiggins, H. S., 1981, Conservation of mannitol, lactulose and raffinose by the human colon, *Am. J. Physiol.* **241**:G397–G402.

Smith, A. N., 1982, Effects of fibre on colonic function and motility, in: *Colon and Nutrition* (M. Kasper and M. Goebell, eds.), MTP, Lancaster, England, pp 181–188.

Snape, W. J., Shiff, S., and Cohen, S., 1980, Effect of deoxycholic acid on colonic motility in the rabbit, *Am. J. Physiol.* **288**:G321–325.

Soltoft, J., Gudmand-Hoyer, E., Krag, B., Kristensen, E., and Wulff, H. R., 1976, A double blind trial of the effect of wheat bran on symptoms of irritable bowel syndrome, *Lancet* **1**:270–272.

Stephen, A. M., and Cummings, J. H., 1979, Water holding by dietary fibre *in vitro* and its relationship to faecal output in man, *Gut* **20**:722–729.

Stephen, A. M., and Cummings, J. H., 1980, Mechanisms of actions of dietary fibre in the human colon, *Nature* **284**:283–284.

Summers, R. W., and Dusdieker, N. W., 1981, Patterns of spike burst spread and flow in the canine small intestine, *Gastroenterology* **81**:742–780.

Summers, R. W., Anuras, S., and Green, J., 1983, Jejunal manometry patterns in health, partial intestinal obstruction and pseudo-obstruction, *Gastroenterology* **85**:1290–1300.

Sundberg, A.-S., Anderson, H., Hallgren, B., Hasselblad, K., Isaakson, B., and Hulten, L., 1981, Experimental model for *in vivo* determination of dietary fibre and its effect on the absorption of nutrients in the small intestine, *Br. J. Nutr.* **45**:283–294.

Topping, D. C., and Visek, W. J., 1976, Nitrogen intake and tumorigenesis in rats injected with 1,2-dimethylhydrozine, *J. Nutr.* **106:**1583–1590.

Walters, R. L., Baird, I. M., Daines, P. S., Hill, M. J., Drasar, B. S., Southgate, D. A. T., Green, J., and Morgan, B., 1975, Effects of two types of dietary fibre on faecal steroid and lipid excretion, *Br. Med. J.* **2:**536–538.

Wiggins, H. S., and Cummings, J. H., 1976, Evidence for the mixing of dietary residue, *Gut* **17:**1007–1011.

Wrick, K. L., Robertson, J. B., Van Soest, P. J., Lewis, B. A., Rivers, J. M., Roe, D. A., and Hadder, L. R., 1983, The influence of dietary fibre source on human intestinal transit and stool output, *J. Nutr.* **113:**1464–1479.

8

The Ecology of the Colon

KATHLEEN FADDEN

1. INTRODUCTION

The gastrointestinal tract and its contents constitute a dynamic ecosystem, the existence and relative stability of which is very important to the well-being of the host. By definition, ecology of the gut implies the inter- and intraspecific relations among host, microflora, and their environment, with special reference to species distribution and abundance. Interactions within the gastrointestinal tract are numerous and intricate; however, the major interacting components may be considered as: (1) those relating to host physiology, i.e., absorptive and secretory mechanisms and intestinal motility; (2) nutrient supply; and (3) flora.

This delicately balanced ecosystem is easily and constantly influenced by many internal and external factors, the consequences of which may include, e.g., alteration in pH, redox potential, metabolism of exogenous and/or endogenous compounds, the binding capacity of solid digesta particles for micronutrients, or gut transit of digesta.

Evidently the intestinal ecosystem attains a high degree of complexity and consequently is by no means fully understood or often appreciated. The situation was succinctly summarized by Luckey (1977), who stated that "Intestinal microecology will not mature until microbiologists, histologists, geneticists, virologists and immunologists, physiologists, nutritionists, biophysicists, veterinarians and physicians are working together."

Nevertheless, an understanding of the dynamics and metabolic capabilities of the intestinal ecosystem is of fundamental importance in many instances, especially with regard to the study of human and animal nutrition

KATHLEEN FADDEN • PHLS Centre for Applied Microbiology and Research, Bacterial Metabolism Research Laboratory, Salisbury, Wiltshire SP4 OJG, United Kingdom.

and to the understanding of gastrointestinal disorders, especially when at times there is a transition from the commensal nature of the flora to a pathogenic status of part of the flora. Of particular interest is the relationship between the "state" of the intracolonic environment and the presence of colonic adenomas.

A wealth of circumstantial evidence strongly suggests a positive relationship between colonic cancer incidence and a high-fat, low-fibre diet (Walker, 1976; IARC, Intestinal Microecology Group, 1977; Reddy et al., 1978), high fecal pH (Thornton, 1981; Pietroiusti et al., 1983; Van Dokkum et al., 1983), high fecal secondary bile acid levels (Reddy and Wynder, 1977; Hill, 1981)— more specifically, high levels of lithocholic acid with respect to deoxycholic acid (Owen et al., 1983)—and finally elevated ratios of strictly anaerobic to facultatively anaerobic microorganisms within the gut (Legakis et al., 1981). Clearly, then, with respect to colon cancer, elucidation of factors influencing the intestinal milieu are paramount.

A major obstacle to the study of any intestinal ecosystem is its inaccessibility. Sampling by means of nasointestinal tubes and colonoscopes is of limited value, because in the former case sampling cannot be undertaken beyond the ileocecal junction and in the latter the bowel is normally cleansed prior to examination. Consequently, much knowledge has been gained about the intestinal ecosystem by using model systems. Many model systems are much more simplistic than the habitat they have been designed to represent. However, advancing the understanding of important metabolic interactions among the various species of an ecosystem is often dependent on studies of the individual species. Studies of this nature frequently reveal associations that are otherwise masked when examining a more complex mixed culture.

2. MODEL SYSTEMS FOR STUDYING THE ECOLOGY OF THE INTESTINE

Model systems for ecological studies are useful in that generally the range of experimental manipulations possible is much wider than in intact man. The types of model system that have been employed successfully are summarized in Table I.

2.1 Batch Culture

Batch culture is a technique used frequently to investigate species–species interaction. For example, Hirano and Masuda (1982) demonstrated enhanced 7α-hydroxysteroid dehydroxylase activity of a *Eubacterium lentum*-like intestinal anaerobe by a *Bacteroides* species, and Booth et al. (1977) have

TABLE I. Model Systems for Studying the Ecology of the Intestine

In vitro models	Batch culture	
	Continuous culture (chemostat)	
In vivo models	Animal model systems	Gnotobiotic animals
		Conventional cannulated animals
	Human model systems	Ileostomies + colostomies
		Infant studies

shown that *Bacteroides* species isolated from the human intestine are capable of bacteriocin production. It is not clear what advantage this confers on the organism, since bacteriocin-suspectible strains of *Bacteroides* actually outnumbered the producing strains in the feces of the subject studied. This simultaneous presence of susceptible and producing strains has also been demonstrated with *Escherichia coli* (Cooke *et al.*, 1972).

In addition to species–species interactions, batch culture has been used to examine several other types of interactive situations. Both Minato and Suto (1978) and Latham *et al.* (1978) have demonstrated attachment of various rumen isolates to cellulose powder and cell walls in leaves of Perennial Ryegrass *(Lolium perenne)* under batch culture conditions. There are many independent observations on cells that are immobilized or bound to a surface, that infer that such cells can behave differently from those that are free in solution (Mattiasson and Hahn-Hägerdal, 1982). However, such observations remain unexplained. It is certainly difficult to explain how a physical attachment could influence metabolism to such an extent as to cause changed metabolic patterns.

An alteration in the pH of the colonic environment undoubtedly has diverse consequences for the colonic ecosystem, including the solubility of various organic salts, and the binding capacity of certain fractions of the digesta for bile acid salts and possible carcinogens (Eastwood and Hamilton, 1968; Smith-Babaro *et al.*, 1981). A more acidic pH tends to favor the lactic acid-producing organisms, e.g., *Lactobacillus* and *Bifidobacterium* species, and suppress the lactic acid-utilizing organisms. Perhaps more importantly, in addition to influencing the balance of the flora, pH may influence the metabolic patterns of the flora. Certainly the bacterial hydrolysis of urea is pH-dependent (Suzuki, 1979). Since a high fecal pH may be of significance in the etiology of colorectal cancer (Thornton, 1981; Pietroiusti *et al.*, 1983; Van Dokkum *et al.*, 1983), the effect of pH particularly on hydroxysteroid dehydroxylases has been investigated in batch culture by MacDonald *et al.* (1978). Using a fecal inoculum, these studies demonstrated that at a higher culture pH (8.0 and 9.0) the percentage of secondary bile acids formed from primary bile acids was much greater; since it is well documented that secondary bile acids have comutagenic activity (Narisawa *et al.*, 1974; Wilpart *et al.*, 1983), this is an important observation.

A recent study by Fadden *et al.* (1984) on the effect of wheat bran fiber on the anaerobic metabolism of cholic acid by fecal bacteria substantiates the observations of MacDonald *et al.* (1978) (Fig. 1). The 7α-dehydroxylation of cholic acid to produce deoxycholic acid was affected by the addition of wheat bran fiber. Addition of 1% fiber retarded the 7α-dehydroxylase enzyme and addition of 2.5% fiber completely inhibited 7α-dehydroxylation. Inhibition of cholic acid metabolism appeared to be related to culture pH, which was reduced by fermentative breakdown of the fiber, liberating volatile fatty acids.

Clearly batch culture is a useful technique for the initial study of colonic ecology. The obvious limitations are that during an incubation there may be accumulation of unfavorable compounds in the culture medium and that within any particular incubation there is little scope for flexibility.

2.2 Continuous Culture (Chemostat)

Continuous culture is a natural progression from batch culture. As the name implies, there is a continuous flow or replenishment of nutrient to the system and continuous removal of waste products, similar to the human colon. The chemostat model is inherently more complex than a batch culture system. The system consists of a glass culture vessel with several portholes. The culture medium is maintained at constant temperature (37°C) by a thermocouple and continually stirred with a magnetic stirrer. Medium is administered at a chosen dilution rate with a peristaltic pump and the culture volume maintained by an overflow weir to waste. The headspace, culture, and fresh medium are kept in a reduced atmosphere by continual sparging with an oxygen-free gas mix and the culture pH maintained by suitable acid and alkali additions. A typical system for modeling the colon is shown in Fig. 2.

A most useful facet of continuous culture systems is the ability to alter the dilution rate and nutrient availability, thereby enabling one to achieve the low growth rates of organisms seen *in vivo* (Gibbons and Kapsimalis, 1967). The chemostat was initially used to model rumen ecosystems in the early 1960s with varying degrees of success (Rufener *et al.*, 1963; Slyter and Putnam, 1964). It is only comparatively recently that the system has been used to model monogastrics and indeed the human colon.

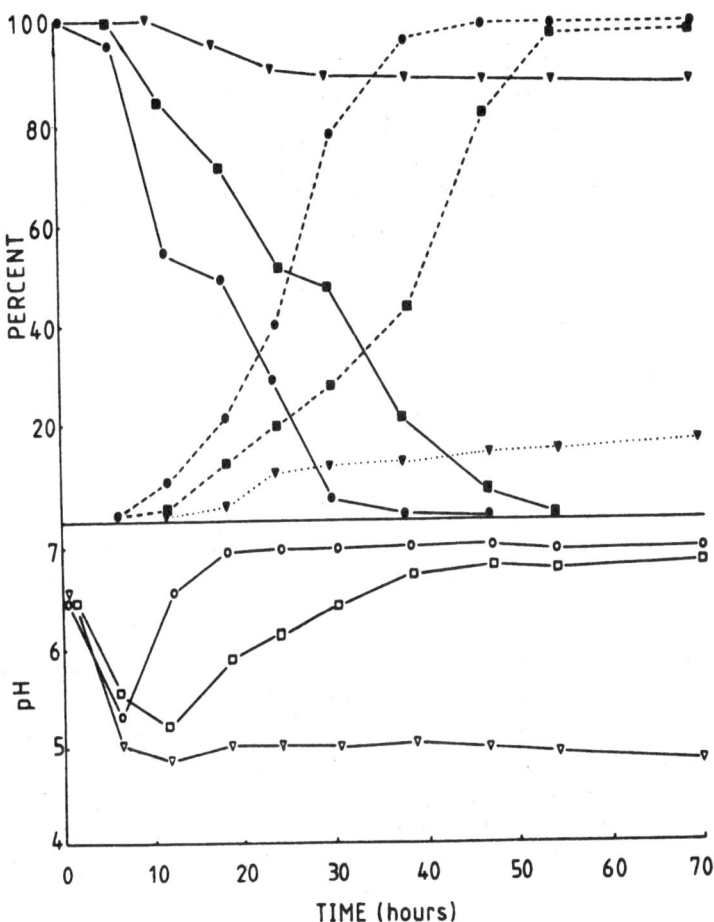

FIGURE 1. The effect of wheat bran fiber on pH and cholic acid metabolism by mixed fecal bacteria in anaerobic batch culture. (—) Cholic acid, (- - -) deoxycholic acid, (...) $3\alpha,12\alpha$-dihydroxy-7-oxo-1 5β-cholanic acid; (O,●) fiber-free, (□,■) 1% fiber, (∇,▼) 2.5% fiber.

The chemostat can be used in two different ways. First, the culture vessel can be innoculated with several known strains previously isolated, purified, and characterized from the habitat one aims to model, e.g., colonic contents or feces (if the former are not easily accessible). Or, second, the chemostat can be seeded with a colonic digesta or fecal inoculum. The application of the former type of study is similar to that discussed for batch culture, that is, to examine interactions between a limited number of populations that may be otherwise masked in a complex mixture of populations. Nevertheless, when studying an ecosystem with such species diversity as the

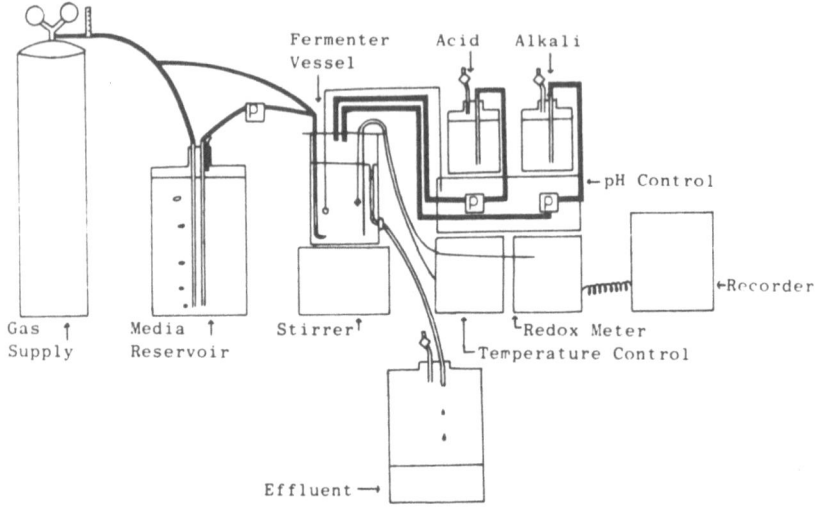

FIGURE 2. Diagrammatic representation of continuous culture scheme.

human colon, it is often more relevant to use the chemostat in the latter way, i.e., as a microcosm, and seed the chemostat with fecal or colonic inocula. Although the rumen has been quite extensively modeled in this manner, there has been comparatively less work on models of the colon.

Freter *et al.* (1983) used continuous culture to simulate the mouse large intestine, using both approaches mentioned above. The culture inoculum consisted of either (1) 37 representative strains isolated from a conventional mouse, or (2) part of the cecal contents and a small part of the cecal wall of a conventional mouse. The flora balance in the former type of culture was compared to that in a cecal homogenate of a mouse associated with the same 37 strains, and the flora balance in the latter type of culture compared to a cecal homogenate of a normal mouse. Comparability between the continuous flow cultures and cecal homogenates was quite acceptable. Importantly, there was no instance of one or a limited number of strains outgrowing any of the others.

Freter *et al.* (1983) also used a strain of *E. coli* C25 as an indicator of the function of the indigenous microflora *in vivo* and in continous culture. This organism typically attains levels of 5×10^9 cells/cecum in monoassociated mice, whereas in conventional mice such populations range from 5×10^6 to 0 cells/cecum. When identical floras were established *in vitro* and in gnotobiotic mice, the mean population level for *E. coli* C25 at equilibrium was very similar in both. In addition, when *E. coli* C25-infected mice were inoculated with a sample of continous flow culture initially from a conventional mouse, the *E. coli* population and cecal size reverted to normal. It seems, then, that this particular model did at least succeed in reproducing some of the ecological control mechanisms present *in vivo*.

Veilleux and Rowland (1981) and Mallett *et al.* (1983) have simulated the rodent ecosystem by using a two-stage continous culture. These workers compared the *in vivo* and *in vitro* flora on the basis of the relative proportions of the main bacterial groups present and their species composition at steady state conditions. Unlike Freter *et al.* (1983), these workers found that simulation of the rodent hindgut ecosystem using a single-stage continous flow culture was not possible. Progression to a two-stage model employing pH 5.1 (or 5.5) and 7.1, respectively, in the two stages and recycling cells from stage two back to stage one (to mimic coprophagy) was successful in simulating the proportion of bacterial groups found in feces (see Table II).

The metabolic activity of a rat fecal microflora maintained in a similar two-stage culture with respect to a limited range of substrates was examined by Mallett *et al.* (1983). These workers concluded that the metabolic activity of the microbial population from stage two of the culture was similar to that of the cecal microflora. Although nitrate reductase and nitroreductase activities were greater *in vitro* and β-glucosidase was more active in cecal contents, all activities were within the same order of magnitude.

Studies concerning continuous flow models of the human intestine are limited to three, all of which used feces as the initial inoculum. Early work by Zubrzycki and Spaulding (1957) reported that the numerical relationships between genera *in vitro* resembled those observed *in vivo* and that the manner in which various species appeared and reappeared was also similar to that observed *in vivo*. A more recent study by Miller and Wolin (1981) using a semicontinuous flow culture of the human large intestine with pulsed nutrient entry of large volumes once or twice a day, in order to mimic the manner in which ileal fluid enters the large intestine, was also successful in terms of the major groups of organisms cultured and the proportions of volatile fatty acids generated.

Edwards *et al.* (1983), using a synthetic medium but including bile, were able to culture all the major groups of organisms occurring in feces, and the model has been successfully used to simulate carbohydrate metabolism in the colon by incorporating starch into the medium. This produced acetate, propionate, and butyrate in similar proportions to those observed in the colon.

In general, evidence from the literature points to the fact that *in vitro* continuous culture models have definite potential for producing reasonable facsimiles of the large intestine of both rodent and man. There are, neverthe-

TABLE II. Comparison of the Most Common Microorganisms in Fecal Samples and in Continuous Culture Samples from Wistar Rats[a]

		Abundance of species,[b] %	
Bacterial group and species		Feces	Continuous culture
Staphylococci:	Staphylococcus aureus	<1	ND
Enterobacteria:	Esherichia coli	95	78
	Proteus mirabilis	4	18
	Klebsiella pneumoniae	<1	ND
Lactobacilli:	Lactobacillus acidophilus	64	79
	L. delbrueckii	18	4
	L. plantarum	5	10
	L. lactis	<1	2
	L. brevis	<1	<1
	L. fermentum	<1	<1
Streptococci:	Streptococcus salivarius	98	92
	S. faecalis	<1	8
	S. mitis	<1	ND
	S. sanguis	<1	<1
	S. viridans	<1	ND
	S. bovis	ND	<1
	S. durans	ND	<1
Anaerobes:	Bacteroides fragilis (subsp. vulgatus)	75	90
	Bacteroides melaninogenicus	10	3
	Bacteroides sp. a (?)	5	4
	Bifidobacterium bifidum	<1	2
	Bacteroides oralis	<1	<1
	Fusobacterium sp. (?)	<1	<1
	Bacteroides sp. b (?)	<1	ND
	Bifidobacterium sp. (?)	ND	<1
	Clostridium sp. (?)	ND	<1

[a] Adapted from Vielleux and Rowland (1981). Isolates followed by (?) were tentatively identified. Organisms unidentified at the species level are distinguished from other unidentified species of the same genus by a and b.
[b] Percentage of the total viable count for each bacterial group. ND, not detected.

less, a number of salient points to bear in mind when using the chemostat as a model of the intestine. Primarily, the purpose of a chemostat is to produce a homogeneous stirred environment; yet, in reality, homogeneity rarely occurs and of course the colon is no exception. Consequently, there is little scope for the establishment of gradients and specific niches, which undoubtedly occur both within the intestinal lumen and on the intestinal wall (Hartley et al., 1979; Croucher et al., 1983) [although the Gradostat developed by Lovitt and Wimpenny (1981) is an attempt to overcome this problem]. In practice, chemostat cultures are not homogeneous, due to the presence of wall growth, which may or may not be similar to the composition of cells in suspension.

A further problem is that, although there is continual (or semicontinual) input and output to and from chemostat models, there is no opportunity for absorption or secretion of compounds, including water; consequently, chemostat cultures are much more dilute than colonic contents. It is true that various bile salts and electrolytes can be incorporated into the medium in order to mimic secretion, but *in vivo* secretion is carefully controlled through extrinsic nerves, intrinsic nerves, and hormones; thus it is unlikely that the homeostatic nature of the colon can be mimicked precisely for long periods of time. There is obviously no mucin or immunoglobulin secretion, both of which may have a bearing on the flora balance in the *in vivo* situation, especially since it is known that certain enteric species degrade mucin (Miller and Hoskins, 1981).

Finally, the chemostat cannot model any aspect of colonic motility, the main purpose of which is not only to transport digesta in an aboral direction, but to mix the digesta thoroughly by a combination of haustral shuttling, propulsion, and peristalsis.

2.3. Gnotobiotic Animals

In order to progress from examining the contrived environments that are established in *in vitro* culture one must consider study using animal models. A "gnotobiote" (derived from the Greek *gnotos,* well known, and *biota,* all life) is an animal that contains a defined flora, and therefore, strictly speaking, may be germ-free, mono-, di-, tri-, or polyassociated with various organisms. Techniques for production and rearing of gnotobiotic animals are now well established. The method is based on the fact that almost without exception embryos *in utero* are sterile; in order to maintain sterility of the new born, birth is by Ceasarian section (just prior to parturition) into a sterile environment.

The variety of studies conducted using gnotobiotes to examine various aspects of species–species and species–host relationships is immense and a plenary review is beyond the scope of this chapter [see review by Gordon and Pesti (1971)]. However, in order to put this model in perspective with the other model systems described, it is useful to note the potential and limitations of gnotobiotes.

The major advantages of gnotobiotic study are that a particular species or number of species of organisms can be examined in their "natural" habitat, i.e., the habitat encompasses all those intestinal facets that cannot be mimicked *in vitro.* The effect, then of specific species on some aspect of host physiology or metabolism can be examined with relative ease. Unfortunately, several anomalies must be borne in mind when interpreting results from any gnotobiotic study. The physiology of the digestive tract in germ-free animals is frequently different, especially in rodents, which tend to develop an enlarged cecum. The villus structure is more regular and the brush border more clearly defined. Additionally, the immune system is almost insensitive and mucin secretion is greatly enhanced, although the mucin remains undegraded. It is well established that enteric bacteria degrade intestinal mucins, especially the carbohydrate moieties and to a lesser extent the mucin protein. Miller and Hoskins (1981) concluded that mucin glycoproteins in the human gut are degraded by bacterial subpopulations that comprise approximately 1% of the total flora. Given the gel-forming properties and viscous nature of mucin, variations in its abundance could undoubtedly affect the gut ecosystem.

Since there is no bacterial metabolism in germ-free animals, the intestinal pH tends toward alkaline and the redox potential of the gut is high. Consequently, establishment of a mix of strictly anaerobic gut bacteria is difficult to achieve and it is usually necessary to infect the host with a facultative anaerobe first in order to reduce the E_h. Once a limited flora has become established, quite often the numbers of a particular species may be far in excess of those normally achieved in the conventional animal. For example, Berg (1978) reported that the population level of a *Bacteroides* species was 100-fold greater in monoassociated mice than in equivalent mice also associated with strains of a *Eubacterium* species and a *Fusobacterium* species. The mechanism of this apparent *in vivo* antagonism is unknown. Due to the lack of bacterial metabolic activity in germ-free animals, there are inevitably differences in the pattern of metabolites present within the lumen. In germ-free animals bile acids remain in the conjugated form to either taurine or glycine, since the carbon–nitrogen bond in these conjugates cannot be cleaved by mammalian enzymes (Tazume, 1979; Sacquet *et al*, 1982). There is no capacity, therefore, for formation of comutagenic secondary bile acids (lithocholic acid and deoxycholic acid) by 7α-hydroxysteroid dehydroxylases. Consequently, the gnotobiote can be an extremely valuable tool for assessing microbe–bile acid and bile acid–host interactions, and could conceivably be a useful model to use in studies relating to colonic carcinogenesis.

Bearing in mind the differences between germ-free and conventional animals, the difficulty in obtaining suitable control animals can be appreciable. Ideally, control animals should be from the same litter, isolator-housed, and fed the same purified diet. The problem that then arises is how to conventionalize animals and avoid a "locked flora" (Reyniers *et al.*, 1960). This has proved to be a somewhat controversial matter. The use of gnotobiotic animals to study not only aspects of intestinal ecology but also nutrient and drug metabolism and for disease research (possibly the most significant field) has been invaluable, especially when used as an adjunct to studies with conventional animals.

2.4. The Gastrointestinal Cannulated Pig

As previously stated, one of the major obstacles to ecological studies of the intestine is the inaccessibility of the colon, and hence in the majority of studies the ecosystem is only examined at sacrifice. By using conventional swine with simple gut cannulas at selected sites along the small and/or large intestine, the gut can be sampled at time intervals for an indefinite period while the animal leads a "normal" life. Pigs will consume an omnivorous diet and they have a similar gut physiology to man, although the pig gut is slightly larger, with a better defined cecal area. The proximal gut tends to be colonized to a greater extent than the human gut, but colonization of the large intestine in terms of the major bacterial genera is similar to man (although some species differences do occur). The pig is considered to be a more suitable model than any other laboratory animal for ecological studies relating to the human colon. The model is obviously not as amenable to such precise pH and E_h control as a chemostat, but it lends itself to studies involving dietary manipulation and perhaps more importantly realizes the opportunity to monitor events in the region of the proximal colon, which may be quite different from those manifest in feces. A number of workers have examined bacterial populations from feces and various sites along the gastrointestinal tract (at autopsy) of swine (Allison et al., 1979; Russell, 1979; Robinson et al., 1981). It is difficult to draw definitive conclusions relating sampling site to flora observed, because there is considerable variation among pigs and few studies have made a comprehensive comparison between fecal flora (from fresh fecal or rectal sample) and samples obtained from higher up in the gastrointestinal tract.

Gastrointestinal cannulation of the pig has been used in studies by Decuypere et al. (1977), Sambrook (1979), and Fadden et al. (1984). Sambrook (1979) used single reentrant cannulas to monitor the flow of total lipid, acid detergent fiber, and volatile fatty acids in the intestines of growing pigs. Important observations from this study in terms of intestinal ecology were that the apparent absorption of acid detergent fiber in the different regions of the gut studied was influenced by diet, and that diet did not affect the molar proportions of acetate, propionate, and butyrate in ileal digesta, but did have an effect on these fatty acids in feces.

There are evidently both gross and discrete compositional changes of the digesta along the length of the gastrointestinal tract. This is further supported by data on the relative proportions of steroids along the gastrointestinal tract (Table III). The percentage of free bile acids as opposed to conjugated bile acids and the percentage of secondary bile acids as opposed to primary bile acids may have an important bearing on the flora within the lumen, since it is well documented that bile acids are inhibitory toward some components of the enteric flora (Floch *et al.*, 1971).

The cannulated pig, then, appears to be a particularly promising model to use in an attempt to elucidate some of the factors influencing the intestinal ecosystem. The model would be even more valuable if it could be used in conjunction with gnotobiotic animals, but the technical difficulties may be insurmountable. The cannulated pig has one major disadvantage, in that the cannulas *in situ* may have unknown effect(s) on this ecosystem, and such effects might be difficult to detect.

2.5. Ileostomy and Colostomy Patients

The study of ileostomy and colostomy patients affords a unique opportunity to examine easily bacterial interactions higher up the human gastrointestinal tract. The flora may be studied either by inserting a catheter into the stoma and sampling the contents by intubation or by simply collecting effluent from the ileostomy or colostomy appliance. Once an ileostomy or colostomy is established, the majority of patients lead a "normal" life and can consume a "normal" diet. Nevertheless, careful interpretation of results is required because studies by Gorbach *et al.* (1967) suggest that production of an ileostomy stoma upsets the ecology of the ileum and hence the microecology of ileostomy effluent becomes quite unique. Gorbach *et al.* (1967) reported that the number of organisms in ileostomy fluid was 80-fold greater than in the terminal ileum but 25-fold fewer than in feces. The precise reasons for the difference observed between ileostomies and normal ileum are unknown. Surprisingly, these authors did not observe any significant differences in total anaerobes, coliforms, lactobacilli, or anaerobic lactobacilli between ileostomy effluent and feces. Only staphylococci, strepto-

TABLE III. Steroid Profile along the Gastrointestinal Tract of the Cannulated Pig[a]

Substrate	Enzyme	Product	Percentage conversions			
			Ileum	Cecum	Colon	Feces
Cholesterol	Cholesterol reductase	Coprostanol	2.0	53.3	77.3	78.0
Chenodeoxycholic acid	7α-Hydroxysteroid dehydroxylase	Lithocholic acid	2.4	64.2	84.3	92.9

[a] Adapted from Fadden *et al.* (1984b).

cocci, and fungi were significantly increased in feces. Studies by Finegold *et al.* (1970) comparing ileostomy, transverse colostomy, and fecal floras also showed higher fecal counts of organisms, 10^{10}/g as opposed to 10^8/g for ileostomy and transverse colostomy effluents. However, in contrast to Gorbach *et al.* (1967), these workers found a considerable difference between the number of anaerobes in ileostomy fluid and feces. The ratio of anaerobes to aerobes was approximately 1000:1 in feces, 10:1 in transverse colostomy effluent, and 1:1000 in ileostomy effluent. This study also revealed a patient to patient variation in flora composition and highlighted the need to study as many patients as possible.

Despite the fact that the ileostomy flora may be different from the normal terminal ileal flora, useful information can still be gained regarding the effect of diet on this ecosystem. Recent studies by Fernandez *et al.* (1983) have compared ileostomy flora of patients when they were consuming a control diet, a low-protein diet (40–50 g/day), a high-protein diet (100–120 g/day), a low-fat diet (40–50 g/day), and a high-fat diet (120 g/day). The flora during the control, low-protein, and low-fat periods was similar. However, the high-protein and high-fat diets did produce some changes in the major groups of organisms examined (Table IV). Hori *et al.* (1983) investigated the effects of diets high (~22 g/day) and low(~13 g/day) in unrefined carbohydrates on the bacterial flora of ileostomy fluid. In contrast to the effects of increased levels of protein and fat, the relative proportions of organisms did not differ between the two diets, but the number of organisms/gram was higher on the unrefined carbohydrate diet (6.85 ± 1.15 vs. 5.45 ± 1.68, $p < 0.02$). This finding is contrary to the effect of fiber on feces, Stephen and Cummings (1980) observed that a high fiber intake actually decreased the number of organisms/g although the total excretion/day was increased.

In conclusion, it is apparent that a different set of control mechanisms must operate in the terminal ileal region as compared to, for example, the midcolon, and the study of ileostomy and colostomy patients must play a major role in elucidation of these mechanisms.

2.6. Infant Studies

Although not strictly a model system as such, several workers have examined sequentially fecal samples from infants' meconium through to the first years of life (Ellis-Pegler *et al.*, 1975; Rotomi and Duerden, 1981; Tomkins *et al.*, 1981; Stark and Lee, 1982). Studies of this nature are particularly useful when attempting to delineate which factors are responsible for the eventual climax flora established in adults.

At parturition the infant gut is subjected to vast numbers of organisms, primarily from the mother's vaginal flora and other environmental sources,

TABLE IV. Effect of Diet on Ileostomy Flora[a]

	Control vs. low protein	Control vs. high protein	Low protein vs. high protein	Low fat vs. high fat
Total aerobes	—	inc. $p < 0.01$	—	—
Total anaerobes	—	—	—	inc. $p < 0.05$
Enterobacteria	—	inc. $p < 0.05$	inc. $p < 0.05$	—
Streptococci	—	inc. $p < 0.05$	—	
Enterococci	—	—	—	—
Lactobacilli	—	inc. $p < 0.001$	inc. $p < 0.01$	inc. $p < 0.05$
Bacteroides	—	—	—	—
Veillonella	dec. $p < 0.05$	—	inc. $p < 0.05$	—
Clostridia	—	—	—	—

[a]Data of Fernandez *et al.* (1983). Results indicate statistically significant changes only.

some of these organisms are short-lived in the gut and do not colonize. Over recent years much attention has focused on the relationships between breast-fed and formula-fed infants, stool pH, stool buffering capacity, and fecal flora (Stark and Lee, 1982).

Soon after birth, irrespective of diet, the neonate gut is colonized by facultative anaerobes; e.g., *Enterobacterium* and *Streptococcus* species. In infants receiving breast milk the biota rapidly becomes dominated by *Bifidobacterium* species and a low pH. This pattern is not observed in formula-fed infants, who frequently have higher counts of the facultative anaerobes and are colonized by other anaerobes in addition to *Bifidobacterium*; e.g., *Bacteroides* species, *Clostridium* species, and anaerobic *Streptococcus* species. With the introduction of solid food to the infant diet there is a rise in the numbers and diversity of strictly anaerobic species colonizing the gut, especially in infants that have been breast-fed. The introduction of solid food to the formula-fed infants does not elicit such a marked change in the flora, since the intestines of these infants are frequently already colonized by high numbers of strictly anaerobic (putrefactive) species. After weaning and up to the age of 12 months the infant fecal flora develops, and by 12–48 months tends to closely resemble that of adults.

It is clear that diet seems to play a fundamental role in determining the development of the fecal flora, but the exact mechanisms are uncertain. It is interesting to note that while in infants there are such pronounced changes in the fecal flora balance between breast-fed and formula-fed infants (Stark and Lee, 1982) and between pre- and post-weaning (Tomkins *et al.*, 1981), it appears particularly difficult to elicit a change in the fecal flora of adults even after drastic dietary changes (Fuchs *et al.*, 1976; Hentges *et al.*, 1977). It has been suggested by Tomkins *et al.* (1981) that diet during infancy and childhood may determine the fecal flora of adulthood. Studies concerning the development of fecal flora over childhood years (including detailed dietary data) and subsequent adult follow-up would greatly increase our understanding of the role of dietary factors in flora development and final flora composition.

3. CONCLUSIONS

This chapter has by no means provided an exhaustive discussion on colonic ecology. It has, however, attempted to highlight the various ways in which the colonic ecosystem can be studied and the limitations and inadequacies of each method. One of the major problems in studying the colonic ecosystem is the enormous diversity of species. It is evident from comparisons of microscopic counts and plate counts that microbiologists still cannot account for all the fecal flora (of course a proportion of the organisms observed under a microscope may not be viable). As a result of the vast numbers of species present, it is impossible to distinguish such indirect interactions between species as competition, commensalism, and mutualism, hence the necessity to study limited numbers of species in model systems. One important aspect of colonic ecology hitherto not mentioned because it is not particularly amenable to study by model systems is that of mucosa-associated growth. Mucosa-associated microorganisms must be studied either by taking biopsy specimens (which are often criticized for being unrepresentative because they are so small) or alternatively at *postmortem*. In several animal species there would appear to be a distinct flora associated with the gut epithelium and mucus layer (Savage, 1969). This does not appear to be so in the human, where the diversity of species isolated tends to reflect that of luminal contents (Croucher *et al.*, 1983).

In conclusion, there is an increased need to understand the intricate workings of the colonic ecosystem, especially in terms of disease and drug research and also in the field of nutrition research. It is also apparent that feces is not necessarily a good index of the character of the colonic ecosystem, and so there is a real need to appreciate and understand events occurring from cecum to sigmoid colon. This can be achieved to some degree by the use of appropriate model systems.

REFERENCES

Allison, M. J., Robinson, I. M., Bucklin, J. A., and Booth, G. D., 1979, Comparison of bacterial populations of the pig caecum and colon based upon enumeration with specific energy sources, *Appl. Environ. Microbiol.* **37**:1142–1151.

Berg, R. D., 1978, Antagonism among the normal anaerobic bacteria of the mouse gastrointestinal tract determined by immunofluorescence, *Appl. Environ. Microbiol.* **35**:1066–1073.

Booth, S. J., Johnson, S. S., and Wilkins, T. D., 1977, Bacteriocin production by strains of *Bacteroides* isolated from human faeces and the role of these strains in the bacterial ecology of the colon, *Antimicrob. Agents Chemother.* **11**:718–724.

Cooke, E. M., Hettiaratchy, I. G. T., and Buck, A. C., 1972, Fate of ingested *Escherichia coli* in normal persons, *J. Med. Microbiol.* **5:**361–369.

Croucher, S. C., Houston, A. P., Bayliss, C. E., and Turner, R. J., 1983, Bacterial populations associated with different regions of the human colon wall, *Appl. Environ. Microbiol.* **45:**1025–1033.

Decuypere, J. A., Vervaeke, I. J., Henderick, H. K., and Dierick, N. A., 1977, The gastrointestinal cannulation in pigs: A simple technique allowing multiple replacements, *J. Anim. Sci.* **46:**463–468.

Eastwood, M. A., and Hamilton, D., 1968, Studies on the adsorption of bile salts to nonabsorbed components of diet, *Biochim. Biophys. Acta* **152:**165–173.

Edwards, C. A., Duerden, B. I., and Read, N. W., 1983, Continuous culture model of the human colon, *J. Med. Microbiol.* **16:**xiii.

Ellis-Pegler, R. B., Crabtree, C., and Lambert, H. P., 1975, The faecal flora of children in the United Kingdom, *J. Hyg. Camb.* **75:**135–142.

Fadden, K., Owen, R. W., Hill, M. J., and Mason, A. N., 1984a, The effect of wheat bran fibre on the anaerobic metabolism of cholic acid by mixed faecal bacteria, *Biochem. Soc. Trans.* **12:**860.

Fadden, K., Owen, R. W., Hill, M. J., Latymer, E., Low, A. G., and Mason, A. N., 1984b, Steroid degradation along the gastrointestinal tract—the use of the cannulated pig as a model system, *Biochem. Soc. Trans.* **12:**1105–1106.

Fernandez, F., Hill, M. J., Kennedy, H., Todd, E. A., and Truelove, S., 1983, Effect of changes in amount of dietary protein and fat on composition of ileostomy bacterial flora, *J. Med. Microbiol.* **16:**xv.

Finegold, S. M., Sutter, V. L., Baule, J. D., and Shmida, K., 1970, The normal flora of ileostomy and transverse colostomy effluents, *J. Infect. Dis.* **122:**376–381.

Floch, M. H., Gershengoren, W., Elliot, S., and Spiro, H. M., 1971, Bile acid inhibition of the intestinal microflora a function for simple bile acids? *Gastroenterology* **61:**228–233.

Freter, R., Stauffer, E., Clevan, D., Holdeman, L. V., and Moore, W. E. C., 1983, Continuous-flow cultures as *in vitro* models of the ecology of large intestinal flora, *Infect. Immun.* **39:**666–675.

Fuchs, H. M., Dorfman, S., and Floch, M. H., 1976, The effect of dietary fibre supplementation in man II. Alteration in fecal physiology and bacterial flora, *Am. J. Clin. Nutr.* **29:**1443–1447.

Gibbons, R. J., and Kapsimalis, B., 1967, Estimates of the overall rate of growth of the intestinal microflora of hamsters, guinea pigs, and mice, *J. Bacteriol.* **93:**510–512.

Gorbach, S. L., Nahas, L., Weinstein, L., Leviton, R., and Patterson, J. F., 1967, Studies of intestinal microflora iv. The microflora of ileostomy effluent: A unique microbial ecology, *Gastroenterology* **53:**574–580.

Gordon, H. A., and Pesti, L., 1971, The gnotobiotic animal as a tool in the study of host microbial relationships, *Bacteriol. Rev.* **35:**390–429.

Hentges, D. J., Maier, B. R., Burton, G. C., Flynn, M. A., and Tsutakawa, R. K., 1977, Effect of a high beef diet on the fecal bacterial flora of humans, *Cancer Res.* **37:**568–571.

Hill, M. J., 1981, Bile acids in colorectal carcinogenesis, in: *Banbury Report 7, Gastrointestinal Cancer: Endogenous Factors,* Cold Spring Harbor Laboratory, Cold Spring Harbor, New York, pp. 365–380.

Hirano, S., and Masuda, N., 1982, Enhancement of the 7α-dehydroxylase activity of a Gram positive anaerobe by *Bacteroides* and its significance in the 7-dehydroxylation of ursodeoxycholic acid, *J. Lipid Res.* **29:**1152–1158.

Hori, S., Berghouse, L., Hill, M. J., Hudson, M. J., Rodgers, E., and Lennard-Jones, J. E.,

1983, The effect of dietary fibre on the bacterial flora of ileostomy fluid, *J. Med. Microbiol.* **162**:vii.

International Agency for Research on Cancer, Intestinal Microecology Group, 1977, Dietary fibre, transit time, fecal bacteria, steroids and colon cancer in two Scandinavian populations, *Lancet* **2**:207–211.

Latham, M. J., Brooker, B. E., Pettipher, G. L., and Harris, P. J., 1978, *Ruminococcus flavefaciens* cell coat and adhesion to cotton cellulose and to cell walls in leaves of perennial ryegrass *(Lolium perenne), Appl. Environ. Microbiol.* **35**:156–165.

Legakis, N. J., Ioannides, H., Tzannetis, S., Golematis, B., and Papavassiliou, J., 1981, Fecal bacterial flora in patients with colon cancer and control subjects, *Zentrabl. Bakteriol. Mikrobiol. Hyg.* **251**:54–61.

Lovitt, R. W., and Wimpenny, J. W. T., 1981, The gradostat: A bidirectional compound chemostat and its application in microbiological research, *J. Gen. Microbiol.* **127**:261–268.

Luckey, T. D., 1977, Bicentennial overview of intestinal microecology 1. New concepts of the anaerobic intestinal flora, *Am. J. Clin. Nutr.* **30**:1753–1762.

MacDonald, I. A., Singh, G., Mahony, D. E., and Meier, C. E., 1978, Effect of pH on bile salt degradation by mixed fecal cultures, *Steroids* **32**:245–256.

Mallett, A. K., Bearne, C. A., and Rowland, I. R., 1983, Metabolic activity and enzyme induction in rat fecal microflora maintained in continuous culture, *Appl. Environ. Microbiol.* **46**:591–595.

Mattiasson, B., and Hahn, Hägerdal, B., 1982, Microenvironmental effects on metabolic behaviour of immobilized cells. A hypothesis, *Eur. J. Appl. Microbiol. Biotechnol.* **16**:52–55.

Miller, R. S., and Hoskins, L. C., 1981, Mucin degradation in human colon ecosystems, *Gastroenterology* **81**:759–765.

Miller, T. L., and Wolin, M. J., 1981, Fermentation by the human large intestine microbial community in an *in vitro* semi-continuous culture system, *Appl. Environ. Microbiol.* **42**:400–407.

Minato, H., and Suto, T., 1978, Technique for fractionation of bacteria in rumen microbial ecosystem. II. Attachment of bacteria isolated from bovine rumen to cellulose powder *in vitro* and elution of bacteria attached therefrom, *J. Gen. Appl. Microbiol.* **24**:1–16.

Narisawa, T., Magadia, N. E., Weisburger, J. H., and Wynder, E. L., 1974, Promoting effect of bile acids on colon carcinogenesis after intrarectal instillation of *N*-methyl-*N*-nitro-*N*-nitroso-guanidine in rats, *J. Nat. Cancer Inst.* **55**:1093–1097.

Owen, R. W., Dodo, M., Thompson, M. H., and Hill, M. J., 1983, The fecal ratio of lithocholic acid to deoxycholic acid may be an important aetiological factor in colorectal cancer, *Eur. J. Cancer Clin. Oncol.* **19**:1307.

Pietroiusti, A., Giuliano, M., Vita, S., Ciarniello, P., and Caprilli, R., 1983, Fecal pH and cancer of the large bowel, *Gastroenterology* **84**:1237.

Reddy, B. S., Hedges, A. R., Laakso, K., and Wynder, E. L., 1978, Metabolic epidemiology of large bowel cancer fecal bulk and constituents of high risk North American and low risk Finnish populations, *Cancer* **42**:2832–2838.

Reddy, B. S., and Wynder, E. L., 1977, Metabolic epidemiology of colon cancer. Fecal bile acids and neutral sterols in colon cancer patients with adenomatous polyps, *Cancer* **39**:2533–2539.

Reyniers, J. A., Wagner, M., Luckey, T. D., and Gordon, H. A., 1960, Survey of germ-free animals: The White Wyndotte bantam and White Leghorn chicken, in: *Lobund Reports*, No. 3, University of Notre Dame Press, Notre Dame, Indiana, pp. 7–159.

Robinson, I. M., Allison, M. J., and Bucklin, J. A., 1981, Characterization of the caecal bacteria of normal pigs, *Appl. Environ. Microbiol.* **41**:950–955.

Rotomi, V. O., and Duerden, B. I., 1981, The developement of the bacterial flora in normal neonates, *J. Med. Microbiol.* **14**:51–62.

Rufener, W. H., Nelson, W. O., and Wolin, M. J., 1963, Maintenance of the rumen population in continuous culture, *Appl Microbiol.* **11**:169–201.

Russell, E. G., 1979, Types and distribution of anaerobic bacteria in the large intestine of pigs, *Appl. Environ. Microbiol.* **37**:187–193.

Saquet, E., Leprince, C., and Riottot, M., 1982, Dietary fibre and cholesterol and bile acid metabolism in axenic and holoxenic rats II. Effects of pectin, *Reprod. Nutr. Dev.* **22**:575–581.

Sambrook, I. E., 1979, Studies on digestion and absorption in the intestines of growing pigs. 8. Measurements of the flow of total lipids, acid-detergent fibre and volatile fatty acids, *Br. J. Nutr.* **42**:279–287.

Savage, D. C., 1969, Localization of certain indigenous microorganisms on the ileal villi of rats, *J. Bacteriol.* **97**:1505–1506.

Slyter, L. L., and Putnam, P. A., 1964, Modification of a device for maintenance of the rumen microbial population in continuous culture, *Appl. Microbiol.* **12**:374–377.

Smith-Barbaro, P., Hanson, D., and Reddy, B. S., 1981, Carcinogen binding to various types of dietary fibre, *J. Nat. Cancer Inst.* **67**:495–497.

Stark, P. L., and Lee, A., 1982, The bacterial colonization of the large bowel of pre-term and low birth weight neonates, *J. Hyg. Camb.* **89**:59–67.

Stephen, A. H., and Cummings, J. H., 1980, Mechanism of action of dietary fibre in the human colon, *Nature* **284**:283–284.

Suzuki, K., Benno, Y., Mitsuoka, T., Takebes, S., Kobashi, K., and Hase, J., 1979, Urease-producing species of intestinal anaerobes and their activities, *Appl. Environ. Microbiol.* **37**:379–382.

Tazume, S., 1979, The role of the intestinal microflora in bile acid metabolism. Comparative studies on the bile acids of germ-free and conventional mice, *Keio Igaku* **56**:103–116.

Thornton, J. R., 1981, High colonic pH promotes colorectal cancer, *Lancet* **I**:1081–1082.

Tomkins, A. M., Bradley, A. K., Oswald, S., and Drasar, B. S., 1981, Diet and the fecal microflora of infants, children and adults in rural Nigeria and urban U.K., *J. Hyg. Camb.* **86**:285–293.

Van Dokkum, W., Deboer, B. C. J., Van Faasen, A., Pikaar, N. A., and Hermus, R. J. J., 1983, Diet fecal pH and colorectal cancer, *Br. J. Cancer* **48**:109–110.

Veilleux, B. G., and Rowland, I., 1981, Simulation of the rat intestinal ecosystem using a two-stage continuous culture system, *J. Gen. Microbiol.* **123**:103–115.

Walker, A. R. P., 1976, Colon cancer and diet with special reference to intakes of fat and fibre, *Am. J. Clin. Nutr.* **29**:1417–1426.

Wilpart, M., Mainguet, P., Maskens, A., and Roberfroid, M., 1983, Mutagenicity of 1,2-dimethylhydrazine towards *Salmonella typhimurium*, co-mutagenic effect of secondary biliary acids, *Carcinogenesis* **4**:45–48.

Zubrzycki, L., and Spaulding, E. H., 1957, Application of the continuous flow culture to studies on the normal fecal flora, *Bacteriol. Proc.* **1957**:101.

9

Diet and the Colonic Environment: Measuring the Response of Human Colonic Bacteria to Changes in the Host's Diet

ABIGAIL A. SALYERS

1. INTRODUCTION

As dietary fiber passes through the human colon, a substantial portion of it is digested by the resident bacteria (Van Soest, 1978; Ehle *et al.*, 1982). Clearly, this digestion by bacteria alters the structure of the fiber itself. It is also possible that dietary fiber affects the bacteria in turn by changing both the metabolic activities and the species composition of the colonic microflora. The question of how and to what extent fiber in the diet affects the colonic microflora is an important one because the metabolic activities of these bacteria largely determine the physicochemical environment of the colon.

The metabolic activities of colonic bacteria and their effects on the host are quite diverse. Some of the effects or products of metabolic activities of colonic bacteria are listed in Table I. Relatively little is known about the metabolic activities of the anaerobes, which are numerically predominant in the colon. Accordingly, the list in Table I should be viewed only as indicative of the variety of reactions that can be carried out by colonic bacteria, and

ABIGAIL A. SALYERS • Department of Microbiology, University of Illinois, Urbana, Illinois 61801.

TABLE I. Some Results of the Metabolic Activites of Intestinal Bacteria

Activity or result	Reference
Low oxidation–reduction potential	Wostmann and Bruckner-Kardoss (1966)
Production of short-chain fatty acids (especially acetate, propionate, butyrate)	McNeil et al. (1978), Wolin and Miller (1983)
Production of gases (CO_2, H_2, CH_4)	Wolin and Miller (1983)
Production of ammonia from protein, polysaccharides that contain hexosamines, or other nitrogenous compounds	Hespell and Smith (1983), A. A. Salyers (unpublished results)
Alteration of bile salts, steroids, sterols	Hylemon and Glass (1983), Bokkenheuser and Winter (1983)
Alteration of xenobiotics	Goldman (1983)
Production of mutagens	Wilkins et al. (1983)
Production of vitamins	Mackowiak (1982)
Changes in mucosal architecture; increase in rate of epithelial cell turnover	Abrams (1983), Savage (1983)
Catabolism of dietary fiber and mucin	Salyers and Leedle (1983)

not as a complete catalogue of such activities. Changes in one or more of the activities listed in Table I could have a significant effect on the colonic environment and on the host. Thus, the questions we would like to be able to answer are: (1) Does dietary fiber actually cause any changes in the colonic flora or its activities? (2) Are any of these changes significant enough to effect the host? Obviously, the first question must be answered before the second can be addressed.

At present, we are still a long way from being able to answer the first question in a convincing way. The purpose of this chapter is to review some attempts to answer the question of whether dietary fiber actually causes changes in the colonic microflora. Since the main barrier to answering this question is the lack of adequate methods, particular attention will be paid to the methodological difficulties that have to be overcome if answers are to be obtained. Rather than considering all of the work that has been done on the various different activities listed in Table I, I will focus primarily on the breakdown of polysaccharides by intestinal bacteria. I will focus on this area not only because it is the area with which I have had the most experience, but also because the problems encountered in this area are typical of those encountered in other areas, such as bile acid metabolism and production of mutagens.

2. ENUMERATING COLON BACTERIA

To date, most studies of the effect of diet on the colonic flora have been concerned with changes in the concentrations of particular species, i.e., with changes in the species composition of the colonic flora. Some examples of studies of this sort are shown in Table II. The only consistent finding of such studies is that the total number of bacteria can be affected by diet. Although individual studies frequently show significant changes in some species, these changes are not consistent from one study to another (Bornside, 1978; Savage, 1977). In my opinion, there is no convincing evidence that changes in the host's diet produce major changes in the species composition of the colonic microflora. This does not necessarily mean that there are *no* changes in the species composition of the flora, but rather that statistically significant changes, consistent from one study to another, have not been detected.

It is probably the case that only very substantial changes (i.e., changes of at least an order of magnitude) could be detected by current methods for enumerating colon bacteria. To obtain accurate quantitation of colon ana-erobes, one must use fresh specimens and stringent anaerobic techniques. One must also be capable of reliable speciation of the organisms (Finegold *et al.*, 1983; Moore *et al.*, 1978; Holdeman *et al.*, 1977). Even if these basic criteria are met, there are further problems. For example, it is not clear what medium to use for isolation and enumeration. No widely accepted selective or differential media are available for enumerating and identifying colon anaerobes. Moreover, we know very little about the plating efficiencies of the different colonic organisms, i.e., what percent of the viable bacteria actually form colonies on agar medium. These difficulties, together with the difficulty of obtaining fresh specimens and the time needed for classical identification procedures, have deterred research groups that might be interested in trying to measure the effect of diet on the colonic flora from attempting any such undertaking.

There are two possible ways of circumventing the problems mentioned above. One would be to develop new techniques for enumeration of bacteria that do not require growth of the organisms. A second is to avoid the problem by focusing on activities of the bacteria rather than on their relative numbers.

My research group has been working on a new approach to the problem of enumerating colonic bacteria and has developed a method based on DNA–DNA hybridization. We have been interested mainly in enumerating *Bacteroides* species because *Bacteroides* is one of the numerically predominant genera of colon bacteria (Moore and Holdeman, 1974). Moreover, surveys of colonic isolates have shown that most of the polysaccharide-degrading bacteria are members of this genus (Salyers and Leedle, 1983). We have cloned fragments of *Bacteroides* DNA specific for *Bacteroides thetaiotaomicron, B. vulgatus, B. distasonis, B. uniformis,* and *B. fragilis* subsp. a (Salyers *et al.*, 1983; Kuritza and Salyers, unpublished results). These are thought to be the most numerous *Bacteroides* species in the colon (Moore and Holdeman, 1974).

TABLE II. Results of Some Recent Studies of the Effect of Diet on the Species Composition of the Human Fecal Flora [a]

Dietary component(s) tested	Diet	Number of subjects and duration of diet	Summary of results	Reference
Fiber	Diet supplemented with plantain or banana (1 kg/day)	Two to six subjects per group; 2 weeks	Number of bacteria increased with fecal weight; no change in composition of flora	Drasar and Jenkins (1976)
Fiber	Diet supplemented with wheat bran (8 g/day)	Four subjects per group; 3 weeks	Number of bacteria increased with fecal weight; no change in composition of flora	Drasar et al. (1976)
Fiber	Diet supplemented with All-Bran (4 g/day)	Six subjects per group; 3 weeks	Number of bacteria increased with fecal weight; no change in composition of flora	Fuchs et al. (1976)
Protein, meat	Controlled diets with different protein content; also tested meat vs. no-meat diets	Ten subjects per group; 1 month	Some changes at the species level, but no major changes in the composition of flora	Hentges et al. (1977)
—	Absorbable, chemically defined, liquid diet	Three subjects; 8–10 days on liquid diet	Increase in enterobacteria, decrease in enterococci; no change in major genera	Crowther et al. (1973)
—	Absorbable, chemically defined, liquid diet	Fourteen subjects; 12 days on liquid diet	Decrease in enterococci, no change in major genera	Bounous and Devroede (1974)
—	Absorbable, chemically defined, liquid diet	Ten subjects; 7 days on liquid diet	No statistically significant changes in composition of the flora	Bornside and Cohn (1975)

[a] All of the studies listed in this table made some attempt to measure the numerically predominant bacteria, i.e., anaerobes, rather than focusing on the more easily measured but numerically minor facultative bacteria.

DNA from fecal specimens is trapped on nitrocellulose filters, and is then incubated with the cloned DNA fragments, which have been labeled with ^{32}P. The amount of ^{32}P-DNA that hybridizes to the material on the filter is proportional to the number of bacteria belonging to that particular species (Kuritza and Salyers, 1983). This method has the advantage that it allows us to quantitate the concentration of a particular species in a complex mixture without having to grow the bacteria. However, this approach has two serious limitations. First, it can only detect species present in relatively high concentrations, because of the limited amount of DNA that can be trapped on each filter. Second, it employs radioisotopes. This second difficulty can be remedied by labeling the cloned DNA fragments with the newly available biotinylated nucleotides (Enzo Biochem, New York). These nucleotides can be detected colorimetrically by streptavidin that has been conjugated to peroxidase (Leary *et al.*, 1983). We are continuing to investigate methods for improving sensitivity.

3. MEASURING METABOLIC ACTIVITIES OF BACTERIA

In addition to developing new methods for enumerating colonic bacteria, a second way of circumventing the difficulties inherent in determinations of the species composition of the colonic flora is simply to restate the problem. Since we are more interested in what the bacteria are doing in the colon than in what species they belong to, and since different species can share similar metabolic activities, we can ignore species composition and ask instead how diet affects the metabolic activities of the colonic microflora. At first sight, this appears to be an elegant and useful simplification of the problem. However, this approach has its own set of inherent problems.

The first problem one encounters with this approach is that relatively little is known about the metabolic capabilities of the major species of colonic bacteria. For example, when we began to investigate the breakdown of polysaccharides by colonic bacteria, there was no prior body of information to work from. Thus, one must do a considerable amount of basic research on the physiology (i.e., metabolic capabilities) of individual organisms before one can even begin to ask questions about what the organisms are doing in the colon.

A second problem is that each species is capable of a variety of metabolic activities. In addition, although two or more species can be capable of the same metabolic activity, the proteins involved can differ from species to species. These differences cannot be ignored, because they may allow one group of organisms to compete more successfully for a particular substrate than another group with similar metabolic activities. Thus, the array of metabolic activities of colonic bacteria is, if anything, at least as complex as the array of species.

A third problem is that this approach requires a level of technological sophistication that has not yet been attained. It is possible to measure various enzyme activities in feces, but these measurements give no information about which organisms are involved. What we really want to know is whether changes in diet cause certain organisms to change their activities (e.g., to switch from degrading mucins to degrading dietary polysaccharides), or whether the same group of organisms is always responsible for a particular activity. A major challenge for future research is to develop specific probes for detecting a particular activity that is being carried out by a particular species or group.

The next two sections summarize the result of some of our recent attempts to define the metabolic capabilities and limitations of colonic *Bacteroides.* Most of these studies were done, of necessity, with pure cultures growing in laboratory medium. Experiments of this sort are designated *"in vitro"* to emphasize the fact that great caution should be exercized in using the results of such experiments to draw conclusions about what is actually taking place in the colon *("in vivo").* In Section 6, some possible approaches to bridging the *in vitro–in vivo* gap are described.

4. *IN VITRO* STUDIES: THE EFFECT OF GROWTH RATE

We have found previously that almost all the strains of colon bacteria that can degrade polysaccharides are *Bacteroides* (Salyers and Leedle, 1983). Accordingly, we hoped that by studying the catabolism of polysaccharides by pure cultures of *Bacteroides* we could establish the limitations of these organisms. A knowledge of their limitations might then enable us to predict how they would respond to changes in concentrations of dietary polysaccharides in the colon.

Since growth rates in the colon are probably very slow, i.e., longer than 10 h per generation, we first asked whether *Bacteroides* could grow well on polysaccharides if the generation times were longer than 10 h. We found that *B. thetaiotaomicron* can grow very well on polysaccharides, as indicated by high cell yields (i.e., grams of bacteria per gram of substrate consumed), even at generation times as long as 35 h (Salyers *et al.,* 1981, 1982). Recent experiments with other polysaccharide-degrading species, such as *B. ovatus* and *B. fragilis* subsp. a, indicate that cell yields at slow growth rates are comparable to those of *B. thetaiotaomicron* (Salyers *et al.,* unpublished results). The results of these experiments indicate that growth rate alone is not likely to determine which polysaccharides are used.

However, the fact that cell yields of different species are comparable does not necessarily mean that these species are equally efficient at using polysaccharides. Cell yields only measure relatively gross differences in efficiency of utilization. Minor variations in efficiency too small to be detected by cell-yield measurements could become important in a competitive ecosystem. Preliminary results of experiments designed to measure the effects of competition between species indicate that such minor differences do exist and are important. For example, when *B. thetaiotaomicron* and *B. fragilis* subsp. a are first equilibrated separately in medium that contrains polygalacturonic acid as the sole carbon source and are then mixed together, *B. fragilis* subsp. a soon predominates. Thus, although both species have similar cell yields on polygalacturonic acid, one appears to be more efficient than the other with respect to removal of polygalacturonic acid from the medium.

Further competition experiments of this sort may enable us to predict which bacteria will be most likely to utilize various polysaccharides *in vivo*. It is important to note, however, that pure cultures, or even mixtures of pure cultures, growing in a glass vessel that contains laboratory medium may not behave the way they do in the colon. Many characteristics of the colonic milieu, such as absorption of products by the host or high concentrations of bile salts and other lipids, cannot be duplicated in the laboratory.

Although *Bacteroides* grow well on polysaccharides over a wide range of growth rates, there are some parameters that change with growth rate. The relative amounts of end products such as acetate, succinate, and propionate vary with growth rate. Specific activities of some polysaccharide-degrading enzymes also vary with growth rate (Salyers *et al.*, 1982; Salyers and Leedle, 1983). This flexibility probably helps the organisms to survive in the colon. However, we should keep in mind that the metabolic activities of an organism can be affected by a variety of factors.

5. *IN VITRO* STUDIES: ENZYMES AND OTHER PROTEINS

The ability of an organism to utilize polysaccharides might be limited by the location and characteristics of degradative enzymes within the cell. We have now investigated in some depth the catabolism of two polysaccharides, chondroitin sulfate and polygalacturonate, by *Bacteroides*. The results of these investigations are instructive because they give us an idea of the complexity of the systems used by bacteria to degrade polysaccharides.

When *B. thetaiotaomicron* is grown on chondroitin sulfate, it produces two chondroitinases with very similar properties (Linn *et al.*, 1983). These enzymes are soluble and are cell-associated rather than extracellular (Salyers and O'Brien, 1980). Moreover, they are inducible, i.e., high specific activities are detected only when bacteria are grown on chondroitin sulfate or related polysaccharides (Salyers and Kotarski, 1980). There are also outer membrane proteins that appear to be associated with growth on chondroitin sulfate (Kotarski and Salyers, 1984). We do not know the function of these proteins, but they may bind the polysaccharide. Preliminary results obtained with two other species that can utilize chondroitin sulfate, B. ovatus and B. "3452A," indicate that these organisms have systems for degrading chondroitin sulfate that are similar but not identical to the system used by B. thetaiotaomicron.

When B. thetaiotaomicron is grown on polygalacturonic acid, both a polygalacturonate lyase and a polygalacturonate hydrolase are produced. These enzymes are inducibly by polygalacturonic acid or pectin. The hydrolase is located in the inner membrane and the lyase, although it is not an integral membrane protein, appears to associate with membranes under some conditions (McCarthy and Salyers, unpublished data). Thus the enzymes could form a complex in the cell. A number of outer membrane proteins also appear to be associated with growth on polygalacturonic acid. These membrane proteins are not the same proteins as those associated with growth on chondroitin sulfate (Kotarski and Salyers, 1984; Kotarski et al., unpublished results). Preliminary work with three other species of colonic bacteria that can ferment polygalacturonic acid (B. ovatus, B. "3452A," and B. fragilis subsp. a) indicates that these species have similar, but not identical, systems for uptake and breakdown of polygalacturonic acid.

Clearly, the systems used by colonic Bacteroides for degrading polysaccharides are quite complex and are specific for a particular type of polysaccharide. Production of such an array of proteins imposes a serious energy load on the organism. Thus, it is not surprising that the proteins are inducible, i.e., are produced in high amounts only when the appropriate polysaccharide is available for utilization. The complexity and inducibility of the polysaccharide utilization systems may have envolved in such a way as to give the organisms maximum flexibility in a competitive environment where the mixture of available carbon and energy sources is constantly changing. Why are these systems so complex? Are the differences between species more important than the similarities? We are trying to answer these and similar questions by further biochemical and genetic investigations.

6. DEVELOPMENT OF METHODS CAPABLE OF MEASURING *IN VIVO* ACTIVITIES

A number of interesting questions, such as which species is (are) actually degrading a particular polysaccharide in the colon, or whether bacteria switch from one substrate to another as the host's diet changes, cannot be answered by the methods described in the preceding sections. New approaches are needed if we are to learn what organisms are actually doing in the colon. Now that we have some basic information about colonic *Bacteroides* we may be able to develop new methods based on this information. For example, it may be possible to exploit differences in the isoelectric points of the polygalacturonate lyases of *B. thetaiotaomicron* and *B. fragilis* subsp. a to determine which organism, if either, is producing the polygalacturonate lyase activity that can be detected in feces.

It may also be possible to construct specific metabolic probes. For example, we have recently cloned DNA from *B. thetaiotaomicron* that codes for one of the chondroitinases produced by this organism. The cloned DNA fragment is species-specific and could serve as a probe for measuring the concentration of the chondroitinase gene in colon contents. We plan to obtain antibodies to the chondroitinase and to use the antibodies as a species-specific probe for measuring the concentration of gene product in colon contents. The ratio of gene product to gene is an indication of whether the gene is being expressed. A high ratio indicates that *B. thetaiotaomicron* is using chondroitin sulfate.

Of course, the two approaches outlined above are only possible if we have the right kind of basic information about the organism. Basic research on the genetics and physiology of colon bacteria is an essential prerequisite for development of such specific detection methods. Much more research needs to be done before we can construct enough metabolic probes to give us a realistic picture of the metabolic activities that characterize the response of the flora to changes in diet.

7. SAMPLING PROBLEMS

Even if we develop sensitive and specific methods for detecting bacterial activities or for measuring bacterial concentrations, we are still faced with a very serious problem. At present, there is no morally or scientifically acceptable method for obtaining samples of colon contents from healthy human beings. Accordingly, we can only work with fecal specimens and hope that they are representative of colon contents. In some respects, feces may resemble colon contents. For example, concentrations of certain bacterial species appear to be relatively constant throughout the colon (Moore *et al.*, 1978). However, it is likely that growth rates and metabolic activities of bacteria in the ascending colon, where fresh dietary material enters the colon, are different from those of bacteria in other portions of the colon or in feces. Moreover, we cannot learn anything from feces about adherent bacteria or about other special niches (physical or chemical) that may be occupied by colon bacteria. The need for safe and effective sampling techniques is clearly one of the most pressing research needs in the area of human intestinal microecology.

8. CONCLUSIONS

The cumulative result of the research that has been done during the past decade in the area of human intestinal bacteriology is that we have moved from vague hypotheses with very little experimental basis to more specific hypotheses that might be testable if we could develop the right methods. This may seem to be a pessimistic assessment of the results of a tremendous amount of effort. However, given the fact that many researchers have despaired of being able to learn anything meaningful about the colonic microflora due to its complexity, the progress that has been made is, in fact, encouraging. In my opinion, the prospects are quite good for answering certain types of questions, such as which bacteria in feces are degrading a particular polysaccharide and whether this is affected by diet. As mentioned above, a breakthrough in sampling procedures or the development of new methods for monitoring events in the colon interior would expand the horizons of the possible even further.

ACKNOWLEDGMENTS. Experiments described in this chapter were supported by grant AI 17876 from the National Institutes of Health and by grant 59-2171-1-1-664-0 from the Competitive Research Grants Division of the U. S. Department of Agriculture. The author also thanks D. Savage for stimulating discussions of the topics treated in this chapter.

REFERENCES

Abrams, G. D., 1983, Impact of the intestinal microflora on intestinal structure and function, in: *Human Intestinal Microflora in Health and Disease* (D. J. Hentges, ed.), Academic, New York, pp. 292–310.

Bokkenheuser, V. D., and Winter, J., 1983, Biotransformations of steroids, in: *Human Intestinal Microflora in Health and Disease* (D. J. Hentges, ed.), Academic, New York, pp. 214–240.

Bornside, G. H., 1978, Stability of the human fecal flora, *Am. J. Clin. Nutr.* **31**:S141–S144.

Bornside, G. H., and Cohn, I., 1975, Stability of the normal fecal flora during a chemically defined low residue liquid diet, *Ann. Surg.* **181**:58–60.

Bounous, G., and Devroede, G. J., 1974, Effects of an elemental diet on human fecal flora, *Gastroenterology* **66**:210–214.

Crowther, J. S., Drasar, B. S., Goddard, P., Hill, M. J., and Johnson, K., 1973, The effect of a chemically defined diet on the fecal flora and fecal steroid concentration, *Gut* **14**:790–793.

Drasar, B. S., and Jenkins, D. J. A., 1976, Bacteria, diet and large bowel cancer, *Am. J. Clin. Nutr.* **29**:1410–1416.

Drasar, B. S., Jenkins, D. J. A., and Cummings, J. H., 1976, The influence of a diet rich in wheat fiber on the human fecal flora, *J. Med. Microbiol.* **9:**423–431.

Ehle, F. R., Robertson, J. B., and Van Soest, P. J., 1982, Influence of dietary fibers on fermentation in the human large intestine, *J. Nutr.* **112:**158–166.

Finegold, S. M., Sutter, V. L., and Mathisen, G. E., 1983, Normal indigenous intestinal flora, in: *Human Intestinal Microflora in Health and Disease* (D. J. Hentges, ed.), Academic, New York, pp. 3–32.

Fuchs, H.-M., Dorfman, S., and Floch, M. H., 1976, The effect of dietary fiber supplementation in man. II, *Am. J. Clin. Nutr.* **29:**1443–1447.

Goldman, P., 1983, Biochemical pharmacology and toxicology involving the intestinal flora, in: *Human Intestinal Microflora in Health and Disease* (D. J. Hentges, ed.), Academic, New York, pp. 241–264.

Hentges, D. J., Maier, B. R., Burton, G. C., FLynn, M. A., and Tsutakawa, R. K., 1977, Effect of a high beef diet on the fecal bacterial flora of humans, *Cancer Res.* **37:**568–571.

Hespell, R. B., and Smith, C. J., 1983, Utilization of nitrogen sources by gastrointestinal tract bacteria, in: *Human Intestinal Microflora in Health and Disease* (D. J. Hentges, ed.), Academic, New York, pp. 167–188.

Holdeman, L. V., Cato, E. P., and Moore, W. E. C., 1977, *Anaerobe Laboratory Manual,* 4th ed., Anaerobe Laboratory, Virginia Polytechnic Institute and State University, Blacksburg, Virginia.

Hylemon, P. B., and Glass, T. L., 1983, Biotransformations of bile acids and cholesterol by the intestinal microflora, in: *Human Intestinal Microflora in Health and Disease* (D. J. Hentges, ed.), Academic, New York, pp. 189–240.

Kotarski, S. F., and Salyers, A. A., 1984, Isolation and characterization of outer membrane of *Bacteroides thetaiotaomicron* grown on different carbohydrates, *J. Bacteriol.* **158:**102–109.

Kuritza, A. P., and Salyers, A. A., 1983, Simultaneous identification and quantitation of *Bacteroides* species using DNA hybridization, Presented at 83rd Annual Meeting of the American Society for Microbiology, Abstract C402.

Leary, J. T., Brigati, D. J., and Ward, D. C., 1983, Rapid and sensitive colorimetric method for visualizing biotin-labeled DNA probes hybridized to DNA or RNA immobilized on nitrocellulose, *Proc. Nat. Acad. Sci. USA* **80:**4045–4049.

Linn, S. L., Chan, T. C., Lipeski, L., and Salyers, A. A., 1983, Isolation and characterization of two chondroitin lyases from *Bacteroides thetaiotaomicron, J. Bacteriol.* **156:**859–866.

Mackowiak, P. A., 1982, The normal microbial flora, *N. Engl. J. Med.* **307:**83–93.

McNeil, N. I., Cummings, J. H., and James, W. P. T., 1978, Short chain fatty acid absorption by the human large intestine, *Gut* **19:**819–822.

Moore, W. E. C., and Holdeman, L. V., 1974, Human fecal flora, *Appl. Microbiol.* **27:**961–979.

Moore, W. E. C., Cato, E. P., and Holdeman, L. V., 1978, Some current concepts in intestinal bacteriology, *Am. J. Clin. Nutr.* **31:**S33–S42.

Salyers, A. A., and Kotarski, S. F., 1980, Induction of chondroitin sulfate lyase activity in *Bacteroides thetaiotaomicron, J. Bacteriol.* **143:**781–788.

Salyers, A. A., and Leedle, J. Z., 1983, Carbohydrate metabolism in the human colon, in: *Human Intestinal Microflora in Health and Disease* (D. J. Hentges, ed.), Academic, New York, pp. 129–146.

Salyers, A. A., and O'Brien, M., 1980, Cellular location of enzymes involved in chondroitin sulfate breakdown by *Bacteroides thetaiotaomicron, J. Bacteriol.* **143:**772–780.

Salyers, A. A., Arthur, R. A., and Kuritza, A., 1981, Digestion of larch arabinogalactan by a strain of human colonic *Bacteroides* growing in continuous culture, *J. Agric. Food Chem.* **29:**475–480.

Salyers, A. A., O'Brien, M., and Kotarski, S. F., 1982, Utilization of chondroitin sulfate by

Bacteroides thetaiotaomicron growing in carbohydrate-limited continuous culture, *J. Bacteriol.* **150:**1008–1015.

Salyers, A. A., Lynn, S. L., and Gardner, J. F., 1983, Use of randomly cloned DNA fragments for identification of *Bacteroides thetaiotaomicron, J. Bacteriol.* **154:**287–293.

Savage, D. C., 1977, Microbial ecology of the gastrointestinal tract, *Annu. Rev. Microbiol.* **31:**107–133.

Savage, D. C., 1983, Association of indigenous microorganisms with gastrointestinal epithelial surfaces, in: *Human Intestinal Microflora in Health and Disease* (D. J. Hentges, ed.), Academic, New York, pp. 55–78.

Van Soest, P. J., 1978, Dietary fibers: Their definition and nutritional properties, *Am. J. Clin. Nutr.* **31:**S12–S20.

Wilkins, T. D., and Van Tassell, R. L., 1983, Productions of intestinal mutagens, in: *Human Intestinal Microflora in Health and Disease* (D. J. Hentges, ed.), Academic, New York, pp. 265–291.

Wolin, M. J., and Miller, T. L., 1983, Carbohydrate fermentation, in: *Human Intestinal Microflora in Health and Disease* (D. J. Hentges, ed.), Academic, New York, pp. 147–165.

Wostmann, B. S., and Bruckner-Kardoss, E., 1966, Oxidation–reduction potentials in cecal contents of germfree and conventional rats, *Proc. Soc. Exp. Biol. Med.* **128:**137–141.

10

Fermentation and the Production of Short-Chain Fatty Acids in the Human Large Intestine

JOHN H. CUMMINGS and
WILLIAM J. BRANCH

1. INTRODUCTION

The principal constituents of dietary fiber are plant cell-wall polysaccharides or dietary nonstarch polysaccharides (NSP). These carbohydrate polymers may be divided chemically into cellulose and noncellulosic polysaccharide (NCP). The latter are a diverse group of substances including hemicelluloses, pectins, and similar molecules from plant tissues other than the cell wall, such as gums (e.g., guar and locust bean gum) and seed mucilages (e.g., ispaghula, sterculia). Fiber is therefore a chemically and physically heterogeneous mixture of substances and it is unwise to generalize about its effect in the human gut. However, it is now clear that all these polysaccharides are potential substrates for fermentation and as such are precursors of short-chain fatty acids (SCFA) in the human colon.

2. FERMENTATION AND THE ORIGIN OF SCFAs

There is now substantial evidence that nonstarch polysaccharides are broken down in the human colon (see review by Cummings, 1981a). This

JOHN H. CUMMINGS and WILLIAM J. BRANCH • MRC Dunn Clinical Nutrition Centre, Cambridge CB2 1QL, United Kingdom.

process is achieved by the concerted action of many species of intestinal microflora, is essentially anaerobic, and is therefore called fermentation. The biochemistry of fermentation is complex. Initially these large polymers are hydrolyzed to monomeric units, principally glucose, galactose, xylose, arabinose, and uronic acids. Fermentation then proceeds via glycolysis to pyruvate, but from there a variety of routes may be followed, depending on the microbial species present. A number of intermediates occur in fermentation, including ethanol, methanol, formate, lactate, and succinate, but these are rarely found in the human colon (Rubinstein *et al.*, 1969), because they are further metabolized, with the eventual production of the short-chain fatty acids acetic, propionic, and butyric acids, together with the gases hydrogen, carbon dioxide, and methane (Smith and Bryant, 1979; Wolin and Miller, 1983a). The pattern of fermentation may be substantially modified by the presence or absence of individual microbial species. Wolin and Miller (1983b) have shown that in the rumen the presence of methanogenic bacteria, which utilize H_2 for the reduction of CO_2 to CH_4, will increase acetate production. Hydrogen uptake by methanogens allows the regeneration of NAD from NADH and ultimately the production of acetate rather than ethanol by *Ruminococcus albus*. In man the significance of individual microbial species in determining fermentation patterns has not been examined, but potentially this could be of great importance in understanding variation in colonic function. Significant methane production is thought to occur in only one-third to one-half of Europeans and North Americans (Pitt *et al.*, 1980; Bjorneklett and Jenssen, 1982).

SCFAs are the predominant anions in human feces (Wrong *et al.*, 1965). Total concentration varies between 60 and 170 mmol/liter, depending on the method of obtaining fecal fluid for analysis (Rubinstein *et al.*, 1969; Bjork *et al.*, 1976; Cummings *et al.*, 1979; Zijlstra *et al.*, 1977). The concentration in colonic contents rather than feces tends to be at the higher end of the range (Pomare, Branch, and Cummings, unpublished results). Table I shows that acetate is the predominant SCFA in the human colon and in the hindgut of a wide variety of other species. The relative proportions (molar ratios) of the three principal SCFAs show a remarkable similarity at approximately 60:25:15 acetate:propionate:butyrate despite the wide variety of sampling techniques and diets of the various animals. In the rumen acetate also predominates (Table I) and the molar ratios are again of the order 60:25:15. Clemens *et al.* (1983) have measured SCFAs in both the rumen and hindgut of 16 East African wild ruminants and overall the values are similar. They have shown, however, that the molar percent of acetate in the large bowel is related to the animals' weight. In animals less than 20 kg it was 59.9% of total SCFA in the cecum and 58.8% in the distal colon, while in the largest species (over 300 kg) it was 72.1% (cecum) and 70.6% (distal colon).

An exception to the general observation that the molar ratios of short-

TABLE I. Molar Ratios (%) of Principal Short-Chain Fatty Acids
in Colon and Feces of Man and Selected Other Species

Species	Site	Molar ratios (%) acetate:propionate:butyrate	Reference
Sheep, Cow	Rumen	62:21:16	Hungate (1966)
Pig	Feces	66:22:7	Sambrook (1979)
	Cecum	56:32:12	Argenzio and Southworth (1974)
Rat	Cecum	61:25:14	Remesy and Demigne (1976)
Greater Glider (*Petauroides volans*)	Cecum	62:23:15	Rubsamen et al. (1983)
Termite (*Reticulitermes flavipes*)	Hindgut	94:3:2	Odelson and Breznak (1983)
Man	Fecal dialyzate	60:22:18	Rubinstein et al. (1969)
	Fecal dialyzate[a]	59:20:21	Cummings et al. (1979)
	Fecal dialyzate	57:28:15	Bjork et al. (1976)
	Whole stool[a]	65:20:15	Spiller et al. (1980)
	Whole stool[a]	54:29:17	Fleming and Rodriguez (1983)

[a] Average of all diets.

chain fatty acids are similar are the lower termites, where acetate accounts for 94–98% of hindgut SCFA. This is probably due to the unusual diet of the termite, which consists almost entirely of wood cellulose and hemicellulose, and also because most of the acetate is produced by flagellate protozoa, which are essential for the degradation of wood polysaccharides in these creatures.

In all species small amounts of other SCFAs, such as isobutyrate, valerate, and isovalerate, are usually present. Concentrations of these fatty acids are usually only 1–2 mmol/liter, although Fleming and Rodriguez (1983) observed greater amounts in fecal samples. These SCFAs originate mainly from the breakdown of protein, particularly branched-chain amino acids, and are not produced in any quantity during carbohydrate fermentation. Their presence may be more dependent on diet than that of other SCFAs (Thomsen et al., 1982).

3. THE EFFECT OF DIET

Dietary change has much less effect on SCFA concentration or molar ratios in the hindgut than might be anticipated. Table II shows SCFA values from a dietary study involving four healthy adult males. During the first

TABLE II. Short-Chain Fatty Acids and Ammonia in Fecal Dialyzate
during Dietary Change[a]

Diet	Total SCFAs, mmol/liter	Molar ratios (%) acetate:propionate:butyrate	Ammonia, mmol/liter
Low protein	65.7 ± 4.6	63:18:19	14.8 ± 1.3
High protein	57.7 ± 4.7	55:23:22	30.4 ± 1.1
High protein + wheat fiber	66.1 ± 4.2	60:19:21	28.2 ± 1.1

[a]From Cummings *et al.* (1979). Values are mean ± SEM.

period they ate a controlled diet containing 63 g/day protein and 23 g/day
dietary fiber, then changed to an equicaloric diet with 136 g/day protein and
22 g/day dietary fiber, and finally a further equicaloric diet with 164 g/day
protein and 53 g/day fiber. Fecal SCFA and NH_4 concentrations were
measured using the dialysis bag technique of Wrong *et al.* (1965). SCFA
concentrations and molar ratios were unchanged despite the large alterations
in fiber and protein intake. By contrast, ammonia concentration increased as
protein intake increased, although it was unchanged with the addition of
fiber. In a larger study of 19 subjects (Fig. 1) no change was again seen in
fecal short-chain fatty acid concentrations with diet, but ammonia and
SCFA levels were related, indicating some common factor in their absorption
from the gut.

In the study of Rubinstein *et al.* (1969), when five healthy subjects
changed from an *ad lib* diet to one containing only carbohydrate (soluble
carbohydrate + methylcellulose, 40 g/day) SCFA concentration in fecal
dialyzate fell from 85 to 46 mmol/liter, but there was little difference in the
molar ratios, 59:22:19 (*ad lib* diet) to 68:17:13 (carbohydrate-only diet). Two
of these subjects then lived on only methylcellulose and water for 4 days.
SCFA concentration fell to 23 mmol/liter, but molar ratios were again
unchanged. When a similar group of subjects were given antibiotics (neo-
mycin, bacitracin, colistin, and gramicidin) in addition to their normal diet,
acetate, propionate, and butyrate all fell to very low levels, while succinate
increased from 4 to 40 mmol/liter.

Therefore, unless dietary intake of fermentable carbohydrate is severely
restricted or antibiotics are given, fecal SCFA concentrations and molar
ratios remain relatively constant in man. From this, one might predict that
fecal output of SCFA should be closely related to total stool weight. This is
in fact the case. Figure 2 shows average daily stool weight (or fecal water
output) and fecal SCFA output from three separate studies of diet and
gastrointestinal function. Figure 2A relates a controlled diet study of six
healthy volunteers taking a standard U.K. diet for 3 weeks and then the same

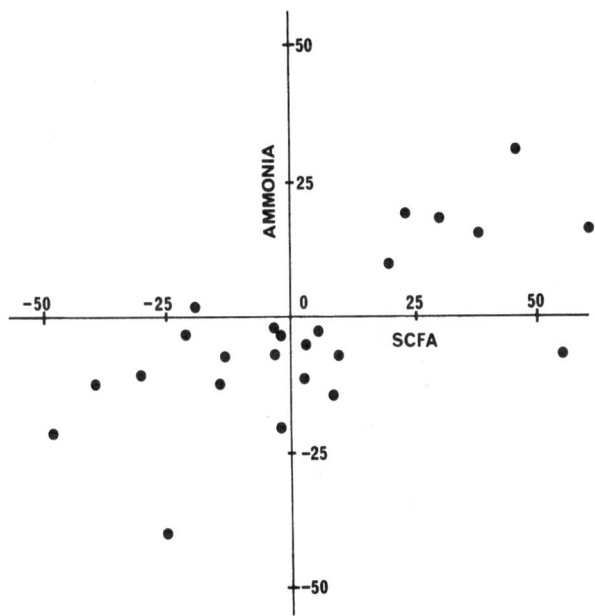

FIGURE 1. Change in mean fecal dialyzate ammonia and total SCFA concentrations in 19 healthy volunteers when going from a control diet to one supplemented with 15–20 g dietary fiber from either bran, cabbage, carrot, apple, or guar gum; $r = 0.69$; $p < 0.001$. [From Cummings *et al.* (1978).]

diet with the addition of about 30 g dietary fiber from wheat, added by exchanging white bread for whole meal (whole wheat) bread, and cornflakes for All-Bran, and giving a bran biscuit and raw bran. The dietary changes led to a threefold increase in stool output and a threefold increase in short-chain fatty acid output (Cummings *et al.*, 1976). In the study in Figure 2B the subjects were given varying doses of the nonabsorbable carbohydrates mannitol, lactulose, or raffinose as a single dose and feces were collected over the ensuing 48 h. Stool weight increased threefold and short-chain fatty acid excretion twofold (Saunders and Wiggins, 1981). Perhaps more significantly in this context is the study of Grove *et al.* (1929/1930), in which four healthy subjects were given magnesium sulfate. Stool weight increased substantially, as did SCFA output, an observation confirmed by Saunders and Wiggins (1981). Other studies have been reported in which the effect on stool and SCFA output of bran pentosan (Olmsted *et al.*, 1935), a variety of vegetable and cereal foods (Williams and Olmsted, 1936), cellulose and pectin (Spiller *et al.*, 1980) and cellulose, xylan, corn bran, or pectin (Fleming and Rodriguez, 1983) have been observed. In general, therefore, SCFA output rises in conjunction with fecal output, even in subjects with diarrhea (Cummings *et al.*, 1973). Only limited information can thus be gained from the study of

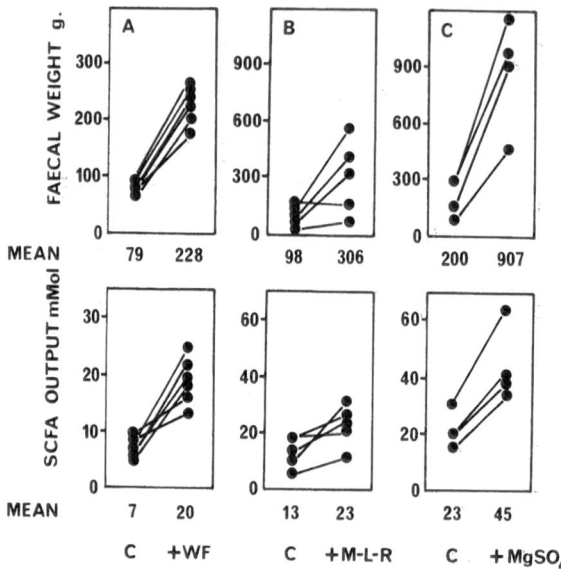

FIGURE 2. Mean daily stool weight (g/day) and total short-chain fatty acid output (mmol/ day). C, Control diet. (A) The effect of wheat bran (WF). Six healthy subjects ate a controlled diet typical of that eaten in the U.K. and then the same diet with 36 g dietary fiber from wheat added. (B) The effect of nonabsorbable sugars. Four healthy volunteers were studied on either an *ad lib* diet or after a single test dose containing approximately 150 mmol of either mannitol (M), lactulose (L), or raffinose (R). Values are the mean of two days of fecal collection. [From Saunders and Wiggins (1981).] (C) The effect of catharsis. Four healthy medical students were studied while eating controlled high-carbohydrate diets for 7 days and were then given about 30 g MgSO$_4$ for 2–7 days. [From Grove *et al.* (1929/1930).]

fecal SCFA, since no specific patterns of SCFA excretion in human stools have emerged that relate to events occurring within the large intestine. The role of SCFA in the colon would be much clearer if production rates were known.

4. SCFA PRODUCTION RATES

Knowledge of the amounts of SCFA produced in the hindgut would facilitate a much clearer understanding of colonic function and of the significance of fermentation. Measuring production rates, however, has proved to be exceedingly difficult and accurate data are few even in ruminant physiology. In animals where fermentation occurs mainly in the foregut, SCFA production and metabolism have been assessed by two methods. The first uses concentration differences among portal, hepatic, and arterial blood together with estimates or assumptions about blood flow to calculate net absorption. The second general approach is the use of isotope dilution methods to measure turnover (Bergman, 1975). The problem with these studies is that each fatty acid is metabolized differently and at a number of sites in the body, for example, in colonic epithelium, liver, and muscle. Moreover, the picture is further complicated by endogenous production of acetate. This type of study has not been attempted in man and the prospects of being able to obtain blood from the relevant sites in a person eating a reasonably normal diet over several weeks are not good.

An alternative approach (Cummings, 1981b) is to measure the supply of substrate for fermentation and from this, using fermentation balance equations derived for the ruminant, calculate theoretical production rates. The substrate available for fermentation in the human colon will include dietary carbohydrate that escapes digestion in the small intestine and endogenous carbohydrate from both the small and large bowel. The principal dietary carbohydrates that pass into the large bowel are the cell wall polysaccharides of plants (NSP). Much work remains to be done in conclusively demonstrating that the small intestine is not a major site of breakdown of NSP in the human gut. However, preliminary studies have shown that NSP can be substantially recovered in ileostomy effluent when taken as part of a normal diet (Holloway et al., 1978; Sandberg et al., 1981, 1983). The amount available for fermentation in the colon will therefore depend largely on dietary intake. This varies from between 15 and 30 g/day in the U. K., Scandinavia, and Japan (Bingham et al., 1979; Englyst et al., 1982; Minowa et al., 1983) to probably in excess of 100 g/day in parts of Africa (Bingham and Cummings, 1980).

Starch may also escape breakdown in the small bowel, although at the moment the degree to which and why this failure of digestion occurs are not clear. I. H. Anderson et al. (1981), using breath hydrogen excretion as a marker of fermentation in man, have suggested that 10–20% of the carbohydrate in white flour is malabsorbed. Using a very different approach, but with the same end in view, Stephen et al. (1983) measured the amount of starch reaching the terminal ileum in seven healthy volunteers through whom they had passed a multilumen tube by mouth and positioned it close to the ileocecal valve. Between 6 and 9% of the carbohydrate in a liquidized meal of banana, rice, and other vegetables reached the ileum. If from these studies one concludes that 5–10% of dietary starch is available for fermentation in subjects living on Western type diets, then this would add another 15–20 g to that available from NSP. In addition to this, small amounts (5 g/day) of soluble carbohydrate may also pass into the colon (Bond et al., 1980; McNeil et al., 1982). The only other source of carbohydrate available to the colonic microflora will be that derived from intestinal mucus. Although mucus-degrading bacteria are present in the colon (Salyers *et al.*, 1977; Hoskins and Boulding, 1981), the amounts degraded can only be surmised at present. An overall figure for total carbohydrate entering the large intestine in those living on Western type diets may be something between 40 and 50 g/day.

If the amount of carbohydrate fermented is known, then some idea of SCFA production can be obtained using equations derived from rumen metabolism (Hungate, 1966) or proposed for man (Miller and Wolin, 1979). From the equation

$$10 \text{ g hexose fermented} \rightarrow 100 \text{ mmol SCFA} + 850 \text{ ml CH}_4 + 1200 \text{ ml CO}_2$$

it can be predicted that 40–50 g of carbohydrate will yield theoretically 400–500 mmol SCFA, which, given the molar ratios in Table I, would include 240–300 mmol acetate and 80–100 mmol of both propionate and butyrate. However, a number of assumptions have to be made in doing these calculations, not all of which may be appropriate. For example, it is believed that a close parallel between rumen and hindgut fermentation exists, although in man there is apparently much less CH_4 produced in the hindgut then there is in the rumen and the hindgut also contains few if any protozoa. Furthermore, the carbon to nitrogen ratio in available substrate is likely to be different in the rumen and the hindgut. It is also supposed that carbohydrate breakdown in the colon is entirely an anaerobic process. While the great majority of the colonic flora are anaerobic (99.9%), some areobes are present and could exert an important effect on SCFA production. Finally, the overall efficiency of fermentation in the large bowel is unknown.

What other substrates could potentially be fermented and produce SCFAs in the colon? Long-chain fatty acids are not fermented, but proteolysis is known to occur in the large intestine and many species of microflora can break down amino acids (Hespell and Smith, 1983). In man, ileostomy effluent contains 2–3 g/day of nitrogen, most of which must be protein (equivalent to 12–18 g/protein), since ileal effluent contains little urea or ammonia (Gibson, 1977; McNeil *et al.*, 1982). Fecal nitrogen, which is usually less than ileostomy nitrogen (1–2 g/day), is present largely in microbial cells (Stephen and Cummings, 1979). Protein is therefore available for fermentation in the colon and during passage through this organ some protein nitrogen is probably incorporated into microbial nitrogen. Only 7% of total fecal nitrogen comes from urea diffusion into the gut (Wrong *et al.*, 1982). It is likely that after deamination the carbon skeletons of amino acids are fermented by the microflora and used as an energy source while nitrogen is available for microbial protein synthesis. The carbon skeletons will yield acetate and propionate together with the branched-chain fatty acids isobutyrate and isovalerate. The relative contribution of proteolytic fermentation in man is unknown and may well be influenced by the concomitant availability of carbohydrate for fermentation.

5. EFFICIENCY OF FERMENTATION

The amount and type of SCFA produced by the anaerobic breakdown of a given amount of carbohydrate in the colon will depend partly on the prevailing conditions in the lumen of the bowel. In the rumen overall fermentation balance is of considerable importance since energy lost as methane rather than absorbed as SCFA diminishes the potential value to the host of a particular forage. Furthermore, a substantial amount of protein is synthesized in the rumen during fermentation by the anaerobic flora from simple nitrogen sources such as urea. The efficiency of growth of microbial cells during fermentation (and therefore of protein synthesis) is of major importance and has been extensively studied. In practice the efficiency of fermentation is measured as the yield of bacterial cells (grams dry weight) from a given amount of carbohydrate utilized. Fermentation is usually studied by a continuous culture technique in chemostats. The method involves inoculating a single or multiple species of bacteria into a vessel in which microbial growth is limited by a single nutrient, such as glucose. Nutrient medium is infused into the vessel at a uniform rate and volume is maintained constant by use of an overflow. When steady state conditions are reached, bacterial growth rate, i.e., the amount of microbial material produced per unit of substrate consumed, can be measured. Typically in rumen studies cell yields are of the order of 25–40 g bacteria/100 g carbohydrate fermented (Isaacson et al., 1975; Owens and Isaacson, 1977; Hespell and Bryant, 1979).

Chemostat studies have shown that fermentation efficiency is affected by chemical factors such as pH, redox potential, or osmotic pressure and by metabolic factors like the availability of energy substrates and of preformed monomers such as amino acids, and by the transfer of intermediates between cells. Perhaps most important in determining cell yields is the maintenance energy requirement of the bacteria, which can be defined as the net "diversion of energy substrate to processes not leading directly to an increase in cell mass" (Hespell, 1979). This in effect means energy used for motility, maintenance of cellular integrity, turnover of cell macromolecules such as protein, active transport, synthesis of extracellular enzymes, and resynthesis of cells in the system due to cell loss through lysis. A major factor determining maintenance energy is dilution rate or turnover time of the system, which in the parlance of hindgut function is equivalent to transit time. In man it has been shown that turnover time affects microbial cell yields for given substrate loads (Stephen, 1980). The slower the transit time, the greater are maintenance energy requirements and therefore the lower is the efficiency of fermentation.

Thus a number of host and microbial factors combine to set the pattern of fermentation at any particular time. How these various influences affect anaerobic metabolism in man is unknown at present, although, by using single species of *Bacteroides* obtained from human feces grown in continuous culture Salyers and colleagues (Kotarski and Salyers, 1981; Salyers *et al.*, 1981) have shown that this organism responds in a similar fashion to energy supply and dilution rate as those isolated from the rumen. When fermentation efficiency is calculated for human studies cell yields are remarkably close to those predicted from the rumen, at 25–36 g bacteria/100 g carbohydrate fermented (Cummings, 1983). However, most of the work defining the control of anaerobic metabolism in man remains to be done.

6. ABSORPTION

The reason so little information about SCFA production and metabolism can be obtained from examination of feces is that these acids are rapidly absorbed from the colonic lumen. The mode of production and that of absorption have important effects on large bowel function. The absorption of acetate, propionate, and butyrate from the colonic lumen has been shown in man using a number of techniques (McNeil *et al.*, 1978, 1979; Ruppin *et al.*, 1980; Roediger and Moore, 1981). The characteristics of this absorptive process are listed in Table III. A striking feature is the rapidity of absorption, the rate exceeding that of sodium. In McNeil's studies (McNeil *et al.*, 1978, 1979) net absorption of acetate from a solution containing equimolar amounts of acetate and sodium (97 mmol/liter) was 8.1 ± 0.8 (SEM) $\mu mol/cm^2/per$ h for acetate and 4.7 ± 0.8 $\mu mol/cm^2/per$ h for sodium. These rates of total SCFA absorption in man are similar to those measured in animals, such as the horse, 8 $\mu mol/cm^2/per$ h (Argenzio *et al.*, 1974), and pig, 8–10 $\mu mol/cm^2$ per h (Argenzio and Whipp, 1979), and from the rumen, 10.5 $\mu mol/cm^2/per$ h (Stevens and Stettler, 1966a,b). In man little secretion of SCFA occurs into control solutions perfused through the healthy colon. The early studies of

TABLE III. Characteristics of Short-Chain Fatty Acid Absorption in Man

Concentration-dependent
Associated with bicarbonate "secretion"
Associated with pH rise and pCO_2 fall
Associated with stimulation of sodium and water
Occurs probably both as anion and undissociated acid

The early studies of Dawson (Dawson *et al.*, 1964) indicated that absorption rates were proportional to the chain length of the fatty acids and were a function of lipid solubility. However, subsequent studies have not confirmed this difference (McNeil, 1980; Ruppin *et al.*, 1980).

The mechanism by which SCFAs cross the colonic mucosa is thought to be principally by passive diffusion of the un-ionized acid into the mucosal cell, although recently Rechkemmer and Von Engelhardt (1982) have suggested that in the guinea pig proximal colon SCFA anions may permeate in part by the paracellular pathway. At the pH of both colonic luminal contents (pH 6–7) and the epithelial cells (pH 7.4) SCFAs are dissociated. However, Sallee and Dietschy (1973) have shown that the mucosa is relatively impermeable to anions, the apparent permeability coefficient for acetate and butyrate increasing fivefold when the pH of the absorption solution was changed from 7.4 to 6.0. Acetate transport into isolated rat colonic epithelial cells is also greater at more acid pH (Umesaki *et al.*, 1980). *In vitro* studies of the horse colon show that acetate transport is unaffected by transmucosal potential difference, in keeping with the view that the mucosa provides a diffusion barrier to the anion. Furthermore, the appearance of bicarbonate in the lumen during acetate transport and the stimulation of sodium absorption are both explicable on the basis that acetate is carrying hydrogen from the lumen into the mucosal cell. Nevertheless, these arguments over the form in which SCFAs are absorbed are by no means resolved. Studies in both the rumen and colon indicate that simple diffusion is insufficient to explain the rapid transport rates of these acids. The proportion of these acids that crosses the mucosa as the anion or undissociated acid is clearly important to the overall control of electrolyte absorption from the colonic lumen, since the movement of such large amounts of hydrogen ion will materially affect several epithelial transport processes.

6.1. Bicarbonate

Bicarbonate consistently appears in the colonic lumen during SCFA absorption. This process is independent of the chloride–bicarbonate exchange, since it occurs in the absence of luminal chloride (McNeil *et al.*, 1979) and is independent of chloride absorption (Argenzio and Whipp, 1979). The amount of bicarbonate that accumulates is equivalent to about half that of acetate absorbed. Bicarbonate appearance in the lumen could be explained by the presence of an acetate–bicarbonate exchange at the cell surface, were the cell to be readily permeable to the anion. In fact, the associated change in luminal pCO_2 and pH does not accord with such an anion exchange. CO_2 and bicarbonate in body fluids are related through the equation

$$H_2O + CO_2 \underset{\text{carbonic anhydrase}}{\overset{}{\rightleftharpoons}} H_2CO_3 \underset{\text{pK}_a\ 6.4}{\overset{}{\rightleftharpoons}} H^+ + HCO_3^-$$

Any increase in luminal bicarbonate due to secretion or ionic exchange by the mucosa will push the reaction in this equation to the left, resulting in a rise in pH and pCO_2. In experimental studies in the pig (Argenzio and Whipp, 1979), rumen (Stevens, 1970), and man (Ruppin et al., 1980), pH rises but pCO_2 falls during acetate absorption. The explanation that has been advanced for this is that luminal or juxtamucosal hydration of CO_2 occurs and that hydrogen ion is used to protonate SCFA anion prior to crossing the mucosa as undissociated acids. Thus absorption of the acid leads to bicarbonate accumulation, a rise in pH, and fall in pCO_2. The presence of carbonic anhydrase in colonic epithelium (Carter and Parsons, 1968) suggests that it plays some part in fermentation, most likely in providing the principal buffer for SCFAs. In the rat, however (Umesaki et al., 1979), pCO_2 does not fall during SCFA absorption and the manner of bicarbonic accumulation will not be resolved without further in vitro studies.

6.2. Sodium

The generation of intracellular hydrogen ion either by hydration of CO_2 or the transport of undissociated SCFAs into the cell may well be important in explaining the effects of SCFAs on sodium absorption. Short-chain fatty acids stimulate sodium absorption from the colonic lumen. This has been demonstrated in the rat (Parsons and Paterson, 1965), goat (Argenzio et al., 1975), pig (Crump et al., 1980), sheep (Rubsamen and von Engelhardt, 1981), and in man with butyrate (Roediger and Moore, 1981) and propionate (Ruppin et al., 1980). The stimulatory effect of short-chain fatty acids on sodium absorption is quite considerable. In Roediger and Moore's (1981) study of the isolated perfused human colon, net sodium absorption (nmol/min per $cm^2 \pm SEM$) increased from 320 ± 10 in the control perfusion to 1960 ± 480 with the addition of 20 mmol/liter butyrate to the perfusate. In the rat colon it is notable that neither succinate nor lactate, which are poorly absorbed anions, stimulates sodium absorption, whereas acetate does (Umesaki et al., 1979, 1980).

The link between SCFA and Na^+ absorption has been postulated by Von Engelhardt's group to be the recycling of hydrogen ions (Fig. 3) (von Engelhardt and Rechkemmer, 1983; Rechkemmer and von Engelhardt, 1982; Rubsamen and von Engelhardt, 1981). The un-ionized acid crosses into the cell, where it dissociates and hydrogen ion is moved back into the lumen in exchange for sodium. In the studies of pig colon (Argenzio and Whipp, 1979), marked differences in luminal pCO_2 and pH were observed when

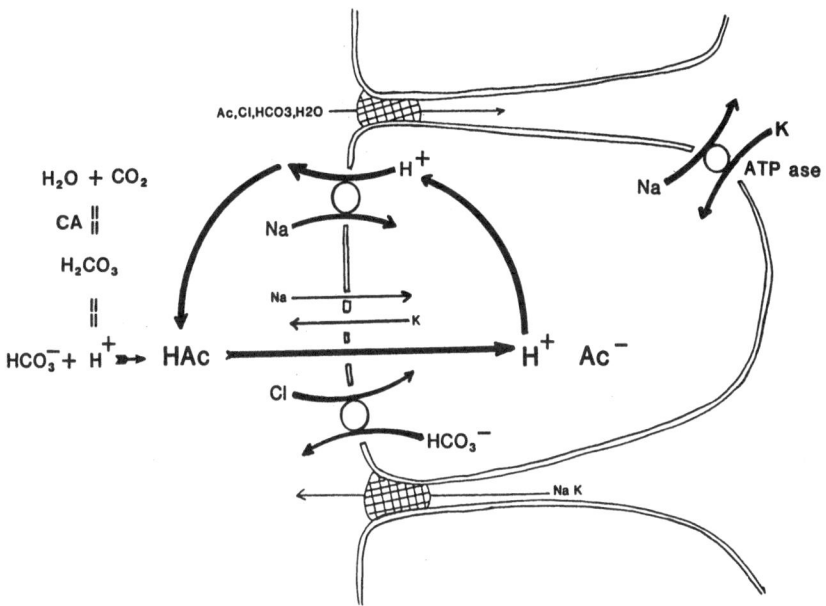

FIGURE 3. Overview of colonic epithelial transport of electrolytes and short-chain fatty acids. CA, carbonic anhydrase. [Modified from Cummings (1984).]

Na_2SO_4 or CH_3COONa were perfused. When Na_2SO_4 was perfused sodium absorption occurred, pCO_2 rose, bicarbonate fell, the pH changed from 7.4 to 6.95. This is consistent with the addition of hydrogen to the lumen in exchange for sodium and a shift in the equation to the left. By contrast, CH_3COONa perfusion caused a marked increase in sodium absorption, a rise in pH from 7.05 to 7.6, and a rise in HCO_3^-. The pCO_2 fell to below plasma levels, indicating that the equation was shifted to the right, and providing hydrogen ion for the absorption of protonated acid and on intracellular source of H^+ to drive the Na^+/H^+ exchange.

This mechanism depends on the presence of a sodium–hydrogen ion exchange, which has been demonstrated in animals (Binder and Rawlins, 1973) and the human ileum (Turnberg *et al.*, 1970), but not the human colon (Hawker *et al.*, 1978). Furthermore, perfusion of Na_2SO_4 solutions through the colon in man does not lead to luminal acidifiction (Bown *et al.*, 1972). Ruppin *et al.* (1980) suggested that stimulation of sodium transport relates to ionic diffusion of short-chain fatty acids, which occurs simultaneously with absorption of the undissociated acid. A monocarboxylate anion carrier has been demonstrated in the rat small intestine by Lamers (1975).

Whatever the mechanism, the principal effect of short-chain fatty acid absorption is to stimulate sodium absorption and thus provide a powerful mechanism for the movement of water out of the colonic lumen. In this context SCFAs must be seen as antidiarrheal agents and failure in their production could lead to alterations in salt and water metabolism. SCFA production and absorption will also affect luminal pH, which in turn may alter microbial metabolism.

7. THE FATE OF SCFAs

Once absorbed, SCFAs are metabolized in colonic epithelial cells, liver, or peripheral tissues. As such, they contribute to normal energy metabolism. They represent 60–70% of the potential energy available had the carbohydrate been absorbed intact in the small intestine.

Mucosal metabolism of SCFA, especially butyrate, may be of critical importance in maintaining the integrity of the colonic epithelium. In the ruminant, butyrate is almost entirely metabolized in the epithelium, while about 50% of propionate and some acetate are also utilized (Bergman and Wolff, 1971; Bergman, 1975). In guinea pig isolated colonocyte it has been shown, using ^{14}C-labeled substrate, that all three acids are metabolized, with butyrate > propionate > acetate (Wirthensohn, 1981). Using the rat isolated coloncyte, Roediger (1982) has shown that SCFAs are substantially metabolized and suppress glucose oxidation through inhibition of pyruvate dehydrogenase. Studies of CO_2 production using mixtures of SCFAs indicate that activation of fatty acids is in the order of butyrate > acetate > propionate, as observed in the rumen.

The main products of short-chain fatty acid metabolism in the colonic epithelium are ketone bodies (acetoacetate, β-hydroxybutyrate), CO_2, and water. In the intact rat Remesy and Demigne (1976) observed that about 12% of butyrate is transformed to ketone bodies in the cecal wall, as evidenced by studies of arteriovenous differences. The cecal artery and cecal vein concentrations are 0.070 ± 0.005 and 0.107 ± 0.005 mmol/liter, respectively, for acetoacetic acid and 0.083 ± 0.006 and 0.133 ± 0.007 mmol/liter, respectively, for β-hydroxybutyrate. Significantly, no evidence of ketogenesis was found in the colon of these rats, a finding similar to that of Henning and Hird for the rabbit and in contrast to the considerable ketogenesis found *in vitro* (Henning and Hird, 1970, 1972).

In isolated human colonocytes (Roediger, 1980) butyrate is actively metabolized to both CO_2 and ketone bodies. When metabolism by cells from proximal and distal colon is compared, acetoacetate production is significantly diminished in the distal colon. Butyrate metabolism accounts for about 80% of oxygen consumption by colonocytes in both regions, but glucose utilization is suppressed to a larger degree in the proximal than distal colon by butyrate. This, together with diminished ketone body production by the distal colon, suggests a greater dependence on butyrate as a fuel in the distal bowel. Butyrate has been shown to have antitumor properties in colonic epithelial and other cell lines *in vitro* (Kim *et al.*, 1982; Kruh, 1982).

Once across the colonic mucosa, SCFAs enter the portal vein and are transported to the liver. All three SCFAs are present in human portal blood (Dankert *et al.*, 1981) but only acetate reaches peripheral tissues (Pomare *et al.*, 1984). The metabolic fate and importance of these acids remain largely unknown in man, although propionate may modify carbohydrate and lipid metabolism in the liver (Anderson and Bridges, 1982; Chen *et al.*, 1984). Potentially, fermentation in the human colon could affect a wide range of metabolic events within the large intestine, in the liver, and in peripheral tissues. However, much remains to be learned about the production and fate of these acids.

REFERENCES

Anderson, I. H., Levine, A. S., and Levitt, M. D., 1981, Incomplete absorption of the carbohydrate in all-purpose wheat flour, *N. Engl. J. Med.* **304**:891.

Anderson, J. W., and Bridges, S. R., 1982, Short chain fatty acid metabolites of plant fiber alter glucose metabolism of isolated rat hepatocytes, *Am. J. Clin. Nutr.* **35**:840.

Argenzio, R. A., Lowe, J. E., Pickard, D. W., and Stevens, C. E., 1974, Digesta passage and water exchange in the equine large intestine, *Am. J. Physiol.* **226**:1035.

Argenzio, R. A., Miller, N., and von Engelhardt, W., 1975, Effect of volatile fatty acids on water and ion absorption from the goat colon, *Am. J. Physiol.* **229**:997.

Argenzio, R. A., and Southworth, M., 1974, Sites of organic acid production and absorption in gastrointestinal tract of the pig, *Am. J. Physiol.* **228**:454.

Argenzio, R. A., and Whipp, S. C., 1979, Inter-relationship of sodium, chloride, bicarbonate and acetate transport by the colon of the pig, *J. Physiol.* **295**:365.

Bergman, E. N., 1975, Production and utilization of metabolites by the alimentary tract as measured in portal and hepatic blood, in: *Digestion and Metabolism in the Ruminant* (I. W. McDonald, and A. C. I. Warner, eds.), University of New England Publishing Unit, Biddeford, Maine, p. 292.

Bergman, E. N., and Wolff, J. E., 1971, Metabolism of volatile fatty acids by liver and portal-drained viscera in sheep, *Am. J. Physiol.* **221**:586.

Binder, H. J., and Rawlins, C. C., 1973, Electrolyte transport across isolated large intestinal mucosa, *Am. J. Physiol.* **225**:1232.

Bingham, S., and Cummings, J. H., 1980, Sources and intakes of dietary fiber in man, in: *Medical Aspects of Dietary Fiber* (G. A. Spiller and R. M. Kay, eds.), Plenum, New York, p. 261.

Bingham, S., Cummings, J. H., and McNeil, I., 1979, Intakes and sources of dietary fiber in the British population, *Am. J. Clin. Nutr.* **32**:1313.

Bjork, J. T., Soergel, K. H., and Wood, C. M., 1976, The composition of "free" stool water, *Gastroenterology* **70**:A-6/864.

Bjorneklett, A., and Jenssen, E., 1982, Relationships between hydrogen (H_2) and methane (CH_4) production in man, *Scand. J. Gastroenterol.* **17**:985.

Bond, J. H., Currier, B. E., Buchwald, H., and Levitt, M. D., 1980, Colonic conservation of malabsorbed carbohydrate, *Gastroenterology* **78**:444.

Bown, R. L., Sladen, G. E., Rousseau, B., Gibson, J. A., Clark, M. L., and Dawson, A. M., 1972, A study of water and electrolyte transport by the excluded human colon, *Clin. Sci.* **43**:891.

Carter, M. J., and Parsons, D. S., 1968, Carbonic anhydrase activity of mucosa of small intestine and colon, *Nature* **219**:176.

Chen, W.-J. L., Anderson, J. W., and Jennings, D., 1984, Propionate may mediate the hypo-cholesterolemic effects of certain soluble plant fibers in cholesterol-fed rats (41791), *Proc. Soc. Exp. Biol. Med.* **175**:215.

Clemens, E. T., Maloiy, G. M. O., and Sutton, J. D., 1983, Molar proportions of volatile fatty acids in the gastrointestinal tract of East African wild ruminants, *Comp. Biochem. Physiol.* **76A**:217.

Crump, M. H., Argenzio, R. A., and Whipp, S. C., 1980, Effects of acetate on absorption of solute and water from the pig colon, *Am. J. Vet. Res.* **41**:1565.

Cummings, J. H., 1981a, Dietary fibre, *Br. Med. Bull.* **37**:65.

Cummings, J. H., 1981b, Short chain fatty acids in the human colon, *Gut* **22**:763.

Cummings, J. H., 1983, Dietary fibre and the intestinal microflora, in: *Nutrition and the Intestinal Flora* (B. Hallgren ed.), Swedish Nutrition Foundation, Stockholm, p. 77.

Cummings, J. H., 1984, Colonic absorption: The importance of short chain fatty acids in man, *Scand. J. Gastroenterol.* **19**:93.

Cummings, J. H., Hill, M. J., Bone, E. S., Branch, W. J., and Jenkins, D. J. A., 1979, The effect of meat protein and dietary fiber on colonic function and metabolism. II. Bacterial metabolites in feces and urine, *Am. J. Clin. Nutr.* **32**:2094.

Cummings, J. H., Hill, M. J., Jenkins, D. J. A., Pearson, J. R., and Wiggins, H. S., 1976, Changes in fecal composition and colonic function due to cereal fiber, *Am. J. Clin. Nutr.* **29**:1468.

Cummings, J. H., James, W. P. T., and Wiggins, H. S., 1973, Role of the colon in ileal-resection diarrhoea, *Lancet* **i**:344.

Cummings, J. H., Southgate, D. A. T., Branch, W., Houston, H., Jenkins, D. J. A., and James, W. P. T., 1978, Colonic response to dietary fibre from carrot, cabbage, apple, bran, and guar gum, *Lancet* **i**:5.

Dankert, J., Zijlstra, J. B., and Wolthers, B. G., 1981, Volatile fatty acids in human peripheral and portal blood: Quantitative determination by vacuum distillation and gas chromatography, *Clin. Chim. Acta* **110**:301.

Dawson, A. M., Holdsworth, C. D., and Webb, J., 1964, Absorption of short chain fatty acids in man, *Proc. Soc. Exp. Biol. Med.* **117**:97.

Englyst, H. N., Bingham, S. A., Wiggins, H. S., Southgate, D. A. T., Seppanen, R., Helms, P., Anderson, V., Day, K. C., Choolun, R., Collinson, E., and Cummings, J. H., 1982, Non-starch polysaccharide consumption in four Scandinavian populations, *Nutr. Cancer* **4**:50.

Fleming, S. E., and Rodriquez, M. A., 1983, Influence of dietary fiber on fecal excretion of volatile fatty acids by human adults, *J. Nutr.* **113**:1613.

Gibson, J. A., 1977, Studies of Urea and Ammonia Metabolism, M. D. Thesis, University of Cambridge, Cambridge, England.

Grove, E. W., Olmsted, W. H., and Koenig, K., 1929/1930, The effect of diet and catharsis on the lower volatile fatty acids in the stools of normal men, *J. Biol. Chem.* **85**:127.

Hawker, P. C., Mashiter, K. E., and Turnberg, L. A., 1978, Mechanisms of transport of Na, Cl and K in the human colon, *Gastroenterology* **74**:1241.

Henning, S. J., and Hird, F. J. R., 1970, Concentration and metabolism of volatile fatty acids in the fermentative organs of 2 species of kangaroo and the guinea-pig, *Br. J. Nutr.* **24**:145.

Henning, S. J., and Hird, F. J. R., 1972, Ketogenesis from butyrate and acetate by the cecum and the colon of rabbits, *Biochem. J.* **130**:785.

Hespell, R. B., 1979, Efficiency of growth by ruminal bacteria, *Fed. Proc. Fed. Am. Soc. Exp. Biol.* **38**:2707.

Hespell, R. B., and Bryant, M. P., 1979, Efficiency of rumen microbial growth: Influence of some theoretical experimental factors of ATP, *J. Anim. Sci.* **49**:1640.

Hespell, R. B., and Smith, C. J., 1983, Utilization of nitrogen sources by gastrointestinal tract bacteria, in: *Human Intestinal Microflora in Health and Disease* (D. J. Hentges, ed.), Academic, New York, p. 167.

Holloway, W. D., Tasman-Jones, C., and Lee, S. P., 1978, Digestion of certain fractions of dietary fiber in humans, *Am. J. Clin. Nutr.* **31**:927.

Hoskins, L. C., and Boulding, E. T., 1981, Mucin degradation in human colon ecosystems: Evidence for the existence and role of bacterial subpopulations producing glycosidases as extracellular enzymes, *Am. J. Clin. Invest.* **67**:163.

Hungate, R. E., 1966, *The Rumen and Its Microbes,* Academic, New York. Isaacson, H. R., Hinds, F. C., Bryant, M. P., and Ownes, F. N., 1975, Efficiency of energy utilization by mixed rumen bacteria in continuous culture, *J. Dairy Sci.* **58**:1645.

Kim, Y. S., Tsao, D., Morita, A., and Bella, A., 1982, Effect of sodium butyrate and three human colorectal adenocarcinoma cell lines in culture, in: *Colonic Carcinogenesis* (R. A. Malt and R. C. N. Williamson, eds.), Falk Symposium 31, MTP, Lancaster, England, p. 317.

Kotarski, S. F., and Salyers, A. A., 1981, Effect of long generation times on growth of *Bacteroides thetaiotaomicron* in carbohydrate-limited continuous culture, *J. Bacteriol.* 853.

Kruh, J., 1982, Effects of sodium butyrate, a new pharmacological agent, on cells in culture, *Mol. Cell Biochem.* **42**:65.

Lamers, J. M. J., 1975, Some characteristics of monocarboxylic acid transfer across the cell membrane of epithelial cells from rat small intestine, *Biochem. Biophys. Acta* **413**:265.

McNeil, N. I., 1980, Short Chain Fatty Acid Absorption from the Human Gut, M. D. Thesis, University of Cambridge, Cambridge, England.

McNeil, N. I., Bingham, S., Cole, T. J., Grant, A. M., and Cummings, J. H., 1982, Diet and health of people with an ileostomy. 2. Ileostomy function and nutritional state, *Br. J. Nutr.* **47**:407.

McNeil, N. I., Cummings, J. H., and James, W. P. T., 1978, Short chain fatty acid absorption by the human large intestine, *Gut* **19**:819.

McNeil, N. I., Cummings, J. H., and James, W. P. T., 1979, Rectal absorption of short chain fatty acids in the absence of chloride, *Gut* **20**:400.

Miller, T. L., and Wolin, M. J., 1979, Fermentations by saccharolytic intestinal bacteria, *Am. J. Clin. Nutr.* **32**:164.

Minowa, M., Bingham, S., and Cummings J. H., 1983, Dietary fibre intake in Japan, *Hum. Nutr. Appl. Nutr.* **37A**:113.

Odelson, D. A., and Breznak, J. A., 1983, Volatile fatty acid production by the hindgut microbiota of xylophagous termites, *Appl. Environ. Microbiol.* **45**:1602.

Olmsted, W. H., Curtis, G., and Timm, O. K., 1935, Stool volatile fatty acids. IV. The influence of feeding bran pentosan and fiber to man, *J. Biol. Chem.* **108**:645.

Owens, F. N., and Isaacson, H. R., 1977, Ruminal microbial yields: Factors influencing synthesis and bypass, Fed. Proc. Fed. Am. Soc. Exp. Biol. **36**:198.

Parsons, D. S., and Paterson, C. R., 1965, Fluid and solute transport across rat colonic mucosa, *Q. J. Exp. Physiol.* **50**:220.

Pitt, P., de Bruijn, K. M., Beeching, M. F., Goldberg, E., and Blendis, L. M., 1980, Studies on breath methane: The effect of ethnic origins and lactulose, *Gut* **21**:951.

Pomare, E. W., Branch, W. J., and Cummings, J. H., 1985, Carbohydrate fermentation in the human colon and its relation to acetate concentrations in venous blood, *J. Clin. Invest.,* **75**:448.

Rechkemmer, G., and von Engelhardt, W., 1982, Absorptive processes in different colonic segments of the guinea-pig and the effects of short-chain fatty acids, in: *Colon and Nutrition* (H. Kasper and H. Goebell, eds.), Falk Symposium 32, MTP. Lancaster, England, p. 61.

Remesy, C., and Demigne, C., 1976, Partition and absorption of volatile fatty acids in the alimentary canal of the rat, *Ann. Rech. Vet.* **7**:39.

Roediger, W. E. W., 1980, Role of anaerobic bacteria in the metabolic welfare of the colonic mucosa in man, *Gut* **21**:793.

Roediger, W. E. W., 1982, Utilization of nutrients by isolated epithelial cells of the rat colon, *Gastroenterology* **83**:424.

Roediger, W. E. W., and Moore, A., 1981, Effect of short-chain fatty acid on sodium absorption in isolated human colon perfused through the vascular bed, *Dig. Dis. Sci.* **26**:100.

Rubinstein, R., Howard, A. V., and Wrong, O. M., 1969, *In vivo* dialysis of faeces as a method of stool analysis. IV. The organic anion component, *Clin. Sci.* **37**:549.

Rubsamen, K., and von Engelhardt, W., 1981, Absorption of Na, H ions and short chain fatty acids from the sheep colon, *Pfluegers Arch.* **391**:141.

Rubsamen, K., Hume, I. D., Foley, W. J., and Rubsamen, U., 1983, Regional differences in electrolyte, short-chain fatty acid and water absorption in the hindgut of two species of arboreal marsupials, *Pfluegers Arch.* **399**:68.

Ruppin, H., Bar-Meir, S., Soergel, K. H., Wood, C. M., and Schmitt, M. G., 1980, Absorption of short chain fatty acids by the colon, *Gastroenterology* **78**:1500.

Sallee, V. L., and Dietschy, J. M., 1973, Determinants of intestinal mucosal uptake of short- and medium-fatty acids and alcohols, *J. Lipid. Res.* **14**:475.

Salyers, A. A., Vercellotti, J. R., West, S. E. H., and Wilkins, T. D., 1977, Fermentation of mucin and plant polysaccharides by strains of *Bacteroides* from the human colon, *Appl. Environ. Microbiol.* **33**:319.

Salyers, A. A., Arthur, R., and Kuritza, A., 1981, Digestion of larch arabinogalactan by a strain of human colonic *Bacteroides* growing in continuous culture, *J. Agric. Food Chem.* **29**:475.

Sambrook, I. E., 1979, Studies on digestion and absorption in the intestines of growing pigs. 8. Measurements of the flow of total lipid, acid-detergent fibre and vilatile fatty acids, *Br. J. Nutr.* **42**:279.

Sandberg, A.-S., Andersson, H., Hallgren, B., Hasselblad, K., Isaksson, B., and Hulten L., 1981, Experimental model for *in vivo* determination of dietary fibre and its effect on the absorption of nutrients in the small intestine, *Br. J. Nutr.* **45**:283.

Sandberg A.-S., Ahderinne, R., Andersson, H., Hallgren, B., and Hulten, L., 1983, The effect of citrus pectin on the absorption of nutrients in the small intestine, *Hum. Nutr. Clin. Nutr.* **37C**:171.

Saunders, D. R., and Wiggins, H. S., 1981, Conservation of mannitol, lactulose and raffinose by the human colon, *Am. J. Physiol.* **24**:G397.

Smith, C. J., and Bryant, M. P., 1979, Introduction to metabolic activities of intestinal bacteria, *Am. J. Clin. Nutr.* **32**:149.

Spiller, G. A., Chernoff, M. C., Hill, R. A., Gates, J. E., Nassar, J. J., and Shipley, E. A., 1980, Effect of purified cellulose, pectin, and a low-residue diet on fecal volatile fatty acids, transit time, and fecal weight in humans, *Am. J. Clin. Nutr.* **33**:754.

Stephen, A. M., 1980, Dietary Fibre and Human Colonic Function, Ph. D. Thesis, University of Cambridge, Cambridge, England.

Stephen, A. M., and Cummings, J. H., 1979, The influence of dietary fiber on fecal nitrogen excretion in man, *Proc. Nutr. Soc.* **38**:141A.

Stephen, A. M., Haddad, A. C., and Phillips, S. F., 1983, Passage of carbohydrate into the colon. Direct measurements in humans, *Gastroenterology* **85**:589.

Stevens, C. E., 1970, Fatty acid transport through the rumen epithelium, in: *Physiology of Digestion and Metabolism in the Ruminant* (A. T. Phillipson, ed.), Oriel, Newcastle on Tyne, p.101.

Stevens, C. E., and Stettler, B. K., 1966a, Factors affecting the transport of volatile fatty acids across rumen epithelium, *Am. J. Physiol.* **210**:365.

Stevens, C. E., and Stettler, B. K., 1966b, Transport of fatty acid mixtures across rumen epithelium, *Am. J. Physiol.* **211**:264.

Thomsen, L. L., Tasman-Jones, C., Lee, S. P., and Robertson, A. M., 1982, Dietary factors in the control of pH and volatile fatty acid production in the rat caecum, in: *Colon and Cancer* (H. Kasper and H. Goebell, eds.), Falk Symposium 32, MTP, Lancaster, England, p. 47.

Turnberg, L. A., Bieberdorf, F. A., Morawski, S. G., and Fordtran, J. S., 1970, Interrelationships of chloride, bicarbonate, sodium, and hydrogen transport in the human ileum, *J. Clin. Invest.* **49**:557.

Umesaki, Y., Yajima, T., Yokokura, T., and Mutai, M., 1979, Effect of organic acid absorption on bicarbonate transport in rat colon, *Pfluegers Arch.* **379**:43.

Umesaki, Y., Yajima, T., Tohyama, K., and Mutai, M., 1980, Characterization of acetate uptake by the colonic epithelial cells of the rat, *Pfluegers Arch.* **388**:205.

Von Engelhardt, W., and Rechkemmer, G., 1983, The physiological effects of short chain fatty acids in the hind gut, in: *Fibre in Human and Animal Nutrition* (G. Wallace and L. Bell, eds.), Royal Society of New Zealand, p. 149.

Williams, R. D., and Olmsted, W. H., 1936, The effect of cellulose, hemicellulose and lignin on the weight of the stool: A contribution to the study of laxation in man, *J. Nutr.* **11**:433.

Wirthensohn, K., 1981, Der Stoffwechsel Kurzkettiger Fettsauren im Colonepithel des Meerschweinchens und seine Bedeutung fur die Natriumresorption, Thesis, University of Hohenheim.

Wolin, M. J., and Miller, T. L., 1983a, Carbohydrate fermentation, in: *Human Intestinal Microflora and Health and Disease* (D. J. Hentges, ed.), Academic, New York. p. 147.

Wolin, M. J., and Miller, T. L., 1983b, Interactions of microbial populations in cellulose fermentation, *Fed. Proc.* **42**:109.

Wrong, O., Metcalfe-Gibson, A., Morrison, B. I., Ng, S. T., and Howard, V., 1965, *In vivo* dialysis of faeces as a method of stool analysis. 1. Technique and results in normal subjects, *Clin. Sci.* **28**:357.

Wrong, O. M., Vince, A. J., and Waterlow, J. C., 1982, The origins and bacterial metabolism of faecal ammonia, in: *Colon and Cancer* (H. Kasper and H. Goebell, eds.), Falk Symposium 32, MTP, Lancaster, England, p. 133.

Zijlstra, J. B., Beukema, J., Wilthers, B. F., Byrne, B. M., Groen, A., and Donkert, L., 1977, Pretreatment methods prior to gas chromatographic analysis of volatile fatty acids from faecal samples, *Clin. Chim. Acta* **78**:243.

11

Methane Production and Excretion: A Marker of Cecal Fermentation

MARTIN A. EASTWOOD, LINDA F. MCKAY, W. GORDON BRYDON

1. INTRODUCTION

Dietary fiber is a complex heterogeneous material increasingly used in the management of colorectal and other disease. Dietary fiber can be defined as that component of plant cells resistant to human alimentary enzyme action (Trowell, 1974). Some studies of fiber have shown a degree of hydrolysis by colonic bacteria. However, which components of fiber are hydrolyzed and the extent of their breakdown in the human colon are not clear. Not enough is known of the metabolism of fiber in the colon. The effect of dietary fiber on gastrointestinal function in man depends on the type of fiber (Royal College of Physicians, 1981). It is now appreciated that cereals, bran, and vegetable fiber behave differently along the gastrointestinal tract (Stephens and Cummings, 1980). Indirect evidence suggests that the cecum is a major site for metabolism of certain fibers. Anaerobic bacteria in the colon produce methane, hydrogen, volatile fatty acids, and carbon dioxide. It has been suggested that the fiber affects stool weight either directly (Smith *et al.*, 1981), by bacterial mass (Stephens and Cummings, 1980), or by volatile fatty

MARTIN A. EASTWOOD, LINDA F. MCKAY, and W. GORDON BRYDON • Wolfson Gastrointestinal Laboratories, Department of Medicine, Western General Hospital, Edinburgh EH4 2XU, United Kingdom.

acids (VFA) derived therefrom (Hellendoorn, 1978). Retention of water by
the fiber matrix as with cereal bran influences stool weight (Smith *et al.*,
1981).

The effect of wheat bran on stool weight is predictable. The higher the
water-holding capacity, the more effective is the wheat bran. Similarly,
increasing the dietary intake of wheat bran results in an orderly increase in
stool weight. Figure 1 shows the increase in stool weight when eight normal
young males increased at monthly intervals their intake of wheat bran (6, 12,
24 g, as Primus Bar) in a regular manner. Fiber from fruit and vegetables is
hydrolyzed in the cecum, leading to increased bacterial metabolic activity
and growth. Such metabolic activity is difficult to measure directly. However, the evolution of hydrogen and methane can be monitored. Carbon
dioxide and volatile fatty acids are for various reasons difficult to measure
and such measurements may be unrepresentative of cecal metabolic activity.

2. HYDROGEN

Hydrogen is excreted in the breath and flatus, the latter being the
principal route. Breath hydrogen excretion varies throughout the day and is
influenced by food ingestion. It has been shown that unabsorbed sugars are
important stimulants of hydrogen production (Tadesse *et al.*, 1980). The
time interval between ingesting an oligosaccharide and the evolution of
breath hydrogen from the cecum depends upon the type of sugar. The
interval for disaccharides is 90 min, for trisaccharides 120 min, and for tetra-
saccharides $\geq$ 180 min. However, if these oligosaccharides are placed directly
in the cecum, their hydrogen evolution begins immediately (Tadesse *et al.*,

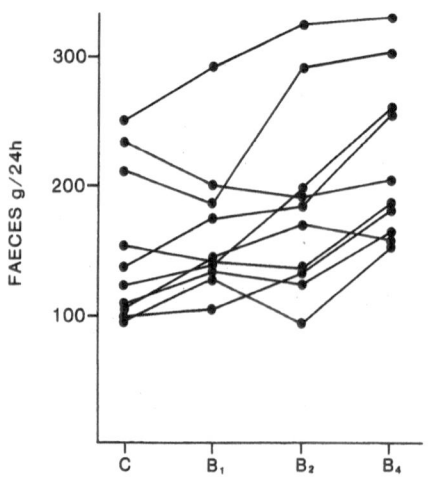

FIGURE 1. Fecal wet weight/24 h for each individual during control period, (C); 6 g wheat bran/24 h, B_1; 12 g wheat bran/24 h, B_2 and 24 g wheat bran/24 h, B_4. The time interval in each case was 1 month.

1980). Polysaccharides, e.g., gum arabic or carrot fiber, if ingested as a single dosage do not result in an increase in breath hydrogen. Yet after 3 weeks of daily intake there is an increase in breath-hydrogen response to a single dosage (McLean Ross *et al.*, 1984; Robertson *et al.*, 1979;). This implies the development of bacterial enzymatic systems capable of hydrolyzing the polysaccharide and stimulating hydrogen production.

3. METHANE

An interest in methane has developed from several different areas, including ruminology, the study of possible fuel production from anaerobic digestion processes, and problems related to manned space flights. The accumulation of flatus, with high concentrations of hydrogen and methane, in a confined space can create an explosive hazard. Gas chromatographic measurements of breath hydrogen and methane were applied as part of the investigation into the effect and the role of intestinal gas in manned space flight (Calloway and Murphy, 1968).

The bean industry has sponsored research into the origin and nature of bean-related flatulence. Beans were found to be rich in oligosaccharides, e.g., stachyose and raffinose, which are fermented by the colonic flora (Steggerda, 1968). The gas-forming potential of a variety of fruits, legumes, and cereals has been investigated (Calloway, 1966; Hickey *et al.*, 1972). Hydrogen production was found to be substrate-related, but the factors influencing methane production have yet to be identified. A recent finding that 80% of patients with colonic carcinoma excrete breath methane compared to 40% of control patients (Haines *et al.*, 1977) has stimulated further research into potential applications of breath methane measurements.

Methanogenic bacteria are a morphologically diverse group of organisms, which share the common metabolic capacity to produce methane. *Methanobacterium ruminantium*, the most common species in ruminants, has been isolated from human feces (Nottingham and Hungate, 1968). Formate and carbon dioxide are the substrate for methanogens in ruminants.

Hydrogen and carbon dioxide are present in human colonic gas. Methane is not an invariable component of the colonic gas of man (Levitt and Ingelfinger, 1968). The methane content of flatus can vary from 0 to 54% (Calloway, 1968). Gases produced in the bowel as a result of bacterial activity can also be excreted in expired air. The diffusion rate varies directly with surface area and inversely with membrane thickness. The removal of gas from the intestine is affected by the rate of blood flow in the gut and also the lungs. Decreased absorption from the intestinal lumen may be due to a reduced gut perfusion rate, mucosal thickness, or impaired contact with gut membranes. Colonic distension decreases the rate of gas removal. When intestinal motility is stimulated, the gas in the lumen will be expelled in flatus. Even if some methane is passed as flatus, there is ample evidence to show that the amount of gas excreted in the breath is proportional to the intestinal production, (Calloway, 1968; Levitt 1969; Levitt and Bond 1970). Reports of the proportion of subjects excreting methane in healthy populations range from 30% (Calloway 1968; Levitt and Bond 1970; Bond et al., 1971) to 58% (Pitt et al., 1980). The reason only some subjects excrete breath methane is uncertain and many factors that influence methane production and excretion have still to be elucidated. Hydrogen and methane production are related in ruminants and in bacterial cultures (Hungate, 1968; Wolfe, 1971; Hungate, 1976; Prins, 1979). It seems that the factors that influence methane formation in man are more complex and different from those in ruminants or in vitro. A number of factors may be acting together to bring about methane formation and a single factor such as diet or bacteria may not be the sole determinant. The following investigations attempt to answer the questions, (1) why do all subjects not excrete methane in the breath, and (2) what factors influence the production and excretion of methane? To this end, human investigations on factors affecting methane production are presented, including work on breath and flatus analysis, diet, fecal components, and bowel function in healthy subjects and clinical patients. Supportive evidence has been obtained from in vitro work with pure methanogens and other intestinal bacteria and also investigations with animals.

3.1 Factors Influencing Methane Excretion in Normal Populations

A group of subjects consisting of 142 hospital staff, students, and local volunteers (74 men, 68 women) aged 16–79 (mean 35 years) was investigated. Local volunteers were selected by their family doctor and all subjects were considered to be free of gastrointestinal disease.

3.2 Breath Analysis

All subjects provided two nonfasting end expiratory breath samples of 40 ml each using a modified Haldane Priestly sampling tube (Metz et al., 1976). The room air was also sampled. No subjects smoked prior to breath sampling (Tadesse and Eastwood, 1977). Methane concentrations were determined by gas chromatography (Tadesse et al., 1979). Breath methane concentrations were taken as the difference between the mean of two breath samples and the room air concentrations. Methane producers were defined as those subjects producing at least 0.09 μmol/liter of methane above room air concentrations. This criterion was based on the sensitivity and reproducibility of the methods used and the results of previous investigations (McKay *et al.*, 1981; Tadesse *et al.*, 1980). There was no significant difference between the prevalence of methane excretion in males and females—58 and 50%, respectively. The breath methane concentration was not influenced by age ($r = 0.09$).

3.3 Intestinal Transit Measurements and Fecal Analysis

Seventy-one subjects from this group (41 men, 30 women) collected stools for intestinal transit and other measurements. Stools were collected individually and stored at $-20°$ C. Intestinal transit time was measured using barium-impregnated markers, as described by Hinton *et al.* (1969). Markers in the frozen stool were identified under a fluoroscope. Transit time was assessed as time taken for the passage of 80% of the swallowed markers. Five-day fecal collections were thawed, pooled, and homogenized, and a weighed aliquot was freeze-dried. Freeze-dried feces were analyzed for bile acids (Evrard and Janssen, 1968), fat (Varley, 1967), and electrolytes (flame photometry and atomic absorption spectrophotometry after charring with nitric acid). Table I shows details of fecal constituents and transit time for breath methane excretors and nonexcretors in these 71 subjects. There were no significant differences between methane excretors and nonexcretors and no associations between the concentration of excreted methane and any fecal constituent.

3.4 Dietary Analysis

Fifty-six of the local volunteers were visited at home by a dietitian and a detailed diet history was taken. The subjects were shown how to complete a diet diary, which was kept for 7 days. Daily visits were made during this period. The daily intakes of energy, protein, fat, carbohydrate, cholesterol,

TABLE I. Fecal Constituents and Transit Time for Methane Excretors ($n = 42$) and Nonexcretors ($n = 29$)

	Methane excretors		Nonexcretors	
	Mean	SD	Mean	SD
Wet weight, g/day	101	39	128	44
Dry weight, g/day	27	8	33	10
Fat, mmol/day	11.4	5.2	13.3	7.1
Total bile acids, mmol/day	0.70	0.29	0.81	0.30
Total electrolytes, mmol/day[a]	35.5	16.4	39.3	18.2
Total neutral sterols, mmol/day	1.82	0.94	1.79	0.61
Transit time, h	72	30	62	28

[a]Na^+, K^+, Ca^{2+}, Mg^{2+}

total fiber, cellulose, noncellulosic polysaccharides (hexose, pentose, and uronic acid residues), and lignin were calculated (Paul and Southgate, 1978; Southgate *et al.*, 1976). The results of the dietary analysis are shown in Table II.

Breath methane concentrations in breath methane excretors were significantly correlated with intakes of the pentose fraction of noncellulosic polysaccharide ($r = 0.44$, $p < 0.01$) and lignin ($r = 0.40$, $p < 0.05$). The intakes of lignin and pentose were strongly correlated ($r = 0.82$, $p < 0.001$). Methane excretion was not associated with the intake of any other food category.

Subsequently test meals were given to 12 healthy subjects, all of whom were methane excretors. The test meals given contained 5 g of pentose (approximately twice the average daily intake), and consisted of (1) 350 g orange, (2) 22.1 g coarse bran, and (3) 200 g boiled sprouts or parsnips, 200 g boiled carrots, and 110 g stewed apple. Test meals containing 25 g L-xylose, 25 g D-xylose, 20 g D-arabinose, 20 g L-arabinose, and 10 g xylan were also given to methane-producing subjects in 250 ml of water. All subjects provided a baseline breath sample after fasting for 12 h. After the ingestion of the test meals, breath samples were collected every $1/2$ h for a period of 5 h. The test meals consisting of fruit, bran, cooked vegetables, fruit, and xylan had no significant effect on breath methane production during 5 h. After the administration of D-xylose and L-arabinose, there was a significant increase in methane excretion at 90–120 min compared to baseline ($p < 0.01$ and $p < 0.025$, respectively, Wilcoxon signed rank test) and at 210–240 min compared to the measurement 1 h previously ($p < 0.01$, $p < 0.025$) (Fig. 2). Both L-

TABLE II. Daily Dietary Intake in 34 Methane-Producing Subjects and Correlation with Breath Methane Concentration

Food Category	Mean	SD	r
Protein, g	70	19	−0.13
Carbohydrate, g	228	85	−0.24
Fat, g	99	33	−0.13
Energy, MJ	8.9	2.9	−0.20
Unsaturated fat, g	5.2	1.7	−0.28
Saturated fat, g	94	32	−0.12
Cholesterol, g	0.4	0.2	−0.12
Total dietary fiber, g	13.1	5.5	−0.22
Cellulose, g	3.2	1.4	−0.18
Noncellulosic polysaccharide, g	9.3	3.9	−0.20
Hexose, g	5.3	2.4	−0.09
Pentose, g	2.3	1.6	0.44 $p < 0.01$
Uronic acid, g	1.9	0.7	0.11
Lignin, g	0.8	0.6	0.40 $p < 0.05$

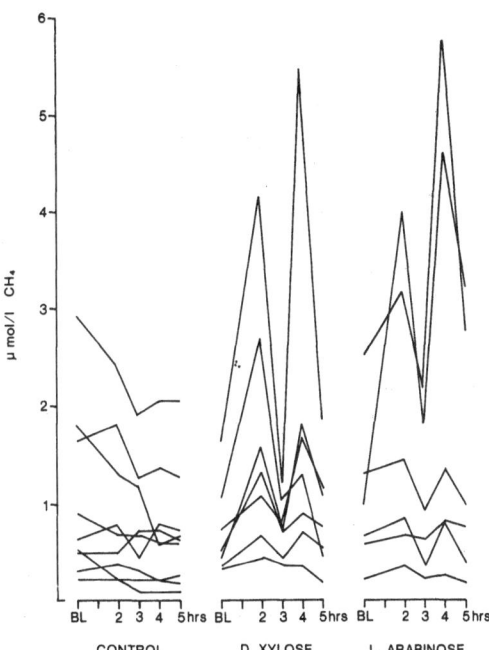

FIGURE 2. Breath methane concentration (μmol/liter) at 0, 2, 3, 4, and 5 h after an overnight fast and following the ingestion of D-xylose and L-arabinose.

xylose and D-arabinose caused diarrhea in the methane-producing subjects tested. There were no significant changes in methane production before this.

3.5 Factors Influencing Breath Methane Excretion in Clinical Populations

The clinical population consisted of 245 patients attending the Gastrointestinal Unit, Western General Hospital, 104 men and 141 women, aged 16–73 (mean 49 years). The clinical diagnoses in this group were as follows: unresected colonic carcinoma (20), Crohn's disease (40), ulcerative colitis (40), irritable bowel syndrome (42), and pneumatosis cystoides intestinalis (9). A group with diarrhea (94) of various etiologies is outlined in Table III. A second clinical group consisted of 64 patients, 35 men and 29 women, aged 17–86 (mean 48 years), from general hospital wards who were considered free of gastrointestinal disease as assessed by routine clinical history and examination. Patients taking antibiotics or laxatives or who had received enemas or intestinal washouts within the previous month or who were on elemental diets as part of their preoperative bowel preparation were excluded from this study. Breath analysis was performed on these patients and results are shown in Table IV. The overall proportion of methane producers is 32% in these patients and 53% in the known gastrointestinal patients. Within the gastrointestinal patient group there were differences in the prevalence of

TABLE III. Details of Nonspecific Diarrheal Patients

Diagnosis	Number of patients	Diagnosis	Number of patients
Post-vagotomy/gastro-enterostomy	24	Giardia	1
		Laxative abuse	2
Diarrhea of unknown etiology	15	Rectal ulcer	1
		Jejunal diverticulosis	2
Postcholecystectomy diarrhea	6	Milk sensitivity	1
Lactase deficiency	9	Duodenal pseudo-obstruction	1
Diverticular disease	5	Shigella infection	1
Celiac disease	5	Total gastrectomy/gastric lymphoma	1
Polygastrectomy	5		
Postradiation ileitis	3	Ileocolic tuberculosis/ileal resection	1
Small intestinal colonization	5	Autonomic neuropathy	1
Pancreatic carcinoma	1	Disordered small intestinal motor activity	1
Diarrhea secondary to ileal resection	1	Ileal resection	1

methane production. Patients with Crohn's disease, ulcerative colitis, and pneumatosis cystoides intestinalis had a significantly decreased prevalence of methane excretion compared with nongastrointestinal patients ($p < 0.001$, $p < 0.001$, and $p < 0.025$, respectively, χ^2 test).

Patients with colonic carcinoma and diarrhea who were methane excretors produced significantly more methane ($p < 0.005$ and $p < 0.001$, respectively) than the nongastrointestinal patients. The prevalence and concentration of methane from patients with Crohn's disease and ulcerative colitis were independent of disease distribution.

3.6 Rectal Gas Analysis

In 20 subjects from the clinical group [Crohn's disease (five), ulcerative colitis (eight), irritable bowel syndrome (six), colonic carcinoma (one)] rectal gas was also sampled in the rectosigmoid area between 7 and 10 cm at sigmoidoscopy by passing a rubber tube attached to a syringe through the sigmoidoscope. The sigmoidoscope was passed up to 7–10 cm without inflation. The end of the sigmoidoscope was sealed in such a manner that the rubber tube could be inserted without room air contaminating the colonic gas. A concentration of hydrogen in excess of 11 μmol/liter confirmed that colonic gas was being measured. Room air contains up to 0.09 μmol/liter hydrogen. The presence or absence of methane in breath and colonic gas was concordant in 15 patients. Patients excreting detectable concentrations of

methane in the breath ($n = 3$) excreted high concentrations in the colonic gas
(>30 μmol/liter). Methane was not detected in either the breath or the
colonic gas from all of the ulcerative colitis patients and two patients with
Crohn's disease. The mean methane concentration detected in the colonic
gas of three patients with Crohn's disease and two with irritable bowel
syndrome, who did not excrete methane in the breath, was 1.48 μmol/liter
(McKay *et al.*, 1984).

3.7. Colonic Function in the Elderly

Colonic function and methane-producing status were investigated in a
population of elderly subjects. Sixty-six patients, 17 men and 49 women,
aged 67–98 years (mean 79 years), newly admitted to the Geriatric Assessment wards were studied (McKay *et al.*, 1983a,b). Following an overnight
fast, breath samples were taken from each patient and abdominal radiographs were obtained in the following 2 h. Patients were classified into two
groups determined by the presence or absence of feces in the cecum suggested
by stippling or the presence of gas alone. For the purpose of this study
patients with mixtures of gas and feces in the cecum were not included, so
only the extremes were compared. The analysis of breath samples and the
classification of the radiographs were performed independently in a double
blind manner. The overall proportion of methane production in these elderly
subjects was 53%. A higher proportion of subjects with a feces-filled cecum
excreted methane (65%) than those with a gas-filled cecum (30%) ($p < 0.01$).
Methane producers with a gas-filled cecum produced higher concentrations
of methane ($p < 0.005$).

TABLE IV. Incidence and Concentration of Breath Methane
in Control and Patient Groups

Diagnosis	Percent methane excretors	Breath methane, μmol/liter		
		Range	Mean	SD
Colonic carcinoma ($n = 20$)	50	0.18–3.42	0.99	0.90
Crohn's disease ($n = 40$)	13	0.23–1.03	0.43	0.33
Ulcerative colitis ($n = 40$)	15	0.2–1.08	0.47	0.33
Pneumatosis cystoides intestinalis ($n = 9$)	11	1.5[a]	—	—
Irritable bowel syndrome ($n = 42$)	40	0.28–2.25	0.60	0.52
Diarrhea ($n = 94$)	42	0.09–5.40	1.12	1.08
Nongastrointestinal disease (controls) ($n = 64$)	53	0.09–1.84	0.54	0.45

[a] One patient.

3.8. Breath Methane and Peripheral Vascular Disease

The incidence of breath methane excretion has also been investigated in a group of patients with peripheral vascular disease (McKay *et al.*, 1983).

Sixty patients were studied, 44 men and 16 women, aged 45–77 years (mean 62 years), attending the peripheral vascular clinical for vascular investigation. Peripheral vascular patients were divided into two groups by vascular radiology: group 1, patients in whom the disease was confined to the aortoiliac region, and group 2, patients in whom the disease was confined to the femoral popliteal region. Classification of the patients and breath analysis were performed independently. Thirty control patients, free from gastrointestinal disorders and peripheral vascular disease, 13 men and 17 women, aged from 19–78 years (mean 46 years), were obtained from General Medical wards. The proportion of subjects excreting methane in the control hospital group (43%) was significantly less than in patients with aortoiliac disease (83%, $p < 0.05$), but not significantly different from patients with femoral popliteal disease (30%). The proportions of methane-excreting subjects with the aortoileac and femoral popliteal diseases were significantly different ($p < 0.001$). There were no significant differences in the concentrations with breath methane excreted in the three patient groups.

3.9. Animal Investigations

Several series of animal experiments in which expired methane was measured have been reported (McLean Ross *et al.*, 1981, 1984; McKay and Eastwood, 1983, 1984). These studies were designed to investigate the effect of diet on bacterial metabolism in the rat cecum. In one study 18 Wistar rats were divided into three groups consisting of three males and three females each, which were given one of three diets from weaning (3 weeks) until 14 weeks of age: Diet 1 (bran diet) (high in fiber and carbohydrate but low in fat) was designed to be a herbivorous type of diet, which consisted of equal weights of fine bran and powdered Spiller's Laboratory Small Animal Diet. Diet 2 (meat diet) contained equal weights of raw mince and chopped boiled egg and was a low-fiber, high-fat carnivorous diet. The control diet was Spratt's Laboratory Small Animal Diet, which contained protein from fish, yeast, and plant sources and carbohydrates from fish and yeast. All diets were fed *ad lib* and the daily intakes were measured. Water intake was unrestricted. Production of methane was measured weekly using a closed circuit apparatus, a modification of the method used by Gumbmann and Williams (1971). Methane was not detected at any time from rats in the two test groups receiving bran and meat diets. Measurable quantities of methane were detected (>0.094 ml/h per rat) at 12 weeks and thereafter in rats given the control diet, with no significant differences between males and females (mean and standard deviation 0.73 ± 0.15 and 0.591 ± 0.13 ml/h per kg, respectively).

In a similar experiment the metabolism in the rat intestine of a chemically defined, readily identifiable polysaccharide, gum arabic, was studied. Gum arabic is a water-soluble polysaccharide (molecular weight approximately 850,000), which contains rhamnose, arabinose, glucuronic acid, and galactose. Wistar rats (3 months old) were fed on gum arabic, incorporated into pellets of reconstituted Oxoid breeder's diet, at doses of 0–200 g/kg, for a period of 4 weeks. Other rats were fed on a complete elemental diet (residue-free) containing gum arabic (220 g/kg dry weight) in jelly form administered over the same time period. Gum arabic could be detected from the stomach to the ileum but not in the colon. In three rats the cecum was excised with subsequent reconstitution of intestinal continuity. In these rats gum arabic was recovered from stomach to rectum. Excreted methane was measured as an indicator of bacterial activity in the cecum and colon. Methane excretion increased significantly ($p < 0.001$) on the gum arabic pellet diet. Methanogenesis ceased on elemental diets alone and following cecal excision. When the animals were given the elemental diet plus gum arabic, methane was produced after 28 days.

3.10. *In Vitro* Incubation of Anaerobic Bacteria of the Human Intestine in Single and Mixed Cultures

Single strains of common human bacteria were grown in Brain Heart Infusion Broth (Oxoid) gassed with oxygen-free nitrogen. *Bacteroides* species that require carbon dioxide for good growth were gassed with carbon dioxide. All bottles were incubated at 37°C, usually for 48 h (McKay *et al.*, 1982). After inoculation and incubation, the headspace gas was analyzed for methane by gas chromatography. Most strains of bacteria tested produced only trace amounts of methane. *Clostridium perfringens* (strain 690) produced 1.08 μmol/liter methane, but the remaining four strains of *C. perfringens* produced no methane. Two other *Clostridia*, a strain of *C. septicum* (strain 558) and of *C. histolyticum* (strain RIE 2), produced 0.9 and 1.08 μmol/liter respectively. Increased methane production was noted with the test strain of *C. histolyticum* after incubation for 5 days (mean 4.77). Preliminary studies of the effect of single carbohydrates on methane production by pure cultures *in vitro* have so far failed to give consistent results.

Incubation experiments were also performed with fresh feces. Sixteen healthy subjects provided freshly passed stool. One gram of fresh stool was homogenized with 10 ml of 0.2 M phosphate-buffered saline (PBS), pH 7.0. One milliliter of homogenate was added to 10 ml Brain Heart Infusion Broth (BHI) (i.e., 10^{-3} g feces/ml BHI). Inocula consisting of 10^{-2} g feces/ml PBS were also prepared. All incubations were left at 37°C for 48 h, after which time headspace gas was analyzed for methane. Preliminary studies showed that 10^{-3} g feces/ml BHI yielded significant concentrations of methane gas from slow-growing methanogens after 48 h with the substrate-rich growth. However, with a weak buffer (PBS) and no additional substrate a dilution of 10^{-2} g feces was required to yield measurable concentrations of methane gas. There were no significant differences in headspace gas percentage methane between inocula from breath methane excretors ($n = 10$; range 0.012–0.015%) and nonexcretors ($n = 6$; range 0.012–0.013%) in PBS alone. However, in the presence of BHI broth, inocula from methane excretors yielded significantly more methane (range 2.37–5.97%) than nonexcretors (range 0.95–1.78%), p 0.001.

The ability of fresh fecal microflora to produce methane while incubated at 37°C in phosphate-buffered saline for 24 h was also investigated from a range of animals divided into carnivores, herbivores, and primates, including man (McKay and Eastwood, 1984). Methane concentrations were found to be greatest in herbivores, followed by primates and then man. No methane was detected in headspace gas from incubations with feces from carnivores.

4. DISCUSSION AND CONCLUSIONS

There are wide variations reported in the proportion of methane-excreting subjects in different healthy adult populations, ranging from 33% (Bond et al. 1971) to 58% (Pitt et al. 1980) in North America, 40% (Haines et al. 1977) to 61% (McKay et al., 1981) in Britain, and 75 to 80% in Nigeria (Cummings, 1981). The incidence of methane excretion in our surveys was not dependent upon age or sex in either the nonclinical or clinical populations. It has been suggested that intestinal transit time is an important factor in the production of methane (Mah et al., 1977). There were no significant differences in stool weight or gut transit time in our studies between methane-producing and nonproducing subjects. The concentration of breath methane excreted was not related to stool weight or transit time.

In a healthy population with a stable dietary intake, breath methane concentrations were found to be associated with the intake of the pentose fraction of noncellulosic polysaccharide. When pentoses were taken in monomeric form, D-xylose and L-arabinose, significant increases in breath methane were observed during the periods at 1.5–2 and 3.5–4 h after ingestion. The first peak of the biphasic methane response is probably caused by the fermentation of this unabsorbed fraction of pentose passing into the cecum. The reason for the two increases in gas excretion is uncertain, but may result from the activity of two different methanogenic bacterial species, which reflects the complexity of bacterial metabolism in the cecum. The increases in breath methane excretion were related to the initial baseline concentrations; the higher the initial concentration, the greater the increase. This may reflect a larger methanogenic bacterial population. The association between breath methane concentration and the estimated intake of pentose-containing fiber in the population study may require a steady metabolic state in the cecum. The production of methane after the acute administration of free pentoses and the lack of methane production after the ingestion of polysaccharide sources may indicate that the release and availability of free pentose monomers from plant polysaccharides may be rate-limiting steps in this process.

Within the clinical gastroenterology populations investigated the only subgroups with significantly different prevalences of methane excretion were patients with pneumatosis cystoides intestinalis (11%), Crohn's disease (13%), and ulcerative colitis (15%). These conditions are chronic diarrheal states with rapid colonic transit times. However, variations in transit time in patients within the normal range of 68.4–29.5 h did not influence methane excretion status. Also, patients with diarrhea from other causes do not have a significantly different prevalence of methane excretion (42%) compared to nongastrointestinal patients (53%). The absence of methane excretion with inflammatory bowel disease and pneumatosis cystoides intestinalis may result from an altered epithelial mucosa. Analysis of colonic gas showed a lack of methane production in patients with inflammatory bowel disease, and, in addition, several patients ($n = 5$) with no detectable methane in the breath had low concentrations in the colonic gas. Patients with inflammatory bowel disease may lack the capacity for significant methane production or excretion due to differences in relative oxygen tension, blood flow, or membrane condition and permeability. A group of patients with possible reduced colonic blood flow have been shown to have an increased incidence of breath methane. Impaired colonic arterial circulation from atherosclerosis of the abdominal aorta may alter the colonic environment by reducing oxygen tension, making it more conducive to methanogensis. The aortoiliac patient group and the control hospital patients without peripheral vascular disease showed a highly significant ($p < 0.005$) difference in the proportion of methane-excreting subjects. This difference does not appear to be due to the presence of peripheral vascular disease in general, since the proportion of methane excretors in the group of patients with fermoral popliteal disease is similar to that of the patients without peripheral vascular disease. Increased concentrations of breath methane were observed in methane excretors with colonic carcinoma and diarrhea. These patients may have a greater population of methanogenic bacteria, fewer methane-utilizing bacteria that oxidize methane, yielding carbon dioxide, or altered colonic mucosal absorption.

It is possible that methane-producing bacteria colonize the mucosa of the distal intestine, where there is a complex microbial ecology. This will affect their response to different intestinal diseases. Several inflammatory colonic diseases, however, significantly reduce the prevalence of methane production. We tentatively conclude that methane production in the colon is the norm. For a person to excrete methane in the breath, a sufficient volume and hence concentration must be generated in the colon to be absorbed and pass to the lungs. A number of individuals do not excrete methane in the breath possibly because insufficiently high concentrations are generated in the colon.

Animal experiments show that all rats over the age of 3 months produce methane. Cecectomy abolished methane production, which suggests that the cecum is the main site of bacterial activity; cecectomy results in loss of bacteria and failure of gum arabic metabolism. Methanogenic bacteria appear to colonize the cecum and require a fibrous residue, possibly to assist in colonization and to provide a potential source of substrates. There may be a critical period during which time anaerobic methanogens colonize the gastrointestinal tract (Savage, 1977, 1978). However, methane excretion was undetectable from rats on both high-wheatbran-fiber and low-fiber test diets. An increased fiber content, although providing substrate, may alter bacterial fermentation patterns, changing the cecal environment, which may prevent or delay colonization by methanogens. Similarly, a lack of fibrous residue may also prevent or delay bacterial colonization. The lack of methane production from incubation of carnivore feces also supports this.

During bacterial fermentation experiments species variation and even strain variation were apparent. Small but significant amounts of methane were produced by three test strains (*Clostridium histolyticum, C. perfringens, C. septicum*). Methane production was a reproducible finding in these strains where it was detected, but was not a constant finding within all strains. It is still not clear whether the much smaller volume of methane produced in humans is the result of the metabolic activity of a few methanogens or of the production of small amounts of methane by large numbers of gut organisms such as clostridia. Although all fecal incubations yielded methane, incubations with Brain Heart Infusion Broth, a complex growth medium, produced significantly more methane using stool from breath methane excretors. This may reflect differences in bacterial populations, increased activity of methanogens, or greater numbers of methanogens in stool from breath methane excretors. Differences in methane absorption from the colon into the blood stream and transport to the lungs may also exist. The similarity in methane production during fecal fermentation both in healthy methane excretors and nonexcretors would indicate that methane is produced by all subjects but in varying concentrations, and that only when the production reaches a threshold level does methane appear in the breath. It appears that diet and the fiber component of the diet are contributing factors to the volume and composition of gas produced.

ACKNOWLEDGMENTS. This work was supported by the Medical Research Council.

REFERENCES

Bond, J. H., Engel, R. R., and Levitt, M. D., 1971, Factors influencing pulmonary methane excretion in man, *J. Exp. Med.* **133**:572–588.

Calloway, D. H., 1966, Respiratory hydrogen and methane as affected by consumption of gas-forming foods, *Gastroenterology* **51**:383–389.

Calloway, D. H., 1968, Gas in the alimentary canal, in: *Handbook of Physiology,* Section 6, *Alimentary Canal,* Volume V, *Bile, Digestion, Ruminal Physiology* (C. Code, and W. Heidel, eds.), American Physiological Society, Washington, D.C.

Calloway, D. H., and Murphy, E. L., 1968, The use of expired air to measure intestinal gas formation, *Ann. N. Y. Acad. Sci.* **150**:82–95.

Cummings, J. H., 1981, Short chain fatty acids in the human colon, *Gut* **22**:763–779.

Evrard, E., and Janssen, G., 1968, Gas-liquid chromatographic determination of human faecal bile acids, *J. Lipid Res.* **9**:226–236.

Gumbmann, H. R., and Williams, S. N., 1971, The quantitative collection and determination of hydrogen gas from the rat and factors affecting its production, *Proc. Soc. Exp. Biol. Med.* **136**:1171–1175.

Haines, A., Metz, G., Dilawari, J., Blendis, L., and Wiggins, H., 1977, Breath methane in patients with cancer of the large bowel, *Lancet* **2**:481–483.

Hellendoorn, E. W., 1978, Fermentation as the principle cause of the physiological activity of indigestible food residue, in: *Topics in Dietary Fiber Research,* (G. A. Spiller, ed.), Plenum, New York, pp. 127–168.

Hickey, C. A., Calloway, D. H., and Murphy, E. L., 1972, Intestinal gas production following ingestion of fruits and fruit juices, *Am. J. Dig. Dis.* **17**:383–389.

Hinton, J. M., Lennard-Jones, J. E., and Young, A. C., 1969, A new method for studying gut transit times using radio-opaque markers, *Gut* **10**:842–847.

Hungate, R. E., 1968, Ruminal fermentation, in: *Handbook of Physiology,* Section 6, *Alimentary Canal,* Volume V, *Bile, Digestion, Ruminal Physiology* (C. Code and W. Heidel, eds.), American Physiological Society, Washington, D. C., p. 2725.

Hungate, R. E., 1976, Microbial activities related to mammalian digestion and absorption of food, in: *Fibre in Human Nutrition* (G. Spiller and R. J. Amen, eds.), Plenum, New York, p. 131.

Levitt, M. D., 1969, Hydrogen gas in man, *N. Eng. J. Med.* **281**:122–127.

Levitt, M. D., and Bond, J. H., 1970, Volume, composition and source of intestinal gas, *Progr. Gastroenterol.* **59**:921–929.

Levitt, M. D., and Ingelfinger, F. J., 1968, Hydrogen and methane production in man, *Ann. N. Y. Acad. Sci.* **150**:75–81.

Mah, R. A., Ward, D. M., Baresi, L., and Glass, T. L., 1977, Biogenesis of methane, *Annu. Rev. Microbiol.* **31**:309–341.

McKay, L. F., and Eastwood, M. A., 1983, The influence of dietary fibre on caecal metabolism in the rat, *Br. J. Nutr.* **50**:679–684.

McKay, L. F., and Eastwood, M. A., 1984, A comparison of bacterial fermentation endproducts in carnivores, herbivores and primates including man, *Proc. Nutr. Soc.* **43**:35A.

McKay, L. F., Brydon, W. G., Eastwood, M. A., and Smith, J. H., 1981, The influence of pentose on breath methane, *Am. J. Clin. Nutr.* **34**:2728–2733.

McKay, L. F., Holbrook, W. P., and Eastwood, M. A., 1982, Methane and hydrogen production by human intestinal anaerobic bacteria, *Acta. Pathol. Immunol. Scand. B.* **90**:257–260.

McKay, L. F., Brydon, W. G., Eastwood, M. A., and Housley, E., 1983a, The influence of peripheral vascular disease on methanogenesis in man, *Atherosclerosis* **47**:77–81.

McKay, L. F., Smith, R. G., Eastwood, M. A., Walsh, S. D., and Cruikshank, J. G., 1983b, An investigation of colonic function in the elderly, *Age Ageing* **12**:105–110.

McKay, L. F., Eastwood, M. A., and Brydon, W. G., 1985, Methane excretion in man—A study of breath, flatus and faeces, *Gut,* **26**:69–74.

McLean Ross, A. H., McKay, L. F., Busuttil, A., Anderson, D. M. W., Brydon, W. G., and Eastwood, M. A., 1981, Gum arabic metabolism in the rat colon, *Proc. Nutr. Soc.* **40**:73A.

McLean Ross, A. H., Eastwood, M. A., Brydon, W. G., Busuttil, A., McKay, L. F., and Anderson, D. M. W., 1984, A study of the effects of dietary gum arabic in the rat, *Br. J. Nutr.* **51**:47–56.

McLean Ross, A. H., Eastwood, M. A., Brydon, W. G., Anderson, J. R., and Anderson, D. M. W., 1983, A study of the effects of dietary gum arabic in humans, *Am. J. Clin. Nutr.* **37**:368–375.

Metz, G., Gassull, M. A., Leeds, A. R., Blendis, L. M., and Jenkins, D. J. A., 1976, A simple method of measuring breath hydrogen in carbohydrate malabsorption by end-expiratory sampling, *Clin. Sci. Molec. Med.* **50**:237–240.

Nottingham, P. M., and Hungate, R. E., 1968, Isolation of methanogenic bacteria from faeces of man, *J. Bacteriol.* **96**:2178–2179.

Paul, A. A., and Southgate, D. A. T., 1978, *McCance and Widdowson's: The Composition of Foods,* 4th ed., Her Majesty's Stationery Office, London.

Pitt, P., de Bruijn, K. M., Beeching, M. F., Goldberg, E., and Blendis, L. M., 1980, Studies on breath methane: The effect of ethnic origins and lactulose, *Gut* **21**:951–959.

Prins, R. A., 1979, Methanogenesis in the gastrointestinal tract of ruminants and man, *Antonie van Leeuwenhoek* **45**:339–345.

Robertson, J. A., Brydon, W. G., Tadesse, K., Wenham, P., Walls, A., and Eastwood, M. A., 1979, The effect of raw carrot on serum lipids and colon function, *Am. J. Clin. Nutr.* **32**: 1889–1892.

Royal College of Physicians, 1981, *Medical Aspects of Dietary Fibre,* Pitman Medical, London.

Savage, D. C., 1977, Interaction between the host and its microbes, in: *Microbial Ecology of the Gut* (R. T. J. Clarke and T. Buachop, eds.), Academic, New York, pp. 277–310.

Savage, D. C., 1978, Factors involved in colonization of the gut epithelial surface, *Am. J. Clin. Nutr.* **31**:S131–S135.

Smith, A. N., Drummond, E., and Eastwood, M. A., 1981, The effect of coarse and fine Canadian red spring wheat and French soft wheat bran on colonic motility in patients with diverticular disease, *Am. J. Clin. Nutr.* **34**:2460–2463.

Southgate, D. A. T., Bailey, B., Colinson, E., and Walker, A. F., 1976, A guide to calculating intakes of dietary fibre, *J. Hum. Nutr.* **30**:303–313.

Steggerda, F. R., 1968, Gastrointestinal gas following food consumption, *Ann. N. Y. Acad. Sci.* **150**:57–66.

Stephens, A. M., and Cummings, J. H., 1980, Mechanisms of action of dietary fibre in the human colon, *Nature* **284**:283–284.

Tadesse, K., and Eastwood, M. A., 1977, Breath hydrogen tests and smoking, *Lancet* **2**:91.

Tadesse, K., Smith, A., Brydon, W. G., and Eastwood, M. A., 1979, Gas chromatographic technique for combined measurement of hydrogen and methane using thermal conductivity detector, *J. Chromatogr.* **171**:416–418.

Tadesse, K., Smith, D., and Eastwood, M. A., 1980, Breath hydrogen and methane excretion patterns in normal man and in clinical practice, *Q. J. Exp. Physiol.* **65**:85–97.

Trowell, H., 1974, Definitions of fibre (letter), *Lancet* **i**:503.

Varley, H., 1967, *Practical Clinical Biochemistry,* Heinemann, London, Chapter XVI, p. 325.

Wolfe, R. S., 1971, Microbial formation of methane, *Adv. Microb. Physiol.* **6**:107–146.

12

The Glycemic Index: Blood Glucose Response to Foods

DAVID J. A. JENKINS,
THOMAS M. S. WOLEVER,
ALEXANDRA L. JENKINS,
LILIAN U. THOMPSON,
A. VENKETESHWER RAO, and
THOMAS FRANCIS

1. INTRODUCTION

Much of the current interest in the blood glucose responses to food evolved as a natural consequence of earlier dietary fiber studies. Considerable impetus has also come from the need to find sustained release or lente carbohydrate foods that would fit the requirements for the diabetic diet, where an increase in carbohydrate intake has been recommended [Committee of the American Diabetes Association on Food and Nutrition, 1979; Special Report Committee, 1981 (Canadian Diabetes Association); Nutrition Sub-Committee of the British Diabetic Association's Medical Advisory Committee, 1982)]. Such studies, therefore, have focused attention on the differences among foods and on those factors, including fiber, that were

DAVID J. A. JENKINS, THOMAS M. S. WOLEVER, and ALEXANDRA L. JENKINS • Department of Nutritional Sciences, Faculty of Medicine, and Division of Endocrinology and Metabolism, St. Michael's Hospital, University of Toronto, Toronto M5S 1A8, Canada. LILIAN U. THOMPSON, A. VENKETESHWER RAO, and THOMAS FRANCIS • Department of Nutritional Sciences, Faculty of Medicine, University of Toronto, Toronto M5S 1A8, Canada.

responsible for these differences. Investigation of the physiological effect of foods has proceeded in a similar fashion to what was applied to the screening of dietary fibers. Foods have been tested to determine whether there were in fact differences in digestibiity and whether the rate of nutrient release from the gastrointestinal tract might be a factor in determining the glycemic response (Jenkins *et al.*, 1982, 1984c; O'Dea *et al.*, 1981). In turn, the glycemic responses to a range of foods have been studied in both normal and diabetic individuals and the foods analyzed for fiber, macronutrients, and selected antinutrients to assess whether these could account for the observed differences. Studies of carbohydrate malabsorption have also been undertaken. Finally, longer term studies, although primarily focusing on fiber, have also allowed exploration of the possible clinical use of lente carbohydrate diets in diabetes and hyperlipidemia.

2. DIFFERENCES IN DIGESTIBILITY

A number of studies now indicate that different foods are digested at different rates (Jenkins *et al.*, 1982, 1984c; O'Dea *et al.*, 1981). Thus, when selected individual carbohydrate foods (12 foods, 2-g available carbohydrate portions) were submitted to digestion via human enzymes in a dialysis tube, the rates of digestion varied by as much as threefold (Jenkins *et al.*, 1984c), as reflected by the rates of release of the digestion products glucose, maltose, and maltotriose into the dialyzate. The most rapidly digested food was whole meal (whole wheat) bread, while some of the starchy foods digested most slowly were the legumes (Jenkins *et al.*, 1982, 1984c) (Fig. 1). Other studies have indicated that ground rice is digested more rapidly than whole rice (O'Dea *et al.*, 1981) and, in general, legumes are digested more slowly than cereals (Jenkins *et al.*, 1982, 1984c). Although the dietary fiber content may be one of the factors involved, many other factors, such as the amounts and types of antinutrients present, are also likely to play a determining role. In addition to the nature of the starch, the content of amylose and amylopectin, the starch–protein interaction and other factors concerned with the physical form and gelation characteristics of the starch can be expected to be important factors. Nevertheless, the large differences in the rates of digestion observed made it important to determine whether equally large differences might result in terms of the blood glucose response to these different types of starchy foods. To this end, large-scale comparative studies were undertaken.

3. DIFFERENCES IN GLYCEMIC RESPONSE

In order to allow the glycemic effects of different foods to be compared, tables of "biological equivalence" (Otto *et al.*, 1973) or "glycemic index"

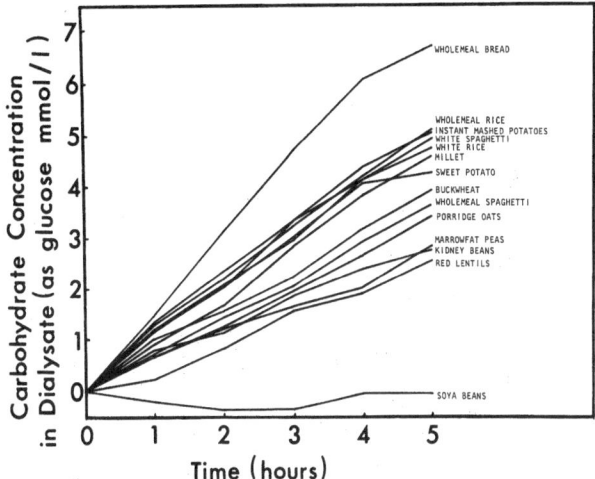

FIGURE 1. The increase in concentration over 5 h of the products of starch digestion, measured as glucose after acid hydrolysis, subsequent to incubation of 2-g available carbohydrate portions of foods with pooled human saliva and pancreatic juice.

(Jenkins *et al.*, 1984a), which ascribe a numerical value to each food, have been constructed. Estimation of the glycemic index of a food requires that the blood glucose response area resulting from ingestion of that food be compared with the blood glucose response to a reference food containing the same amount of carbohydrate. In the past, glucose has been used as the reference food (Jenkins *et al.*, 1981a), although it is now probably better to use bread as a more representative physiological standard (Jenkins *et al.*, 1983c, 1984a). The glycemic index (GI) is calculated as

$$GI = \frac{\text{blood glucose response area for food}}{\text{blood glucose response area for bread (or glucose)}} \times 100$$

In a study where a group of over 60 foods and sugars were compared in normal volunteers, fourfold differences were seen between the highest and lowest blood glucose responses among the starchy foods (Jenkins *et al.*, 1981a). Figure 2 shows these differences, which were observed both within food groups, such as root vegetables, breakfast cereals, and cereal products, and between groups, such as root vegetables and dried legumes, where large differences were found (Jenkins and Wolever, 1981). As already mentioned, large differences existed in the rates at which different foods were digested. Construction of a digestibility index, whereby the rate of digestion of a food was standardized against the rate of digestion of bread, showed that digesti-

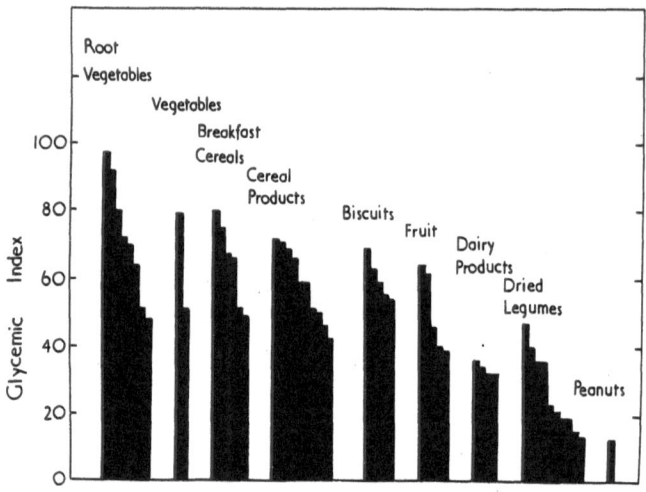

FIGURE 2. The glycemic index of foods (i.e., area under the 2-h blood glucose response curve of a 50-g available carbohydrate portion, 50 g glucose itself being 100). Each bar in each block represents the mean result for one food tested by 5–10 individuals. (From Jenkins and Wolever, 1981.)

bility related positively to the glycemic index (Jenkins *et al.*, 1982, 1984c). This suggested that, as in the dietary fiber story, the rate of digestion and absorption of nutrients from foods is also important in determining the glycemic response. Furthermore, comparison of the glycemic index in diabetics with the glycemic index tested in normal individuals also showed a good correlation (Fig. 3) (Jenkins *et al.*, 1983c).

Over the past 25 years, several studies have highlighted major differences among different starchy foods. The original systematic classification of a number of foods was undertaken by Otto and co-workers (Otto *et al.*, 1973). The approach was similar to that used currently in the glycemic index classification (Jenkins *et al.*, 1984a) and was termed the "biological equivalence" of foods (Otto *et al.*, 1973). In general, the glycemic indices agree well among different laboratories (Otto *et al.*, 1973; Jenkins *et al.*, 1981a, 1983c, 1984a; Crapo *et al.*, 1977, 1981; Walker and Walker, 1984), with mean differences about 10% (Jenkins *et al.*, 1984a).

4. FACTORS RESPONSIBLE FOR DIFFERENCES IN GLYCEMIC RESPONSE

Many factors may be responsible for the differences seen in glycemic responses to different foods. For example, fat is known to delay gastric emptying and may therefore reduce the glycemic response (Thomas, 1957).

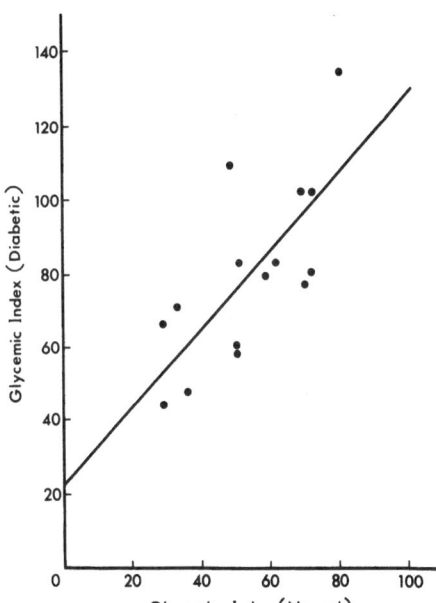

FIGURE 3. The relationship between the glycemic index of 15 foods tested in normal volunteers and the same foods tested in diabetics ($r = 0.756$, $p < 0.01$). (From Jenkins *et al.*, 1983c.)

Protein, too, through increasing insulin secretion, may reduce the glycemic response (Fagans *et al.*, 1967). Simple sugars are considered to cause higher rises than starches. Fiber may delay the absorption of carbohydrate and therefore reduce the glycemic response (Jenkins *et al.*, this volume, Chapter 6; Leeds and Judd, this volume, Chapter 22; Anderson, this volume, Chapter 23), as may starches rich in amylose or where there is a particularly strong starch–protein interaction (Anderson *et al.*, 1981). The form in which the food is eaten is also of importance. Apples eaten whole as opposed to apple juice produce flatter glucose and insulin responses (Haber *et al.*, 1977), as do meals of whole rice when compared to ground rice (O'Dea *et al.*, 1980). Additional components of foods, not generally listed in food tables, such as lectins, saponins, phytates, and tannins, may all contribute to a reduced rate of intraluminal digestion or absorption.

So far, studies have indicated that both the fat and the protein content of a food may reduce the glycemic response (Fig. 4) (Jenkins *et al.*, 1981a). However, this is not necessarily the case with added fat and protein, as, for example, when butter or cheese is added to a bread meal (Jenkins *et al.*, 1984b). In this situation, the addition of fat causes a small initial reduction in the rate of blood glucose rise but no overall change in area, while addition of protein causes little difference at all (Jenkins *et al.*, 1984b). The effects of sugars are variable and depend upon the proportion of fructose and galactose involved, since these sugars raise the blood glucose level minimally.

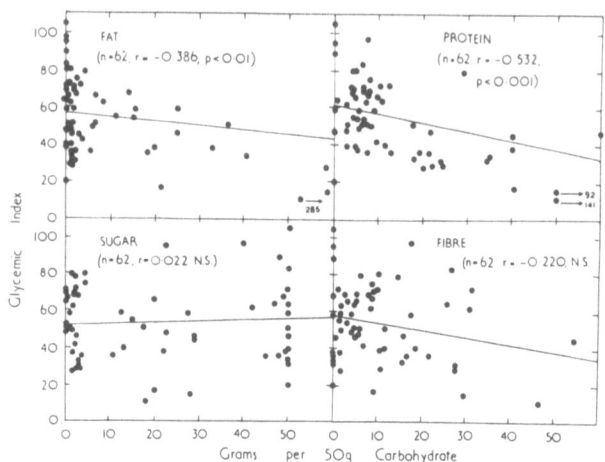

FIGURE 4. Relationship of fat, protein, sugars, and fiber content of 62 foods to the glycemic index of 50-g available carbohydrate portions. (From Jenkins *et al.*, 1981a.)

Overall, there is therefore no significant correlation between total sugar content and the glycemic response (Jenkins *et al.*, 1981a). Likewise, in comparisons such as this, because the majority of the fiber in foods is of cereal origin, which has minimal effect on the blood glucose response, no significant relationship between fiber and reduction in blood glucose was seen (Jenkins *et al.*, 1981a). The lack of effect of fiber is further borne out both in normal and diabetic volunteers by the lack of glycemic effects of white versus whole wheat bread, of white rice versus brown rice, and of white spaghetti as opposed to whole wheat spaghetti (Jenkins *et al.*, 1981b, 1983b). Nevertheless, such studies do illustrate the importance of food form, as shown by the fact that spaghetti produces much lower responses than bread, despite the close similarity of their macronutrient profiles. This clearly shows that factors other than fiber can be major determinants of the physiological effects of foods.

5. PREDICTIVE VALUE OF THE GLYCEMIC INDEX

If use is to be made of the glycemic index, then it should be able to answer a number of questions. Do foods tested singly, when mixed in equal proportions, give a glycemic index that is the mean of the two constituent foods? Does knowledge of the glycemic indices of individual foods in a mixed meal allow the relative glycemic response of that meal to be predicted even in the presence of such confounding variables as fat and protein? Finally, does selection of diets with known glycemic index characteristics result in long-term metabolic changes that reflect the physiological effects of short term testing?

To answer these questions in noninsulin-dependent diabetics, a meal of bread was given with white pea beans; the resulting glycemic index of the meal was intermediate between that of bread and beans given singly (Fig. 5) (Jenkins *et al.*, 1984b). In addition, the glycemic index of a half bread meal was approximately 50% that of the full bread meal (Jenkins *et al.*, 1984b). This relationship was not so clear in insulin-dependent diabetics, since many other factors affect their glycemic responses. Furthermore, their results are generally not stable, as evidenced by more varied starting blood glucose values (Jenkins *et al.*, 1984b). Even so, the glycemic index values for the legume meals always fell below that of bread, and the half bread meal fell below that of the full bread meal, with a glycemic index of 65 (Jenkins *et al.*, 1984b)

When it came to predicting the comparative blood glucose responses to different mixed meals of normal composition, current glycemic index data again appeared to stand up well. Figure 6 shows the result of assessing meals from two studies in the recent literature (Bantle *et al.*, 1983; Nuttall *et al.*, 1983) and comparing the estimated glycemic index of the meal with the observed blood glucose rise (Wolever *et al.*, 1985). As can be seen, both insulin-dependent and noninsulin-dependent diabetics who took the same series of meals, and also the normal volunteers, showed a good proportionality between the glycemic index, estimated for the meal from the individual

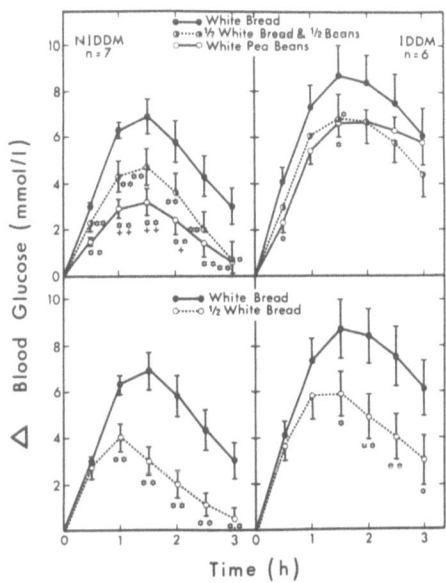

FIGURE 5. Mean (± SEM) blood glucose rise in non-insulin-dependent (NIDDM) and insulin-dependent diabetics (IDDM) after meals containing either 50 g available carbohydrate from white bread, white pea beans, or bread and beans, or bread (25 g available carbohydrate) alone. Significance from mean bread value: ★ $p < 0.05$; ★★ $p < 0.01$. Significance from bread and beans value: †$p < 0.05$; ††$p < 0.01$. (From Jenkins *et al.*, 1984.)

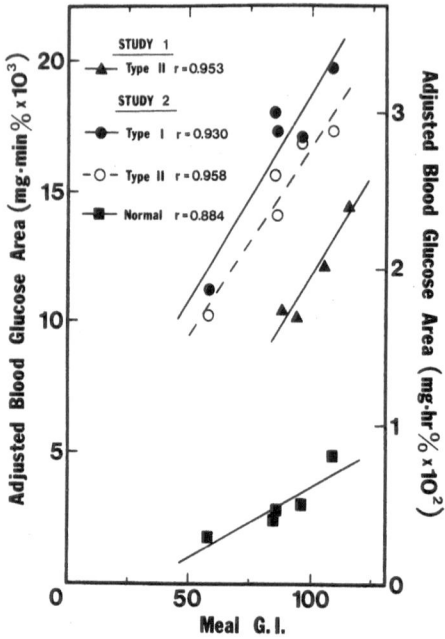

FIGURE 6. Adjusted (0–3 H) blood glucose areas in response to mixed meals from two studies reported in the literature (Bantle et al., 1983; Nuttal et al., 1983) involving IDDM, NIDDM, and normal volunteers, plotted against calculated meal glycemic indices (mean GI). (From Wolever et al., 1985.)

constituents, and the adjusted blood glucose areas as observed. Such data support the contention that, even in the presence of fat and protein, the glycemic index is a useful predictor of metabolic effect. The final test, however, came from using the glycemic index in the selection of foods to be incorporated into the diets of those with disordered carbohydrate metabolism, for example, patients with diabetes or those with hyperlipidemia.

6. DIABETES

Although diabetics have not been the subject of any studies specifically designed to test the effects of low-glycemic-index foods, a number of high-fiber studies have been undertaken in which the diets were coincidentally of low glycemic index. One such study used legumes as the major source of carbohydrate in the diet (Simpson et al., 1981). In 6-week studies using these foods, significant improvement in all aspects of diabetic control, including 24-h blood glucose profiles, hemoglobin$_{AIC}$ and serum cholesterol, were noted (Simpson et al., 1981). These improvements were seen despite the fact that the high-legume diet contained 20% more carbohydrate than the control diet (Simpson et al., 1981). In addition, the studies of Anderson and co-workers (Kihem et al., 1978; Anderson and Ward, 1978, 1979), who pioneered the use of the high-fiber, high-carbohydrate diets in diabetics, achieved therapeutic success with diets containing many low-glycemic-index foods, including legumes, corn, and other low-glycemic-index cereal products. Similar results have been reported by others (Rivellese *et al.*, 1980). Although it has been suggested that the effects of such diets were due largely to their high fiber and carbohydrate contents, some of the benefits may have resulted from the fact that such diets were also low-glycemic-index diets. It seems important, then, that studies be undertaken to distinguish between the effects of high fiber and high carbohydrate and where the emphasis is on the exchange of low- for high-glycemic-index foods.

7. HYPERLIPIDEMIA

A number of studies have indicated the hypolipidemic effect of legumes, especially in the older age group (Grande *et al.*, 1965; Bingwen *et al.*, 1981; Jenkins *et al.*, 1983a; Albrink *et al.*, 1979; Anderson *et al.*, 1984). Some recent studies have focused attention on their potential therapeutic effects in hyperlipidemic individuals. Work in Seshwan, China indicated a lowering of serum cholesterol levels using diets incorporating an average of 30 g of dried beans per day (Bingwen *et al.*, 1981). In studies on predominantly type IV hyperlipidemic men, it was found that when 25% of their total calories were replaced by legumes without altering macronutrient intakes, decreases were seen in both serum cholesterol and serum triglyceride levels (Fig. 7) (Jenkins *et al.*, 1983a). Such studies confirmed what had already been suggested as a possible use for such foods as hypolipidemic agents, since they cause minimal rises in blood glucose and insulin. In this way, it was suggested that they reduced the stimulus to hepatic triglyceride synthesis and so may lower

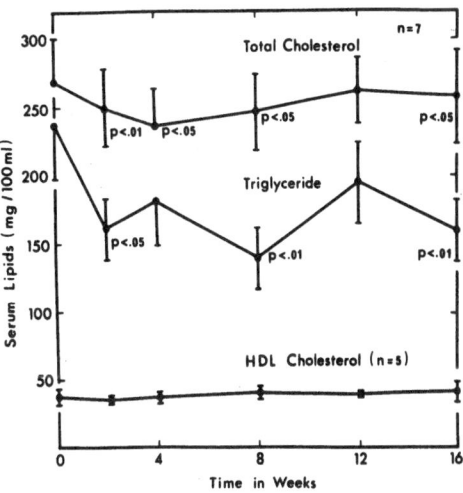

FIGURE 7. Total serum cholesterol, triglyceride (seven patients), and high-density lipid cholesterol (five patients) over the 16-week bean supplementation period. Significance levels refer to differences from the mean of the previous five control samples. (From Jenkins *et al.*, 1983a.)

serum triglyceride levels (Potter *et al.*, 1981). These studies have been extended using a range of low-glycemic-index foods, including specific breads, vegetables, and breakfast cereals, where both the dietary fiber and macronutrient composition of the diet remained unchanged. In studies of type IV hyperlipidemic patients, it has been possible again to demonstrate falls in both serum cholesterol and triglyceride during the middle or test month of 3-month studies (Fig. 8). These studies were specifically designed to test the metabolic effects of low-glycemic-index foods. They demonstrated that an action is seen irrespective of changes in dietary fiber content. Nevertheless, the effect of alteration in the nature of the fiber, including the exchange of leguminous seed and oat fiber for wheat fiber, may be responsible for some of the effects, especially those on serum cholesterol (Kirby *et al.*, 1981). Further work in this area should be undertaken where not only the fiber amount but also the fiber type remains constant in control and low-glycemic-index diets.

8. CONCLUSION

Studies of the glycemic effect of foods represent a logical extension of dietary fiber studies of carbohydrate metabolism. They have demonstrated that large differences indeed exist in terms of blood glucose response to different starchy carbohydrate foods. Not all the explanation for these

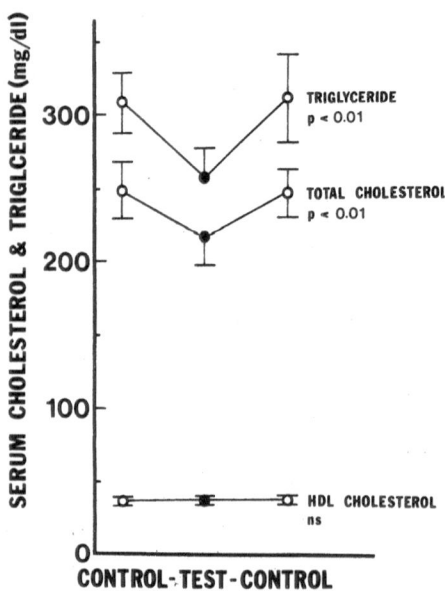

FIGURE 8. Mean total serum cholesterol, triglyceride, and high-density lipid cholesterol levels (ten patients) during a 3-month study during the middle month of which low-glycemic-index foods were substituted into the diet without altering the fiber or macronutrient composition. The values represent the mean of the fasting samples taken at the end of the second and fourth weeks of each month. (Jenkins *et al.*, 1985.)

findings can be ascribed to fiber, although the nature of fiber and its interaction with the starch may be of great importance in determining the response. Other factors, such as the nature of the starch, the food form, protein–starch interaction, and the antinutrient content, may also be important. All these factors relate to the digestibility of the food, which in turn influences its metabolic effect. Clinical studies, many of which were not specifically aimed at testing the effects of low-glycemic-index foods but did so incidentally, indicate that the range of therapeutic use of low-glycemic-index foods may be similar to the spectrum of activity of dietary fiber. In addition, the physiological principles involved appear to have similarities. Further studies, however, are required for a more complete classification of foods in order to uncover and clarify the diversity of the food factors involved and to provide the variety in terms of diet required for clinical studies and therapeutic regimens.

ACKNOWLEDGMENT.   Work by the authors was supported by funds from the Natural Sciences and Engineering Research Council.

REFERENCES

Albrink, M. J., Newman, T., and Davidson, P. C., 1979, Effect of high and low-fiber diets on plasma lipids and insulin, *Am. J. Clin. Nutr.* **32**:1486–1491.

Anderson, I. H., Levine, A. S., and Levitt, M. D., 1981, Incomplete absorption of the carbohydrate in all purpose wheat flour, *N. Engl. J. Med.* **304**:891–892.

Anderson, J. W., and Ward, K.,1978, Long term effects of high carbohydrate, high fiber diets on glucose and lipid metabolism: A preliminary report on patients with diabetes, *Diabetes Care* **1**:77–82.

Anderson, J. W., and Ward, K., 1979, High carbohydrate, high fiber diets for insulin treated men with diabetes mellitus, *Am. J. Clin. Nutr.* **32**:2312–2321.

Anderson, J., Story, C., Sibling, B., and Chen, W.-J. L., 1984, Hypocholesterolemic effects of high fiber diets rich in water-soluble plant fibers: Long term studies with oatbran and bean supplemented diets for hypercholesterolemic men, *Can. Dietet. J.* **45**:140–148.

Bantle, J. P., Laine, D. C., Castle, G. W., Thomas, J. W., Hoogwerf, B. J., and Goetz, F. C., 1983, Postprandial glucose and insulin responses to meals containing different carbohydrates in normal and diabetic subjects, *N. Engl. J. Med.* **309**:7–12.

Bingwen, L., Zhaofeny, W., Wanshen, L., and Rongjue, Z., 1981, Effects of bean meal on serum cholesterol and triglycerides, *Chinese Med. J.* **94**:455–8.

Committee of the American Diabetes Association on Food and Nutrition, 1979, Special Report: Principles of nutrition and dietary recommendations for individuals with diabetes mellitus, *Diabetes Care* **2**:520–523.

Crapo, P. A., Reaven, G., and Olefsky, J., 1977, Post-prandial plasma-glucose and insulin responses to different complex carbohydrates, *Diabetes* **26**:1178–1183.

Crapo, P. A., Insel, J., Sperling, M., and Kolterman, O. G., 1981, Comparison of serum glucose, insulin and glucagon responses to different types of complex carbohydrate in non-insulin-dependent diabetic patients, *Am. J. Clin. Nutr.* **34**:184–190.

Fagans, S. S., Floyd, J. C., Knopf, R. F., and Conn, J. W., 1967, Effect of amino acids and proteins on insulin secretion in man, *Rec. Prog. Horm. Res.* **23**:617-656.

Grande, F., Anderson, J. T., and Keys, A., 1965, Effect of carbohydrates of leguminous seeds, wheat and potatoes on serum cholesterol in man, *J. Nutr.* **86**:313-317.

Haber, G. B., Heaton, K. W., Murphy, D., and Burroughs, L. F., 1977, Depletion and disruption of dietary fibre: Effects on satiety, plasma-glucose, and insulin *Lancet* **2**:679-682.

Jenkins, D. J. A., and Wolever, T. M. S., 1981, Slow release carbohydrate and the treatment of diabetes, *Proc. Nutr. Soc.* **40**:227-235.

Jenkins, D. J. A., Wolever, T. M. S., Taylor, R. H., Barker, H. M., Fielden, H., Baldwin, J. M., Bowling, A. C., Newman, H. C., Jenkins, A. L., and Goff, D. V., 1981a, Glycemic index of foods: A physiological basis for carbohydrate exchange, *Am. J. Clin. Nutr.* **34**:362-366.

Jenkins, D. J. A., Wolever, T. M. S., Taylor, R. H., Barker, H. M., Fielden, H., and Gassull, M. A., 1981b, Lack of effect of refining on the glycemic response to cereals, *Diabetes Care* **4**:509-513.

Jenkins, D. J. A., Ghafari, H., Wolever, T. M. S., Taylor, R. H., Barker, H. M., Fielden, H., Jenkins, A. L., and Bowling, A. C., 1982, Relationship between the rate of digestion of foods and post-prandial glycemia, *Diabetologia* **22**:450-455.

Jenkins, D. J. A., Wong, G. S., Patten, R., Bird, J., Hall, M., Buckley, G. C., McGuire, V., Reichert, R., and Little, J. A., 1983a, Leguminous seeds in the dietary management of hyperlipidemia, *Am. J. Clin. Nutr.* **38**:567-573.

Jenkins, D. J. A., Wolever, T. M. S., Jenkins, A. L., Lee, R., Wong, G. S., and Josse, R., 1983b, Glycemic response to wheat products: Reduced response to pasta but no effect of fiber, *Diabetes Care* **6**:155-159.

Jenkins, D. J. A., Wolever, T. M. S., Jenkins, A. L., Thorne, M. J., Lee, R., Kalmusky, J., Reichert, R., and Wong, G. S., 1983c, The glycaemic index of foods tested in diabetic patients: A new basis for carbohydrate exchange favouring the use of legumes, *Diabetolgia* **24**:257-264.

Jenkins, D. J. A., Wolever, T. M. S., Jenkins, A. L., Josse, R. G., and Wong, G. S., 1984a, The glycaemic response to carbohydrate foods, *Lancet* **2**:388-391.

Jenkins, D. J. A., Wolever, T. M. S., Wong, G. S., Kenshole, A., Josse, R. G., Thompson, L. U., and Lam, K. Y., 1984b, Glycemic responses to foods: Possible differences between insulin-dependent and non-insulin-dependent diabetics, *Am. J. Clin. Nutr.,* **40**:971-981.

Jenkins, D. J. A., Wolever, T. M. S., Thorne, M. J., Jenkins, A. L., Wong, G. S., and Josse, R. G., 1984c, The relationship between glycemic response, digestibility and factors influencing the dietary habits of diabetics, *Am. J. Clin. Nutr.,* **40**:1175-1191.

Jenkins, D. J. A., Wolever, T. M. S., Buckley, G., Hall, M., Wong, G. S., Bird, J., Patten, R., Kalmusky, J., Guiduchi, S., Giordeno, C., Little, J. A., 1985, Effect of low glycemic index diet in hyperlipidemic patients. Unpublished Observations, *Am. J. Clin. Nutr.,* (in press).

Kiehm, T. G., Anderson, J. W., and Ward, K., 1978, Beneficial effects of a high carbohydrate high fiber diet in hyperglycemic men, *Am. J. Clin. Nutr.* **29**:895-899.

Kirby, R. W., Anderson, J. W., Sieling, B., Rees, E. D., Chen, W.-J. L., Miller, R. E., Kay, R. M., 1981, Oat-bran intake selectively lowers serum low-density lipoprotein cholesterol concentrations of hypercholesterolemic men, *Am. J. Clin. Nutr.* **34**:824-829.

Nutrition Sub-Committee of the British Diabetic Association's Medical Advisory Committee, 1982, Dietary recommendations for diabetics for the 1980s—A Policy Statement by the British Diabetic Association, *Hum. Nutr. Appl. Nutr.* **36A**:378-394.

Nuttall, F. Q., Mooradian, A. D., DeMarais, R., and Parker, S., 1983, The glycemic effect of different meals approximately isocaloric and similar in protein, carbohydrate, and fat content as calculated using the Ada exchange lists, *Diabetes Care* **6**:432-435.

O'Dea, K., Nestol, P. J., and Antonoff, L., 1980, Physical factors influencing postprandial glucose and insulin responses to starch, *Am. J. Clin. Nutr.* **33**:760-765.

O'Dea, K., Snow, P., and Nestel, P., 1981, Rate of starch hydrolysis *in vitro* as a predictor of metabolic responses to complex carbohydrate *in vivo*, *Am. J. Clin. Nutr* **34**:1991–1993.

Otto, H, Bleyer, G., Pennartz, M., Sabin, G., Schauberger, G., and Spaethe, K., 1973, Kohlenhydrataustausch nach Biologischen Aquivalenten, in: *Diatetik bei Diabetes Mellitus* (H. Otto and R. Spaethe, eds.), Hans Huber, Bern, pp. 41–50.

Potter, J. G., Coffman, K. P., Reid, R. L., Krall, J. M., and Albrink, M. J., 1981, Effect of test meals of varying dietary fiber content on plasma insulin and glucose response, *Am. J. Clin. Nutr.* **34**:328–334.

Rivellese, A., Riccardi, G., Giacco, A., Pacioni, D., Genovese, S., Mattioli, P. L., and Mancini, M., 1980, Effect of dietary fibre on glucose control and serum lipoproteins in diabetic patients, *Lancet* **2**:447–450.

Simpson, H. C. R, Simpson, R. W, Lousley, S., Carter, R. D., Geekie, M., Hockaday, T. D. R., and Mann, J. I., 1981, A high carbohydrate leguminous fibre diet improves all aspects of diabetic control, *Lancet* **1**:1–5.

Special Report Committee, 1981, Guidelines for the nutritional management of diabetes mellitus: A special report from the Canadian Diabetes Association, *J. Can. Dietet. Assoc.* **42**:110–118.

Thomas, E. J., 1957, Mechanics and regulation of gastric emptying, *Physiol. Rev.* **37**:453–474.

Walker, A. R. P., and Walker, B. F., 1984, Glycaemic index of South African foods determined in rural blacks—A population at low risk to diabetes, *Hum. Nutr. Clin. Nutr.,* **36C**:215–222.

Wolever, T. M. S., Nuttall, F. Q., Lee, R., Wong, G. S., Josse, R. G., Csima, A., and Jenkins, D. J. A., 1985, Prediction of the relative blood glucose response to mixed meals using the white bread glycemic index, *Diabetes Care* (in press).

Yoon, J. H., Thompson, L. U., and Jenkins, D. J. A., 1983, The effect of phytic acid on *in vitro* rate of starch digestibility and blood glucose response, *Am. J. Clin. Nutr.* **38**:835–842.

13

Dietary Fiber and Intestinal Adaptation

GEORGE V. VAHOUNY and MARIE M. CASSIDY

1. INTRODUCTION

It is well recognized that the structure and function of the small intestine can be significantly modified by manipulation of dietary patterns (Creamer, 1974; Dworkin et al., 1976; Hageman and Stragand, 1977; Maudsley et al., 1976). There is also considerable evidence to suggest that modifications of the enterohepatic circulation of bile acids and/or increased luminal concentrations of unconjugated bile acids can result in morphological damage to the intestine (Dawson and Isselbacher, 1960; Low-Beer et al., 1970; Teem and Phillips, 1972) and cause abnormalities in water and salt transport (Mekhijian and Phillips, 1970; Mekhijian et al., 1971; Sladen and Harries, 1972).

The acute or chronic effects of dietary fiber intake on gastric filling and emptying, on delayed or modified nutrient bioavailability, and on bile acid sequestration have been extensively documented throughout this volume and elsewhere (Roth and Mehlman, 1978; Spiller and Kay, 1980; Kay, 1982; Vahouny and Kritchevsky, 1982; Heaton, 1983). It might be expected that any or all of these effects could alter the overall nutrition and characteristics of the small intestine and colon. Accordingly, there is accumulating evidence that the acute and prolonged ingestion of foods high in dietary fiber or

GEORGE V. VAHOUNY • Department of Biochemistry, George Washington University School of Medicine and Health Sciences, Washington, D.C. 20037. MARIE M. CASSIDY• Department of Physiology, George Washington University School of Medicine and Health Sciences, Wahington, D.C. 20037.

administration of specific fiber derivatives can alter many aspects of intestinal structure and function, as well as modulating certain aspects of extra-intestinal metabolism.

In the present chapter, we have concentrated on the potential effects of dietary fiber derivatives on specific aspects of structural and functional adaptations of the gastrointestinal tract.

2. EFFECTS ON INTESTINAL AND COLONIC MORPHOLOGY

There are numerous reports implying a relationship between dietary fiber intake and morphological patterns in the small intestine. In the human, the jejunal villi in the fetus are fingerlike and regular, and this pattern is also typical of adults in Western societies (Baker *et al.*, 1962; Cook *et al.*, 1969; Chacko *et al.*, 1969). In contrast, the intestinal villi of individuals in developing countries (Owen and Brandborg, 1977) and in healthy vegetarians (Chacko *et al.*, 1969) are broad and leaf-shaped, with numerous ridges and convolutions.

These patterns have largely been reproduced in experimental animals. Tasman-Jones and co-workers (Tasman-Jones *et al.*, 1978; Tasman-Jones, 1980) have reported that rats fed a fiber-free diet maintain an immature, finger-shaped villus pattern. Rats on a standard laboratory diet containing fiber or given diets containing pectin develop mucosal ridges and a decrease in the total number of jejunal villi. We have conducted similar studies with rats weaned onto defined diets (Cassidy *et al.*, 1981b), which were either fiber-free or contained 10% cellulose or 5% pectin. As shown in Fig. 1, the immature, finger-shaped villus pattern of the jejunum is maintained in animals weaned onto the fiber-free diet, while the villus structure in rats given the fiber supplements is more typical of that observed in rats fed laboratory chow (Cassidy *et al.*, 1981b). Thus, the collective evidence clearly demonstrates that the morphological development of the small intestine can be dramatically influenced by dietary patterns. These modifications are clearly related to altered patterns of DNA, RNA, and protein content of the mucosa, and to specific enzyme activities associated with the mucosal cell and mucosal brush border. The overall influence of these differences in villus structure and function on transport processes and the overall economy of the organism has yet to be assessed. It is also unclear as to whether these fiber-related modifications in intestinal structure and function are reversible.

In addition to the effects of dietary fiber supplements on the development of the small intestine, it is also clear that dietary fiber supplements given to adult animals can influence intestinal length and weight (Younoszai *et al.*, 1978; R. C. Brown *et al.*, 1979; Schneeman, 1982) and intestinal

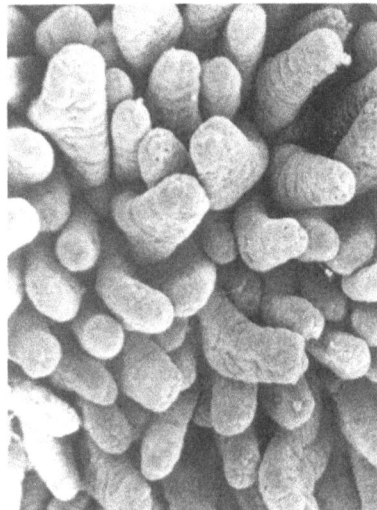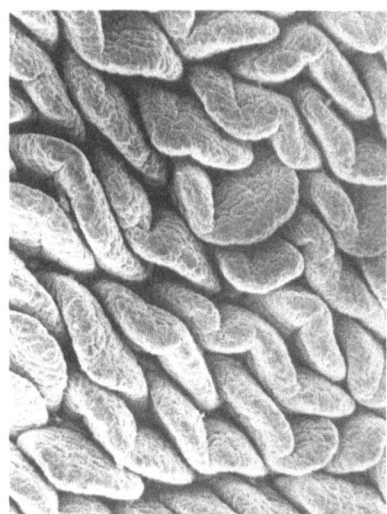

FIGURE 1. Scanning electron micrographs of small intestinal villi from rats weaned onto (left) fiber-free defined diets or (right) diets containing 10% cellulose.

morphology at the light (Schneeman, 1982; Tasman-Jones, 1980; Sigleo *et al.*, 1984) and electron microscopic levels (Cassidy *et al.*, 1981b, 1982). In the studies of Cassidy *et al.* (1981b) a variety of insoluble and soluble fiber derivatives were included in defined diets and fed to rats for 4–6 weeks. The feeding of 15% levels of white wheat bran or purified cellulose had little apparent effect on the ultrastructural morphology of either jejunum or colon, except that there was evidence of increased mucus and an apparent increase in goblet cell activity. The feeding of diets containing pectin or alfalfa was associated with significant morphological abnormalities in both the small and large intestine compared to animals fed fiber-free diets or those given cellulose or bran. These abnormalities were also observed in animals fed diets containing 2% levels of cholestyramine, colestipol, or DEAE–Sephadex, all of which are used as hypocholesteremic agents, presumably due to their ability to sequester intraluminal bile acids (Cassidy *et al.*, 1980, 1982).

Certain dietary fiber derivatives are also reported to sequester bile acids and other micellar components *in vitro* or to cause increased bile acid excretion *in vivo* (Story, 1980; Vahouny *et al.*, 1980c, 1981; Kay, 1982; Story and Thomas, 1982). As shown in Table I, it appears that there is at least a qualitative relationship between the apparent extent of bile acid sequestration by dietary fibers or ion-exchange resins and the degree of morphological or topographic abnormalities observed by feeding these materials. More recent

TABLE I. Comparison of Bile Acid Sequestration by Dietary
Fiber Derivatives and Morphological Changes in Rat Small
Intestine and Colon Following Feeding[a]

Test material	Apparent bile acid sequestration, %	Percentage of villi or ridges with structural deviations	
		Jejunum	Colon
Control	0	7.1 ± 2.3	5.0 ± 0.8
Wheat bran	5[b,c]	5.0 ± 1.1	15.0 ± 4.9
Cellulose	0[c]	7.5 ± 2.1	22.1 ± 4.1
Pectin	Extensive[d]	30.7 ± 4.7	29.4 ± 8.0
Alfalfa	15[b,c]	32.8 ± 7.2	58.6 ± 4.3
DEAE–Sephadex	30–40[e]	13.0 ± 3.6	40.6 ± 9.1
Colestipol	50—60[b,e]	35.9 ± 12.6	55.0 ± 10.1
Cholestyramine	80—100[b,a,e]	64.2 ± 4.7	39.5 ± 10.5

[a] From Cassidy *et al.* (1982). Values are means ± SEM for 259 intestinal villi or colonic folds.
[b] From Kritchevsky and Story (1974).
[c] From Vahouny *et al.* (1978, 1980b).
[d] Not measurable *in vitro*; extrapolated from the *in vivo* data of Leveille and Sauberlich (1966).
[e] From Cassidy *et al.* (1980).

studies (Cassidy *et al.*, 1982; Vahouny *et al.*, 1984) suggest that the morphological abnormalities in the colon are a result of the increased colonic bile acid concentrations, rather than being due to the bile acid-sequestering agent *per se*. This observation may be of considerable significance, since increased colonic bile acid concentrations are purported to act as promoters in chemically induced carcinogenesis of the large bowel (e.g., Hill, 1982), and that this promotion will occur whether the bile acids are unbound or remain bound to the sequestering agent (Asano *et al.*, 1975). Similarly, there is evidence (Hill, 1982) that fiber additives that increase colonic (and fecal) bile acid concentrations may also adversely affect the extent of chemically induced tumorigenesis of the large bowel. These types of findings raise important questions regarding specific fiber supplements, which are outside the scope of this review.

3. MORPHOLOGICAL CORRELATIONS

3.1 Intestinal Cytokinetics and Mucin Production

Irrespective of mechanisms, the studies described above collectively suggest that specific dietary fiber components can express adaptive morphological changes in the small and large bowel, and that these adaptations may be a function of the overall nutriture of the organ. These morphological changes also expressly imply the possibility of modified cytokinetics of the organ (Sprinz, 1971). It is generally accepted that cell turnover in the crypts of Lieberkühn is an important determinant of villus morphology (Lipkin, 1981; Loehry and Creamer, 1968), and that this process is regulated in part by the gastrointestinal peptide hormones (Lipkin, 1981). It is of interest to note that fiber feeding has been shown to modify the secretions of several of these peptides (e.g., Leeds, 1982), suggesting that the structural responses, particularly in the small intestine, may be at least in part hormonally mediated.

Evidence that feeding of dietary fiber supplements can modify intestinal cell turnover has recently been demonstrated. Jacobs and White (1983) reported that the incorporation of [³H]thymidine into DNA in the cecum and colon, but not in the proximal jejunum, was increased in animals fed a 20% wheat bran-supplemented diet for 4 weeks. These studies, which are further elaborated in Chapter 14 of this volume, are difficult to conduct and require additional attention to other types of fiber derivatives.

We have recently completed studies on modifications in intestinal cytokinetics and mucin turnover in animals fed defined diets supplemented with either 10% cellulose or 10% wheat bran for 15 weeks. The interest in intestinal synthesis and secretion of mucins was based on several factors. As indicated previously, our earlier studies (Cassidy et al., 1981a,b) with cellulose- and wheat bran-supplemented diets suggested an increased goblet cell secretory activity as assessed by scanning electron microscopy. Others (Schneeman, 1982) have suggested that dietary fiber may increase the relative number of intestinal goblet cells. These cells are responsible for the secretion of mucins lining the intestinal epithelium (Cassidy et al., 1981a).

Among the putative functions ascribed to these intestinal surface constituents are cytoprotection, antigenic responses, and antiviral and antibacterial activities (Cassidy et al., 1981a). The mucins have also been implicated as an important constituent of the unstirred water layer (Smithson et al., 1981), and have been suggested to be a rate-limiting diffusion barrier for nutrient absorption (Smithson et al., 1981; Williams and Turnberg, 1980). Thus, changes in the mucin content or composition at the mucosal surface might be involved in the mechanism by which dietary fibers modify nutrient absorption in the small intestine.

In our studies, intestinal cytokinetics were assessed by autoradiographic analysis of jejunal sections following incorporation of [³H]thymidine via the jugular vein. All studies were conducted between 10:00 A.M. and noon to avoid diurnal affects on labeling indices (Sigdestad et al., 1969). Animals were killed at 1 and 24 h postinjection. Tissue samples from the midjejunum were fixed in 10% neutral formalin, dehydrated, mounted on slides, and stained with hematoxylin. These were then processed for autoradiography. Data on labeled and unlabeled cell counts, migration rates, and labeling indices were obtained by Apple 2 computer-assisted analyses. Additional sections were used for histological assessment of mucin-staining cells. These were stained with PAS-alcian blue at pH 2.5, and total numbers of cells, goblet cells, and stained cells were determined by light and phase contrast microscopy.

To estimate mucin synthesis and secretion, animals in each group were fasted for 24 h and the duodenum was perfused with phosphate-buffered saline (PBS, pH 7.2). A mixture of [^{3}H] glucose and $Na_2^{35}SO_4$ was injected into the jugular vein and after 90 min, blood was obtained by cardiac puncture. The middle one-fifth of intestine was removed and perfused with 10 ml cold PBS to obtain a "wash" fluid. The intestine was everted and shaken with 25 ml PBS to obtain a "rinse" fluid. The mucosa was scraped and homogenized in PBS. Samples of the rinse and wash fluids and the mucosal homogenate were centrifuged at $20,000 \times g$ for 30 min, and glycoproteins, including mucins, were precipitated with 1% cetyltrimethylammonium bromide (CTAB) (Ofuso et al., 1978). The $20,000 \times g$ precipitates were washed with 0.1% CTAB, suspended in saline, and counted. Data are expressed as labeling indices [(dpm/mg protein ÷ dpm/μl serum) $\times$ 100]

Data on intestinal cell numbers and cytokinetics for animals fed the fiber-free, cellulose, and bran-supplemented diets are shown in Table II. The numbers of total intestinal cells, enterocytes, and mucin-staining cells on the left villus column (Fig. 2) were comparable in all three dietary groups. There

TABLE II. Intestinal Cell Numbers and Cytokinetics in Rats
Fed Fiber-Free or Fiber-Supplemented Diets[a]

Measurement	Control	Cellulose	Bran
Total cells/left villus column	107.0 ± 7.2	102.1 ± 6.1	111.8 ± 8.7
Goblet cells, %	$13.2 \pm 0.8*$	$9.7 \pm 1.4*†$	$13.6 \pm 1.1†$
Mucin stained cells, %	31.4 ± 2.4	31.4 ± 2.6	32.8 ± 2.5
Crypt cells, number	$38.4 \pm 3.4*$	$39.8 \pm 2.2†$	$31.7 \pm 1.6*†$
Labeling index, 1 h (percent crypt cells labeled)	$27.1 \pm 2.1*$	$33.9 \pm 3.0*†$	$51.7 \pm 1.5*$
Position of uppermost labeled cell (24 h)	$17.5 \pm 3.2*$	$24.1 \pm 1.8*†$	$40.6 \pm 2.4*†$
Cell migration rate, h	$0.73 \pm 0.13*$	$1.00 \pm 0.10*†$	$1.70 \pm 0.10*†$

[a] Rats were fed *ad libitum* for 15 weeks on defined diets containing no fiber, 10% wheat bran, or 10% cellulose. At 9:00 A.M. each animal was given an intravenous injection of [^{3}H]thymidine (1 μCi/g body weight) and animals were killed at 1 or 24 h later. Tissue samples from midjejunum were fixed in formalin, sectioned, stained with hematoxylin, and processed for autoradiography. Values for cell numbers represent means ± SEM for six animals where at least 20 villi from each section were observed. Value for [^{3}H]thymidine incorporation are means ± SEM for two animals at each time in which at least ten villi were assessed on the autoradiographs. Figures in rows with the same superscript are significantly different ($p < 0.05$).

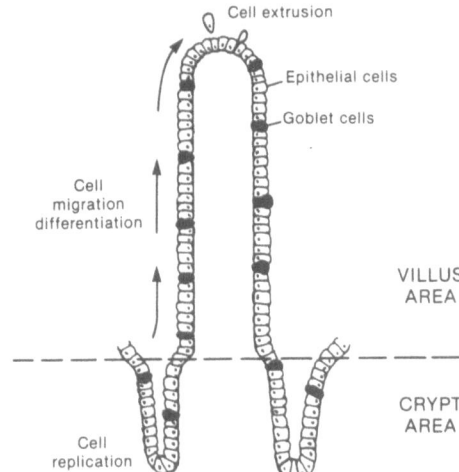

FIGURE 2. Schematic representation
of a small intestinal villus column indicating the crypt area of cell renewal
and the cell transit up the villus column.

appeared to be fewer goblet cells in the cellulose-fed group, and the apparent
number of crypt cells in bran-fed rats was statistically less than for the fiber-
free and cellulose-fed groups. However, the studies with [^{3}H]thymidine
clearly demonstrated that animals on the fiber-supplemented diets had increased crypt cell turnover and a faster transit of cells up the villus column in
the mid-small intestine (Fig. 2).

The goblet cells are derived from undifferentiated crypt cells, and
during cell migration and differentiation these cells are clearly differentiated
from enterocytes, representing about one of every eight cells on the villus
column (Moe, 1955). Assuming that cells are differentiated at the same rate
during transit up the villus column (Fig. 2), then one could expect the
increased crypt cell turnover and cell migration rates observed in fiber-fed
animals to be reflected in changes in either enterocyte or goblet cell function.
Sulfated carbohydrates are typical of the sulfomucins (Belanger, 1954) and
represent a major component of goblet cell secretions (Belanger, 1954;
Forstner et al., 1973). In earlier studies (Cassidy et al., 1981a) we demonstrated that the technique of measuring ^{35}S incorporation into CTAB-
precipitable intestinal glycoproteins was appropriate for assessing acute
responses in mucin turnover to either aspirin or prostaglandin E_1 treatment
of rats. In the present study, however, it was expected that the level of
response to dietary manipulation might be blunted.

The incorporation of total isotope and of [^{3}H]glucose and $Na_2^{35}SO_4$
into CTAB-precipitable glycoproteins of intestinal mucosa is shown in Fig.
3. Animals fed the cellulose- or bran-supplemented diets exhibited increased
incorporation of both isotopes into intestinal glycoproteins. The labeling
indices for ^{3}H and ^{35}S incorporation are shown in Table III, and clearly

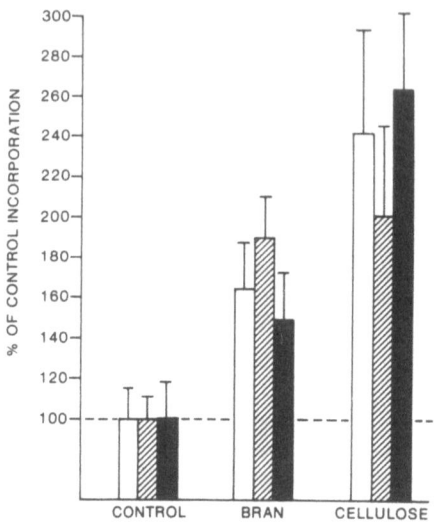

FIGURE 3. Incorporation of intrave-
nously administered [³H]glucose and
$Na_2{}^{35}SO_4$ into intestinal glycoproteins
that are precipitable with cetyltrimethylammonium bromide. (□) Total radioactivity: (□) [³H]glucose; (□) $Na_2{}^{35}SO_4$.
Figures represent means ± SEM for six
animals.

demonstrate increases in rats fed either of the fiber-supplemented diets. This
was particularly evident for the ${}^{35}S$ labeling index in rats given the bran diet.

Although arbitrary, the release of glycoproteins during initial perfusion
of the intestine might be taken to represent loosely adherent mucins. The
release of radioactivity during subsequent incubation of the everted intestine
is taken to represent more tightly adherent, but still noncellular glycoprotein.
Homogenates of the scraped mucosa were taken to represent cellular glycoproteins.

Analysis of the ${}^{35}S$ radioactivity in the CTAB-precipitable glycoproteins
in each of these arbitrary fractions (Table III) suggested that, with animals
fed either the cellulose- or bran-containing diets, a greater percentage of the
${}^{35}S$ was less tightly associated with the mucosal surface and more extensively
released into the rinse fluid. Similar results were obtained on ${}^3H$ distribution
in the cellulose-fed rats.

There was no evidence for the nature or source of the glycoprotein
analyzed by the isotope incorporation method. This could represent membrane glycoproteins whose turnover is modified in association with the
altered cytokinetics observed during fiber feeding. However, the data with
${}^{35}S$ provide some confidence that at least a portion of the changes in isotope
turnover could be associated with the sulfomucins of goblet cells.

These data provide some preliminary evidence that specific dietary fiber
components not only can modify intestinal cell turnover rates, but may also
alter the expressed activities of the goblet cells (and the enterocytes?) on the
villus column.

TABLE III. Incorporation of $Na_2{}^{35}SO_4$ and [^{3}H]Glucose into
Intestinal Glycoproteins[a]

Measurement	Control	Cellulose	Bran
Labeling index^{35}S[b],			
percent of control	16.5 ± 3.0*	24.7 ± 4.0*†	43.7 ± 1.0*†
Distribution of ^{35}S, %			
Wash	51.7 ± 12.0	44.2 ± 8.0	31.7 ± 9.1
Rinse	12.1 ± 2.4*†	26.5 ± 4.0*	29.2 ± 4.0†
Homogenate	36.2 ± 2.4	29.2 ± 4.0	30.6 ± 9.1
Labeling index [^{3}H]glucose,			
percent of control	9.2 ± 1.0*†	17.5 ± 2.0*	18.6 ± 4.0†
Distribution of [^{3}H]glucose, %			
Wash	48.1 ± 4.4*†	35.7 ± 4.7*	25.0 ± 4.3†
Rinse	11.4 ± 2.2*†	22.3 ± 5.7*	22.0 ± 10.8†
Homogenate	40.4 ± 4.4	41.9 ± 2.3	52.9 ± 21.6

[a] Animals were fasted for 24 h and given a single intravenous injection of $Na_2{}^{35}SO_4$ and [^{3}H]glucose. After 90 min, blood was obtained and the entire small intestine was perfused with 10 ml phosphate-buffered saline, pH 7.2 (wash solution). The intestine was everted and shaken for 10 min in 25 ml PBS (rinse solution). The mucosa was scraped and homogenized in 10 ml PBS. Glycoproteins in each solution were precipitated with cetyltrimethylammonium bromide (CTAB) overnight, washed with 0.1% CTAB suspended in saline, and, together with serum samples, analyzed for radioactivity. Data represent means from six animals ± SEM. Figures with common superscripts are significantly different ($p < 0.05$).
[b] Labeling index = (cpm/mg protein ÷ cpm/μl serum) × 100.

3.2 Villus Marker Enzymes

Reports on the responses of mucosal surface-associated marker enzyme activities to dietary fiber intakes have not been entirely consistent. In the studies of R. C. Brown et al. (1979) the activities of intestinal peptidase and alkaline phosphatase, which are surface markers of mature enterocytes, were reduced in pectin-fed rats. The extent to which tissues were freed of residual fiber, however, was not described.

Elsenhans et al. (1981) assessed the effect of guaran on the intestinal surface hydrolysis of D-maltose and L-phenylalanylglycine using everted segments of rat jejunum. The presence of guar gum (5 g/liter) inhibited hydrolysis of the substrates in a competitive manner, and this was not affected by the shaking rate. There were, however, no differences in hydrolytic rates of substrates when mucosal homogenates were studied in the absence and presence of guaran. It was suggested that the fiber increased the thickness of the unstirred water layer, resulting in an apparent competitive inhibition of surface enzyme activity. Based on kinetic analyses, however, there was no actual competition for substrate binding sites on the maltases or peptidases.

Recent studies by Schwartz et al. (1983) suggest that 6-week feeding of pectin, but not cellulose, caused an apparent increase in the activities of intestinal surface disaccharidases compared to the levels in fiber-free controls.

Thus, the specific activities of lactase, maltase, and invertase in mucosal homogenates from the distal jejunum of pectin-fed rats were between 119 and 140% of those levels in either fiber-free controls or cellulose-fed rats.

Thus, the evidence (Table IV) has been obtained from rats fed cellulose-, pectin-, or guar-containing diets. Cellulose-supplemented diets had little effect on the activities of mucosal surface peptidase or disaccharidase activities. Pectin-containing diets, however, appeared to influence intestinal enzyme activities in a variable way, depending on the age of the animals, the amount fed, and the intestinal site of measurement.

We have recently assessed (Calvert et al., 1984) whether the morphological responses observed in adult rats fed various dietary fiber supplements (Cassidy et al., 1981b) could be associated with changes in the functional activity of the small intestine. Rats were fed for 4 weeks on defined diets (Cassidy et al., 1981b) containing no fiber, 10% levels of insoluble fibers (cellulose or alfalfa), or 5% levels of gel-forming materials (pectin, guar gum, or Metamucil). The entire small intestine was removed, carefully flushed with phosphate-buffered saline, divided into equal thirds, and everted. Mucosal scrapings were homogenized and assayed for protein, for thymidine kinase as a crypt cell activity, and for alkaline phosphatase and sucrase activities as villus cell surface markers.

As shown in Fig. 4, the activities of the two villus cell markers sucrase and alkaline phosphatase in control rats were highest in the proximal third of the small intestine and progressively decreased in the middle and distal intestine. The crypt cell marker activity (thymidine kinase), in contrast, was lowest in the proximal third of the small intestine and highest in the middle and distal intestine. Feeding of any of the fiber derivatives for 4 weeks did

TABLE IV. Effect of Dietary Supplementation with Fiber Derivatives on Intestinal Surface Enzymes

Supplement	Change in intestinal enzyme activity			Reference
	Peptidase	Disaccharidases	Phosphatase	
Cellulose (weanling rats)		→		Thomsen and Tasman-Jones (1982)
Cellulose		→		Schwartz et al. (1983)
Pectin	↘		↘	R. C. Brown et al. (1979)
Pectin	↘		↘	Schwartz et al. (1983)
Pectin (weanling rats)		↘		Thomsen and Tasman-Jones (1982)
Pectin (weanling rats)		→		Thomsen et al. (1983)
Galactomannan (weanling rats)		→		Thomsen et al. (1983)

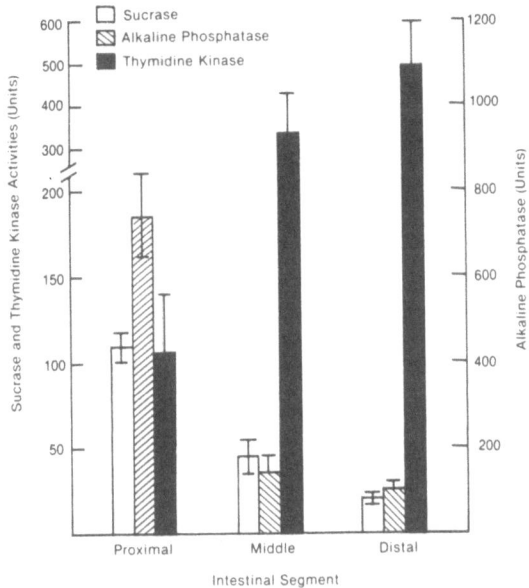

FIGURE 4. Distribution of intestinal villus marker enzymes (sucrase and alkaline phosphatase) and crypt marker thymidine kinase among the proximal, middle, and distal segments of rat small intestine. Figures represent means ± SEM for four animals.

not result in significant changes in total intestinal length (Table V). There was, however, a significant decrease in the mucosal protein levels in the proximal intestine of animals on all of the fiber-supplemented diets compared to levels in rats fed the fiber-free diet. Mucosal protein levels in the middle and distal intestinal segments were largely unaffected by fiber supplementation, except with guar gum- and Metamucil-fed rats, in which mucosal protein content in these segments was increased.

None of the fiber derivatives had consistent effects on either the total activity or the specific activity (activity/mg protein) of the villus marker enzymes in the middle and distal segments of the small intestine. In the proximal intestine, the total activities of sucrase and alkaline phosphatase were similar for all dietary groups. However, because of the decreased mucosal protein content, the specific activities of the villus market enzymes were significantly greater than in the fiber-free group (Table VI). Furthermore, these changes were parallel for the specific activities of both enzymes, with a correlation coefficient of 1.08 ± 0.08.

Thymidine kinase activities were highly variable in all small intestinal segments and were largely unaltered in the proximal and middle segments.

TABLE V. Effect of Fiber Supplementation on Intestinal
Length and Mucosal Protein Content

Group	Intestinal length, cm	Mucosal protein, mg		
		Proximal	Middle	Distal
Fiber-free	124 ± 6	58 ± 7	65 ± 6	41 ± 5
Cellulose	120 ± 3	31 ± 8^a	62 ± 5	38 ± 9
Alfalfa	121 ± 2	38 ± 3^a	40 ± 4^a	31 ± 7
Bran–pectin (3:1)	121 ± 3	34 ± 6^a	63 ± 3	43 ± 2
Pectin	127 ± 2	29 ± 6^a	53 ± 6	49 ± 6
Guar gum	118 ± 2	33 ± 2^a	87 ± 2^a	70 ± 6^a
Metamucil	127 ± 7	25 ± 2^a	74 ± 4	64 ± 6^a

[a] Significantly different from fiber-free, $p < 0.05$.

In the distal segment of the small intestine (Table VII), the largely insoluble fiber supplements (cellulose and bran–pectin) had no significant effect on thymidine kinase, while the soluble fiber derivatives and alfalfa caused significant elevations in the specific activity of this crypt cell marker.

These studies largely serve to point out differences in the distributions of crypt and villus marker enzymes and problems in the methods of expression of data. However, they also suggest that dietary supplementation with various fiber derivatives can affect specific morphofunctional parameters in the small intestine. The data also suggest that viscous fiber derivatives, which are purported to delay nutrient transport in the upper small intestine (Leeds, 1982), may also influence the nutriture of the distal small intestine and alter cell turnover, as indicated by increases in the crypt cell marker activity.

TABLE VI. Changes in Villus Marker Enzyme Specific Activities
in the Proximal Small Intestine of Rats Fed Dietary
Fiber Supplements

Group	Enzyme specific activities, percent of fiber-free	
	Sucrase	Alkaline Phosphatase
Fiber-free	100 ± 7	100 ± 25
Cellulose	230 ± 50^a	244 ± 21^a
Alfalfa	200 ± 23^a	146 ± 11^a
Bran–pectin (3:1)	221 ± 46^a	230 ± 41^a
Pectin	208 ± 44^a	193 ± 15^a
Guar gum	221 ± 26^a	226 ± 17^a
Metamucil	279 ± 44^a	293 ± 24^a

[a] $p < 0.05$ from fiber-free control.

TABLE VII. Effect of Fiber Supplementation on the Relative Activity of Thymidine Kinase in Distal Small Intestine

Group	Thymidine kinase specific activity, percent of fiber-free
Fiber-free	100 ± 23
Cellulose	135 ± 34
Alfalfa	239 ± 30[a]
Bran–pectin (3:1)	136 ± 28
Pectin	337 ± 102[a]
Guar gum	430 ± 103[a]
Metamucil	495 ± 136[a]

[a] $p < 0.05$ from fiber-free control.

3.3 Secretory Immunoglobulin A (IgAs)

In addition to the cytoprotective role of the mucins lining the intestinal tract, other important components of host defense at the epithelial surface are the intestinal antibodies (Walker and Isselbacher, 1977).

Evidence suggests that the immunoglobulins, and particularly IgA, in the intestine are derived from at least two sources, the intestine *per se* and bile. The production of IgA in the intestine is mediated by plasma cells located in the lamina propria near the epithelial surface (Fig. 5). It appears that these cells may be originally derived from intestinal lymphoid tissues (e.g., Peyer's patches) and are predestined to secrete IgA prior to their "homing" within the lamina propria (Fig. 5) (Lamm, 1976). Although all classes of immunoglobulins are represented in the intestinal secretions, the predominant antibody is secretory IgA (sIgA), which exists in a dimeric form.

The secretory antibodies, such as IgA, appear to be assembled within the local plasma cells, and the joining chain (J chain) participates in the formation of polymeric antibodies, such as IgM. These are released from the plasma cells in the crypt region of the villi and transported through the intestinal epithelium via a specific intracellular glycoprotein carrier system (W. R. Brown *et al.*, 1976). As part of the diffusion mechanism, the IgA is linked to a secretory component (SC) and the completed secretory IgA is transported from the epithelial cell to the mucosal surface.

Although secretory antibodies are apparently not present in goblet cells, there does appear to be a relationship between the secreted antibody and the secreted mucins. Secretory IgA is largely retained at the mucosal surface or epithelial cells, and it is suggested that this localization is in part due to interaction with cysteine residues of the surface-associated mucins (Walker and Isselbacher, 1977).

It has also been demonstrated that sIgA is secreted into bile against a strong concentration gradient (Lemaitre-Coelho *et al.*, 1977, 1978; Oku *et al.*, 1982), and that the liver may have an important role in providing sIgA to the upper intestinal tract.

The findings that dietary fiber supplements could modify intestinal cell turnover and mucin secretory patterns suggested the possibility that the levels of intestinal sIgA associated with the surface mucins might also be affected by the changing dietary pattern. To test this possibility, groups of rats were fed for 4 weeks on defined diets (Cassidy *et al.*, 1980) that were fiber-free or contained either 10% wheat bran or 5% guar gum. After a 24-h fast, animals were anesthetized and the middle one-fifth of the small intestine and the entire colon were removed. Each segment was washed with 5 ml phosphate-buffered saline (PBS, pH 7.2), everted, and rinsed with PBS. The mucosa was scraped with a glass slide and sonicated in the combined wash and rinse solution. This was centrifuged at $4000 \times g$ for 10 min and the supernatant was centrifuged at $50,000 \times g$ for 20 h. The precipitate was dissolved in 0.5 ml of 0.54% taurocholate in saline. Aliquots of each sample (9 μl) were subjected to analysis of sIgA by radial immunodiffusion according to Vaerman (1981). Immunoreactive IgA was determined by ring sizes measured on a calibrating viewer and compared to standards of authentic rat myeloma IgA (kindly provided by Dr. J. P. Vaerman, Catholic University of Louvain Brussels) using commercial sheep anti-rat α-chain antiserum (Pel-Freez, Rogers, Arkansas). Under these conditions, rat bile generally gave a single radial immunodiffusion band, representing sIgA composed of α chains, L chains, and secretory component (Oku *et al.*, 1982). Samples of small intestine and colon, in contrast, gave 2–3 rings, suggesting the presence of multiple forms of immunoreactive IgA. This included the proteolytic-resistant sIgA (Oku *et al.*, 1982), monomeric IgA, and partial degradation products of mIgA (Oku *et al.*, 1982). For purposes of comparison, these were calculated as a single value for total immunoreactive IgA and its products.

As summarized in Table VIII, rats fed diets supplemented with 10% wheat bran had decreased levels of total immunoreactive IgA in the mid-small intestine and a slight but insignificant increase in colonic IgA. In contrast, animals fed diets containing 5% guar gum showed a significant increase in midintestinal IgA and a marked decrease in colonic IgA. The changes in measurable IgA in colonic samples of rats fed wheat bran- or guar gum-supplemented diets appear to correlate with the reported morphological observations in rats fed wheat bran or viscous fiber derivatives (Cassidy *et al.*, 1981b). The levels for IgA in the mid one-fifth of the small intestine were, however, unexpected, based on the information derived from the cytokinetic studies. Nevertheless, these data indicated that measurable levels of intestinal and colonic IgA were modified by the type of fiber supplement included in the diet.

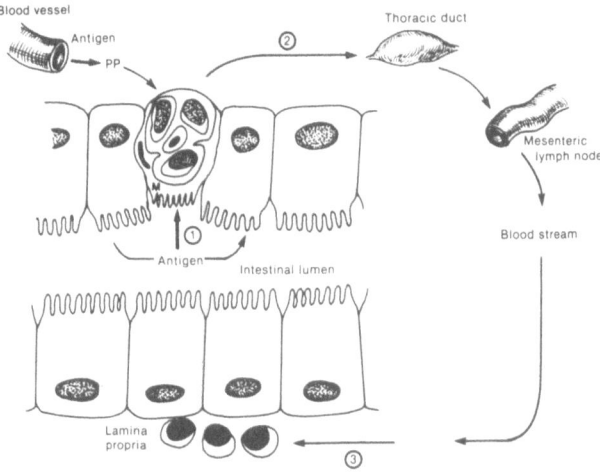

FIGURE 5. Schematic representation of the cell cycle for IgA-producing plasma cells of the intestinal mucosa. (1) Antigens in the intestinal lumen stimulate lymphocytes within the Peyer's patches (PP) via specialized epithelium (M cells). (2) Across absorptive cells or via the systemic circulation, lymphoblasts migrate to lymph nodes, enter the systemic circulation, and (3) are distributed along the intestinal submucosa. These produce secretory IgA in response to absorbed antigens. (Modified from Walker and Isselbacher, 1977.)

It has been suggested (Lemaitre-Coelho *et al.*, 1978) that biliary sIgA contributes to the levels of intestinal IgA, particularly in the proximal jejunum. Thus, the levels of IgA in the wash fluid of the proximal intestine of bile-diverted rats were only about 10% of the levels observed in rats with intact biliary recirculation (Table IX). Using a similar approach in animals fed the fiber supplements, we assessed IgA levels in bile samples of bile-duct cannulated rats and the IgA levels in the first 20 cm of intestine (combined rinse, wash, and mucosa) of these same rats with biliary diversion for 24 h. As shown in Table X, diets supplemented with wheat bran, but not with guar gum, caused significant increases in levels of biliary IgA and of IgA in proximal intestinal samples that were free from the influence of biliary IgA secretions.

These findings, albeit preliminary, suggest that different dietary fiber supplements may have complex effects on various physiological and immunologic aspects of the intestine (and bile) that have not yet been considered. At least two of these possibilities relating intestinal mucins and immunoglobulin concentrations in the intestine are worth mention.

It is now well recognized that diets high in dietary fibers or supplemented with viscous fiber derivatives can influence the intestinal secretions of gastric inhibitory peptide and enteroglucagon (e.g., Jenkins, 1980). Effects on other intestinal hormones, such as secretin or pancreozymin, that influence the

TABLE VIII. Intestinal and Colonic IgA Levels in Rats
Fed Defined Diets[a]

Group	IgA levels, mg/ml	
	Small intestine	Colon
Fiber-free (6)	3.1 ± 0.3*†	0.8 ± 0.1*
Wheat bran, 10% (6)	2.0 ± 0.2 ‡	1.0 ± 0.04 †
Guar gum, 5% (6)	5.1 ± 0.3 ‡	0.4 ± 0.02*†

[a]Animals were fed for 4 weeks on defined diets. The entire small and large intestines were washed with 5 ml phosphate-buffered saline, and the mucosa scraped and added to the washings. Figures in parenthesis represent the number of animals per group. Figures with the same superscript are significantly different ($p < 0.05$).

intestine, pancreas, and bile flow have not yet been assessed. Secretin, for example, can stimulate mucin secretion by Brunner's glands (Stenning and Grossman, 1969) and promote secretion of mucosal and glandular fluids (Dreiling and Messer, 1978). These hormones have also been reported to influence IgA and IgM levels in human duodenal fluid (Lebenthal and Clark, 1981). Thus, administration of secretin to children with no gastrointestinal disease caused a significant increase in both IgA and IgM levels of duodenal aspirates under conditions known to influence intestinal mucin secretion. Pancreozymin, in contrast, caused a decrease in duodenal IgA and an increase in IgM levels. Although these immunoglobulins could be derived from either intestinal, hepatic, or pancreatic sources, the findings do suggest the possibility that modification of intestinal hormone secretion by, for example, dietary fiber supplements might have important influences on the immunologic status of the gastrointestinal tract.

A second important consideration in relating intestinal mucins and immunoglobulins is the formation of immune complexes in the intestine. Studies by Walker and Isselbacher (1977) suggest that certain immune complexes can stimulate mucin release from the rat small intestine (presumably goblet cell-derived), and that this response could be associated with clearing the intestinal surface of these complexes.

TABLE IX. Intestinal IgA Levels in Control and Bile-Diverted Rats[a]

Group	Intestinal IgA, μg/ml[b]
Control (5)	59.8 ± 3.0
Bile-Diverted (5)[c]	6.3 ± 0.3

[a]Modified from Lemaitre-Coelho et al. (1978).
[b]IgA levels in 5 ml of wash fluid from the first 20 cm of small intestine.
[c]Bile diversion was for 48 h.

TABLE X. Biliary and Intestinal IgA Levels in Bile-Diverted
Rats Fed Defined Diets[a]

| Group | Bile | | Intestine (20 cm) |
	Volume, ml	IgA, mg/ml	IgA, mg/ml
Fiber-free (5)	14.8 ± 5.2	0.8 ± 0.2*	1.0 ± 0.1*
Wheat bran (5)	11.5 ± 5.5	1.4 ± 0.1*	2.0 ± 0.3*†
Guar gum (4)	13.8 ± 5.6	1.0 ± 0.2	0.9 ± 0.2†

[a] Animals were fed for 4 weeks on defined diets and subjected to cannulation of the common bile duct. Bile was collected for 24 h prior to removal of the first 20 cm of small intestine. The intestine was handled as described in Table VIII. Figures with the same superscript are significantly different ($p < 0.05$).

These types of relationships have not yet been investigated with respect to dietary fibers (and their associated substances, including lectins), and serve to emphasize the complexity of potential intestinal and biliary responses to modifications of the diet.

4. FUNCTIONAL CORRELATIONS

4.1 In Vitro Nutrient Flux

The acute effects of viscous dietary fiber substances such as pectins or guar gum (guaran) on reducing postprandial glucose and insulin concentrations are well recognized (Jenkins, 1980). Among the mechanisms suggested for these observations are delayed gastric emptying, decreased small intestinal transit time, and effects on intestinal motility.

Recent in vitro and perfusion studies have suggested that the fiber gelling agents may directly inhibit certain digestive and transport functions in the rat intestine (Elsenhans et al., 1980, 1981, 1984; Johnson and Gee, 1981). In general, inhibition of nutrient transport and hydrolysis of disaccharides and dipeptides in these systems is directly related to the viscosity of the medium, and therefore to the concentration of the fiber gelling agent (Johnson and Gee, 1981). Thus, washing the tissue free of the fiber prior to transport studies in vitro (Elsenhans et al., 1980) or in vivo (Elsenhans et al., 1984) completely reverses the inhibitory effect of the gelling fiber. This acute effect of the viscous fiber derivatives on hydrolytic and transport characteristics of the intestine has been suggested to be due to an increased resistance or thickness of the unstirred water layer barrier to intestinal diffusion (Elsenhans et al., 1981, 1984; Johnson and Gee, 1981; Gerencser et al., 1984).

In addition to these acute effects of viscous fiber derivatives on modifying bulk phase diffusion and intestinal transport of nutrients, the effects of prolonged ingestion of dietary fibers on adaptive changes in mucosal transport functions require attention. Schwartz and Levine (1980) reported that sustained supplementation with cellulose or pectin resulted in impaired glucose transport and also modified the sodium and chloride fluxes in rat jejunal mucosa (Schwartz et al., 1982). Our own studies on impaired or delayed lipid absorption in fasted rats previously fed fiber supplements for 4–6 weeks also suggested a modification of intestinal function in response to sustained intake of various fiber derivatives.

We have recently investigated the possibility that prolonged fiber feeding could modify not only morphological characteristics of the intestine (Cassidy et al., 1980, 1982), but also nutrient absorptive functions of the intestinal epithelium (Sigleo et al., 1984). Animals were fed for 4 weeks on defined fiber-free diets or diets supplemented with either cellulose or pectin. In addition to assessing changes in villus height and width and the distance between villi, functional characteristics of the intestinal epithelium were determined by examination of the in vitro unidirectional influxes of a hexose (3-O-methylglucose, 3-O-MG) the amino acid α-aminoisobutyric acid (AIB), and sodium (Na). As shown in Table XI, sustained intake of either cellulose or pectin resulted in increases in intestinal villus height and width compared to fiber-free controls. This was attributed to an increase in the total numbers of enterocytes and goblet cells on the villus column. Studies on the unidirectional fluxes of the three nutrients by washed segments of jejunal mucosa are summarized in Table XII. As is evident, sustained intake of either fiber supplement resulted in dramatic increases in the unidirectional flux of 3-O-MG and AIB, and, to a lesser, but still significant extent, of Na^+. Kinetic analyses of the influx data (Table XII) suggested changes in K_m associated with fiber feeding, and that these changes were not simply ascribed to changes in the surface area of the intestinal mucosa.

The results of these studies confirm the earlier observations that certain dietary fiber components may modify intestinal architecture, and indicate that these structural changes may be correlated, at least in part, with altered transport characteristics of the small intestine even in the absence of the fiber source.

TABLE XI. Dietary Effects on Villus Morphology[a]

Group	Villus length (mm)	Villus width (mm)	Distance between villi (mm)
Control (18)	0.40 ± 0.01*†	0.10 ± 0.002*†	0.02 ± 0.001
Cellulose (22)	0.44 ± 0.01*	0.11 ± 0.004*	0.02 ± 0.001
Pectin (24)	0.46 ± 0.02†	0.11 ± 0.005†	0.02 ± 0.001

[a]Values are means ± SE. Animals were fed ad libitum for 4 weeks on defined diets with the inclusions indicated. Weight gains and food intake were monitored weekly, and the data (number of analyses shown in parentheses) represent means for all animals for the entire feeding period. Figures with the same superscript are significantly different from control.

TABLE XII. Dietary Effects on Intestinal Influxes of Nutrients in Vitro[a]

Group	Unidirectional influx mmol/100 mg dry wt^{-1}/min^{-1}		
	3–0–MG 1 mM	AIB 1 mM	Na$^+$ 143 mM
Control (9)	1.4 ± 0.1*†	0.7 ± 0.1*†	276 ± 22*†
Cellulose (8)	2.8 ± 0.2*	1.9 ± 0.1*	343 ± 20*
Pectin (7)	2.8 ± 0.2†	1.9 ± 0.2†	349 ± 19†

[a] Values are means ± SE. Number in parentheses represents number of animals studied. Feeding regimens are described in Table XI. AIB, α–aminoisobutyric acid: 3–0–MG, 3–0–methyglucose. Figures with the same superscripts are significantly different ($p < 0.05$).

4.2. Absorption of Lipids

There is a considerable literature on the overall effects of dietary fibers and their derivatives on general aspects of lipid metabolism, including circulating lipid and lipoprotein levels and fecal steroid levels (Kay, 1982; Vahouny, 1982). These approaches, however, do not distinguish direct or indirect effects of dietary fibers on intestinal absorption of lipids from secondary effects due to modified sugar metabolism or other responses to fiber supplementation of diets.

Hyun et al. (1963) first demonstrated that the addition of citrus pectin to an intragastrically administered lipid emulsion could inhibit the lymphatic absorption of cholesterol in rats. In these studies, the fiber supplement was included in the test meal, and it was not possible to distinguish the effect of the pectin on delayed gastric emptying from a direct effect on intestinal absorption of cholesterol.

The direct effect of viscous fiber derivatives on intestinal absorption of water-soluble and water-insoluble "nutrients" has recently been demonstrated. In the presence of guar gum or pectin, the *in vitro* transport of water-soluble molecules is retarded (Elsenhans et al., 1980; Johnson and Gee, 1981). This effect is lost if the intestinal tissue is washed prior to transport studies (Elsenhans et al., 1980), and it has been suggested that these fiber derivatives influence nutrient flux by modifying the resistance of the surface-associated unstirred water layer (Elsenhans et al., 1980; Johnson and Gee, 1981; Gerencser et al., 1984).

Similar studies have been reported on the effects of guar gum on intestinal transport of micellar cholesterol by intestinal segments *in vitro* or intestinal loops *in situ* (Gee et al., 1983). Thus, in the presence of the viscous fiber derivative, cholesterol transport was reduced in both preparations. When segments were preincubated with guar gum, cholesterol uptake was also reduced, but a lesser extent than when the fiber was present. These and other studies (Imaizumi *et al.*, 1982) suggest that viscous fibers like guar gum may interfere with bulk phase diffusion of lipids, but may also have a residual effect in limiting transmural transport of cholesterol.

In earlier studies from this laboratory (Vahouny *et al.*, 1978, 1980b), we reported that either short- or long-term feeding of defined diets containing fiber supplements or bile acid sequestrants showed a persistent influence on the absorbability of both cholesterol and triolein into thoracic duct lymph of rats. In these studies, animals were surgically provided a thoracic duct lymph drainage catheter and were fasted overnight prior to study. The lipid test emulsion was introduced directly into the stomach in the absence of additional fiber supplementation, and the results suggested that the feeding of specific fiber derivatives could have effects on intestinal lipid absorption without being present in the test meal.

These observations have been confirmed and extended by Imaizumi *et al.* (1982) using guar gum-supplemented diets prior to studies on triolein absorption into mesenteric lymph. It was also reported that absorption of the lipid was delayed in the proximal intestine and improved in the distal small intestine. However, this should result in larger chylomicrons (Sabesin *et al.* (1975), which, unfortunately was not determined. Schwartz *et al.* (1983) have also reported on modified cellular synthesis of cholesterol and phospholipid in the rat jejunum in response to feeding diets containing pectin. Phospholipids are an integral component of chylomicron membranes. If their intestinal synthesis is sufficiently altered, it is conceivable that chylomicron formation and/or secretion in the upper small intestine could be impaired.

These studies collectively suggest that certain fiber derivatives could have influences on intestinal metabolism and on the absorption of lipids, including cholesterol and triglycerides. In general, however, they do not distinguish effects of prefeeding the fibers on gastric emptying of the lipids, on possible effects of prolonged feeding on pancreatic lipase activities, or on the size and composition of intestinal chylomicrons during impaired or delayed lipid absorption.

We have recently extended our original observations (Vahouny *et al.*, 1980b, 1982), in an attempt to further elucidate the "adaptive" responses in the gastrointestinal tract in response to feeding diets supplemented with various dietary fiber derivatives. Rats were fed *ad libitum* for 4 weeks on defined diets containing no fiber or one of several "soluble" or "insoluble" fiber derivatives. These were surgically provided with a thoracic duct lymph drainage catheter and were fasted overnight.

In order to circumvent possible influences of the fibers on gastric emptying, the lipid test emulsion was introduced via an infusion catheter directly into the duodenum. The possible effect of prolonged fiber feeding on pancreatic enzyme activities, including lipase (Schneeman, 1982), was avoided by including oleic acid rather than triolein in the lipid test emulsion. Lymph was collected for 4 h to assess effects on the rapid phase of lipid absorption and from 4 to 24 h to assess total recovery of absorbed lipids. Finally, chylomicron sizes in the initial 4-h collection were assessed by scanning electron microscopy and lipoprotein lipid compositions were determined.

As shown in Fig. 6A, the absorption of oleic acid into lymph during the initial 4 h after duodenal administrations of the test emulsion was not significantly different between animals fed the fiber-free diet and those fed diets supplemented with 10% levels of insoluble fiber preparations (cellulose or alfalfa). Prefeeding diets containing viscous fiber derivatives, however, all resulted in reduced recovery of oleic acid in thoracic duct lymph. This included 10% bran–pectin (3:1), 5% pectin, 5% guar gum, 5% Metamucil, and 2% cholestyramine (a bile acid-phospholipid sequestrant). This effect was largely due to delayed absorption of the fatty acid, since, as shown in Fig. 6B, the total 24-h recoveries of absorbed fatty acid were, with one exception, the same for all dietary groups. The persistent effect of prefeeding Metamucil-containing diets on oleic acid absorption may be due to the drastic effects of this material on the morphology, and likely the function, of the small intestine.

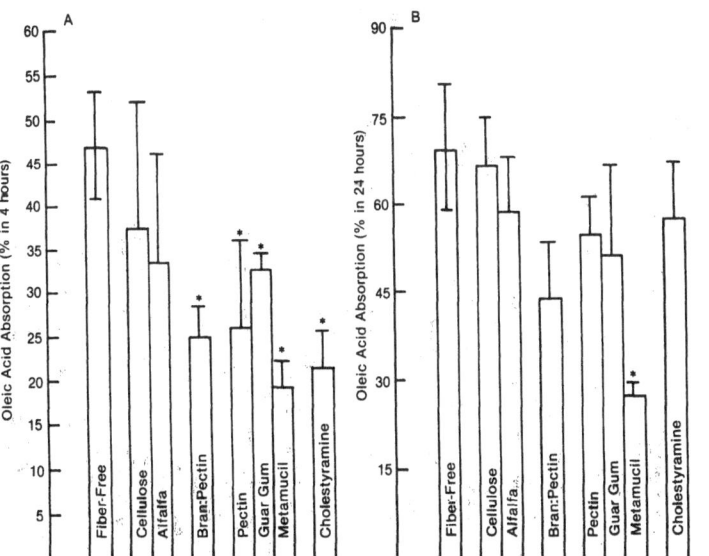

FIGURE 6. Absorption of oleic acid (145 mg) in the thoracic duct lymph of fasted rats fed for 4 weeks ad libitum on defined diets containing: no fiber; 10% cellulose, alfalfa, or a bran–pectin (3:1) mixture; 5% pectin, guar gum, or Metamucil; or 2% cholestyramine. (A) Recovery during the first 4 h after an intraduodenal lipid test dose. (B) Recovery by 24 h after the lipid dose. Asterisks indicate significant differences ($p < 0.05$) from fiber-free group.

These data suggest that viscous fiber derivatives delay, but do not impair, fatty acid absorption in the rat, and are in contrast to the inhibition of triglyceride digestion and absorption observed earlier with these same feeding approaches (Vahouny *et al.*, 1982).

The effect of prefeeding diets containing these fiber supplements on sebsequent cholesterol absorption in fasted rats is shown in Fig. 7. All of the isoluble and soluble fiber derivatives had a dramatic effect on the absorption of cholesterol into lymph during the initial 4 h of collection (Fig. 7A). However, in contrast to fatty acid absorption, the overall 24-h recoveries, improved only with the insoluble fiber derivatives (Fig. 7B). With the soluble fiber derivatives, cholesterol absorption, as assessed by 24-h lymph recoveries, not only was delayed, but was impaired.

Despite these effects of fiber supplementation on either delayed or impaired absorption of fatty acid and cholesterol, there were no differences in chylomicron sizes for any of the dietary groups when assessed by morphometric analysis of scanning electron micrographs.

The distributions of absorbed oleic acid and cholesterol among the major lymph lipoprotein fractions are summarized in Tables XIII and XIV. In general, absorbed oleic acid was largely (90%–95%) recovered in lymph

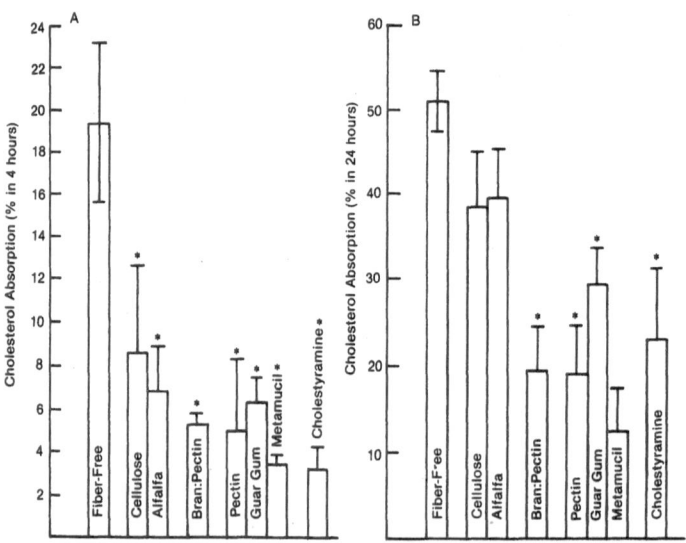

FIGURE 7. Absorption of cholesterol (25 mg) in the thoracic duct lymph of fasted rats fed for 4 weeks *ad libitum* on defined diets containing: no fiber; 10% cellulose, alfalfa, or a bran–pectin (3:1) mixture; 5% pectin, guar gum, or Metamucil; or 2% cholestyramine. (A) Recovery during the first 4 h after an intraduodenal lipid test dose. (B) Recovery by 24 h after the lipid dose. Asterisks indicate significant differences ($p < 0.05$) from fiber-free group.

TABLE XIII. Distribution of Absorbed Oleic Acid among the Lymph
Lipoproteins of Rats Prefed Diets Containing Various
Fiber Derivatives

Dietary group	Distribution of oleic acid[a], %			
	Chylomicrons	VLDL	LDL	HDL
Fiber-free	77.9	18.3	2.6	1.1
Cellulose, 10%	73.9	17.4	7.6	1.1
Alfalfa, 10%	85.4[b]	10.2[b]	2.2	2.2
Bran–pectin (3:1) 10%	77.6	18.9	2.5	0.9
Pectin, 5%	63.3[b]	25.8[b]	7.8[b]	3.1
Guar gum, 5%	86.1[b]	11.3[b]	1.4	0.9
Metamucil, 5%	83.5	11.8	3.1	1.2
Cholestyramine, 2%	80.0	15.5	3.9	0.7

[a] Abbreviations: VLDL, very low-density lipoproteins; LDL, low-density lipoproteins; HDL, high-density lipoproteins.
[b] $p < 0.05$ from fiber-free controls.

chylomicrons and very low-density lipoproteins (VLDL), and of this, about 80% associated with the chylomicron fraction, and largely (85%) as triglycerides (Table XV). Similarly, the majority of absorbed cholesterol is associated with chylomicrons and VLDL (Table XIV), but with this lipid, a larger fraction of absorbed cholesterol is associated with the smaller VLDL particles (Vahouny et al., 1980b).

With alfalfa- and guar-containing diets, there appeared to be a greater recovery of oleic acid (and of cholesterol in the case of guar gum) with the chylomicron fractions, while with the pectin-containing diet, there was less recovery of both lipids in this fraction. In no case, however, were there differences in the distribution of oleic acid among the major lipid fractions of of the chylomicrons (Table XV). These lipoprotein separations are based on differential ultracentrifugal flotations at a density of 1.006 g/ml, and differences in distribution of lipids, particularly between slightly larger chylomicrons and smaller VLDLs, are largely arbitrary. If the entire $d < 1.006$ g/ml lipoproteins are combined, there are no significant differences in either lipoprotein or lipid distribution among the dietary groups.

These and the earlier studies (Vahouny et al., 1978, 1980b; Imaizumi et al., 1982; Schwartz et al., 1983) all suggest that the effects of dietary fiber supplementation cannot be simply explained by effects on gastric emptying or by interference with bulk phase diffusion of lipids in the intestinal lumen.

TABLE XIV. Distribution of Absorbed Cholesterol among Lymph Lipoproteins of Rats Prefed Various Fiber Derivatives

Dietary group	Distribution of absorbed cholesterol[a], %			
	Chylomicrons	VLDL	LDL	HDL
Fiber-free	67.7	20.4	7.2	4.7
Cellulose	65.2	24.9	6.2	3.7
Alfalfa	66.2	19.9	6.0	7.9
Bran–pectin (3:1)	69.8	22.0	5.6	2.6
Pectin	50.6[b]	33.7[b]	10.6	5.0
Guar gum	81.1[b]	11.6[b]	4.8	2.5
Metamucil	64.1	17.1	14.5[b]	4.4
Cholestyramine	72.6	17.4	8.7	1.2

[a] For abbreviations see Table XIII.
[b] $p < 0.05$ from fiber-free controls.

The delayed absorption of oleic acid due to fiber prefeeding observed in fasted rats might be a result of altered motility of the intestine and/or modified intestinal transit times, a modification of the intestinal transport diffusion barriers, such as mucins and the unstirred water layer (e.g., Elsenhans *et al.*, 1980), a modification of intestinal phopholipid turnover (Schwartz *et al.*, 1983), or other, as yet unknown effects. In any case, all of these potential mechanisms imply that dietary fiber supplementation may exert effects on lipid transport in the intestine that cannot be accounted for by the acute presence of the fiber derivative in the intestine.

TABLE XV. Distribution of Absorbed Oleic Acid among Major Lymph Chylomicron Lipids

Dietary group	Distribution of oleic acid[a], %				
	TG	MG-DG	FA	PL	CE
Fiber-free	85	4	7	1	3
Cellulose	87	2	7	2	3
Alfalfa	84	3	9	1	3
Bran–pectin (3:1)	84	4	5	3	4
Pectin	89	3	3	3	2
Guar gum	87	2	5	2	4
Metamucil	88	2	4	2	4
Cholestyramine	83	3	7	2	6

[a] Abbreviations: TG, triglycerides; MG-DG, mono- and diglycerides; FA, unesterified fatty acid; PL, phospholipids; CE, cholesterol esters.

5. CONCLUSIONS

It appears likely that dietary fibers in general and specific fiber derivatives in particular can markedly alter various aspects of gastrointestinal physiology. This is at least in part a result of modified gastric emptying, altered rates of availability and transport of intestinal nutrients, and modified cellular metabolism. The range of "adaptive" alterations is apparently even more diverse that are the acute responses to fiber supplements. Effects on intestinal morphology and topography are apparent in both immature and mature animals, and could be expected to be associated with altered cytokinetics and functions of the intestinal tract.

In this chapter we have attempted to review specific aspects of morphological and functional modifications of the small intestine in response to chronic intake of various fiber supplements. The areas discussed are by no means all-inclusive, and are presented largely to indicate the wide range of potential primary and secondary responses to dietary fiber intake. Further studies along these and other lines will improve our understanding of the overall effects of increased dietary fiber intake and of the use of specific fiber supplements for various therapeutic applications.

ACKNOWLEDGMENTS. The authors wish to acknowledge the significant contributions of their colleagues, including Drs. R. Calvert, T. Le, D. Kritchevsky, J. Story, B. Schneeman, and M. Jackson, and S. Satchithanandam, R. Briggs, I. Chen, I. Iffram, and F. Lightfoot.

Portions of these studies were supported by grants from the U.S. Department of Agriculture, the U.S. Public Health Service, ITT Continental Baking Co., Rye, New York, and Farma Foods, McLean, Virginia.

REFERENCES

Asano, T., Pollard, M., and Madsen, D.C., 1975, Effects of cholestyramine on 1,2-dimethylhydrazine-induced enteric carcinoma in germ free rats, *Proc. Soc. Exp. Biol. Med.* **150**:780–785.

Baker, S. J., Ignatino, M., Mathan, V. L., Waich, S. K., and Chacko, C. C., 1962, Intestinal biopsy in tropical sprue, in: *Intestinal Biopsy* (G. E. W. Wolstanholme and M. P. Cameron, eds.), Churchill, London, p. 82.

Belanger, L. F., 1954, Autoradiographic visualization of S^{35} incorporation and turnover by the mucous glands of the gastro-intestinal tract and other soft tissues of rat and hamster, *Anat. Rec.* **118**:755–771.

Brown, R. C., Kelleher, J., and Losowsky, M. S., 1979, The effect of pectin on the structure and function of the rat small intestine, *Br. J. Nutr.* **42**:357–365.

Brown, W. R., Isobe, Y., and Nakane, P. K., 1976, Studies on translocation of immunoglobulin across intestinal epithelium II. Immuno-electron-microscopic localization of immunoglobulins and secretory component in human intestinal mucosa, *Gastroenterology* **71**:985–995.

Calvert, R., Satchithanandam, S., Cassidy, M. M., and Vahouny, G. V., 1984, Dietary fiber and intestinal adaptation: Effect on mucosal protein and specific crypt and villus enzyme activities, *Fed. Proc.* **43**:4561.

Cassidy, M. M., Lightfoot, F. G., Grau, L. E., Roy, T., Kritchevsky, D., and Vahouny, G. V., 1980, Effect of bile salt-binding resin on the morphology of rat jejunum and colon: A scanning electron microscopy study, *Dig. Dis. Sci.* **25**:504–512.

Cassidy, M. M., Lightfoot, F. G., and Vahouny, G. V., 1981a, Structural functional modulation of mucin secretory patterns, in: *Structure and Function in Epithelia* (M. Dinno, ed.), A. R. Liss, New York, pp. 97–127.

Cassidy, M. M., Lightfoot, F. G., Grau, L, Story, J. A., Kritchevsky, D., and Vahouny, G. V., 1981b, Effect of chronic intake of dietary fibers on the ultrastructural topography of the rat jejunum and colon, *Am. J. Clin. Nutr.* **34**:218–228.

Cassidy, M. M., Lightfoot, F. G., and Vahouny, G. V., 1982, Morphological aspects of dietary-fiber in the intestine, *Adv. Lipid Res.* **19**:–229.

Chacko, C. J. G., Paulson, K. A., Mathan, V. I., and Bahu, S. J., 1969, The villus architecture of the small intestine in the tropics. A necroscopy study, *J. Pathol.* **98**:146–151.

Cook, G. C., Kajubi, S. K., and Lu, F. D., 1969, Jejunal morphology of the African in Uganda, *J. Pathol.* **98**:157–169.

Creamer, B., 1974, Intestinal structure in relation to absorption, *Biomembranes* **4A**:1–42.

Dawson, A. M., and Isselbacher, K. J., 1960, Studies on lipid metabolism in the small intestine with observations on the role of bile salt, *J. Clin. Invest.* **39**:730–740.

Dreiling, D. A., and Messer, J., 1978, The secretin story, *Am. J. Gastroenterol.* **70**:455–479.

Dworkin, L. D., Levine, G. M., Farber, J. J., and Spector, N. H., 1976, Small intestinal mass of the rat is partially determined by indirect effects on intraluminal nutrition, *Gastroenterology* **71**:626–630.

Elsenhans, B., Süfke, U., Blume, R., and Caspary, W. F., 1980, The influence of carbohydrate gelling agents on rat intestinal transport of monosaccharides and neutral amino acids *in vitro, Clin. Sci.* **59**:373–380.

Elsenhans, B., Süfke, U., Blume, R., and Caspary, W. F., 1981, *In vitro* inhibition of rat intestinal surface hydrolysis of disaccharides and dipeptides by guaran, *Digestion* **21**:98–103.

Elsenhans, B., Zenker, D., Caspary, W. F., and Blume, R. 1984, Guaran effect on rat intestinal absorption, *Gastroenterology* **86**:645–653.

Forstner, J. F., Fabbal, I., and Forstner, G., 1973, Goblet cell mucin of rat small intestine. Chemical and physical characterization, *Can. J. Biochem.* **51**:1154–1166.

Gee, J. M., Blackburn, N. A., and Johnson, I. T., 1983, The influence of guar gum on intestinal cholesterol transport in the rat, *Br. J. Nutr.* **50**:215–224.

Gerencser, G. A., Cerda, J., Burgin, C., Baig, M. M., and Guild, R., 1984, Unstirred water layers in rat intestine: Effects of pectin, *Proc. Soc. Exp. Biol. Med.* **176**:183–186.

Hageman, R. F., and Stragand, J., 1977, Fasting and refeeding: Cell kinetic response of jejunum, ileum and colon, *Cell Tiss. Kinet.* **10**:3–14.

Heaton, K. W., 1983, Dietary fiber in perspective, *Hum. Nutr. Clin. Nutr.* **37C**:151–170.

Hill, M. J., 1982, Bile acids and human colorectal cancers, in: *Dietary Fiber in Health and Disease* (G. V. Vahouny and D. Kritchevsky, eds.), Plenum, New York, pp. 299–312.

Hyun, S. A., Vahouny, G. V., and Treadwell, C. R., 1963, Effect of hypocholesterolemic agents on intestinal cholesterol absorption, *Proc. Soc. Exp. Biol. Med.* **112**:469–501.

Imaizumi, K., Tominaga, A., Maivatari, K., and Sugano, M., 1982, Effect of cellulose and guar gum on the secretion of mesenteric lymph chylomicrons in meal-fed rats, *Nutr. Rep. Int.* **26**:263–269.

Jacobs, L. R., and White, F. A., 1983, Modulation of mucosal cell proliferation in the intestine of rats fed a wheat bran diet, *Am. J. Clin. Nutr.* **37**:945–953.

Jenkins, D. J. A., 1980, Dietary fiber and carbohydrate metabolism, in: *Medical Aspects of Dietary Fiber* (G. A. Spiller and R. M. Kay, eds.), Plenum, New York, pp. 175–192.

Johnson, I. T., and Gee, J. M., 1981, Effect of gel-forming gums on intestinal unstirred layer and sugar transport *in vitro, Gut* **22:**398–403.

Kay, R. M., 1982, Dietary fiber *J. Lipid Res.* **23:**221–242.

Kritchevsky, D., and Story, J. A., 1974, Binding of bile salts *in vitro* by nonnutritive fiber *J. Nutr.* **104:**458–462.

Lamm, M. E., 1976, Cellular aspects of immunoglobulin A, *Adv. Immunol.* **22:**223–290.

Lebenthal, E., and Clark, B., 1981, Immunoglobulin concentrations in the duodenal fluids of infants and children, *Am. J. Gastroenterol.* **75:**436–439.

Leeds, A. R., 1982, Modification of intestinal absorption by dietary fiber and fiber components, in: *Dietary Fiber in Health and Disease* (G. Vahouny and D. Kritchevsky, eds.), Plenum, New York, pp. 53–71.

Lemaitre-Coelho, I., Jackson, G. D. F., and Vaerman, J. P., 1977, Rat bile as a convenient source of secretory IgA and free secretory component, *Eur. J. Immunol.* **8:**588–590.

Lemaitre-Coelho, I., Jackson, G. D. F., and Vaerman, J. P., 1978, Relevance of biliary IgA antibodies in rat intestinal immunity, *Scand. J. Immunol.* **8:**459–463.

Leveille, G. A., and Sauberlich, H. E., 1966, Mechanism of the cholesterol-depressing effect of pectin in the cholesterol-fed rat, *J. Nutr.* **88:**209–214.

Lipkin, M., 1981, Proliferation and differentiation of gastrointestinal cells in normal and disease states, in: *Physiology of the Gastrointestinal Tract* (L. R. Johnson, J. Christensen, M. I. Grossman, E. D. Jacobson, and S. G. Schulz, eds.), Raven, New York, pp. 145–168.

Loehry, C. A., and Creamer, B., 1968, Three-dimensional structure of rat small intestine related to mucosal dynamics, *Gut* **10:**112–120.

Low-Beer, T. S., Schneider, R. E., and Dobbins, W. O., 1970, Morphological changes of the small intestinal mucosa of guinea pig and hamster following incubation *in vitro* and perfusion *in vivo* with unconjugated bile salts, *Gut* **11:**486–492.

Maudsley, D. V., Lief, J., and Kobayashi, Y., 1976, Ornithine decarboxylase in rat small intestine: Stimulation with food or insulin, *Am. J. Physiol.* **231:**1557–1561.

Mekhijian, H. S., and Phillips, S. F., 1970, Perfusion of the canine colon with unconjugated bile acids: Effect on water and electrolyte transport, morphology and bile acid absorption, *Gastroenterology* **59:**120–129.

Mehijian, H. S., Phillips, S. F., and Hofmann, A. F., 1971, Colonic secretion of water and electrolytes induced by bile acids: Perfusion studies in man, *J. Clin. Invest.* **50:**1569–1577.

Moe, H., 1955, On goblet cells, especially of the intestine of some mammalian species, *Int. Rev. Cytol.* **4:**299–334.

Ofuso, F., Forstner, J., and Forstner, G., 1978, Mucin degradation in the intestine, *Biochim. Biophys. Acta* **543:**476–483.

Oku, T., Akamatsu, A., and Hosoya, N., 1982, Property and physiological role of biliary secretory IgA in rats, *J. Nutr. Sci. Vitaminol.* **28:**643–653.

Owen, R. L., and Brandborg, L. L., 1977, Jejunal morphologic consequences of vegetarian diet in humans, *Gastroenterology* **72:**A88–A88.

Roth, H. P., and Mehlman, M. A. (eds.), 1978, Symposium on Role of Dietary Fiber in Health, *Am. J. Clin. Nutr.* **31** (Suppl.).

Sabesin, S. M., Holt, P. R., and Clark, S. B., 1975, Intestinal lipid absorption: Evidence for an intrinsic defect of chylomicron secretion by normal rat distal intestine, *Lipids* **10:**840–846.

Schneeman, B. O., 1982, Pancreatic and digestive function, in: *Dietary Fiber in Health and Disease* (G. V. Vahouny and D. Kritchevsky, eds.), Plenum, New York, pp. 73–83.

Schwartz, S. E., and Levine, G. D., 1980, Effects of dietary fiber on intestinal glucose absorption and glucose tolerance in rats, *Gastroenterology* **79:**833–836.

Schwartz, S. E., Levine, G. D., and Starr, C. M., 1982, Effect of dietary fiber on intestinal ion fluxes in rats, *Am. J. Clin. Nutr.* **36:**1102–1105.

Schwartz, S. E., Starr, C., Bachman, S., and Holtzapple, P. G., 1983, Dietary fiber decreases cholesterol and phospholipid synthesis in rat intestine, *J. Lipid Res.* **24:**746–752.

Sigdestad, C. P., Bauman, J., and Lesher, S., 1969, Diurnal fluctuations in the number of cells, mitosis and DNA synthesis in the jejunum of the mouse, *Exp. Cell Res.* **58:**159–162.

Sigleo, S., Jackson, M. J., and Vahouny, G. V., 1984, Effects of dietary fiber constituents on intestinal morphology and nutrient transport, *Am. J. Physiol.* **246:**G34–39.

Sladen, G. E., and Harries, J. T., 1972, Studies on the effects of unconjugated dihydroxy bile salts on rat small intestinal function *in vivo, Biochim. Biophys. Acta* **288:**443–456.

Smithson, K. W., Millar, D. B., Jacobs, L. R., and Gray, G. M., 1981, Intestinal diffusion barrier: Unstirred water layer or membrane surface mucus coat?, *Science* **214:**1241–1244.

Spiller, G.A., and Kay, R. M. (eds.), 1980, *Medical Aspects of Dietary Fiber,* Plenum, New York.

Sprinz, H., 1971, Factors influencing intestinal cell renewal, *Cancer* **28:**71–74.

Stenning, G. F., and Grossman, M. I., 1969, Hormonal control of Brunner's glands, *Gastroenterology* **56:**1047–1052.

Story, J. A., 1980, Dietary fiber and lipid metabolism: An update, in: *Medical Aspects of Dietary Fiber* (G. A. Spiller and R. M. Kay, eds.), Plenum, New York, pp. 137–152.

Story, J. A., and Thomas, J. N., 1982, Modification of bile acid spectrum by dietary fiber, in: *Dietary Fiber in Health and Disease* (G. V. Vahouny and D. Kritchevsky, eds.), Plenum, New York, pp. 193–201.

Tasman-Jones, C., 1980, Effects of dietary fiber on the structure and function of the small intestine, in: *Medical Aspects of Dietary Fiber* (G. A. Spiller and R. M. Kay, eds.), Plenum, New York, pp. 67–74.

Tasman-Jones, C., Jones, A. L., and Owen, R. L., 1978, Jejunal morphological consequences of dietary fiber in rats, *Gastroenterology* **74:**1102.

Teem, M. V., and Phillips, S. F., 1972, Perfusion of hamster jejunum with conjugated and unconjugated bile acids: Inhibition of water absorption and effects on morphology, *Gastroenterology* **62:**261–267.

Thomsen, L. L., and Tasman-Jones, C., 1982, Disaccharidase levels in rat jejunum are altered by dietary fibre, *Digestion* **23:**253–258.

Thomsen, L. L., Tasman-Jones, C., and Maher, C., 1983, Effects of dietary fat and gel-forming substances on rat jejunal disaccharidase levels, *Digestion* **26:**124–130.

Vaerman, J.-P., 1981, Single radial immunodiffusion, *Meth. Enzymol.* **73:**291–305.

Vahouny, G. V., 1982, Dietary fiber, lipid metabolism and atherosclerosis, *Fed. Proc. Fed. Am. Soc. Exp. Biol.* **41:**2801–2806.

Vahouny, G. V., and Kritchevsky, D. (eds.), 1982, *Dietary Fiber in Health and Disease,* Plenum, New York.

Vahouny, G. V., Roy, T., Gallo, L. L., Story, J. A., Kritchevsky, D., Cassidy, M. M., Grund, B., and Treadwell, C. R., 1978, Dietary fiber and lymphatic absorption of cholesterol in the rat, *Am. J. Clin. Nutr.* **31:**S208–212.

Vahouny, G. V., Blendermann, E. M., Gallo, L. L., and Treadwell, C. R., 1980a, Differential transport of cholesterol and oleic acid in lymph lipoproteins: Sex differences in puromycin sensitivity, *J. Lipid Res.* **21:**415–424.

Vahouny, G. V., Roy, T., Gallo, L. L., Story, J. A., Kritchevsky, D., and Cassidy, M. M., 1980b, Dietary fibers III. Effect of chronic intake on cholesterol absorption and metabolism in the rat, *Am. J. Clin. Nutr.* **33:**2182–2191.

Vahouny, G. V., Tombes, R., Cassidy, M. M., Kritchevsky, D., and Gallo, L. L., 1980c, Dietary fibers V. Binding of bile salts, phospholipids and cholesterol from mixed micelles by bile acid sequestrants and dietary fibers, *Lipids* **15:**1012–1018.

Vahouny, G. V., Tombes, R., Cassidy, M. M., Kritchevsky, D., and Gallo, L. L., 1981, Dietary fiber VI. Binding of fatty acids and monolein from mixed micelles containing bile salts and lecithin, *Proc. Soc. Exp. Biol. Med.* **166:**12–16.

Vahouny, G. V., Satchithanandam, S., Lightfoot, F., Grau, L., Haas-Smith, S., Kritchevsky, D., and Cassidy, M. M., 1984, Morphological disruption of colonic mucosa by free or cholestyramine-bound bile acids, *Dig. Dis. Sci.* **29:**432–442.

Walker, W. A., and Isselbacher, K. J., 1977, Intestinal antibodies, *N. Engl. J. Med.* **297:**767–773.

Williams, S. E., and Turnberg, L. A., 1980, Retardation of acid diffusion by pig gastric mucins, *Gastroenterology* **79:**299–304.

Younoszai, M. K., Adedoyin, M., and Ranshaw, J., 1978, Dietary components and gastrointestinal growth in rats, *J. Nutr.* **108:**341–350.

14

Dietary Fiber and Gastrointestinal Epithelial Cell Proliferation

LUCIEN R. JACOBS

1. INTRODUCTION

The use of high-fiber diets in the treatment and prevention of gastrointestinal disorders has markedly increased in recent years. In view of this widespread popularity for consuming diets rich in fiber, it has become increasingly important to determine what effects the different forms of dietary fiber have on the epithelial lining of the gastrointestinal tract. Older studies mostly concluded that consumption of diets high in bulk or fiber produced little or no change in the gastrointestinal epithelium. However, with the advent of newer, more sensitive techniques, recent studies have demonstrated that dietary fibers produce marked alterations in the morphology and cell renewal of the gastrointestinal epithelium. These morphological and cytokinetic changes appear to have important implications for maintaining a normal healthy epithelium and preventing mucosal disease. The development and refinement of techniques that measure the mucosal topography, cell size and number, rates of cell mitoses and migration, DNA synthesis, and cell cycle times have all enhanced our ability to study dietary perturbations of gut epithelial cell proliferation. This chapter will review principles and

LUCIEN R. JACOBS • Department of Internal Medicine, Division of Gastroenterology, School of Medicine, University of California, Davis, California 95616.

techniques for measuring cell proliferation and their application to studying the effects of the fiber on the gastrointestinal mucosa.

2. PRINCIPLES OF GASTROINTESTINAL EPITHELIAL CELL PROLIFERATION

Turnover of the gastrointestinal epithelium involves the proliferation, migration, differentiation, and eventual exfoliation of epithelial cells. Epithelial cell renewal begins within the proliferative zone of the gastrointestinal mucosal layer (Fig. 1). Within these zones stem cells divide, providing a constant source of new cells, many of which migrate toward the gut lumen, into which they are eventually exfoliated. As the cells migrate they mature, becoming more differentiated, while at the same time losing their capacity to proliferate. During the process of cell division, cells undergo a sequence of phases, which together constitute the cell cycle (Fig. 2). Following completion of mitosis (M phase), proliferating cells enter the first portion of the interphase, or the postmitotic–presynthetic gap (G_1 phase), during which cells contain their normal ($2N$) diploid DNA content. DNA synthesis occurring during the S phase results in a variable content of DNA per cell. This is then followed by another interval, the postsynthetic–premitotic gap or G_2 phase, during which cells contain twice the diploid DNA content ($4N$) in preparation for mitosis. As shown in Fig. 2, cells that have undergone mitosis do not necessarily continue the cyclic process of cell division. Some cells may enter a dormant or prolonged G_1 phase called the G_0 phase, during which DNA synthesis and mitosis are temporarily suspended, but the potential for cell

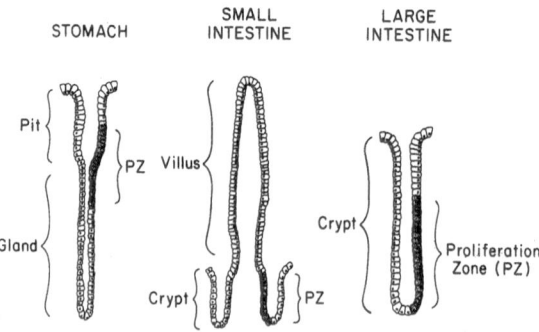

FIGURE 1. The proliferation zone (PZ) in the stomach, small, and large intestine. The PZ is illustrated by the shaded cells, which are the site of [³H]thymidine incorporation and can be identified by autoradiographic techniques. The PZ of the stomach extends from the isthmus and neck of the glands up into the base of the pits. In the small intestine the PZ is confined to the crypts. In the large bowel the PZ occupies the lower two-thirds of the crypt.

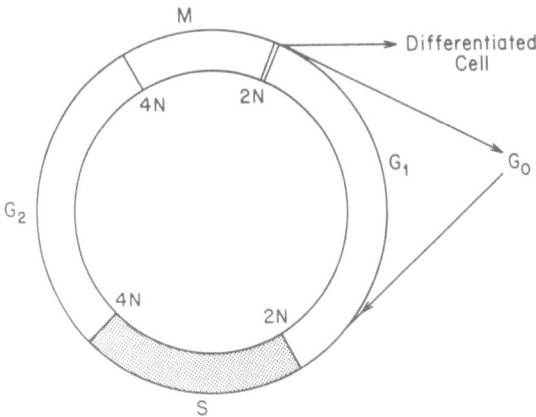

FIGURE 2. Phases of the cell cycle. M, mitosis; G_1, postmitotic-presynthetic gap; G_0, dormant, prolonged G_1; S, DNA synthesis; G_2, postsynthetic-premitotic gap; normal diploid (2N) DNA content.

proliferation remains. Other cells, on completion of mitosis, enter a non-proliferative phase, migrate out of the proliferative zone, and differentiate into mature cells.

The duration of the cell cycle phase can be estimated using autoradiographic techniques to count the percentage of mitoses that are labeled at various times after a pulse label of [³H]thymidine. For example, if the first labeled mitosis does not appear until 1 h after injection of the thymidine, then the minimum duration of the G_2 phase is 1 h. This is because for a mitotic figure to be labeled, the radioisotope must be incorporated into DNA during the time new DNA is being synthesized. Other cells that are in mid or early S phase at the time of the thymidine pulse label will demonstrate labeled mitosis at a later time. Thus, over a period of time the fraction of labeled mitoses rises, falls, and then rises again as the events of the cell cycle recur. Estimates for the durations of the other phases of the cell cycle can be made by analyzing the configuration and duration of the first wave of labeled mitoses and the time between the first and second waves. The total duration of the cell renewal cycle in human gastric and intestinal epithelium varies from 1 to 2 days. In general the S phase requires about 10 h, G_2 phase 1–6 h, and the M phase approximately 1 h.

2.1 Stomach

The proliferative zone of the stomach is located in the upper portion of the glands (isthmus and neck) and the contiguous portion of the base of the pits (Fig. 1). Cells migrate upward into the pits and onto the mucosal surface to replace the exfoliated surface cells. The turnover of this population varies from one area of the stomach to another, which may explain the variation in migration times from 2 to 3 days for rodents and from 2 to 6 days for humans. Other dividing cells appear to replenish cell loss occurring within the glands.

2.2 Small Intestine

Proliferation here is confined to the crypts (Fig. 1). Four major epithelial cell types, including columnar, mucus, Paneth, and enteroendocrine cells, are present. The columnar cells originate at the base of the crypts and differentiate as they migrate up the crypts, onto the villi, and then up to the villus tips, from where they are finally extruded into the bowel lumen. This process requires 2–3 days in rodents and approximately 5–6 days in man.

2.3 Large Intestine

This is composed of closely spaced crypts, which open onto a flat surface. The proliferative zone comprises the basal two-thirds of the crypt (Fig. 1). Cells migrate up from the proliferative zone toward the gut lumen and are eventually extruded from the mucosal surface between the crypts. As in the small intestine, the three main types of epithelial cells are columnar, mucus, and enteroendocrine. All three types probably arise from common stem cells located in the base of the crypts. Epithelial cell migration in the large intestine of rodents takes 2–3 days, whereas in humans estimates range from 3 to 8 days. For a more detailed review and bibliography of gastrointestinal epithelial cell proliferation, the reader is referred to Eastwood (1977) and Appleton et al. (1980).

3. TECHNIQUES FOR EVALUATING MUCOSAL CELL PROLIFERATION

The simplest and probably still most widely used group of methods to evaluate epithelial cell proliferation utilize light microscopic techniques. By examining intact histological sections, overall villus and/or crypt architecture can be assessed. In addition, any mucosal damage or presence of inflammatory cells can be determined. Histological measurements provide a measure of the number of epithelial cells within the intestinal crypt and on the villus. Such measurements have been found to be useful for detecting changes in total cell number, such as occur with the development of mucosal hyperplasia or atrophy. Estimation of the number of crypt cells in mitosis provides a measure of mitotic activity, usually expressed as the mitotic index. However, due to the low levels of mitotic activity present within the colon, this measurement alone may be relatively insensitive and subject to considerable variation. The sensitivity of this measurement can be enhanced by prior administration and incorporation of [^{3}H]thymidine into DNA. Incorporation of this isotope can then be measured either chemically or by autoradiography.

Biochemical measurements of DNA synthesis by liquid scintillation counting of extracted DNA is simple and quick, but subject to certain errors (Al-Muktar *et al.*, 1982; Maurer, 1981). Because the entire mucosal layer is removed and then subjected to DNA extraction, no anatomic localization of DNA-synthesizing cells is obtained. Thus, if there are changes in the nonproliferation compartment equal to those occurring in the proliferation zone, then no alteration in the specific activity of the DNA will be detected. On the other hand, if the size of the nonproliferating compartment increases while the proliferation zone remains constant, specific activity of DNA will decrease and could be misinterpreted as showing a decrease in DNA synthesis. Thymidine uptake into DNA is also influenced by the activity of DNA salvage pathway enzymes, changes in thymidine pool sizes, and the transport of thymidine through the cell membrane and incorporation into nonepithelial cell populations (which will be included in scintillation counting of whole tissue).

Autoradiography provides a significant improvement over this technique by permitting localization and measurement of those cells that are synthesizing DNA (S phase). In addition, the number of cells in the nonproliferative compartment can also be estimated. The major shortcoming of this technique is that it is time-consuming and two-dimensional. Since the intestine is a three-dimensional structure, changes that occur in the crypt–villus ratio and the number of villi or crypts per unit area of intestine are unlikely to be detected by two-dimensional autoradiography unless combined with stereological techniques (Elias and Hyde, 1980). Under these circumstances, scanning electron microscopy is an extremely useful methodology, since it provides topographic information about the intestinal epithelial structure. However, routine electron microscopy does not provide reliable quantitative information about the rates of cell proliferation. If this is required, then more than one technique may be needed. Al-Muktar *et al.* (1982) have strongly advocated measuring the crypt cell production rate, which can be achieved by combining the metaphase arrest method with crypt microdissection.

A more recent approach to measuring intestinal cell proliferation utilizes the technique of flow cytometry (Cheng and Bjerknes, 1982). In this procedure individual cells are isolated from the mucoal epithelium and suspended in solution. The cells are then stained for DNA content using propidium iodide, a fluorescent marker, following which the amount of fluorescence in each individual cell is measured by passing the cell suspension through a flow cytometer. Using this technique, 5000 cells/sec can be counted and the number of cells in the whole epithelial population that are in S phase estimated. In addition, as illustrated in Fig. 3, the percentage of cells in G_1, G_0, and $G_2 + M$ can also be estimated. However, one of the drawbacks of flow cytometery is that it does not provide anatomic localization of proliferative changes. For example, if there is a change in the location of the proliferative zone within the crypt, then this will not be detected by flow cytometry. By combining this technique with measurements of bromodeoxyuridine incorporation (Dolbeare *et al.*, 1983), cell cycle traverse rates can also be estimated.

In summary, it would appear that most of these techniques have their strengths and weaknesses and that they should therefore be selected according to the nature of the question to be asked. In many situations we have found that a combination of different methodologies will together provide a more global picture of the morphological and proliferative changes occurring in the mucosal epithelium.

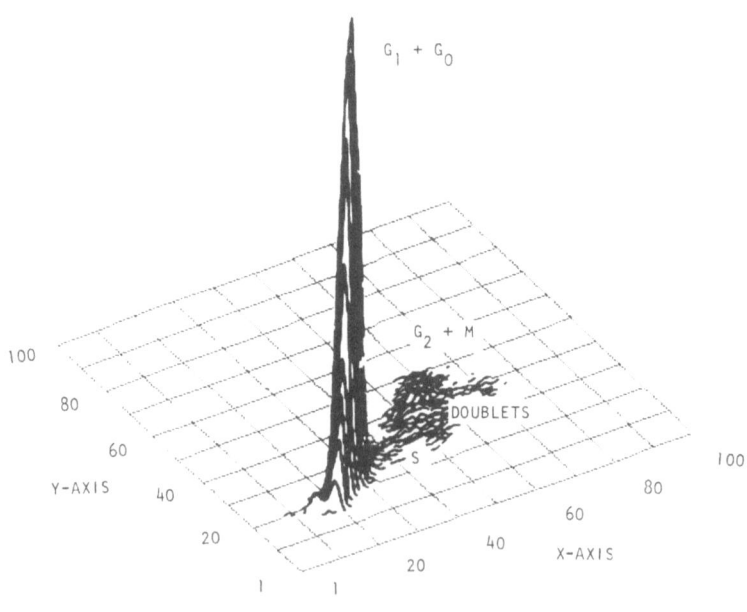

RED-FL, PEAK/Y VS AREA/X

FIGURE 3. Bivariate DNA histogram of rat colonic epithelial cells stained with propidium iodide. DNA pulse area is represented on the x-axis, DNA pulse height on the y-axis, and cell number in the third dimension. G_1, G_0, G_2, and M phase are defined in the legend to Fig. 2. Doublets refer to paired clumps of cells.

4. DIETARY FIBER AND GASTRIC EPITHELIAL CELL PROLIFERATION

Consumption of diets high in fiber correlates directly with the incidence of gastric cancer (Mirvish, 1983). However, it has not yet been established whether this relationship is one of cause and effect. Since most cancer-promoting agents stimulate cell replication in the target organ, the possibility arises of whether dietary fiber might produce such an effect in the stomach. A recent study (Lupton and Jacobs, 1983) examined this question, measuring the effect on gastric mucosal proliferation of several experimental diets, including a control fiber-free diet, or the same diet uniformly diluted by the addition of either 20% oat bran, 20% wheat bran, 10% pectin, or 10% guar. These diets were fed to rats for a minimum of 4 weeks, following which cell proliferation studies were carried out on the gastric mucosa. Measurements of DNA, RNA, and DNA synthesis revealed no differences among the dietary treatments. However, autoradiographic studies showed that all dietary fibers stimulated cell replication within the gastric mucosal glands when compared with the fiber-free control diet. Expansion of the proliferation zone in the fiber-fed animals resulted in the proliferation zone occupying a larger percentage of the total mucosal thickness than in the fiber-free control.

The proliferation zone of the groups fed fiber-supplemented diets showed evidence of increased mitogenic activity together with a decrease in mucosal thickness when compared to the control group ($p < 0.01$). For example, the mucosal thickness of the guar-fed group was only three-quarters of that found in the control group ($p < 0.01$). The higher proliferative activity in the presence of mucosal atrophy suggests that fiber increases the rate of gastric mucosal cell exfoliation. The implications of these results for the pathogenesis of gastric cancer remains to be more fully evaluated. Nevertheless, based on these preliminary data, a promoter effect by dietary fiber on gastric tumorigenesis appears to be a distinct possibility. However, further experimental studies incorporating carcinogen administration need to be performed before this question can be considered any further.

5. FIBER AND SMALL BOWEL MUCOSAL EPITHELIAL CELL PROLIFERATION

A number of recent studies have shown that certain dietary fibers alter small intestinal mucosal morphology, in contrast to many earlier reports, which indicated that supplemental dietary bulk or fiber had no effect on small intestinal growth. Ultrastructural investigations have demonstrated that dietary fibers such as bran, cellulose, pectin, and alfalfa all produce topographic alterations, some of which are consistent with increased desquamation (Cassidy *et al.*, 1981; Tasman-Jones *et al.*, 1982). Brown *et al.* (1979) showed that dietary pectin produced deeper jejunal crypts, while Schwartz and Levine (1980) noted a trend toward shorter villi. Elsenhans *et al.* (1981) found that guar, when compared to other gelling agents, produced the greatest increase in small intestinal mucosal mass. However, none of these studies examined the effects of dietary fiber on intestinal cytokinetics. Earlier investigations using bulk agents such as agar (Fischer, 1957) and kaolin (Dowling *et al.*, 1967) found no evidence of any effect on small intestinal growth, whereas feeding of chemically defined diets (Morin *et al.*, 1980; Ecknauer *et al.*, 1981) is associated with the development of small intestinal mucosal hypoplasia. After a period of fasting, refeeding with a low-residue diet produces a depressed response in jejunal proliferative activity when compared to a normal diet (Hagemann and Stragand, 1977). These reports provide evidence that exclusion of dietary fiber from the diet leads to decreased proliferative activity and cell hypoplasia.

We have recently compared the effects of three different forms of dietary fiber—oat bran, pectin, and guar—with total fiber deprivation and studied the response to these diets on small intestinal morphometrics and epithelial cell proliferation (Jacobs, 1983a). The diet containing 10% guar by weight was the only diet to produce a significant increase in small bowel mucosal mass when compared to the controls fed the fiber-free diet ($p < 0.05$). The diet containing 10% pectin by weight produced a slight but significant reduction in villus height and an increase in crypt column length when compared to the control group ($p < 0.05$). The labeling index distribution curves for pectin and guar were shifted to the right of the control curve (Fig. 4), while the labeling index distribution for oat bran was shifted to the left, indicating an increase and decrease, respectively, in labeling index. A high rate of epithelial cell migration in the pectin- and guar-fed groups shortened their estimated villus cell transit times to 36.4 ± 0.7 and 37.0 ± 1.4 h, respectively, when compared with 42.6 ± 1.2 h in the oat bran and 41.1 ± 1.0 h in the control ($p < 0.05$). The addition of cellulose to the diet has been found to stimulate small bowel mitotic activity (Gordon *et al.*, 1983) and increase the rate of cell renewal (Ecknauer *et al.*, 1981). These results show that modulation of small intestinal mucosal structure and growth by dietary fiber appears to be mediated through alterations in epithelial proliferation and that these changes depend not only on the quantity but also the quality of the fiber present in the diet.

6. DIETARY FIBER AND LARGE BOWEL MUCOSAL CELL PROLIFERATION

Among the most frequent reasons for implementing high-fiber diets has been the treatment of colonic disorders, including constipation, irritable

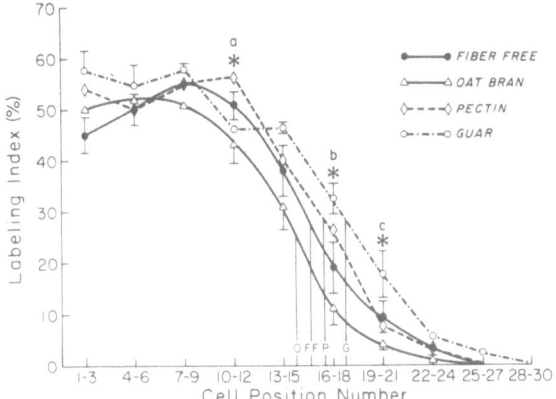

FIGURE 4. Effect of dietary fiber on the 1-hour labeling index distribution curve for rat jejunal crypts, as expressed for every three cell positions. The perpendicular lines represent the upper limit of the proliferation zone and are drawn at the cell positions of the 50% peak value for the fiber-free (FF) diet and for those containing oat bran (O), pectin (P), and guar (G). Each point on a curve is the mean ±SEM of five animals. (a) Pectin > oat bran and guar ($p < 0.05$); (b) guar > oat bran and fiber-free; pectin > oat bran ($p < 0.05$); (c) guar > oat bran and pectin ($p < 0.05$). [Reprinted from Jacobs 1983a by permission.]

bowel syndrome, and diverticular disease, and in the prevention of colonic cancer. Despite this broad range of indications for using dietary fiber, there is still a relative lack of information concerning its effect upon the large intestinal epithelium. Jacobs and Schneeman (1981) demonstrated that the feeding of a wheat bran diet for 2 weeks produces colonic mucosal cell hyperplasia. In order to investigate the mechanism for this observed increase in colonic cell number, cytokinetic studies were subsequently carried out (Jacobs and White, 1983). Male Sprague-Dawley rats were fed a diet containing a 20% wheat bran supplement for a minimun of 4 weeks. At the end of this time there was no change in small intestinal mucosal DNA or DNA synthesis. In contrast, large intestinal mucosal DNA was increased by 59.1% in the cecum ($p < 0.001$), by 28.3% in the proximal colon ($p < 0.001$), and by 35.6% in the distal colon ($p < 0.02$) when compared with the controls fed the fiber-free diet. Measurements of mucosal cell DNA synthesis, cell proliferation, and migration demonstrated evidence of decreased cell exfoliation in the cecum, with a 45.2% decrease in cell migration ($p < 0.05$), whereas in the proximal colon cell proliferation was significantly enhanced, with a cell migration rate that was 114.3% greater than that observed in the control group ($p < 0.005$). In the proximal colon (Fig. 5) the wheat bran diet produced little change in the labeling index at 1 h except for a 21.2% decrease at cell positions 4–6 when compared with the control ($p < 0.05$). However, 23 h

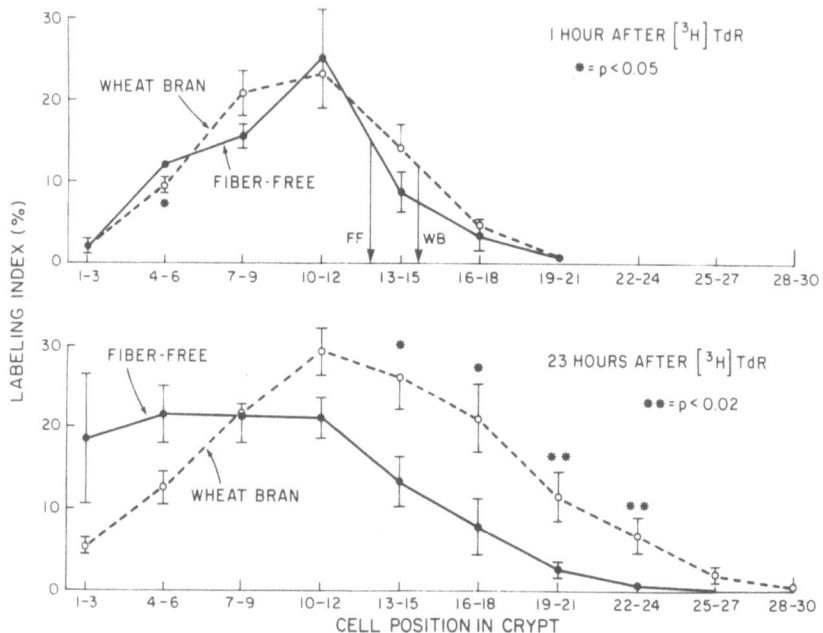

FIGURE 5. Effect of dietary wheat bran on the labeling index distribution curve for rat proximal colonic crypts, as expressed for every three cell positions 1 and 23 h after [³H]thymidine (³[H]TdR). The perpendicular lines in the upper panel represent the upper limit of the proliferation zone and are drawn at the cell positions of the 50% peak value for the fiber-free (FF) and wheat bran (WB) diets. Each point on the curves is the mean ± SEM of five control and 10 bran-fed animals. * $p < 0.05$; ** $p < 0.02$. [Reprinted from Jacobs and White, 1983 by permission.]

following the pulse label of [³H]thymidine (Fig. 5) the bran diet had produced a significant shift in the labeling index distribution curve to the right, indicating an increased labeling index in the upper half of the crypt as compared with the control group ($p < 0.05$ to $p < 0.02$). This increase in labeling index was associated with an upward shift of the proliferation compartment, which was 16.1% larger than that seen in the control group.

In order to explore which properties of wheat bran might be important in stimulating colonic mucosal cell turnover, a further study was carried out in which the colonic cell proliferative response to three other forms of fiber were compared (Jacobs and Lupton, 1984). The three fibers studied were oat bran, pectin, and guar. Compared with the other two fibers, a 10% guar diet produced the largest stimulation of mucosal growth, an effect that was greater in the cecum than in the colon. Indices of epithelial cell proliferation showed evidence of increased mitotic activity and a longer cell turnover time.

The combination of an increase in cell production and slowing in cell turnover (Fig. 6) and hence a decreased rate of cell exfoliation must result in an accumulation of mucosal epithelial cells, as confirmed by the observed increase in mucosal mass. Although pectin was also fed at a 10% level by weight, its effect on mucosal growth was significantly less than that observed with guar. Nevertheless, pectin produced a considerable simulus to large intestinal mucosal cell number, as measured by an increase in total DNA, which again, like guar, was more marked in the cecum that in the colon. Measurements of cell proliferation revealed that pectin feeding was associated

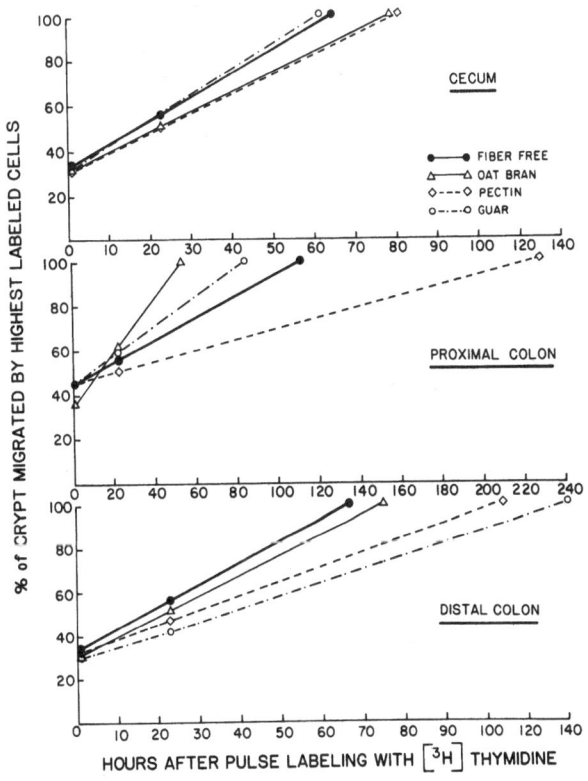

FIGURE 6. Effect of dietary fiber on epithelial cell migration in cecum, proximal, and distal colon. Points at 1-h are the leading edge of labeled cells per mean crypt height. Points at 23 h are the leading edge of labeled cells at 23 h per mean crypt height. The hour at which the leading edge is projected to reach the top of the crypt was calculated by subtracting 23-h values from the crypt height and dividing by the migration rate. This number was then added to 23. The slope of the line is the migration rate. The time taken for the leading edge of labeled cells to migrate 100% of the crypt length was defined as the turnover time. [Reprinted with permission from Jacobs and Lupton, 1984.]

with a longer colonic cell turnover time (Fig. 6), which suggests that the major reason for the observed increase in mucosal DNA was a slowing of cell migration and hence, as with the guar-fed group, an accumulation of epithelial cells within the mucosa. In contrast with the other two fibers, the diet containing oat bran produced no effect on total mucosal growth. However, there was evidence of a change in colonic crypt epithelial cytokinetics, with a shorter turnover time (Fig. 6) and an increase in labeling of cells within the proliferation zone. With oat bran the increased epithelial cell replication appears to have been equal in magnitude to the increase in exfoliation, thereby resulting in no overall change in total mucosal cell growth.

In contrast to dietary wheat bran, which produced a greater hyperplastic response in the distal colonic mucosa (Jacobs and White, 1983), guar and pectin produced their greater effect proximally (Jacobs and Lupton, 1984). Furthermore, the mechanism of cell hyperplasia appears to be different with individual fibers. An increase in proliferative activity and epithelial cell migration was observed in the proximal colon of the wheat bran-fed rats (Jacobs and White, 1983), whereas with pectin and guar, there was a slowing of migration time. This suggests that, although a number of fibers may produce colonic hyperproliferation, the mechanisms of action can be very different.

The finding that pectin and guar, even when fed in equal amounts, produce marked differences in large bowel proliferative response is of considerable interest. Both pectin and guar share many physiochemical properties. Both are water-soluble and form gels, in addition to being highly degradable by intestinal bacteria (Kay and Strasberg, 1978). A comparable degree of mechanical distension of the intestine is therefore likely to have occurred with the feeding of these two fibers. The observed differences in proliferative response by the intestine therefore suggests that distension alone is not a major factor in the regulation of large-bowel cell proliferation. Further evidence to support this view comes from studies in which kaolin, an inert form of bulk, failed to prevent the mucosal atrophy that develops in rodents fed a fiber-free diet (Goodlad and Wright, 1983), in contrast to dietary cellulose, which does prevent mucosal atrophy and stimulates colonic mucosal DNA synthesis (Sircar et al., 1983).

Pectin and guar both produced the greatest increase in mucosal cell growth within the cecum, a lesser effect occurring in the more distal colon. This may mean that fiber is most trophic while it remains intact, and that as bacterial fermentation proceeds, this action is dissipated (Elsenhans et al., 1981). However, the absence of effects or the presence of relatively minor effects of dietary fibers on small bowel proliferation tends to discount this theory. Another explanation is that the trophic effects of fiber are mediated through its fermentation products, which are produced maximally in the cecum (Kay and Strasberg, 1978). Pectin and guar are almost completely fermented within the large intestine (Nyman and Asp, 1982), although fermentation of pectin may be reduced in the more highly methoxylated forms, as used in our own experiment (Nyman and Asp, 1982), which could explain why its trophic effects were less than that of guar. Fermentation of pectin and guar results in significant production of volatile fatty acids (Cummings, 1981), which have been shown to produce a hyperproliferative effect on the colonic epithelium (Sakata *et al.*, 1980). Differences in the types as well as the amount of acids produced may also influence the trophic response to dietary fibers. For example, pectin does not produce branch-chain volatile fatty acids (Thomson *et al.*, 1982). If these volatile fatty acids stimulate cell proliferation, then this may explain in part why guar produced a greater hyperproliferative response than pectin.

Fermentation of fiber and the production of volatile fatty acids also result in acidification of luminal contents and feces (Jacobs and Lupton, 1982). In order to evaluate the relative role of colonic luminal acidification on mucosal cell proliferation, we recently carried out an experiment (Lupton *et al.*, 1984) in which experimental fiber-free diets were fed to rats in order to obtain a range of pH values by acidifying and alkalinizing large bowel contents. This was achieved by feeding either lactulose or sorbitol, two poorly digested carbohydrates, or magnesium sulfate, which raises colonic pH. Cell proliferation was examined by flow cytometry and it was shown that there was a direct relationship between the level of cell proliferation, as measured by the percentage of cells in S phase, and the pH of colonic contents. This relationship was most marked in the cecum, where, as pH was lowered, cell proliferation increased. In the more distal regions of the large bowel it was more difficult to achieve acidification by these dietary modifications and therefore no relationship between luminal pH and epithelial cell proliferation could be demonstrated. Of the various volatile fatty acids produced from poorly digested substrates such as fiber, butyrate appears to be the most effective stimulant to cell proliferation, possibly because it is preferentially metabolized by the colonic epithelium (Sakata *et al.*, 1980).

Dietary fibers may also influence intestinal cell growth through the binding of luminal factors known to influence epithelial cell proliferation. For example, fibers bind inorganic ions (James, 1980) such as calcium, which is known to play an important part in the control of cell proliferation (Durham and Walton, 1982). In addition, binding can also occur with bile acids that have been shown to produce mucosal cell surface damage (Chadwick *et al.*, 1979) and, in turn, higher rates of cell exfoliation, resulting in a compensatory stimulation of cell synthesis (Deschner *et al.*, 1981). Oat bran, pectin, and guar absorb bile acids (Kay and Strasberg, 1978), thereby increasing fecal bile excretion. Guar, a neutral storage polysaccharide, has a greater bile acid binding capacity than pectin, which is an acidic polysaccharide and therefore would be expected to produce a greater stimulation of cell proliferation, as has been observed.

Any alteration in exfoliation must be mediated through the factors that regulate mucosal cell loss or extrusion. The intestinal mucus coat has long been considered to protect the mucosal surface (Florey, 1955). Recent evidence suggests that the intestinal mucus coat may be effectively increased by feeding fiber, such as wheat bran. Ultrastructural studies (Cassidy et al., 1981) have demonstrated a qualitative increase in goblet cell activity and secreted mucin in the colon of bran-fed animals, while quantitative studies have revealed a significant increase in large intestinal mucosal goblet cells of wheat bran-fed rats (Schneeman et al., 1982). These findings may therefore explain why cell exfoliation appears to be decreased in the cecum of wheat bran-fed rats.

7. DIETARY FIBER, CELL PROLIFERATION, AND COLON CANCER

Recent investigations have shown that consumption of a number of different fibers, including wheat bran, pectin, guar, and cellulose, produces colonic epithelial cell hyperplasia and associated changes in cell proliferation. These growth-stimulating properties of certain fibers are of some theoretical concern, since a hyperplastic response, due to nondietary perturbations, has previously been associated with an increased incidence of experimentally induced cancer, both in the colon and other tumor model systems. For example, small bowel resection (Oscarson et al., 1979) and diversion of pancreatic and biliary secretions to the large intestine (Williamson et al., 1979) produce colonic mucosal hyperplasia and enhancement of experimental colon carcinogenesis. Mice inoculated with the bacterium *Citrobacter freundii* develop mucosal hyperplasia and increased expression of chemical-induced focal atypia (Barthold and Beck, 1980). Feeding of bile acids such as cholic acid also produces enhancement of colonic epithelial cell proliferation and a greater frequency of colonic tumors (Cohen et al., 1980). On the other hand, the feeding of ascorbic acid and butylated hydroxyanisole decreases colonic epithelial cell proliferation (Deschner and Wattenberg, 1982; Deschner et al., 1983) and inhibits colon carcinogenesis (Wattenberg and Sparnens, 1979; Reddy et al., 1982).

These observations have led to the proposal that any dietary component that stimulates intestinal cell proliferation, such as wheat bran, could enhance colon tumor development. Evidence to support this comes from the recent demonstration that colon carcinogenesis is enhanced in those rats fed wheat bran during the period of 1,2-dimethylhydrazine (DMH) administration

(Jacobs, 1983b). In a more recent followup study, it was found that dietary wheat bran produced a stimulation of colonic crypt cell proliferative activity (Fig. 7) that was most marked in the proximal colon and was greatest when wheat bran was consumed during the stage of carcinogenic exposure (Jacobs, 1984). This suggests that wheat bran acts by modifying the stage of tumor initiation. A possible mechanism of action is a greater susceptibility of colonic cells to DNA damage, due to the stimulation of proliferative activity and/or a reduction in the DNA repair mechanisms of the cell, occurring as a result of the increased rate of cell turnover and hence a reduction in the time available for effective DNA repair. Pectin, another fiber that stimulates large-bowel cell proliferation, has in one report been found to increase colonic tumor yield (Bauer *et al.*, 1979), and in another study (Freeman *et al.*, 1980) to increase the number of small bowel tumors.

These studies also illustrate how dietary fiber may be used as a probe for examining the effects of diet-induced colonic cell hyperplasia and hyperproliferation on colon carcinogenesis. Recent evidence (Jacobs, 1983b) suggests that the timing of these actions relative to the different stages of the carcinogenic process is critical in determining what the overall modifications to tumor development will be. It is important to define these mechanisms and interactions in order to understand more clearly how diet affects colon tumorigenesis. Furthermore, it is of paramount importance to determine which of the many actions of dietary fiber might enhance and which might

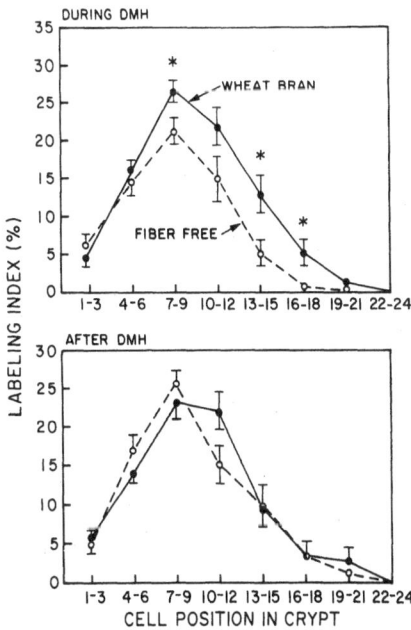

FIGURE 7. Effect of dietary wheat bran on the 1-h labeling index distribution curve for rat proximal colonic crypts, as expressed for every three cell positions. (Above) Effect of diet during stage of 1,2-dimethylhydrazine (DMH) administration. (Below) Effect of diet following stage of DMH administration. Points are means of at least ten animals; bars, SEM; * $p < 0.05$. [Reprinted with permission from Jacobs, 1984.]

protect. This will greatly aid in prospectively identifying specific dietary fibers that have a much greater protective action and avoiding those that may have tumor-promoting properties. A greater understanding of the mechanisms whereby diet modulates colon carcinogenesis appears to be essential before prospective dietary intervention studies are implemented for human population groups known to be at high risk for colon cancer.

ACKNOWLEDGMENTS. The author wishes to acknowledge the valuable assistance of Francie A. White, Joanne R. Lupton, David M. Coder, and Donald A. Martinich, without whose assistance this work could not have been fully accomplished. This work was supported in part by NCI grant CA 35627.

REFERENCES

Al-Muktar, M. Y. T., Polak, J. M., Bloom, S. R., and Wright, N. A., 1982, The search for appropriate measurements of proliferative and morphological status in studies on intestinal adaptation, in: *Mechanisms of Intestinal Adaptation* (J. W. L. Robinson, R. H. Dowling, and E.-O. Riecken, eds.), MTP, Boston, pp. 3–25.

Appleton, D. R., Sunter, J. P., and Watson, A. J., 1980, *Cell Proliferation in the Gastrointestinal Tract,* Pitman, Tunbridge Wells, England.

Barthold, S. W., and Beck, D., 1980, Modification of early dimethylhydrazine carcinogenesis by colonic mucosal hyperplasia, *Cancer Res.* **40**:4451–4455.

Bauer, H. G., Asp, N.-G., Oste, R., Dahlqvist, A., and Fredlund, P.E., 1979, Effect of dietary fiber on the induction of colorectal tumors and fecal β-glucuronidase in the rat, *Cancer Res.* **39**:3752–3756.

Brown, R. C., Kelleher, J., and Losowsky, M. S., 1979, The effect of pectin on the structure and function of the rat small intestine, *Br. J. Nutr.* **42**:357–365.

Cassidy, M. M., Lightfoot, F. G., Gray, L. E., Story, J. A., Kritchevsky, D., and Vahouny, G. V., 1981, Effect of chronic intake of dietary fibers on the ultrastructural topography of rat jejunum and colon: A scanning electron microscopy study, *Am. J. Clin. Nutr.* **34**:218–228.

Chadwick, V. S., Gaginella, T. S., Carlson, G. L., Debongnie, J.-C., Phillips, S. F., and Hoffman, A. F., 1979, Effects of molecular structure on bile acid-induced alterations in absorptive function, permeability and morphology in the perfused rabbit colon, *J. Lab. Clin. Med.* **94**:661–674.

Cheng, H., and Bjerknes, M., 1982, Whole population cell kinetics of mouse duodenal, jejunal, ileal and colonic epithelia as determined by radioautography and flow cytometry, *Anat. Rec.* **203**:251–264.

Cohen, B. I., Raicht, R. F., Deschner, E. E., Takahashi, M., Sarwal, A. N., and Fazzini, E., 1980, Effect of cholic acid feeding on *m*-methyl-*N*-nitrosourea-induced colon tumors and cell kinetics in rats, *J. Nat. Cancer Inst.* **64**:573–578.

Cummings, J. H., 1981, Short chain fatty acids in the human colon, *Gut* **22**:763–779.

Deschner, E. E., and Wattenberg, L. W., 1982, The proliferative effects of butylated hydroxyanisole on methylazoxymethanol treated colonic mucosa, *Cancer Lett.* **16**:197–202.

Deschner, E. E., Cohen, B. I., and Raicht, R. F., 1981, Acute and chronic effect of dietary cholic acid on colonic epithelial cell proliferation, *Digestion* **21**:290–296.

Deschner, E. E., Alcock, N., Okamura, T., DeCosse, J. J., and Sherlock, P., 1983, Tissue concentrations and proliferative effects of massive doses of ascorbic acid in the mouse, *Nutr. Cancer* **4**:241–246.

Dolbeare, F., Gratzner, H., Pallavicini, M. G., and Gray, J. W., 1983, Flow cytometric measurement of total DNA content and incorporated bromodeoxyuridine, *Proc. Nat. Acad. Sci. USA* **80**:5573–5577.

Dowling, R. H., Riecken, E.-O, Laws, J. W., and Booth, C. C., 1967, The intestinal response to high bulk feeding in the rat, *Clin. Sci.* **32**:1–9.

Durham, A. C. H., and Walton, J. M., 1982, Calcium ions and the control of proliferation in normal and cancer cells, *Biosci. Rep.* **2**:15–30.

Eastwood, G. L., 1977, Gastrointestinal cell renewal, *Gastroenterology* **72**:962–975.

Ecknauer, R., Sircar, B., and Johnson, L. R., 1981, Effect of dietary bulk on small intestinal morphology and cell renewal in the rat, *Gastroenterology* **81**:781–786.

Elias, H., and Hyde, D. M., 1980, An elementary introduction to stereology (quantitative microscopy), *Am. J. Anat.* **159**:411–446.

Elsenhans, B., Blume, R., and Caspary, W. F., 1981, Long-term feeding of unavailable carbohydrate gelling agents. Influence of dietary concentration and microbiological degradation on adaptive responses in the rat, *Am. J. Clin. Nutr.* **34**:1837–1848.

Fischer, J. E., 1957, Effects of feeding diets containing lactose, agar, cellulose, raw potato starch or arabinose on the dry weights of cleaned gastrointestinal tract organs in the rat, *Am. J. Physiol.* **188**:550–554.

Florey, H., 1955, Mucin and the protection of the body, *Proc. R. Soc. London B* **143**:147–158.

Freeman, H. J., Spiller, G. A., and Kim, Y. S., 1980, A double-blind study on the effects of differing purified cellulose and pectin fiber diets on 1,2-dimethylhydrazine-induced rat colonic neoplasia, *Cancer Res.* **40**:2661–2665.

Goodlad, R. A., and Wright, N. A., 1983, Effects of addition of kaolin or cellulose to an elemental diet on intestinal cell proliferation in the mouse, *Br. J. Nutr.* **50**:91–98.

Gordon, D. T., Besch-Williford, C., and Ellersieck, M. R., 1983, The action of cellulose on the intestinal mucosa and elemental absorption by the rat, *J. Nutr.* **113**:2545–2556.

Hagemann, R. F., and Stragand, J. J., 1977, Fasting and refeeding: Cell kinetic response of jejunum, ileum and colon, *Cell Tissue Kinet.* **10**:3–14.

Jacobs, L. R., 1983a, Effects of dietary fiber on mucosal growth and cell proliferation in the small intestine of the rat: A comparison of oat bran, pectin, and guar with total fiber deprivation, *Am. J. Clin. Nutr.* **37**:954–960.

Jacobs, L. R., 1983b, Enhancement of rat colon carcinogenesis by wheat bran consumption during the stage of 1,2-dimethylhydrazine administration, *Cancer Res.* **43**:4057–4061.

Jacobs, L. R., 1984, Stimulation of rat colonic crypt proliferative activity by wheat bran consumption during the stage of 1,2-dimethylhydrazine administration, *Cancer Res.* **44**:2458–2463.

Jacobs, L. R., and Lupton, J. R., 1982, Dietary wheat bran lowers colonic pH in rats, *J. Nutr.* **112**:592–594.

Jacobs, L. R., and Lupton, J. R., 1984, Effect of dietary fibers on rat large bowel mucosal growth and cell proliferation, *Am. J. Physiol.* **246** *(Gastrointest. Liver Physiol.* 9*)*:G378–G385.

Jacobs, L. R., and Schneeman, B. O., 1981, Effects of dietary wheat bran on rat colonic structure and mucosal cell growth, *J. Nutr.* **111**:798–803.

Jacobs, L. R., and White, F. A., 1983, Modulation of mucosal cell proliferation in the intestine of rats fed a wheat bran diet, *Am. J. Clin. Nutr.* **37**:945–953.

James, W. P. T., 1980, Dietary fiber and mineral absorption, in: *Medical Aspects of Dietary Fiber* (G. A. Spiller and R. M. Kay. eds.), Plenum, New York, pp. 239–259.

Kay, R. M., and Strasberg, S. M., 1978, Origin, chemistry, physiological effects and clinical importance of dietary fiber, *Clin. Invest. Med.* **1**:9–24.

Lupton, J. R., and Jacobs, L. R., 1983, Differential response of rat gastric mucosa to dietary oat bran, wheat bran, pectin and guar, *Fed. Proc. Fed. Am. Soc. Exp. Biol.* **42**:1063.

Lupton, J. R., Coder, D. M., and Jacobs, L. R., 1984, Stimulation of rat colonic epithelial cytokinetics by dietary acidification of luminal contents, *Fed. Proc. Fed. Am. Soc. Exp. Biol.* **43**:613.

Maurer, H. R., 1981, Potential pitfalls, of [³H] thymidine techniques to measure cell proliferation, *Cell Tissue Kinet.* **14**:111–120.

Mirvish, S. S., 1983, The etiology of gastric cancer. Intragastric nitrosamide formation and other theories, *J. Nat. Cancer Inst.* **71**:629–647.

Morin, C. L., Ling, V., and Bourassa, D., 1980, Small intestinal and colonic changes induced by a chemically defined diet, *Dig. Dis. Sci.* **25**:123–128.

Nyman, M., and Asp, N.-G., 1982, Fermentation of dietary fiber components in the rat intestinal tract, *Br. J. Nutr.* **47**:357–366.

Oscarson, J. E. A., Veen, H. F., Ross, J. S., and Malt, R. A., 1979, Ileal resection potentiates 1,2-dimethylhydrazine-induced colonic carcinogenesis, *Ann. Surg.* **189**:503–508.

Reddy, B. S., Hirota, N., and Katayama, S., 1982, Effect of dietary sodium ascorbate on 1,2-dimethylhydrazine- or methylnitrosourea-induced colon carcinogenesis in rats, *Carcinogenesis* **3**:1097–1099.

Sakata, T., Hikosaka, K., Shiomura, Y., and Tamate, H., 1980, The stimulatory effect of butyrate on epithelial cell proliferation in the rumen of sheep and its mediation by insulin: Differences between *in vivo* and *in vitro* studies, in: *Cell Proliferation in the Gastrointestinal Tract* (D. R. Appleton, J. P. Sunter, and A. J. Watson, eds.), Pitman, Tunbridge Wells, England, pp. 123–137.

Schneeman, B. W., Richter, B. D., and Jacobs, L. R., 1982, Response to dietary wheat bran in the exocrine pancreas and intestine of rats, *J. Nutr.* **112**:1283–286.

Schwartz, S. E., and Levine, G. D., 1980, Effects of dietary fiber on intestinal glucose absorption and glucose tolerance in rats, *Gastroenterology* **79**:833–836.

Sircar, B., Johnson, L. R., and Lichtenberger, L. M., 1983, Effect of synthetic diets on gastrointestinal mucosal DNA synthesis in rats, *Am. J. Physiol.* **244**(*Gastrointest. Liver Physiol. 7*):G327–G335.

Tasman-Jones, C., Owens, R. L., and Jones, A. L., 1982, Semipurified dietary fiber and small bowel morphology in rats, *Dig. Dis. Sci.* **27**:519–524.

Thomson, L. L., Tasman-Jones, C., Lee, S. P., and Robertson, A. M., 1982, Dietary factors in the control of pH and volatile fatty acid production in the rat cecum, in: *Colon and Nutrition* (H. Kasper and H. Goebell, eds.), MTP, Boston, pp. 47–51.

Wattenberg, L. W., and Sparnens, V. L., 1979, Inhibitory effects of butylated hydroxyanisole on methylazoxy-methanol acetate-induced neoplasia of the large intestine and on nicotinamide adenine dinucleotide-dependent alcohol dehydrogenase activity in mice, *J. Nat. Cancer Inst.* **63**:219–222.

Williamson, R. C. N., Bauer, F. L. R., Ross, J. S., Watkins, J. B., and Malt, R. A., 1979, Enhanced colonic carcinogenesis with azoxymethane in rats after pancreaticobiliary diversion to mid small bowel, *Gastroenterology* **76**:1386–1392.

15

The Effect of Fiber in the Postweaning Diet on Nutritional and Intestinal Morphological Indices in the Rat

MARIE M. CASSIDY, LEO R. FITZPATRICK and GEORGE V. VAHOUNY

1. INTRODUCTION

A number of regulatory or modulating influences have been proposed in the growth of the small and large intestine during the developmental and postnatal periods. These factors include dietary components, hormonal substances (most notably, glucocorticoids), and microbial flora (Johnson, 1981). According to Buts and de Meyer (1981), the mucosal mass of duodenal, jejunal, and ileal segments in rats increases during weaning (15–30 days postbirth) and at 40 days of age was similar to values in adult animals. It was concluded that the mucosal hyperplasia that occurs in the rat small intestine at weaning develops equally in proximal to distal segments of the bowel. In contrast to the small intestine, there is evidence that growth, differentiation, and enzymatic and absorptive characteristics of neonate rat colon undergo adaptation during the first 2 weeks of postnatal life (Helander 1973, 1975; Buts et al., 1983).

MARIE M. CASSIDY and LEO R. FITZPATRICK • Department of Physiology, George Washington University School of Medicine and Health Sciences, Washington, D. C. 20037. GEORGE V. VAHOUNY • Department of Biochemistry, George Washington University School of Medicine and Health Sciences, Washington, D. C. 20037.

Very few studies have been conducted on the effect of dietary fiber on intestinal structure and function in the weanling animal. It is known that rats have regular, finger-shaped small intestinal villi at birth, which becomes leaf-shaped and ridged when the animals mature on a standard laboratory diet. In a study using fiber-free, pectin, and cellulose diets compared to standard chow, the following observations were made. Those animals fed the zero-fiber or cellulose diets did not develop the normal leaf-shaped, ridged pattern, whereas those fed pectin were comparable to the control animals (Tasman-Jones, 1981). Younoszai et al. (1978) found that dietary oat bran and cellulose appeared to enhance the growth of the small intestine and more markedly that of the colon in young rats of weight 50–80 g. It is not known whether the observed effects and possible underlying mechanisms that affect intestinal cell growth and adaptation in the adult animal are similarly operative in the postnatal phase of development. In a series of studies aimed at characterizing the role of dietary fiber in intestinal morphogenesis and biochemical indices of growth and maturation in the weanling rat, we have explored nutritional and morphometric consequences of a liquid diet (Vivo-nex), a zero-fiber diet, regular chow, and a basal diet with either a viscous fiber additive (5% guar gum) or a high-bulk additive (10% cellulose). A particular objective was to determine whether luminal nutrition, i.e., the presence of materials in the intestinal lumen that are not necessarily absorbed, such as dietary fiber derivatives, would exert an adaptational effect on the mucosa of the maturing small and large intestine. Such effects have been previously documented in the adult animal fed these dietary regimens (Cassidy et al., 1981, 1982; Calvert et al., 1984). It was hypothesized that fibers of different sources and physicochemical properties might exhibit or reveal regulatory roles of even greater significance during the neonatal period of ontogeny when lactation is superseded by solid food.

2. MATERIALS AND METHODS

2.1. Animal Maintenance

Lactating female Sprague-Dawley rats with litters of ten male pups were obtained from Zivic-Miller Laboratories (Allison Park, Pennsylvania) or Microbiological Associates (Bethesda, Maryland). On day 12 postnatally, two rats were removed from the litter for morphological studies. The remainder of the litter was weaned at approximately day 21 after birth, on to one of five different diets. The animals were housed four to a cage and were fed either a control (chow) diet or one of four other diets (see below). Thus, equal numbers of littermates of the same age were subjected to different dietary regimens. The rats were fed for a 4-week period and food and water were provided *ad libitum*. All animals were maintained at 25° C, with a 12 h light–dark cycle. Individual body weight measurements were done weekly on rats whose tails had been marked for identification purposes. Food consumption was also monitored on a regular basis by subtracting the weight of food remaining from a known amount that had been presented. Body weight and food consumption measurements were always conducted at approximately the same part of the day to minimize diurnal variation. Figure 1 presents the major features of the experimental design of the project.

2.2. Composition of Diets

Five diets were used during the course of this study. These diets were: (1) Rodent Laboratory Chow 5001 (Ralston Purina Company, St. Louis, Missouri); (2) standard Vivonex, a nutritionally complete elemental liquid diet (Norwich-Eaton Pharmaceuticals, Norwich, New York); (3) a basal diet prepared by Bioserve; (4) the basal diet plus fiber as 10% cellulose; (5) the basal diet plus fiber as 5% guar gum. The compositions of these diets are shown in Table I.

The percent composition of vitamin present in the chow diet was calculated from the available but incomplete information provided with the diet. Vitamins that were listed were calculated to provide approximately the percentage shown in the table. This in fact may be an underestimate of the true composition. The moisture content was then assumed to make up the remainder of the diet, for the purpose of the calculations.

Similarly, the percent composition of salt mix present in the Vivonex diet was calculated from available information provided with the diet. The vitamin content was then calculated as the remaining percentage of the diet.

Lactating female Sprague-Dawley rat with litters of approximately ten male pups

↓

Group I — Male neonates during the suckling period (tissue sampled at day 12 postnatally)

↓

Rats weaned at day 21 postnatally and fed specific diets (chow, fiber-free, Vivonex, cellulose, guar gum) for a 4-week period; body weight and food consumption monitored at regular intervals

↓

Group II — Animals sacrificed at approximately 7 weeks of age; both jejunal and colonic tissues sampled in group I and group II animals for morphological measurements

FIGURE 1. Flow chart depicting experimental design.

TABLE I. Presence of Important Nutritional Components in Various Diets

	Percentage composition of diet, on a weight basis				
	Fiber-free	Cellulose	Guar	Chow	Vivonex
Carbohydrate	55	55	55	49.80	86.50
Protein	25	25	25	23.40	7.72
Fat	14	14	14	4.50	0.98
Salt mix	5	5	5	7.30	3.81
Vitamin	1	1	1	0.20	0.99[a]
Cellulose	—	10	—	—	—
Guar gum	—	—	5	—	—
Fiber	—	—	—	5.00	—
Moisture	—	—	—	9.80[a]	—
Total	100	110	105	100	100

[a]Calculated by difference.

2.3. Evaluation of Caloric Content of Diets

The caloric content of the diets was determined by a summation of the calories provided by each constituent of the diet. For example, each 100 g of the basal fiber-free diet contained 55 g dextrose, 25 g casein, and 24 g corn oil. Guthrie (1975) gives a caloric value of 3.85 cal/g of dextrose, 3.90 cal/g of casein, and 8.66 cal/g for corn oil. It was assumed that the salt mix and vitamin mix did not contribute significantly to the caloric content of the diets. Therefore, each 100 g of fiber-free diet contained (55 g × 3.85 cal/g) + (25 g × 3.90 cal/g) + (14 g × 8.66 cal/g) 430.5 cal.

Calculations of the caloric content of the 5% guar gum and 10% cellulose diets were increased an additional 5% to allow for possible caloric contribution of volatile short-chain fatty acids due to partial enzymatic hydrolysis of the fiber components in the rat cecum. This modification was incorporated based on the studies of Yang et al. (1970), who found that following the feeding of rats a chow diet containing approximately 16% protein, the volatile fatty acids that were produced provided 9.4% of the total energy requirements of the animal. The 5% value was arbitrarily selected as a reasonable estimate of the possible caloric contribution of short-chain fatty acids, since Hove and King (1979) found that with increased protein content in a rat diet the percentage of energy derived from such fatty acid production decreases. The caloric content of these specific fiber diets (cellulose and guar gum) was therefore calculated to provide approximately 451.52 cal/100 g diet.

Using similar calculations, the caloric contents of the chow and Vivonex diets were estimated to provide 358.00 and 406.50 cal/100 g diet, respectively. These diets were slightly hypocaloric to the three diets described above, primarily due to their relatively low fat content (Table I).

2.4. Morphological Measurements

The experiments described in this section were done on pair-fed litter-mates that were randomly assigned to either a control dietary group (chow) or one of four other test dietary groups. Tissue from the midjejunum and the colon from three rats from each dietary group were fixed and processed for light and electron microscopy as previously described (Cassidy *et al.*, 1981). Following the dehydration step, samples for scanning electron microscopy evaluation were critical point-dried with CO_2 and mounted on aluminum stubs (Joel Ltd., Tokyo, Japan).

The embedded tissue was sectioned longitudinally, i.e., in the narrowest dimension of the villus, showing a mucosal lining of single cells, into 500-nm sections with an MT 5000 Sorvall ultra microtome (Dupont). For the jejunal tissue, four blocks were sectioned per animal. Sections were mounted on a clean glass slide, six sections to a slide, and the slide appropriately marked as to dietary group. Four slides per block were routinely obtained; thus, a total of approximately 96 sections per animal were available for analysis.

For colonic tissue, orientation of the sections in a good plane for morphometric analysis proved more difficult, and as a result, fewer sections per animal were available from this organ location. For the colon, four blocks per animal were again sectioned. Sections, however, were mounted one or two per block on a total of four slides. Thus, approximately 24 sections per animal were obtained. Slides were graded for their overall histological quality and rated as either average, good, or excellent. The good and excellent samples were coded so that the morphologist performing the assessment was unaware of the group identification.

A total of 60 jejunal villi (approximately 20 per animal) and 40 colonic folds and crypts (approximately 10–15 per animal) were examined. Length measurements for the jejunal crypt, villus, and crypt–villus column as well as the colonic crypt were examined at a magnification of $25\times$ using a Zeiss microscope. All other measurements were carried out at a magnification of $100\times$ with oil immersion.

3. RESULTS

3.1. Nutritional Data

3.1.1. Effect of Diet on Food Consumption

The effect of the immediate postweaning diet on food consumption over the 4-week feeding period is shown in Fig. 2. Food consumption, in general, increased during the course of the study in all dietary groups, with the exception of the guar gum-fed rats. Table II shows that animals maintained

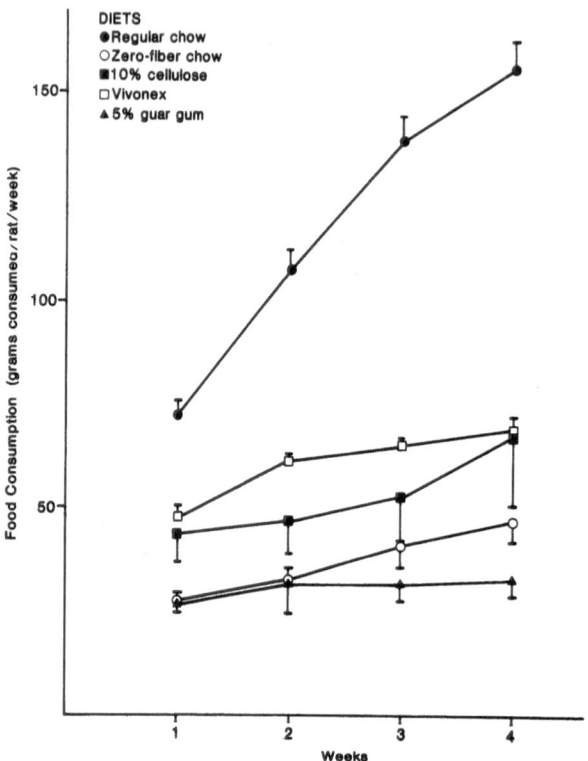

FIGURE 2. Food consumption of rats on different diets: the weekly food consumption values for rats fed different diets over a 1-month period. Points are mean values, with appropriate standard errors bars, representing 31–96 animals per dietary group.

on a chow diet consumed the largest amount of food and correspondingly the largest number of calories. In contrast, these values were lowest in the guar gum-fed rats.

3.1.2. Effect of Diet on Body Weight

Figure 3 shows the rate of body growth of rats maintained on the various postweaning diets. The average initial body weight at the time of weaning was 47 g. The largest weight gains were found in chow-fed animals and the lowest gains in guar gum-fed rats.

3.1.3. Relationship between Food (Caloric)
Consumption and Body Weight

There was a high correlation between mean food (caloric) consumption and body weight for all the diets throughout the feeding period. Correlation

TABLE II. Nutritional Data from Animals Maintained on Various
Postweaning Diets[a]

	Chow (n = 96)	Vivonex (n = 33)	Fiber-free (n = 31)	Ten percent cellulose (n = 34)	Five percent guar gum (n = 32)
Average weekly weight gain per rat	45 ± 3 ‡	16 ± 2 **	13 ± 2 **	24 ± 6 **	9 ± 2 ‡
Average weekly food intake per rat	118 ± 6 ‡	61 ± 2 * ‡	37 ± 2 **	53 ± 10 **	31 ± 2 **
Average weekly calories consumed	423 ± 20 ‡	246 ± 7 ** ‡	160 ± 6 **	238 ± 26 ** ‡	140 ± 7 **
Feed efficiency, percent gain/food	40 ± 2 †	26 ± 1 **	32 ± 3 *	46 ± 2 * ‡	28 ± 2 **
Calories consumed/grams weight gained	11 ± 3	16 ± 2	11 ± 2	10 ± 3	14 ± 3

[a] Values are mean ± SE; major statistical differences are as follows: * $p < 0.05$ from chow-fed animals, ** $p < 0.01$ from chow-fed animals, † $p < 0.05$ from fiber-free-fed animals, ‡ $p < 0.01$ from fiber-free-fed animals.

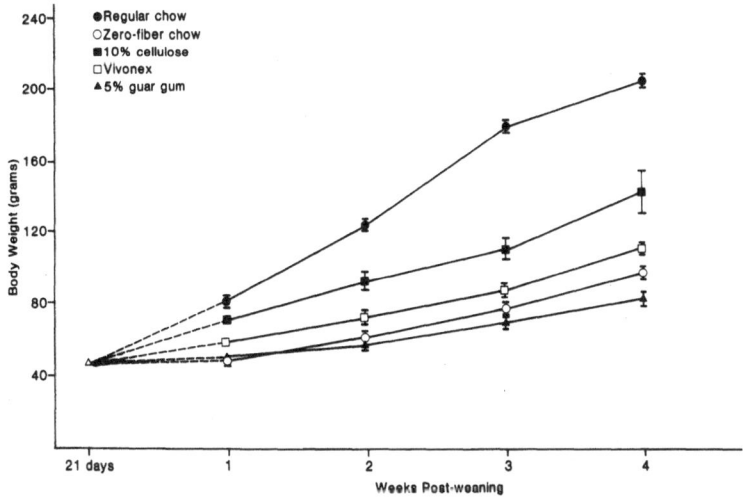

FIGURE 3. Weight gain of rats on various diets: the weekly body weight measurements for rats maintained on the various diets for a 4-week period. Points are mean values, with appropriate standard error bars, representing 31–96 animals per dietary group.

coefficients ranged from 0.82 for guar gum-fed animals to 0.99 for chow-fed rats. The overall correlation coefficient, when all the dietary groups were considered, was 0.91 when based on food consumption and 0.94 when based on caloric consumption.

The data presented in Table II show that the efficiency with which rats gained weight per amount of food consumed was highest in the 10% cellu-lose- and chow-fed rats. It should be noted, however, that approximately the same ratio of calories consumed per gram of body weight gained was found for all the dietary groups.

3.2. Effect of Diet on the Topography of Rat Jejunum by Scanning Electron Microscope

Maturational characteristics of the jejunal villi in rodents were deter-mined by classifying the villi as either finger-shaped (immature) or leaflike/ridged-shaped (mature) An average of 200 villi per condition were examined. Scanning electron micrographs illustrating various degrees of villus matura-tion are presented in Fig. 4. Villi from 12-day-old suckling rats were almost exclusively of the immature, fingerlike type characteristic of the small intes-tine of the preweaned rat. As reported by Tasman-Jones (1981), rats weaned directly onto a 10% cellulose diet exhibited little villus maturation. In the remaining diets tested, including the liquid elemental diet, the majority of the villi were of the mature leaf- or ridge-shaped variety. The chow-fed animals, in particular, showed virtually no retention of the immature, fingerlike villi. Table III is a summary of villar architectural patterns observed in animals ingesting the various diets.

The percent of midjejunal villi exhibiting various degrees of damage to the mucosal surface was determined. An average of 200 villi per condition were again examined. The degree of deviation from normal structure was graded on the following scale:

   1 = apical swelling of cells, disordered microvillar array
   2 = dimpling of swollen cell surface, partial denudation of microvilli
   3 = loss of most microvilli, tears in the apical membrane
   4 = extrusion of cell contents and loss of cells from epithelial layers

Figure 5 illustrates the nature of the necrotic effect on the jejunal villus surface evoked by some of the postweaning diets. The results summarized in Table IV indicate that animals maintained on the Vivonex, fiber-free, or guar gum diets exhibited damage to at least 30% of the villi. Animals maintained on the guar gum diet, in particular, showed the largest percent-age of villi, with moderate to severe damage to the jejunal mucosal surface. Damage to the jejunal mucosal surface with other dietary regimens was

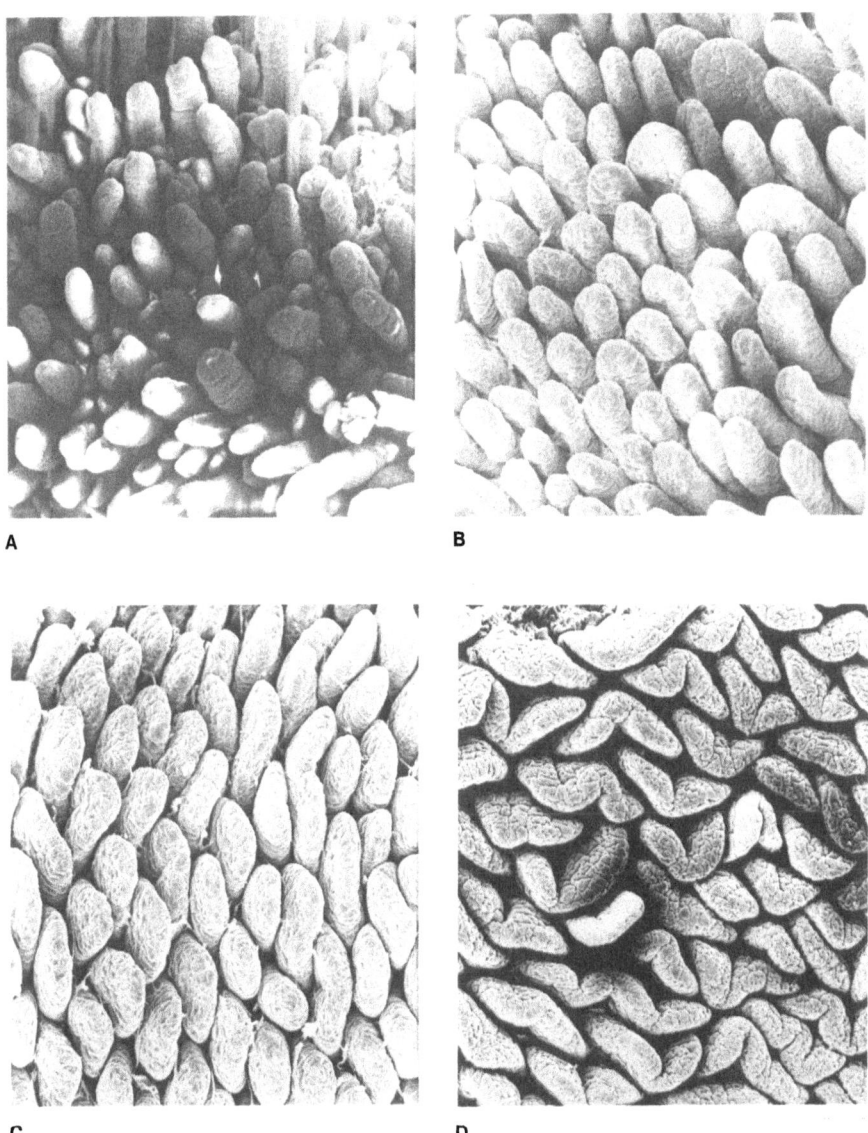

FIGURE 4. Scanning electron micrographs, showing villus maturation in rat jejunum: midjejunal villus maturation. Magnification is 100X. (A) Twelve-day-old suckling; (B) 10% cellulose diet; (C) fiber-free diet; (D) chow diet.

TABLE III. Villus Shape as Characterized by Scanning Electron Microscopy[a]

Dietary condition	Villus maturation, percent of villi of given shape	
	Finger-shaped	Leaf/ridge-shaped
Suckling (12 days old)	98	2
Chow	0	100
Vivonex	1	99
Fiber-free	5	95
10% Cellulose	79	21
5% Guar gum	20	80

[a]These are the results of approximately 200 villi per dietary condition.

minimal and the topographic ultrastructure did not differ essentially from that observed with chow-fed animals.

3.3. Effect of Diet on the Number of Jejunal Villi

Sections of the midjejunum from three rats from the mid-lactational period or maintained on the various dietary regimens were scanned for the determination of number of jejunal villi. Contact prints from sections scanned at 100X were standardized for surface area; the results are shown in Table V. Only villi that were entirely visible within the field of the photograph were counted. Largest numbers of jejunal villi were found in 12-day-old suckling animals and the least number of villi in Vivonex-fed rats.

3.4. Effect of Diet on Jejunal Mucosal Morphometrics

Table V illustrates the major morphometric characteristics of rat jejunal mucosa derived from the small intestines of animals during the lactational period or fed the different diets during the 4-week postweaning period. Crypt length is obviously greater in the chow-fed group compared to the other dietary conditions, as is total crypt plus villus length. The minimal expression of the crypt cell reservoir and villar expansion is seen in the fiber-free, cellulose, Vivonex, and guar gum groups. In the rats fed 10% cellulose, some elaboration of the villus architecture is noted, at the expense of the crypt proliferative zone. The same relationship is seen in Table V when the number of cells in the crypts and villi are compared in animals from the different groups. Figure 6 shows that there is an apparent inverse relationship between the number of villi/cm^2 and the individual villus left column count of actual cell numbers in jejunal mucosa derived from the differently fed animals.

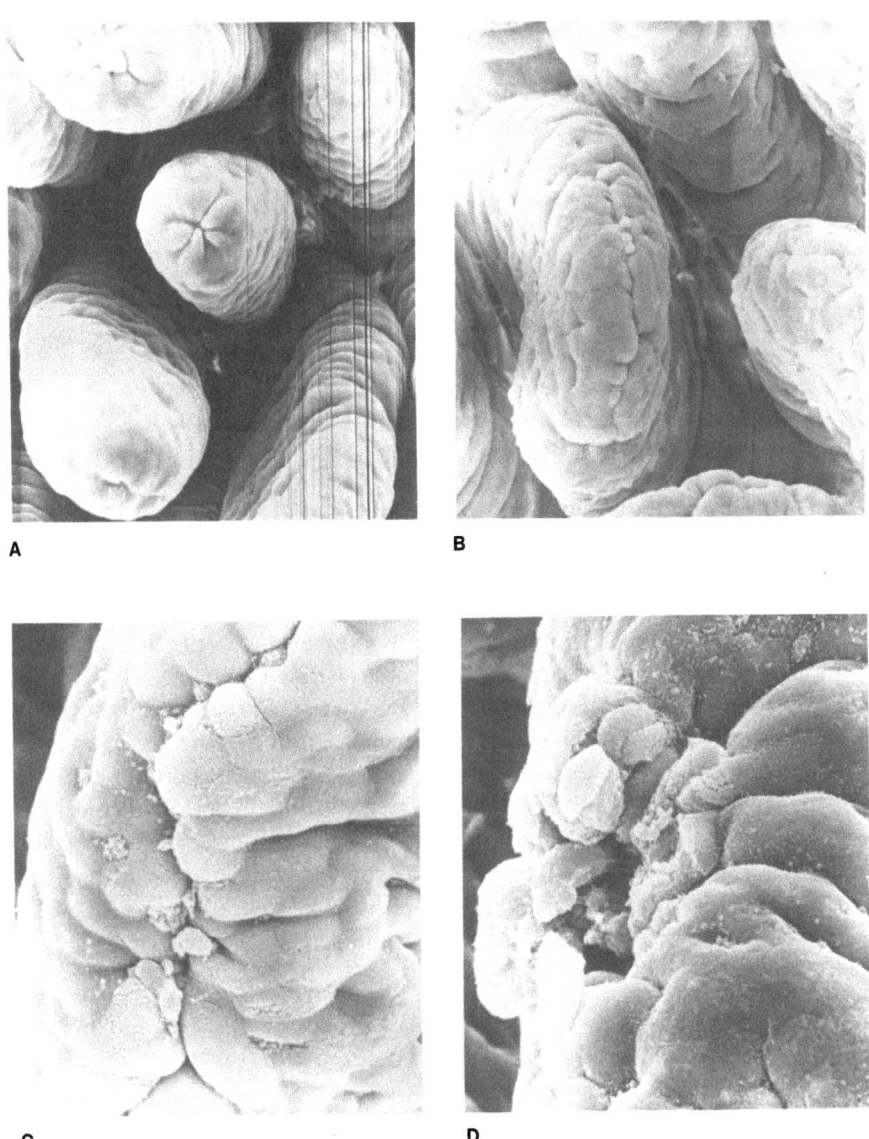

FIGURE 5. Scanning electron micrographs of villus damage in rat jejunum: the effect of the postweaning diet on jejunal morphological deviation. (A) Twelve-day-old suckling, 540×; (B) 10% cellulose diet, 540×; (C) fiber-free diet, 1800×; (D) 5% guar gum diet, 1800×.

TABLE IV. Effect of Dietary Manipulation on Various Degrees of
Damage to the Villi from the Midjejunum[a]

	Percent of villi exhibiting given degree of mucosal damage				
	Graded degree of deviation				
Dietary condition	0	1	2	3	4
Suckling (12 days old)	99	1	0	0	0
Chow	88	9	3	0	0
Vivonex	70	16	11	3	0
Fiber-free	53	34	12	1	0
10% Cellulose	95	5	0	0	0
5% Guar gum	39	30	26	5	0

[a]An average of 200 villi per dietary condition were examined.

3.5 Effect of Diet on the Topography of Rat Colon by Scanning Electron Microscopy

With respect to midcolonic characteristics of the animals on these dietary regimens, Fig. 7 displays the type of mucosal damage occurring in the colon of the neonates exposed to diets of different composition and Table VI numerically documents the varying degrees of cell damage occurring in these animals. Figure 8 shows the number of colonic folds and the number of cells in the left-hand column in the colonic samples of animals on the postweaning diets. There is no obvious statistical relationship between the number of colonic folds (microscopic configuration of the tissue) and the number of cells per fold, except that the general perception pertaining to the jejunal mucosa holds, that is, that the greater the number of microscopic evaginations of this particular epithelial surface, the fewer the number of cells one observes contributing to each particular individual "dome" in the colon. Whether this is a principle of epithelial regeneration in general or occurs only to the small and large intestine remains to be determined.

4. DISCUSSION

4.1. Nutritional Impact of the Postweaning Diet

Neonate animals that were fed either the chow or Vivonex diets, which were slightly hypocaloric in nature due to the low fat content, consumed more food than rats maintained on the other diets. Specifically, chow-fed animals consumed the most food and largest number of calories and had the largest weight gains of any dietary group (Table II). Tasman-Jones *et al.*

TABLE V. Characteristics of Jejunal Villus and Crypt Cells for Various Dietary Conditions[a]

Dietary condition	Number of jejunal villi/cm²	Crypt length, mm	Villus length, mm	Total length, mm	Number of crypt cells	Number of villus cells	Total number[b] of cells
Suckling (12 days old)	10869 ± 539 **††	—	—	—	—	—	—
Chow	4964 ± 247 †	0.073 ± 0.002 ††	0.260 ± 0.006 ††	0.333 ± 0.007 ††	22.31 ± 0.32 ††	59.95 ± 1.22 ††	81.26 ± 1.26 ††
Vivonex	3614 ± 384 *††	0.059 ± 0.001 **	0.251 ± 0.006 ††	0.310 ± 0.006 **††	20.81 ± 0.31 **††	53.60 ± 1.27 **††	74.41 ± 1.36 **††
Fiber-free	6378 ± 481 *	0.061 ± 0.001 **	0.190 ± 0.006 **	0.251 ± 0.006 **	17.13 ± 0.27 **	44.33 ± 1.44 **	61.46 ± 1.56 **
10% Cellulose	8152 ± 154 **†	0.050 ± 0.001 **††	0.276 ± 0.007 **††	0.326 ± 0.007 ††	17.50 ± 0.26 **††	53.76 ± 1.81	74.26 ± 1.82 **††
5% Guar gum	8053 ± 1417 *	0.067 ± 0.001 **††	0.232 ± 0.007 **††	0.299 ± 0.007 **††	22.69 ± 0.28 ††	51.68 ± 1.66 **††	74.37 ± 1.74 **†

[a] Three rats per dietary condition. Results are expressed as mean ± SE; major statistical differences are as follows: * $p < 0.05$ from chow-fed group, ** $p < 0.01$ from chow-fed group, † $p < 0.05$ from fiber-free group, †† $p < 0.01$ from fiber-free group.
[b] The number of cells counted in the left column of each villus and crypt in sections showing a single cell mucosal lining.

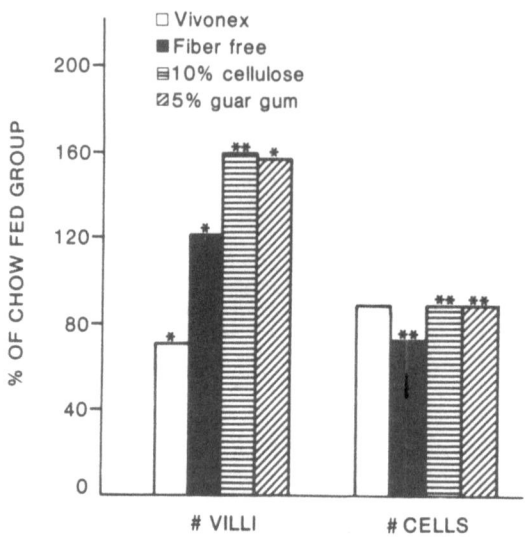

FIGURE 6. Effect of diet on villus and cell number in rat jejunum. Each parameter is expressed as a percentage of the chow-fed dietary group; * $p < 0.05$, ** $p < 0.02$.

(1982) found significantly increased body weight when male rats were weaned onto a standard laboratory diet in comparison to animals fed 10% cellulose-, 10% pectin-, or cholestyramine-supplemented diets.

In the present study, rats fed the 5% guar gum diet had the lowest weekly food and caloric consumption as well as the lowest average body weight gain. Poskay and Schneeman (1983) recently reported a significant decrease in both food intake and body weight for rats fed a 10% guar gum diet compared to either chow- or fiber-free-fed animals. They suggested that the reduced food intake could be explained in part by distension of the gut and slower disappearance of food. In humans, guar gum consumption has been associated with a 10% reduction in appetite and an increased feeling of satiety (Evans and Miller, 1975; Leeds *et al.*, 1975). Delorme and Gordon (1983) found that when another gel-type fiber, pectin, was fed to weanling rats there was a resulting decrease in both food intake and body weight gain.

Interestingly, the present study shows that rats fed the fiber-free diet also consumed lesser amounts of food and correspondingly had reduced weight gains compared to the chow-fed group. A similar observation with regard to body weight gains was reported by Tasman-Jones *et al.* (1982) after feeding weanling rats for a 12-week period. These results taken together

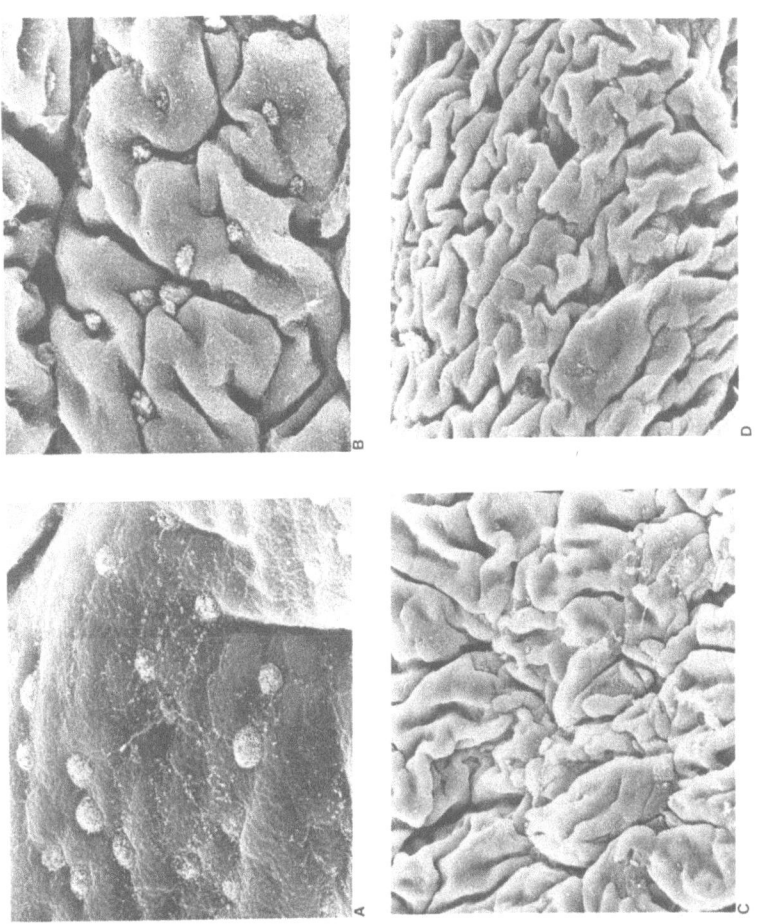

FIGURE 7. Scanning electron micrographs of damage to rat colonic folds: the effect of the postweaning diet on damage to folds of the rat midcolon. (A) Twelve-day-old suckling, 2000×; (B) Vivonex diet, 2000×; (C) chow diet, 1000×; (D) cellulose diet, 1100×.

TABLE VI. Effect of Dietary Condition on Damage to Colonic Folds

| Dietary condition | Percent of colonic folds exhibiting given degree of damage[a] | | | | |
| | Graded degree of deviation | | | | |
	0	1	2	3	4
Suckling (12 days old)	95	5	0	0	0
Chow	70	15	15	0	0
Vivonex	98	2	0	0	0
Fiber-free	95	5	0	0	0
10% Cellulose	50	30	20	0	0
5% Guar gum	87	13	0	0	0

[a]The values shown are average values, graded as described in Section 3.2. Approximately 150 colonic folds per dietary condition were examined.

suggest the need for non-gel-forming, insoluble-type fiber, which is likely to be present in a chow diet, to allow "normal" rates of body growth during the immediate postweaning period. In addition, the results from Table II indicate that the presence in the diet of 10% cellulose, a non-gel-forming, bulk-type fiber, resulted in a significant increase in weight gain, food consumption, and caloric consumption compared to fiber-free-fed animals.

In this study, food consumption and body weight gains were significantly decreased in rats fed the liquid elemental diet Vivonex compared to chow-fed rats. A similar observation has been described recently by Sircar *et al.* (1983) with regard to body weight in adult rats. Feed efficiency was highest in the chow- and 10% cellulose-fed rats. A similar value (42.6%) was reported by Hove and King (1979) for weanling rats fed a 22% casein, 10% cellulose diet to the one found for cellulose-fed animals in Table II (46.1%).

The ratio of calories consumed to weight gain (digestible energy conversion) was not statistically different among the different dietary groups. A value of 16.85 was given for the gel-type fiber pectin when fed at a 4.8% level (Delorme and Gordon, 1983). This is very close to the value (14.0) found in the present study for the gel-type fiber guar gum.

4.2. Effects of the Postweaning Diet on the Structure of the Intestine

4.2.1 Scanning Electron Microscopy: Jejunum

4.2.1a. Villus Shape and Topography. At birth, well-formed, fingerlike villi are present throughout the entire rat small intestine. As the animal grows and matures, the villi become leaf-shaped and gradually broader, so that at maturity the initial fingerlike villus pattern has been transformed into a series of parallel ridges (Baker *et al.*, 1983). The present study showed that at 12 days postnatally, 98% of the midjejunal villi scanned had maintained a fingerlike shape (Table III).

The results presented in Table III also show that animals weaned onto a standard laboratory chow diet, Vivonex, or the fiber-free diet maintained a "normal" topographic pattern of villus development. In contrast, in the jejunum of animals fed a specific form of dietary fiber as either 10% cellulose or 5% guar gum, 79 and 20% of the villi, respectively, retained the fingerlike shape characteristic of early postnatal development. These results are in partial agreement with those of Tasman-Jones *et al.* (1982), who found that compared to control chow feeding, developmental progression from finger-like to leaf- and ridge-shaped villi was delayed or absent in rats fed fiber-free, cellulose, or cholestyramine diets. It was suggested by these investigators that the mechanisms involved in the changes in villus shape with dietary manipulation were due to the additive effect of bile salts, regulatory polypeptides, and microbial composition and function. Of these possibilities, the least likely explanation of the results found in the present study would probably be an effect on villus size due to bacterial flora. Intestinal bacteria would be at lower concentrations in the jejunum than in the more distal intestine and a direct local effect would therefore be unlikely. An interesting hypothesis was originally put forward by Creamer (1967). He found in a study of human intestinal biopsies that finger-shaped villi had comparatively

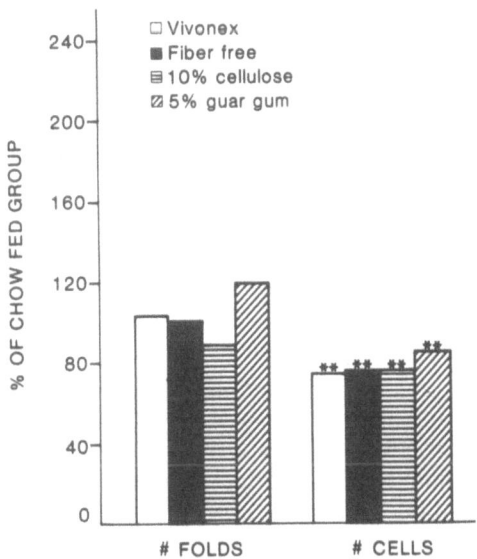

FIGURE 8. Effect of diet on number of colonic folds and cells. Each parameter is expressed as a percentage of the chow-fed group; ** $p <$ 0.01.

TABLE VII. Characteristics of Colonic Crypt Regions with Different
Dietary Regimens[a]

Dietary condition	Crypt height, mm	Number of crypt cells
Suckling (12 days old)	0.159 ± 0.004 *	22.4 ± 0.45 *
Chow	0.249 ± 0.005	40.6 ± 0.93 †
Vivonex	0.214 ± 0.004 * †	30.6 ± 0.73
Fiber-free	0.237 ± 0.004	31.0 ± 0.63
10% Cellulose	0.221 ± 0.006 *	31.0 ± 0.63
5% Guar gum	0.246 ± 0.004	35.0 ± 0.47 * †

[a] * $p < 0.01$ compared to chow-fed group, † $p < 0.01$ compared to fiber-free-fed group.

larger cell populations compared to either leaf-shaped or convoluted (ridge-shaped) villi (Creamer, 1964). He proposed that the shape of the villi was a simple matter of economics; when abundant cells were available, a fingerlike shape was formed, but with fewer cells, leaf- and ridge-like villi were present. *Some* of the adaptational responses in jejunal villi found in the present study could be explained using the Creamer hypothesis. In particular, in the jejunum of cellulose-fed animals, where 79% of the villi retained a fingerlike shape, there is an increased villus/crypt cell ratio (3.35) compared to animals fed chow (2.68) or fiber-free (2.58) diets (Table V). The villus length is also relatively large (Table V). The potential would therefore exist for a large total number of cells on the *three-dimensional surface* of the intestinal villus. In summary, therefore, the different shapes of midjejunal villi found in this work are probably the result of a combination of the effect of various extrinsic factors, such as pancreaticobilary secretions or trophic hormones, as well as a response to the total number of eipthelial cells present. This cell population is thought to be determined by an intrinsic regulation between cell loss and proliferation and can also be modified by the various extrinsic factors just mentioned.

The results presented in Table IV indicate that the structural adaptation of the jejunal mucosa was most severely affected in weanling rats fed a 5% guar gum diet for a 4-week period. Conversely, animals from the 10% cellulose dietary group showed much less intestinal villar structural abnormality. Similar results were presented by Cassidy *et al.* (1982) derived from the midjejunum of adult rats fed either a 5% pectin (gel-type fiber) or 10% cellulose diet. It should be mentioned, however, that the degree of damage with guar gum feeding in this study (61% of villi affected) was greater than that reported for pectin (31%) in adult animals and approached the levels reported for cholestryamine (64%).

4.2.1b. Number of Villi. The results (Table V) show that the largest number of villi were present in the midjejunum of 12-day-old suckling animals. Of the 4-week postweaning dietary groups, 10% cellulose- and 5% guar gum-fed animals had the largest number of villi. Specifically, the number of jejunal villi in 10% cellulose-fed rats was significantly greater than in fiber-free- or chow-fed animals. Similar results were presented by Tasman-Jones et al. (1982) in the ileum of rats fed various diets for a 2-week period after weaning. These investigators found a relatively large number of villi in the small intestine of 10% cellulose- and 5% pectin-fed rats, while the number of villi was less in fiber-free-fed rats and least in chow-fed animals. Figure 6 also demonstrates that regardless of the particular dietary regimen used, there is a consistent inverse correlation between the number of villi per unit square area and the number of cells per villus, at least in the jejunum. That is, the larger the number of villi, the smaller the cell population per villar unit.

4.2.1c. Possible Mechanisms of Structural/Functional Adaptation in the Intestine. Dowling (1982) suggested that intestinal adaptation could be classified as either physiological (type 1) or pathological (type 2). It was proposed that pathological adaptation was a repair process in response to mucosal injury (hyperplasia) or lack of trauma (hypoplasia). With pathological hyperplasia such as occurs in disease states like tropical sprue of celiac disease, the small intestinal mucosa is characterized by an enlarged crypt area with a corresponding decrease in villus size (Creamer, 1967; Williamson, 1982). The results (Table IV) from these studies show that mucosal damage was greatest in the midjejunum of fiber-free- and guar gum-fed animals. Furthermore, the data in Table V indicate increased crypt/villus length ratios in the jejunum of fiber-free- and guar gum-fed animals (0.321 and 0.289) compared to cellulose-fed rats (0.181), which had the least amount of damage to villi, as well as chow-fed rats (0.281). In addition, analysis of the data (Fig. 6) reveals that the crypt cell/villus cell ratios in the jejunum of fiber-free- and guar gum-fed rats (0.386 and 0.439) are larger than in cellulose-fed (0.308) or chow-fed (0.378) animals. Collectively, these results suggest that rats fed either the fiber-free diet or 5% guar gum diet were exhibiting type 2 or pathological small intestinal adaptational hyperplasia, similar to that described by Dowling (1982) for various intestinal disease states.

4.2.2. Colonic Topography

The data from Table VI show that the largest amount of damage to colonic folds appeared to be due to the feeding of the bulk-type fiber cellulose at a 10% level. Interestingly, relatively little damage to the midcolonic mucosa was found with the fiber-free or 5% guar gum diets (5 and 13% respectively), which caused the greatest amount of damage in the jejunum. The results of Cassidy et al. (1982) from the midcolon of adult animals showed that 22% of the folds had some degree of abnormality compared to control-fed animals (5%). This deviation from "normal" of 22% was in comparison to a value of 7.5% reported for the midjejunum in their study. Thus, the feeding of a bulk-type fiber such as cellulose apparently has a more abrasive effect on the large than the small intestine. This effect appears to be more severe during early postnatal development. The mechanisms responsible for the damage to the midcolonic folds in 10% cellulose-fed rats can only be speculated about. It is doubtful, however, that the effect is due to bile salts bound to cellulose, since the bile salt binding capacity is apparently small for cellulose (Vahouny et al., 1980b). Table VII shows that crypt depth and number of crypt cells was greater in the chow-fed animals compared to suckling animals or some of the other weaning diets.

The small and large intestines from animals in this study have also been assayed for biochemical markers of proliferation, e.g., RNA, DNA, DNA synthesis, ornithine decarboxylase activity, and cytokinetic parameters of cell production and migration. The results demonstrate certain correlations between the morphometric indices reported here and the regenerative and repair processes that are a normal and rapid characteristic of these mucosae (Fitzpatrick et al., 1983, 1984). The implication is that both the nutritional growth and the specific architectural or necrotic patterns occurring with these postweaning diets is highly associated with cell proliferation in the crypts and rates of migration of these cells up to the surface of the villi and colonic folds. The use of fiber regimens therefore offers a new means to probe and delineate basic regulatory mechanisms relating to the maintenance and continual regeneration of the mucosal lining of the gut.

5. SUMMARY

1. There was considerable variation in the final average body weight among rats fed the different postweaning diets. This variation was due to corresponding differences in the food and caloric consumption of these animals.
2. It appears that there is a need for insoluble, non-gel-forming dietary fiber to maintain body growth during the immediate postweaning period of the rat.
3. The growth of the rat small and large intestines follows different patterns during postnatal development.
4. The feeding of a specific form of dietary fiber, such as cellulose or

guar gum, had an effect on the shape and number of villi in the midjejunum of the rat during the immediate postweaning period.

5. The jejunum of fiber-free-fed rats appears to be exhibiting pathological adaptational hyperplasia.

6. The jejunum of guar gum-fed rats also appears to be exhibiting pathological adaptational hyperplasia. This adaptational response is probably a repair process in response to rather severe mucosal injury and occurs without an associated increase in proliferative activity.

7. The jejunum of cellulose-fed rats appears to be exhibiting physiological adaptational hypoplasia. This response occurs in association with relatively little damage to the intestinal mucosa.

8. The apparent absence of nutrients in the lumen of the midjejunum, such as occurs with the feeding of a liquid elemental diet, does not appear to adversely affect mucosal growth during the immediate postweaning period.

9. Dietary fibers with different physiochemical properties, such as cellulose and guar gum, caused varying degrees of damage to the mucosal surface of the intestinal tract. Guar gum preferentially caused a larger degree of damage to the jejunum than the colon. In contrast, cellulose had a greater disruptive effect on the colon compared to the small intestine.

10. The colon of cellulose-fed rats appears to be exhibiting hypoplasia. This colonic hypoplasia seems to be occurring despite a significant amount of damage to the colonic mucosa.

11. The colon of fiber-free-fed rats also appears to be in a hypoplastic state.

12. The fiber-free dietary group was unique among the dietary groups tested during the immediate postweaning period, exhibiting jejunal hyperplasia in association with colonic hypoplasia.

ACKNOWLEDGMENTS.   We would like to express our thanks for excellent morphological help on this project to Sally Haas-Smith and Lauretta Grau. This work was supported by USDA grants 82CRCR1-1071 (M. M. C.) and 82CRCR1-1001 (G. V. V.)

REFERENCES

Baker, S. J., Mathan, V. V., and Cherion, V., 1983, The nature of the villi in the small intestine of the rat, *Lancet* 1:860.

Buts, J. B., and de Meyer, R., 1981, Postnatal proximodistal development of the small bowel mucosal mass in growing rats, *Biol. Neonat.* 40:62—69.

Buts, J. P., de Meyer, R., and Kolanowski, J., 1983, Ontogeny of cell proliferation and DNA synthesis in rat colon: Role of glucocorticoids, *Am. J. Physiol.* **244** (*Gastrointest. Liver Physiol.*):6469–6474.

Calvert, R., Satchithanandum, S., Cassidy, M. M., and Vahouny, G. V., 1984, Dietary Fiber and intestinal adaptation: Effect on mucosal protein and specific crypt and villus enzyme activities, *Fed. Proc. Fed. Am. Soc. Exp. Biol.* **43**:1064.

Cassidy, M. M., Lightfoot, F. G., Grau, L., Story, J. A., Kritchevsky, D., and Vahouny, G. V., 1981, Effect of chronic intake of dietary fibers on the ultrastructural topography of rat jejunum and colon: A scanning electron microscopy study, *Am. J. Clin. Nutr.* **34**:218–228.

Cassidy, M. M., Lightfoot, F. G., and Vahouny, G. V., 1982, Dietary fiber, bile acids and intestinal morphology, in: *Dietary Fiber in Health and Disease* (G. V. Vahouny and D. Kritchevsky, eds.), Plenum, New York, pp. 239–264.

Creamer, B., 1964, Variations in small intestinal villous shape and mucosal dynamics, *Br. Med. J.* **2**:1371–1375.

Creamer, B., 1967, The turnover of epitelium of the small intestine, *Br. Med. Bull.* **23**:226–230.

Delorme, C. B., and Gordon, C. L., 1983, The effect of pectin on the utilization of marginal levels of dietary protein by weanling rats, *J. Nutr.* **113**:2432–2441.

Dowling, R. H., 1982, Small bowel adaptation and its regulation, *Scand. J. Gastroenterol.* **17** Suppl. 74):53–74.

Evans, E., and Miller, D. S., 1975, Bulking agents in the treatment of obesity, *Nutr. Metab.* **18**:199–203.

Fitzpatrick, L. R., Cassidy, M. M., Le, T., and Vahouny, G. V., 1983, The effect of diet on intestinal growth in developing rats, *J. Cell Biol.* **97**:400.

Fitzpatrick, L. R., Ekhterae, D., Calvert, R., Vahouny, G., and Cassidy, M. M., 1984, The influence of dietary fiber in the weanling on the development of sucrase activity in rat small intestine, *Fed. Proc.* **43**:1083.

Guthrie, H. A., 1975, *Introductory Nutrition*, C. V. Mosby, St. Louis.

Helander, H. F., 1973, Morphological studies on the development of the rat colonic mucosa, *Acta. Anat.* **85**:153–176.

Helander, H. F., 1975, Enzyme patterns and protein absorption in rat colon during development, *Acta. Anat.* **91**:330–349.

Hove, E. L., and King, S., 1979, Effects of pectin and cellulose on growth, feed efficiency and protein utilization, and their contribution to energy requirement and cecal VFA in rats, *J. Nutr.* **109**:1274–1278.

Joel, Ltd., Tokyo, Japan.

Johnson, L. R., 1981, Regulation of gastrointestinal growth, in: *Physiology of the Gastrointestinal Tract, Vol 1,* Raven, New York. pp. 169–194.

Leeds, A. R., Gassull, M. A., Metz, G. L., and Jenkins, D. J. A., 1975, Food: Influence of form on absorption, *Lancet* **2**:1213–1215.

Poskay, K. S., and Schneeman, B. O., 1983, Pancreatic and intestinal response to dietary guar gum in rats, *J. Nutr.* **113**:1544–1549

Sircar, B., Johnson, L. R., and Lichtenberger, L. M., 1983, Effects of synthetic diets on gastrointestinal mucosal DNA synthesis in rats, *Am. J. Physiol.* **244** (*Gastrointest. Liver Physiol.*):G327–335.

Tasman-Jones, C. T., 1981, Effects of dietary fiber on the structure and function of the small intestine, *Top. Gastroenterol.* **1981**:67–74.

Tasman-Jones, C. T., Owen, R. L., and Jones, A. L., 1982, Semipurified dietary fiber and small bowel morphology in rats, *Dig. Dis. Sci.* **27**:519–524.

Vahouny, G. V., Roy, T., Gallo, L., Story, J., Kritchevsky, D., and Cassidy, M. M., 1980a, Dietary fibers III. Effects of chronic intake on cholesterol absorption and metabolism in the rat, *Am. J. Clin. Nutr.* **33**:2182–2191.

Vahouny, G. V., Tombes, R., Cassidy, M. M., Kritchevsky, D., and Gallo, L. L., 1980b, Dietary fibers: V. Binding of bile salts, phospholipids and cholesterol from mixed micelles by bile acid sequestrants and dietary fibers, *Lipids* **15**:1012–1018.

Williamson, R. C. N., and Chin, M., 1978, Intestinal adaptation II: Mechanisms of control, *N. Engl. J. Med.* **198**:1444–1950.

Williamson, R. C. N., and Chin, M., 1978, Intestinal adaptation II: Mechanisms of control, *N. Engl. J. Med.* **198**:1444–1450.

Yang, M. G., Manoharan, K., and Michelsen, O., 1970, Nutritional contribution of volatile fatty acids from the cecum of rats, *J. Nutr.* **100**:545–550.

Younoszai, M. K., Adedoyin, M., and Ranshaw, J., 1978, Dietary components and gastrointestinal growth in rats, *J. Nutr.* **108**:341–350.

16

Modification of Steroid Excretion in Response to Dietary Fiber

JON A. STORY

1. INTRODUCTION

The interaction between bile acids and dietary fiber has been of interest to nutritionists searching for a mechanism that relates the intake of some sources of dietary fiber to the incidence of diseases related to steroid metabolism. For example, some sources of dietary fiber result in a lowering of serum cholesterol in humans, which some have theorized results from the observed increase in bile acid excretion (Story, 1980; Kritchevsky, 1982). Dietary fiber also alters colonic bile acid concentrations and susceptibility to colon carcinogens in experimental animals (Freeman, 1982) and appears to affect colon cancer in humans (Hill, 1982).

Stimulated by the early work of Heaton and others (Pomare and Heaton, 1973; Pomare et al., 1976; Watts et al., 1978; Miettinen and Tarpila, 1977), which suggested that the relative sizes of the bile acid pools were altered by some sources of dietary fiber and that these changes might alter bile saturation, we began investigations into the effects of dietary fiber on the spectrum of bile acids excreted in experimental animals and in man (Story and Thomas, 1982). Our working hypothesis suggested that these changes involved an increase in the derivatives of chenodeoxycholic acid (CDC), a change reported to alter steroid metabolism in several ways: (1) Increased levels of CDC appear to inhibit cholesterol synthesis by inhibiting 3-hydroxy-

JON A. STORY • Department of Foods and Nutrition, Purdue University, West Lafayette, Indiana 47907.

3-methylglutaryl coenzyme A reductase (Coyne *et al.*, 1976; Cooper, 1976). (2) When CDC replaces cholic acid in bile, cholesterol absorption is decreased in both man and experimental animals (Wilson, 1972; Ponz de Leon *et al.*, 1979). (3) Derivatives of CDC are less readily reabsorbed in the small intestine and thus will appear in the colon and possibly in feces in higher concentrations when their pool sizes increase (Beher *et al.*, 1967). All of the above changes could potentially alter steroid metabolism in a way that would have an effect on susceptibility to atherosclerosis (cholesterol balance), colon carcinogenesis (concentration and spectrum of colonic bile acids), and gallstones (saturation of bile).

The above observations suggest that we need to address two major questions at this time: (1) Are the changes in bile acid metabolism caused by dietary fiber of sufficient magnitude and consistent enough to result in the observed changes in steroid metabolism? (2) What mechanism is responsible for the change in bile acid excretion and spectrum observed in response to some sources of dietary fiber?

2. BILE ACID ADSORPTION

The adsorption of bile acids to dietary fiber and its components has been suggested as a mechanism for increasing steroid excretion for some time (Story and Kritchevsky, 1976). Our early work suggesting that alfalfa, a common source of dietary fiber used in animal diets, bound a substantial amount of bile acids (Kritchevsky and Story, 1974), coupled with reports of its hypocholesterolemic effects (Cookson *et al.*, 1967), led us to a more thorough examination of the component responsible for this adsorption. Initially we employed an extraction scheme that sequentially removed various fractions of the alfalfa to see if the adsorption capacity remained (Story *et al.*, 1982). These data suggested that removal of lignin was the critical step in reducing adsorption capacity, but that a significant ability to adsorb bile acids remained with the holocellulose (cellulose plus hemicellulose). Since isolated cellulose had not been found to have significant adsorption capabilities, we began studies to examine the adsorption capacity of hemicellulose. Some hemicelluloses are water-soluble, necessitating development of a method for measurement of adsorption of bile acids to water-soluble dietary fiber components. As can be seen in Table I, both hemicellulose A (soluble) and B (insoluble) adsorbed much more bile acid than cellulose, suggesting that, together with lignin, they may be responsible for most of the adsorption. Other isolated polysaccharides also seem to interact with bile acids to an extent similar to hemicellulose. Adsorption by oat bran and corn bran, which contain substantial quantities of water-soluble components, were also more accurately measured using this new method.

TABLE I. Bile Acid Adsorption

Adsorbent	Relative adsorption[a]	
	Cholic acid	Deoxycholic acid
Alfalfa	100	303
Oat bran	113	371
Corn bran	117	202
Cellulose[b]	50	15
Hemicellulose A[c]	82	211
Hemicellulose B[c]	99	242
Pectins[b]	14	113
Guar gum[b]	118	315

[a] Five millimolar bile acid solution (5 ml) was incubated with 50 mg of the given adsorbent, and adsorption was measured as percent bound. For these comparisons, the reference level is alfalfa's adsorption of cholic acid, taken as 100. Actual level, 9.8%.
[b] Commercial preparation.
[c] Isolated from corn bran.

These sources of dietary fiber and isolated polysaccharides are capable of interacting with bile acids *in vitro*. However, it should be pointed out that isolation procedures for commercial polysaccharides or for fractionation of dietary fiber sources may cause a modification of their adsorption capabilities. In addition, adsorption by polysaccharides that are subsequently metabolized by colonic bacteria would be of unknown value in modifying steroid balance. Thus, the significance of *in vitro* adsorption in relation to the hypocholesterolemic effects of these materials remains to be demonstrated.

3. CHANGES IN BILE ACID EXCRETION

3.1. Experimental Animals

A first step in demonstrating the importance of bile acid adsorption is the observation of increased bile acid excretion in response to feeding the sources of dietary fiber that adsorb bile acids *in vitro*. Early work suggesting that alfalfa increased fecal steroid excretion in rabbits (Horlick *et al.*, 1967), coupled with its hypocholesterolemic effects and its *in vitro* adsorption properties, have made it an interesting dietary fiber source to examine. The effects of alfalfa are complicated by the presence of saponins, which are known to interact with cholesterol and have been reported to lower serum cholesterol in experimental animals (Malinow *et al.*, 1977, 1979). We have recently reported a series of experiments designed to separate these effects based on our earlier measurement of adsorption of bile acids with various fractions of alfalfa. Rats were fed cholesterol-containing diets with alfalfa or saponin-free alfalfa and compared with those fed a diet containing a similar amount of cellulose (Story *et al.*, 1984). As can be seen in Table II, serum cholesterol was not altered by any of the diet treatments, as has been our experience with this diet in rats. Liver cholesterol was increased threefold by adding cholesterol to the cellulose diet. Alfalfa prevented part of this increase and removal of saponins resulted in an even greater reduction in the increase caused by cholesterol feeding. Interestingly, fecal bile acid concentration was not increased beyond the level observed in cholesterol-fed rats when alfalfa was added to the diet. Removal of saponins did cause some further increase in fecal bile acid concentration. Daily excretion of bile acids changed in a similar fashion. Neutral steroid excretion was increased substantially by alfalfa and saponin-free alfalfa in comparison to cellulose. Combined, these changes in steroid excretion resulted in a significantly higher daily excretion of steroids in response to alfalfa and, to a lesser extent, saponin-free alfalfa. Thus alfalfa did not cause a higher excretion of bile acids than cellulose in spite of the difference in their adsorption capacities. The increase in steroid excretion resulted from a change in neutral steroid excretion. This may have resulted from an adsorption of bile acids in the small intestine, reducing cholesterol absorption and conserving bile acids through colonic reabsorption.

A second change observed in these and other studies was the change in spectrum of bile acids excreted in animals fed alfalfa and other dietary fiber sources, as discussed earlier. We have observed an increase in CDC derivatives in response to alfalfa or whole oats in comparison to cellulose (about 10%), much like the change observed in response to dietary cholesterol

TABLE II. Steroid Excretion in Response to Alfalfa or Saponin-Free Alfalfa in Rats[a]

	Basal	Basal + cholesterol (0.25%)	Alfalfa	Saponin-free Alfalfa[b]
Serum cholesterol	100 (83.3 mg/dl)	105	78	111
Liver cholesterol	100 (1.8 mg/g)	294	194	144
Fecal steroids				
Bile acids	100 (1.38 mg/g)	229	212	279
	100 (7.46 mg/day)	301	294	341
Neutral	100 (2.96 mg/g)	278	403	358
	100 (16.01 mg/day)	365	559	437
Total	100 (23.5 mg/day)	344	474	406

[a] Basal value is set as 100. The actual mean is given in parentheses. Basal diet: 45% sucrose, 25% casein, 10% corn oil, 15% cellulose, alfalfa, or saponin-free alfalfa, 4% AIN salt mix, and 1% AIN vitamin mix.
[b] Saponins removed by exhaustive extraction with ethanol–water (1:1) at 70–C after lipid extraction.

(Kelley *et al.*, 1981). We have also reported a similar change in response to dietary pectin (Thomas *et al.*, 1984).

In a recent study we compared the effects of several sources of dietary fiber and isolated polysaccharides on fecal steroid excretion in rats (Table III). Concentrations of bile acids paralleled adsorption to some extent, with alfalfa causing higher levels than cellulose or wheat bran, but with pectin and guar gum reversed in comparison to their *in vitro* adsorption (Table I). Daily bile acid excretion was increased by all forms of dietary fiber (in comparison to no fiber), except for pectin, but none of the differences between dietary fiber sources was significant. The same was true for neutral steroid excretion. Total steroid excretion was increased by about 50% by the addition of any of the sources of dietary fiber or cholestyramine. Metamucil, which is largely hemicellulose, caused the most dramatic increase in steroid excretion. The spectrum of bile acids excreted was altered significantly only by Metamucil, which had 5-10% more CDC derivatives than the other dietary fiber source.

We have compared the effects of alfalfa, oat bran, and corn bran to cellulose in diets both with and without added cholesterol (0.25%). As before, daily bile acid excretion was increased by the sources of dietary fiber employed in both cholesterol-containing and cholesterol-free diets (Table IV). Little change in neutral steroid excretion in response to these sources of dietary fiber was observed. Small increases in total steroid excretion were observed in the cholesterol-free diet group in response to all sources of dietary fiber, except oat bran; none were statistically significant. In the cholesterol-fed group, all sources of fiber caused increases in total steroid excretion. Corn bran caused the largest increase and, along with cellulose

TABLE III. Fecal Steroid Excretion in Response to Various
Sources of Dietary Fiber in Rats[a]

	Bile acids		Neutral steroids		Total steroids	
	mg/g	mg/day	mg/g	mg/day	mg/g	mg/day
Control	100	100	100	100	100	100
Cellulose[b]	52	182	42	151	45	161
Wheat bran[b]	56	122	69	154	65	146
Alfalfa[b]	65	153	57	145	59	149
Metamucil[b]	90	200	79	182	82	188
Pectin[c]	77	64	94	69	90	68
Guar gum[c]	56	111	79	161	72	147
Cholestyramine[d]	139	200	88	135	103	155

[a] Values given represent results relative to those measured (as mg/g or mg/day) for control.
[b] Ten percent added to diet.
[c] Five percent added to diet.
[d] Two percent added to diet.

TABLE IV. Effects of Oat and Corn Brans, Alfalfa, and Cellulose on Fecal Steroid Excretion in Rats[a]

Diet	Dietary cholesterol (0.25%)	CDC derivatives	Bile acids	Neutral steroids	Total steroids
Basal	−	66	100	100	100
	+	75	155	133	140
Cellulose	−	69	200	71	113
	+	71	350	157	220
Oat bran	−	74	124	82	96
	+	77	243	159	186
Corn bran	−	80	180	83	115
	+	76	400	175	249
Alfalfa	−	71	218	75	122
	+	78	338	147	209

[a] Basal group is set at 100 for comparisons. Basal diet: 60% sucrose (or 45% sucrose, 15% dietary fiber), 25% casein, 10% corn oil, 4% AIN salt mix, and 1% AIN vitamin mix. CDC derivatives were measured as percent; others as mg/day.

and alfalfa, resulted in significantly higher levels of total steroid excretion. The spectrum of bile acids was shifted in the direction of CDC derivatives by oat bran, corn bran, and alfalfa in the absence of cholesterol, but was not changed significantly when cholesterol was included in the diet. One could speculate that these changes are reflected in the higher steroid excretion levels in cholesterol-fed groups and that cholesterol feeding masked the effects of these dietary fibers on bile acid spectrum.

These animal data suggest that adsorption *in vitro* serves in most cases as a predictor of effects on fecal bile acid concentrations, but that daily excretion levels are not always increased concomitantly with concentration.

3.2. Humans

Changes in steroid excretion in response to various sources of dietary fiber in humans agree in general with those effects observed in experimental animals, but with several notable exceptions. Kay (1982) summarized the effects of a wide variety of dietary fiber sources on plasma cholesterol and steroid excretion. Wheat bran generally causes little change in any of these variables, while cellulose causes modest increases in bile acid excretion (25–45%), as we have described in rats. Two materials that have effects in humans unlike those reported for rats are oat bran and pectin. In humans pectin causes a decrease in plasma cholesterol (13–15%) and a concomitant increase in fecal bile acids (33–75%) and thus has been suggested to be one of the more effective isolated polysaccharides (Jenkins *et al.*, 1976; Kay and

Truswell, 1977; Miettinen and Tarpila, 1977). Oat bran also is effective in lowering plasma cholesterol in hyperlipidemic patients and causes a substantial increase in bile acid excretion (Kirby *et al.*, 1981). A recent similar study compared the effects of 100 g of oat bran or beans on plasma cholesterol and steroid excretion in hyperlipidemic patients (Anderson *et al.*, 1984). As is suggested by the data in Table V, both treatments reduced plasma cholesterol levels during the 3-week treatment period, but oat bran caused an increase in bile acid excretion, while beans did not. Thus we have two dietary fiber sources that contain primarily water-soluble polysaccharides and have similar effects on cholesterol levels, but do not have the same effect on steroid excretion. In addition, beans appear to have increased the proportion of CDC derivatives excreted, while oat bran reduced their levels. These data suggest that our hypothesis may be far too simple to explain the changes in steroid metabolism observed in response to these sources of dietary fiber. Changes in steroid excretion are obviously not mandatory in producing changes in serum lipids and an increase in CDC derivatives is also not a necessary part of changes in either variable. It also appears that steroid excretion in rats fed these water-soluble polysaccharides (i.e., from oat bran) does not respond as does human steroid excretion. This may be due to differences in the ability of the intestinal flora to break down these polysaccharides and subsequent effects these differences have on bile acid metabolism. Absorbable products of bacterial action (e.g., short-chain fatty acids) on these polysaccharides may also cause changes in the amount and identity of bile acids synthesized either by direct action on the enzymes involved or through changes in lipoproteins that translate into altered bile acid synthesis.

In another recent study (Spiller *et al.*, 1984) young girls were fed a diet

TABLE V. Effects of Oat Bran or Beans on Plasma Cholesterol Levels and Steroid Excretion in Hyperlipidemic Humans

	Percent change	
	Oat bran[a]	Beans[a]
Serum cholesterol	−19	−19
Fecal Steroids		
Acidic	+65	−30
Neutral	+15	+2
Total	+22	−3
CDC derivatives	−22	+24

[a]One hundred grams/day was added to a diet composed of 20, 43, and 36% of kcal from protein, carbohydrate, and fat, respectively. Serum cholesterol was measured as mg/dl, fecal steroids as g/day, and CDC derivatives as percent.

containing 23 g/day dietary fiber to which 0, 5.7, 17.1, and 28.5 g/day dietary fiber was added as hard red wheat bran (HRWB) incorporated into bread. HRWB had previously been reported to be hypocholesterolemic in adults (Munoz *et al.*, 1979). After 2 weeks of the added HRWB, total and neutral steroid excretion was not significantly altered at any level of consumption (Table VI). However, bile acid excretion was increased significantly by the two higher levels of HRWB intake. This change was coupled with a consistent but not significant increase in CDC derivatives at these higher levels of intake. In all cases, addition of increasing levels of HRWB caused greater dilution of all fecal steroids. These data would suggest that increased bile acid excretion occurs with increases in the proportion of CDC in response to this source of dietary fiber. However, clearly this change in bile acid excretion was not of sufficient magnitude to alter steroid balance at these levels of HRWB intake.

4. CONCLUSIONS

Returning to the first of the two questions posed earlier, are the changes in bile acid metabolism of sufficient magnitude and consistent enough to be the cause of observed changes in cholesterol levels in the blood? It would appear that changes in bile acid excretion alone are neither consistent nor large enough to account for changes in serum cholesterol. In some cases, there appears to be a consistent increase in bile acid excretion in response to a dietary treatment (e.g., cellulose), but no evidence in man or experimental animals of a change in cholesterol levels, while other treatments consistently lower cholesterol levels with about the same change in bile acid excretion (e.g., alfalfa). However, in some cases (e.g., oat bran in hypercholesterolemic humans), a substantial change in bile acid excretion has consistently accompanied the hypocholesterolemic effects. Clearly, this is not the sole mecha-

TABLE VI. Changes in Fecal Steroids in Response to
Hard Red Wheat Bran in Humans

Fecal steroid	Effect of hard red wheat bran[a]			
	0	5.7 g	17.1 g	28.5 g
Acidic	100	138	165	160
Neutral	100	89	86	77
Total	100	93	92	84
CDC derivatives	56	54	61	63

[a] Effect of adding given amount of wheat bran daily to a diet containing 23.3 g dietary fiber per day for 14 days. Zero added wheat bran is taken as 100 for comparisons. Fecal steroids were measured as mg/day, CDC derivatives as percent.

nism involved for all sources of dietary fiber and our initial hypothesis concerning adsorption–excretion is not valid for all situations.

Changes in the spectrum of bile acids excreted in favor of derivatives of CDC occurs in response to many of the sources of dietary fiber that prevent cholesterol accumulation or are hypocholesterolemic. However, some notable exceptions exist, e.g., oat bran in humans. This sort of change could potentially alter several phases of sterol metabolism, which could alter cholesterol levels with or without causing a change in bile acid excretion. Refining this hypothesis may depend on determining if excretion levels of the various bile acids reflect their pool sizes, since one would expect the metabolic effects of changes in relative amounts of bile acids (e.g., alteration of cholesterol or bile acid synthesis) to be affected by the amount of bile acid in each pool, not solely the amount in the intestine.

As was mentioned earlier, changes in sterol metabolism may also be affected by metabolites arising from microbial breakdown of polysaccharides in the intestine. Changes in enzymes regulating both the amount and type of bile acids and cholesterol synthesized could conceivably be induced by these compounds. Much work is needed in order to understand the relative importance and interaction of adsorption, changes in spectrum, and microbial metabolites in determining the net effect of the various dietary fiber sources on steroid metabolism.

What mechanisms are responsible for changes in bile acid excretion? Adsorption still appears to offer a partial explanation for changes in excretion. Bile acid concentrations in feces generally increase when animals are fed sources of dietary fiber that adsorb significant quantities of bile acids. However, this does not translate into higher total steroid excretion in all cases. Adsorption affinities for the different bile acids suggest that the dihydroxy bile acids are better adsorbed than are trihydroxy bile acids. This could partially explain the appearance of larger quantities of this class of bile acids in feces. If that is the case, changes in fecal bile acids would not reflect changes in pool sizes. The relationship between fecal and biliary bile acids and the effects of fiber on each are not well understood.

A second possible explanation involves the possible modification of activities of key enzymes involved in the synthesis of bile acids by absorbable products of the bacterial degradation of dietary fiber in the colon. In rats, preliminary evidence suggests that short-chain fatty acid levels increase in portal blood in response to oat bran and that these fatty acids modify the rate of cholesterol synthesis (Anderson and Bridges, 1981; Chen and Anderson, 1983). A more detailed discussion of current status concerning the feasibility of these changes appears in Chapter 18 of this volume.

Another possible mechanism for changes in bile acid metabolism, which has received minimal attention, relates to changes in lipoprotein metabolism in response to these sources of dietary fiber, which would alter the amount and identity of bile acids synthesized. Chylomicron composition (e.g., lipid-apoprotein ratio) is determined, in part, by the site of absorption along the intestine (Wu *et al.*, 1980). This would suggest that changes in transit time or availability of bile salts in response to certain sources of dietary fiber may alter the site of lipid absorption and, in turn, chylomicron composition. Changes in chylomicron composition could in turn cause changes in hepatic regulation of cholesterol and bile acid metabolism. Little is known about the importance of lipoproteins in determining the rate of bile acid synthesis and the spectrum of bile acids synthesized (Meydani *et al.*, 1983). The exact link from dietary fiber to altered lipoprotein levels and/or clearance to changes in bile acid metabolism remains to be elucidated, but may provide an explanation of the other mechanisms, which seem to fall short of a complete explanation of the observations.

The above mechanisms are speculative. The actual mechanisms involved may lie somewhere within these suggestions or may involve some unknown system. In any case, they suggest a safe and useful role for dietary fiber as part of a diet designed to minimize disease risk.

ACKNOWLEDGMENTS.   This work was supported in part by the Indiana Agricultural Experiment Station (paper no. 10,001), the U. S. Department of Agriculture Competitive Grants Program (83-CRCR-1-1232), and grants-in-aid from the Quaker Oats Company and the Shaklee Corporation.

REFERENCES

Anderson, J. W., and Bridges, S. R., 1981, Plant fiber metabolites alter hepatic glucose and lipid metabolism, *Diabetes* 30:133A.
Anderson, J. W., Story, L., Sieling, B., Chen, W.-J. L., Petro, M. S., and Story, J. A., 1984, Hypercholesterolemic effects of oat bran or bean intake for hypercholesterolemic men, *Am. J. Clin. Nutr.* 40:1146–1155.
Beher, W. T., Beher, M. E., and Rao, B., 1967, Turnover of cholic and chenodeoxycholic acids in normal and hypophsectomized rats, *Life Sci.* 6:868–866.
Chen, W.-J. L., and Anderson, J. W., 1983, Propionate may mediate hypocholesterolemic effects of plant fibers, *Fed. Proc. Fed. Am. Soc. Exp. Biol.* 42:1061.
Cookson, F. B., Altschul, R., and Fedoroff, S., 1967, The effects of alfalfa on serum cholesterol in modifying or preventing cholesterol-induced atherosclerosis in rabbits, *J. Atheroscler. Res.* 7:69–81.
Cooper, A. D., 1976, The regulation of 3-hydroxy-3-methylglutaryl coenzyme A reductase in the isolated purfused rat liver, *J. Clin. Invest.* 57:1461–1470.
Coyne, M. J., Bonouris, G. G., Goldstein, L. I., and Schoenfield, L. J., 1976, Effect of cheno-deoxycholic acid and phenobarbital on the rate limiting enzymes of hepatic cholesterol and bile acid synthesis in patients with gallstones, *J. Lab. Clin. Med.* 87:281–291.
Freeman, H. J., 1982, Studies on the effects of single fiber sources in the dimethylhydrazine rodent model of human colonic neoplasia, in: *Dietary Fiber in Health and Disease* (G. V. Vahouny and D. Kritchevsky, eds.), Plenum, New York, pp. 287–297.

Hill, M. J., 1982, Bile acids and human colorectal cancer, in: *Dietary Fiber in Health and Disease* (G. V. Vahouny and D. Kritchevsky, eds.), Plenum, New York, pp. 299–312.

Horlick, L., Cookson, F. B., and Fedoroff, S., 1967, Effect of alfalfa feeding on the excretion of fecal neutral sterols in the rabbit, *Circulation* **36**:18.

Jenkins, D. J. A., Leeds, A. R., Gassull, M. A., Houston, H., Goff, D. V., and Hill, M. J., 1976, The cholesterol-lowering properties of guar and pectin, *Clin. Sci. Mol. Med.* **51**:8.

Kay, R. M., 1982, Dietary fiber, *J. Lipid Res.* **23**:221–242.

Kay, R. M., and Truswell, A. S., 1977, Effect of citrus pectin on blood lipids and fecal steroid excretion in man, *Am. J. Clin. Nutr.* **30**:171–175.

Kelley, M. J., Thomas, J. N., and Story, J. A., 1981, Modification of spectrum of fecal bile acids in rats by dietary fiber, *Fed. Proc. Fed. Am. Soc. Exp. Biol.* **40**:845.

Kirby, R. W., Anderson, J. W., Sieling, B., Rees, E. D., Chen, W.-J. L., Miller, R. E., and Kay, R. M., 1981, Oat bran intake selectively lowers serum low density lipoprotein concentrations: Studies of hypercholesterolemic men, *Am. J. Clin. Nutr.* **34**:824–829.

Kritchevsky, D., 1982, Fiber and lipid, in: *Dietary Fiber in Health and Disease* (G. V. Vahouny and D. Kritchevsky, eds.), Plenum, New York, pp. 187–192.

Kritchevsky, D., and Story, J. A., 1974, Binding of bile salts *in vitro* by nonnutritive fiber, *J. Nutr.* **104**:458–462.

Malinow, M. R., McLaughlin, P., Kohler, G. O., and Livingston, A. L., 1977, Prevention of elevated cholesterolemia in monkeys by alfalfa saponins, *Steroids* **29**:105–110.

Malinow, M. R., McLaughlin, P., Stafford, C., Livingston, A. L., Kohler, G. O., and Cheeke, P. R., 1979, Comparative alfalfa saponins and alfalfa fiber on cholesterol absorption in rats, *Am. J. Clin. Nutr.* **32**:1810–1812.

Meydani, S. N., Nicolosi, R. J., Sehgal, P. K., and Kayse, K. C., 1983, Altered lipoprotein metabolism in spontaneous vitamin E deficiency of owl monkeys, *Am. J. Clin. Nutr.* **38**:888–894.

Miettinen, T. A., and Tarpila, S., 1977, Effect of pectin on serum cholesterol, fecal bile acids and biliary lipids in normolipidemic and hyperlipidemic individuals, *Clin. Chim. Acta* **79**:471–477.

Munoz, J. M., Sandstead, H. H., Jacob, R. A., Logan, G. M., Reck, S. J., Klevay, L. M., Dintzis, F. R., Inglett, G. E., and Shvey, W. C., 1979, Effects of some cereal brans and textured vegetable protein on plasma lipids, *Am. J. Clin. Nutr.* **32**:580–592.

Pomare, E. W., and Heaton, K. W., 1973, Alteration of bile salt metabolism by dietary fibre (bran), *Br. Med. J.* **4**:262–264.

Pomare, E. W., Heaton, K. W., Low-Beer, T. S., and Espiner, H. J., 1976, The effect of wheat bran upon the lipid composition of bile in gallstone patients, *Dig. Dis.* **21**:521–526.

Ponz de Leon, M., Carulli, N., Loria, P., Lori, R., and Zironi, F., 1979, The effect of chenodeoxycholic acid (CDCA) on cholesterol absorption, *Gastroenterology* **77**:223–230.

Spiller, G. A., Wong, L. G., Nunes, J. D., Story, J. A., Petro, M. S., Furumoto, E. J., Alton-Spiller, N., Whittam, J. H., and Scala, J., 1984, Effect of four levels of hard red wheat bran on fecal composition and transit time in healthy young men, *Fed. Proc. Fed. Am. Soc. Exp. Biol.* **43**:392.

Story, J. A., 1980, Dietary fiber and lipid metabolism: An update, in: *Medical Aspects of Dietary Fiber* (G. A. Spiller and R. M. Kay, eds.), Plenum, New York, pp. 137–152.

Story, J. A., and Kritchevsky, D., 1976, Dietary fiber and lipid metabolism, in: *Fiber in Human Nutrition* (G. A. Spiller and R. J. Amen, eds.), Plenum, New York, pp. 171–184.

Story, J. A., and Thomas, J. N., 1982, Modification of bile acid spectrum by dietary fiber, in: *Dietary Fiber in Health and Disease* (G. V. Vahouny and D. Kritchevsky, eds.), Plenum, New York, pp. 193–201.

Story, J. A., White, A., and West, L. G., 1982, Adsorption of bile acids by components of alfalfa and wheat bran *in vitro*, *J. Food Sci.* **47**:1276–1279.

Story, J. A., LePage, S. L., Petro, M. S., West, L. G., Cassidy, M. M., Lightfoot, F. G., and

Vahouny, G. V., 1984, Interactions of alfalfa plant and sprout saponins with cholesterol *in vitro* and in cholesterol-fed rats, *Am. J. Clin. Nutr.* **39**:917–929.

Thomas, J. N., Kelley, M. J., and Story, J. A., 1984, Alteration of regression of cholesterol accumulation in ratio by dietary pectin, *Br. J. Nutr.* **51**: 339–345.

Watts, J. M., Jablonski, P., and Toouli, J., 1978, The effect of added bran to the diet on the saturation of bile in people without gallstones, *Am. J. Surg.* **135**:321–324.

Wilson, J. D., 1972, The role of bile acids in the overall regulation of steroid metabolism, *Arch. Intern. Med.* **130**:493–505.

Wu, A-L., Clark, S. B., and Holt, P. R., 1980, Composition of lymph chylomicrons from proximal or distal rat small intestine, *Am. J. Clin. Nutr.* **33**:582–589.

17

Dietary Fiber and Atherosclerosis

DAVID KRITCHEVSKY

The influence of any treatment on development of atherosclerosis can be assayed directly in animals by obtaining autopsy data after a suitable experimental period. In man the determination of atherosclerotic involvement is indirect and depends upon measurements of serum or plasma lipid or lipoprotein components. Elevated plasma total cholesterol or low-density lipoprotein (LDL) levels are generally agreed to be positively correlated with the risk of developing cardiovascular disease (Kagan *et al.*, 1962; Gordon *et al.*, 1974). Elevated levels of high-density lipoprotein (HDL), HDL-cholesterol, or ratio of HDL- to LDL-cholesterol are assumed to be negatively correlated (Barr *et al.*, 1951; Miller and Miller, 1975). Thus, in man alteration of risk may be adduced to follow changes in levels of any of these parameters.

Lambert *et al.* (1958) and Malmros and Wigand (1959) demonstrated that atherosclerosis could be induced in rabbits by feeding them a diet devoid of cholesterol but high in saturated fat. The findings seemed paradoxical, since other investigators (Kritchevsky *et al.*, 1954; Hirsch and Nailor, 1955; Steiner *et al.*, 1959) had not found saturated fat alone to be atherogenic. Collation of the existing literature (Kritchevsky, 1964) showed that saturated fat was not atherogenic when added to a stock diet, but did exert an atherogenic effect when fed as part of a semipurified diet (Table I). The amount and type of dietary fiber present in the diet was adduced to be the determining factor. To test this possibility and also to test the suggestion that the fat present in commercial ration (2–4% of an iodine value of

DAVID KRITCHEVSKY • The Wistar Institute of Anatomy and Biology, Philadelphia, Pennsylvania 19104.

TABLE I. Atherogenicity in Rabbits of Saturated Fat
Added to Stock or Semipurified Diet[a]

	Stock diet	Semipurified diet
Number of studies	7	7
Average percent fat added	20.7	17.0
Average duration, months	5.3	7.2
Atherogenicity, 0–4 scale	0.04	1.56

[a] After Kritchevsky (1964).

approximately 115) might be protecting against the atherogenic effects of saturated fat, an experiment was carried out in which rabbits were fed a semipurified diet containing 14% coconut oil; one containing 12% coconut oil plus 2% of the fat extracted from commercial ration; fat-extracted commercial ration plus 14% coconut oil; or commercial ration plus 12% coconut oil. The data (Table II) clearly show that the fat present in the commercial ration exerted no protective effect, whereas the extracted residue did (Kritchevsky and Tepper, 1965, 1968). Moore (1967) fed rabbits semipurified diets containing wheat straw, cellophane, or cellulose and 20% corn oil or 20% butter. Even in the presence of corn oil, the fibers exerted varying effects on cholesterolemia and atherosclerosis (Table III).

Howard et al. (1967) reported that a semipurified diet containing beef tallow and cellophane, when fed to rabbits, resulted in plasma cholesterol levels of 275 mg/dl and average atherosclerosis of 1.60 (based on a 0–3 scale). Dilution of the diet with stock diet totally inhibited atherosclerosis and reduced cholesterolemia to 92 mg/dl, about twice normal. Pectin (5%) added to an atherogenic diet reduced serum cholesterol levels in rabbits by one-third and β- and pre-β-lipoprotein cholesterol levels by 25% (Berenson et al., 1975). When rabbits were fed semipurified diets containing either soy protein or casein and whose fiber was either cellulose, wheat straw, or alfalfa, it was found that cellulose feeding resulted in the highest serum cholesterol levels and most severe atherosclerosis. Wheat straw did not affect cholesterolemia, but reduced atherogenicity, and alfalfa reduced both (Kritchevsky et al., 1977) (Table IV). Rabbits fed the semipurified diet retain more exogenous and endogenous cholesterol in serum and liver than do those fed a stock diet (Kritchevsky et al., 1975a) (Table V).

Chickens were fed a diet containing 0.6% cholesterol and 3% cellulose or pectin. Birds fed cellulose exhibited the highest cholesterol levels and the most severe aortic and coronary atherosclerosis (Fisher et al., 1966)

There have been no direct studies of the effects of fiber on atherosclerosis in rats. Pectin, guar gum, locust bean gum, alfalfa, and lignin all reduce

TABLE II. Effect of Special Diets on Atherosclerosis in Rabbits[a]

Number	Fiber, %	Fat,[b] %	Cholesterolemia,[c] mg/dl ± SEM	Atherosclerosis, arch + thoracic/2
11/15	Cellulose (15)	HCNO (14)	207 ± 36* † ‡	0.85
12/15	Cellulose (15)	HCNO (12) CR (2)	249 ± 41 § ‖ #	0.90
7/15	Stock-R (85)[d]	HCNO (14)	64 ± 9* § ⊥	0.40
14/15	Stock (86)[e]	HCNO (12) CR (2)	35 ± 2 † ‖ ⊥	0.25
6/6	Stock (98)[e]	CR (2)	40 ± 9 ‡ #	0.15

[a] After Kritchevsky and Tepper (1965). Diets fed for 6 months.
[b] HCNO, hydrogenated coconut oil; CR, lipid extracted from commercial ration; iodine value = 115.
[c] Values bearing the same symbol are significantly different.
[d] Residue of commercial diet after lipid extraction.
[e] Commercial ration.

TABLE III. Influence of Dietary Fiber on Cholesterolemia and Atherosclerosis in Rabbits[a]

Fat (20%)	Fiber (19%)	Cholesterol, mg/dl ± SEM	Atherosclerosis (avg ± SEM)
Corn oil	Wheat straw	23 ± 4* †	0.7 ± 0.6‡
Corn oil	Cellulose	61 ± 5*	1.3 ± 0.3§
Corn oil	Cellophane	71 ± 6†	5.0 ± 0.7‡§
Butter fat	Wheat straw	114 ± 12‖	12.7 ± 3.0**
Butter fat	Cellulose	133 ± 10#	20.8 ± 2.9†‖‡‡
Butter fat	Cellophane	216 ± 14‖#⊥	37.5 ± 6.8**‖‖§§
Butter fat	Cellophane–peat, 14:5	141 ± 12⊥	10.7 ± 2.0‡‡§§

[a] After Moore (1967). Values bearing the same symbol are significantly different.

TABLE IV. Interaction of Fiber and Protein in Rabbits Fed Semipurified Diets[a]

Fiber	Casein protein		Soy protein	
	Serum cholesterol, mg/dl ± SEM	Average atherosclerosis	Serum cholesterol, mg/dl ± SEM	Average atherosclerosis
Cellulose	402 ± 40*	1.50	248 ± 44	1.25
Wheat straw	375 ± 42	1.03	254 ± 35	0.91
Alfalfa	193 ± 34*	0.63	159 ± 20	0.73

[a] After Kritchevsky et al. (1977). Rabbits were fed 40% sucrose, 25% protein, 14% coconut oil, and 15% fiber for 10 months. Values bearing the same symbol are significantly different ($p < 0.05$).

TABLE V. Comparison of Cholesterol Disposition in Rabbits Fed
Commercial or Semipurified Diets[a]

	Semipurified diet[b]	Commercial diet
Number	9/10	5/5
Serum lipids, mg/dl		
Cholesterol	215 ± 17	93 ± 5
Triglyceride	131 ± 24	76 ± 24
Average atherosclerosis	1.35	0
Recovery of radioactivity[c]		
Serum		
^3H, dpm $\times 10^5$	4.03 ± 0.36	0.38 ± 0.11
^{14}C, dpm	2757	ND[d]
Liver		
^3H, dpm $\times 10^6$	4.41 ± 0.52	1.34 ± 0.44
^{14}C, dpm $\times 10^4$	3.99 ± 0.59	1.05 ± 0.28
Feces		
^3H, dpm $\times 10^6$	4.70 ± 1.5	19.0 ± 10.5
^{14}C, dpm $\times 10^3$	8.86 ± 1.6	11.2 ± 4.3

[a] After Kritchevsky et al. (1975a). Values ± SEM.
[b] Rabbits were fed 40% carbohydrate, 25% casein, 14% coconut oil, and 15% cellulose for 6 months, then given ip injection of [1,2-^3H]cholesterol and [2-^{14}C]mevalonic acid. ^3H radioactivity = exogenous cholesterol; ^{14}C radioactivity = endogeous cholesterol.
[c] Total serum (body weight × 0.03) and total liver.
[d] ND, Not detectable.

serum and liver cholesterol levels in rats fed semipurified diets containing 0.5–1.0% cholesterol (Wells and Ershoff, 1961; Kiriyama et al., 1969; Kritchevsky et al., 1975b; Story et al., 1981). Cellulose, agar, and pectic or alginic acid increase liver cholesterol levels above those observed in rats fed no fiber (Wells and Ershoff, 1961; Kiriyama et al., 1969; Tsai et al., 1976). Chen and Anderson (1979) fed rats 1% cholesterol, 0.2% cholic acid, and 10% cellulose, pectin, guar gum, or oat bran. Average plasma total cholesterol levels (mg/dl) were: cellulose group 133 ± 4; pectin group 84 ± 3; guar gum group 105 ± 9; and oat bran group 113 ± 3. The ratios of HDL/total cholesterol were 0.14, 0.31, 0.30, and 0.22, respectively.

Baboons fed semipurified diets exhibit significantly higher levels of serum total and LDL-cholesterol than those maintained on bread, peanuts, and fruit (Kritchevsky et al., 1974). Malinow et al. (1978) induced hypercholestolemia and atherosclerosis in female cynomolgous monkeys by feeding a butter-cholesterol diet for 6 months. After cessation of cholesterol feeding, one subgroup maintained on a semipurified diet for 18 months showed a 59% fall in cholesterolemia but a 23% increase in atherosclerosis. A second subgroup fed alfalfa exhibited a 77% reduction in cholesterolemia and 40% reduction in severity of atherosclerosis. Vervet monkeys were fed a semipurifed diet containing 15% cellulose, wheat straw, or alfalfa for 23 weeks (Kritchevsky *et al.*, 1981). Those fed alfalfa exhibited the lowest serum cholesterol levels and those fed wheat straw had the least severe sudanophilia (Table VI). Pectin appears to have no effect on severity of sudanophilia in monkeys fed semipurified diets (Table VII) (Kritchevsky, unpublished material).

Vegetarians habitually ingest a diet high in fiber (Hardinge *et al.*, 1958). Sacks *et al.* (1975) found vegetarians to have significantly lower levels of cholesterol and triglycerides than did matched omnivorous controls (Table VIII). Burselm *et al.* (1978) confirmed Sacks' observation and also found the vegetarians to have significantly lower levels of two apolipoproteins (A1 and B) positively correlated with the risk of coronary heart disease. Knuiman and West (1982) found men on macrobiotic diets to have lower cholesterol levels (147 mg/dl) and higher HDL/total cholesterol ratios than lacto-ovovegetarians (serum cholesterol, 181 mg/dl) or nonvegetarians (212 mg/dl). Another study (Kritchevsky *et al.*, 1985) has shown low cholesterol levels in true vegetarians but little difference in cholesterol levels between lacto-ovovegetarians or nonvegetarians. Burr and Sweetnam (1982) found a significant negative association between vegetarianism and mortality from ischemic heart disease, but there was no significant association with fiber.

TABLE VI. Influence of Fiber on Lipid Metabolism and Aortic Sudanophilia in Vervet Monkeys[a]

	Cellulose	Wheat straw	Alfalfa
Serum lipids, mg/dl ± SEM			
Cholesterol	174 ± 14	167 ± 8	153 ± 9
Triglycerides	213 ± 17	176 ± 24	219 ± 51
Phospholipids	356 ± 27	356 ± 16	301 ± 22
Liver lipids, mg/g ± SEM			
Cholesterol	3.01 ± 0.10	2.56 ± 0.18	2.65 ± 0.16
Percent ester	21.9	19.9	22.2
Triglycerides	3.93 ± 1.10	3.35 ± 0.62	2.70 ± 0.41
Phospholipids	24.1 ± 1.33	26.7 ± 1.38	27.4 ± 1.17
Aortic sudanophilia, % ± SEM	3.8 ± 1.5	1.5 ± 0.4	4.1 ± 2.9

[a] After Kritchevsky *et al.* (1981). Monkeys (six per group) were fed 40% sucrose, 25% casein, 14% coconut oil, and 15% fiber for 23 weeks.

TABLE VII. Influence of Pectin on Lipid Metabolism and Aortic Sudanophilia in Vervet Monkeys[a]

	Cholesterol-free diet		Diet with 0.1% cholesterol	
	Cellulose	Pectin	Cellulose	Pectin
Number	5/6	3/6	5/6	6/6
Serum lipids, mg/dl				
Cholesterol	156 ± 14	173 ± 15	187 ± 27	155 ± 11
HDL/LDL	0.74 ± 0.08	0.48 ± 0.05	0.62 ± 0.09	0.47 ± 0.08
Triglycerides	53 ± 11	57 ± 14	55 ± 13	50 ± 9
Liver lipids, mg/100 g				
Cholesterol	215 ± 13	111 ± 15	110 ± 18	232 ± 23
Triglycerides	435 ± 86	634 ± 120	481 ± 48	553 ± 47
Aorta lipids, mg/g				
Cholesterol	4.23 ± 0.24	5.80 ± 0.95	3.62 ± 0.51	4.07 ± 0.89
Free/ester	12.5 ± 3.9	17.5 ± 7.2	6.5 ± 2.0	6.4 ± 1.3
Triglycerides	18.3 ± 4.7	51.2 ± 15.0	21.9 ± 5.7	16.0 ± 5.9
Sudanophilia, %	7.0 ± 3.2	13.5 ± 9.4	5.8 ± 2.7	21.6 ± 10.3

[a] After Kritchevsky (unpublished data). Values ± SEM. Monkeys were fed 40% lactose, 25% casein, 14% coconut oil, and 15% fiber for 9 months.

TABLE VIII. Lipid Levels of Vegetarians and Matched Controls[a]

	Control	Vegetarians
Number	115	115
Triglycerides, mg/dl	86 ± 4	59 ± 3
Cholesterol, mg/dl		
Total	184 ± 3	126 ± 3
VLDL	17 ± 1	12 ± 0.7
LDL	118 ± 3	73 ± 2
HDL	49 ± 1	43 ± 1
HDL/LDL	0.42	0.59

[a] After Sacks et al. (1975). Values ± SEM.

Stasse-Wolthuis *et al.* (1979, 1980) examined the influence of dietary fiber on cholesterolemia and HDL-cholesterol levels. They found the most significant effects to be in subjects eating low-cholesterol, high-fiber diets. When specific effects of vegetables, bran, and pectin were studied, they found none to influence HDL-cholesterol levels and only pectin to lower significantly serum cholesterol levels. Grande (1974) collated data on changes in cholesterol levels exerted by replacing dietary sucrose with other sources of carbohydrate, such as bread, legumes, fruit, or potatoes. In every case, they were also adding fiber to the diet. Anderson (1982) and his colleagues have shown high-fiber diets to lower plasma cholesterol and glucose levels in diabetics.

There have been recent reviews of the effects of specific fibers on cholesterolemia in man (Kelsay, 1978; Kay, 1980; Story, 1981). In general, only soluble fibers such as pectin, oat gum, or guar gum have a hypocholesterolemic effect. Bran has been studied extensively and findings of its lack of effect have been virtually unanimous (Kay and Truswell, 1980). Guar crispbread (13 g/day) (Jenkins *et al.*, 1980) will reduce total and LDL-cholesterol levels. Pectin (9 g/day) has been shown to reduce serum total cholesterol by 8% and very low-density lipoprotein (VLDL) plus LDL levels by 11% (Nakamura, 1982). Oat bran (Kirby *et al.*, 1981) has been shown to reduce total, LDL-and HDL-cholesterol levels by 13, 14, and 2% respectively (Table IX).

The data relating to fiber ingestion and atherosclerosis suggest only certain types of fiber are effective. Data on cholesterolemia in man show a similar pattern. Further work is needed to elucidate the specific aspects of structure responsible for the hypocholesterolemic effects of certain fibers.

TABLE IX. Influence of Oat Bran on Serum Lipids in Man[a]

	Oat bran	Control
Total cholesterol, mg/dl		
Initial	269 ± 16	256 ± 23
Final	234 ± 19	252 ± 15
LDL-cholesterol, mg/dl		
Initial	184 ± 14	168 ± 22
Final	159 ± 17	169 ± 15
HDL-cholesterol, mg/dl		
Initial	49 ± 3	52 ± 5
Final	48 ± 6	48 ± 4

[a]After Kirby *et al.* (1981). Eight subjects, 10-day study.

REFERENCES

Anderson, J. W., 1982, Dietary fiber and diabetes, in: *Dietary Fiber in Health and Disease* (G. V. Vahouny and D. Kritchevsky, eds.), Plenum, New York, pp. 151–167.

Barr, D. P., Russ, E. M., and Eder, H. A., 1951, Protein–lipid relationships in human plasma. II. Atherosclerosis and related conditions, *Am. J. Med.* **11**:480–493.

Berenson, L. M., Bhandaru, R., R., Radhakrishnamurthy, B., Srinivasan, S. B., and Berenson, G. S., 1975, The effect of dietary pectin on serum lipoprotein cholesterol in rabbits, *Life Sci.* **16**:1533–1544.

Burr, M. L., and Sweetnam, P. M., 1982, Vegetarianism, dietary fiber and mortality, *Am. J. Clin. Nutr.* **36**:873–877.

Burselm, J., Schonfeld, G., Howard, M. A., Werdman, S. W., and Miller, J. P., 1978, Plasma apoprotein and lipoprotein lipid levels in vegetarians, *Metabolism* **27**:711–719.

Chen, W. L., and Anderson, J. W., 1979, Effects of plant fiber in decreasing plasma total cholesterol and increasing high-density lipoprotein cholesterol, *Proc. Soc. Exp. Biol. Med.* **162**: 310–313.

Fisher, H., Soller, W. G., and Griminger, P., 1966, The retardation by pectin of cholesterol-induced atherosclerosis in fowl, *J. Atheroscler. Res.* **6**:292–298.

Gordon, T., Garcia-Palmieri, M. R., Kagan, A., Kannel, W. B., and Schiffman, J., 1974, Differences in coronary heart disease in Framingham, Honolulu and Puerto Rico, *J. Chronic Dis.* **27**:329–344.

Grande, F., 1974, Sugars in cardiovascular disease, in: *Sugars in Nutrition* (H. I. Sipple and K. W. McNutt, eds.), Academic, New York, pp. 401–437.

Hardinge, M. G., Chambers, A. C., Crooks, H., and Stare, F. J., 1958, Nutritional studies of vegetarians, *Am. J. Clin. Nutr.* **6**:523–525.

Hirsch, E. F., and Nailor, R., 1955, Atherosclerosis. III. Fractional distribution of the esterified fatty acids of the blood lipids of rabbits with cream and cholesterol diets, *Arch. Pathol.* **59**:419–428.

Howard, A. N., Gresham, G. A., Jennings, I. W., and Jones, D., 1967, The effect of drugs on hypercholesterolaemia and atherosclerosis induced by semi-synthetic, low cholesterol diets, *Prog. Biochem. Pharmacol.* **2**:117–127.

Jenkins, D. J. A., Reynolds, D., Slavin, B., Leeds, A. R., Jenkins, A. L., and Jepson, E. M., 1980, Dietary fiber and blood lipids: Treatment of hypercholesterolemia with guar crisp-bread, *Am. J. Clin. Nutr.* **33**:575–581.

Kagan, A., Kannel, W. B., Dawber, T. R., and Revotskie, N., 1962, The coronary profile, *Ann. N. Y. Acad. Sci.* **97**:883–894.

Kay, R. M., 1980, Effects of dietary fibre on serum lipid levels and fecal bile acid excretion, *Can. Med. Assoc. J.* **123**:1213–1217.

Kay, R. M., and Truswell, A. S., 1980, Dietary fiber: Effects on plasma and biliary lipids in man, in: *Medical Aspects of Dietary Fiber* (G. A. Spiller and R. M. Kay, eds.), Plenum, New York, pp 153–173.

Kelsay, J. L., 1978, A review of research on effects of fiber intake on man, *Am. J. Clin. Nutr.* **31**:142–159.

Kirby, R. W., Anderson, J. W., Sieling, B., Rees, E. D., Chen, W. J., Miller, R. E., and Kay, R. M., 1981, Oat bran intake selectively lowers serum low density lipoprotein cholesterol concentrations of hypercholesterolemic men, *Am. J. Clin. Nutr.* **34**:824–829.

Kiriyama, S., Okozaki, Y., and Yoshida, A., 1969, Hypocholesterolemic effect of polysaccharides and polysaccharide-rich foodstuffs in cholesterol-fed rats, *J. Nutr.* **97**:382–388.

Knuiman, J. T., and West, C. E., 1982, The concentration of cholesterol in serum and in various serum lipoproteins in macrobiotic, vegetarian and non-vegetarian men and boys, *Atherosclerosis* 43:71–82.

Kritchevsky, D., 1964, Experimental atherosclerosis in rabbits fed cholesterol-free diets, *J. Atheroscler. Res.* 4:103–105.

Kritchevsky, D., and Tepper, S. A., 1965, Factors affecting atherosclerosis in rabbits fed cholesterol-free diets, *Life Sci.* 4:1467–1471.

Kritchevsky, D., and Tepper, S. A., 1968, Experimental and atherosclerosis in rabbits fed cholesterol-free diets: Influence of chow components, *J. Atheroscler. Res* 8:357–369.

Kritchevsky, D., Moyer, A. W., Tesar, W. C., Logan, J. B., Brown, R. A., Davies, M. C., and Cox, H. R., 1954, Effect of cholesterol vehicle in experimental atherosclerosis, *Am. J. Physiol.* 178:30–32

Kritchevsky, D., Davidson, L. M., Shapiro, I. L., Kim, H. K., Kitagawa, M., Malhotra, S., Nair P. P., Clarkson, T. B., Bersohn, I., and Winter, P. A. D., 1974, Lipid metabolism and experimental atherosclerosis in baboons: Influence of cholesterol-free, semi-synthetic diets, *Am. J. Clin. Nutr.* 27:29–50.

Kritchevsky, D., Tepper, S. A., Kim, H. K., Moses, D. E., and Story, J. A., 1975a, Experimental atherosclerosis in rabbits fed cholesterol-free diets. 4. Investigation into the source of cholesteremia, *Exp. Mol. Pathol.* 22:11–19.

Kritchevsky, D., Tepper, S. A., and Story, J. A., 1975b, Non-nutritive fiber and lipid metabolism, *J. Food Sci.* 40:8–11.

Kritchevsky, D., Tepper, S. A., Williams, D. E., and Story, J. A., 1977, Experimental atherosclerosis in rabbits fed cholesterol-free diets. 7. Interaction of animal or vegetable protein with fiber, *Atherosclerosis* 26:397–403.

Kritchevsky, D., Davidson, L. M., Krendel, D. A., Van der Watt, J. J., Russell, D., Friedland, S., and Mendelsohn, D., 1981, Influence of dietary fiber on aortic sudanophilia in vervet monkeys, *Ann. Nutr. Metab.* 25:125–136.

Kritchevsky, D., Tepper, S. A., and Goodman, G., 1985, Diet, nutrient intake and metabolism in populations at high and low risk for colon cancer. 7. Relation of diet to serum lipids, *Am. J. Clin. Nutr.,* 40:921–926.

Lambert, G. F., Miller, J. P., Olsen, R. T., and Frost, D. V., 1958, Hypercholesteremia and atherosclerosis induced in rabbits by purified high fat rations devoid of cholesterol, *Proc. Soc. Exp. Biol. Med.* 97:544–549.

Malinow, M. R., McLaughlin, P., Naito, H. K., Lewis, L. A., and McNulty, W. P., 1978, Effect of alfalfa meal on shrinkage (regression) of atherosclerotic plaques during cholesterol feeding in monkeys, *Atherosclerosis* 30:27–43.

Malmros, H., and Wigand, G., 1959, Atherosclerosis and deficiency of essential fatty acids, *Lancet* 2:749–751.

Miller, G. J., and Miller, N. E., 1975, Plasma high density lipoprotein concentration and development of ischaemic heart disease, *Lancet* 1:16–19.

Moore, J. H., 1967, The effect of the type of roughage in the diet on plasma cholesterol levels and aortic atherosis in rabbits, *Br. J. Nutr.* 21:207–215.

Nakamura, H., Ishikawa, T., Toda, N., Kagami, A., Kondo, K., Myazima, E., and Takeyama, S., 1982, Effect of several kinds of dietary fibres on serum and lipoprotein lipids, *Nutr. Rep. Int.* 26:215–221.

Sacks, F. M., Castelli, W. P., Donner, A., and Kass, E. H., 1975, Plasma lipids and lipoproteins in vegetarians and controls, *N. Engl. J. Med.* 292:1148–1151.

Stasse-Wolthuis, M., Hautvast, J. G. A. J., Hermus, R. J. J., Katan, M. N., Bausch, J. E., Reitberg-Brussnard, J. H., Velma, J. P., Zondervan, J. G., Eastwood, M. A., and Brydon, G. R., 1979, The effect of a natural high fiber diet on serum lipids, fecal lipids and colonic function, *Am. J. Clin. Nutr.* 32:1881–1888.

Stasse-Wolthuis, M., Albers, H. F. F., van Jeveren, J. G. C., Wil de Jong, J., Hautvast, J. G. A. J., Hermus, R. J. J., Katan, M. B., Brydon, G. B., and Eastwood, M. A., 1980, Influence of dietary fiber from vegetables and fruits, bran, citrus pectin on serum lipids, fecal lipids and colonic functions, *Am. J. Clin. Nutr.* **33**:1745–1756.

Steiner, A., Varsos, A., and Samuel, P., 1959, Effect of saturated and unsaturated fats on the concentration of serum cholesterol and experimental atherosclerosis, *Circ. Res.* **7**:448–453.

Story, J. A., 1981, The role of dietary fiber in lipid metabolism, *Adv. Lipid Res.* **18**:229–246.

Story, J. A., Baldino, A., Czarnecki, S. K., and Kritchevsky, D., 1981, Modification of liver cholesterol accumulation by dietary fiber in rats, *Nutr. Rep. Int.* **24**:1213–1219.

Tsai, A. C., Elias, J., Kelley, J. J., Lin, R. S. C., and Robson, J. R. K., 1976, Influence of certain dietary fibers on serum and tissue cholesterol levels in rats, *J. Nutr.* **106**:118–123.

Wells, A. F., and Ershoff, B. H., 1961, Beneficial effects of pectin in prevention of hypercholesterolemia and increase in liver cholesterol in cholesterol-fed rats, *J. Nutr.* **74**:87–92.

18

Hypocholesterolemic Effects of Soluble Fibers

W. J. L. CHEN and JAMES W. ANDERSON

1. INTRODUCTION

Certain high-fiber foods have substantial hypocholesterolemic effects. These effects are related principally to the water-soluble fiber content of these foods (Jenkins *et al.*, 1975; Anderson and Chen, 1979; Aro *et al.*, 1984; Jenkins *et al.*, 1980). Diets supplemented with oat products significantly lower serum cholesterol concentrations of humans (deGroot *et al.*, 1963; Kirby *et al.*, 1981; Judd and Truswell, 1981; Anderson *et al.*, 1984b) and rats (Chen and Anderson, 1979). Since 1977 we have evaluated the hypocholesterolemic effects of oat bran; here we review these results in order to discuss the potential mechanisms involved for the cholesterol-lowering properties of soluble fibers.

2. HUMAN STUDIES

2.1. Hypercholesterolemic Men

2.1.1. Experimental Design

Ten hypercholesterolemic men were admitted to a metabolic ward as previously described (Anderson *et al.*, 1984b). For the first 7 days they

W. J. L. CHEN and JAMES W. ANDERSON• Medical Service, Veterans Administration Medical Center, and Department of Medicine, University of Kentucky College of Medicine, Lexington, Kentucky 40511.

received control diets similar in composition to average Western diets and then received isocaloric oat bran-supplemented diets for 21 days. The carbohydrate, protein, fat, and cholesterol content of the two diets were identical, but the diet with 100 g oat bran daily had more soluble and total fiber (Table I). Oat bran was served as hot cereal and muffins. Fasting serum cholesterol and triglyceride concentrations were measured daily and serum low-density lipoprotein (LDL), very low-density lipoprotein (VLDL), and high-density lipoprotein (HDL) cholesterol concentrations were determined on the last 3 days of each diet. All stools were collected for bile acid and neutral sterol determinations.

2.1.2. Results

Oat bran supplements rapidly lowered serum cholesterol concentrations (Fig. 1). By 11 days values were 25% below control values. During the last week of oat bran use serum cholesterol values averaged 19% below control values (Table II). Oat bran selectively lowered serum LDL-cholesterol but did not significantly affect VLDL-cholesterol or HDL-cholesterol or triglyceride concentrations. Oat bran also increased fecal bile acid excretion by 65%.

2.2. Healthy College Students

2.2.1. Experimental Design

The effects of oat bran intake on serum cholesterol concentrations of healthy young college students maintaining their usual diet and activities

TABLE I. Mean Daily Composition of Foods Consumed[a]

	Control diet	Oat-bran diet
Energy, kcal	1938 ± 63	1948 ± 74
Protein, g	97 ± 3	98 ± 3
Carbohydrate, g	208 ± 7	212 ± 7
Simple	104 ± 4	104 ± 4
Complex	104 ± 4	108 ± 4
Fat, total, g	78 ± 2.6	78 ± 3.3
Saturated	31 ± 1.8	31 ± 2.0
Monounsaturated	31 ± 1.5	28 ± 1.6
Polyunsaturated	15 ± 1.2	16 ± 1.6
Cholesterol, mg	439 ± 4	436 ± 1.5
Total fiber, g	19 ± 0.7	47 ± 0.1
Soluble, fiber, g	6 ± 0.3	17 ± 0.4

[a] From Anderson et al. (1984b). Values are mean ± SEM.

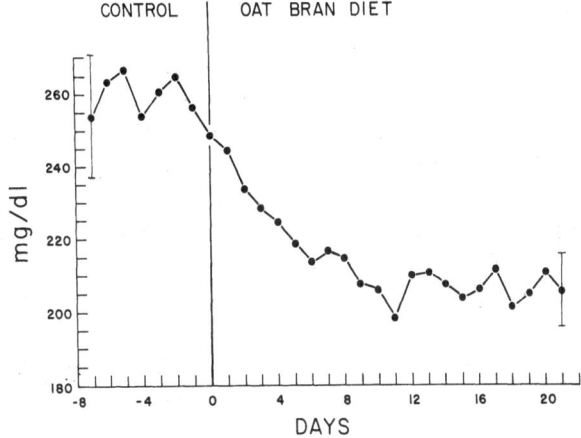

FIGURE 1. Serum cholesterol response of six hypercholesterolemic men fed oat bran-supplemented diet on metabolic ward.

were studied using a random allocation, crossover design with a washout period (Storch *et al.*, 1984). After a 2-week control period six males and six females were randomly allocated to oat bran or wheat bran muffin groups for 6 weeks. Subsequently they continued their usual diet without muffins for 7 weeks and then ate the other muffins for 6 weeks. During the muffin periods they received 50 g of oat or wheat bran daily in four muffins. Throughout the 21-week period they were encouraged to keep meat, egg, and dairy product intake and exercise at the same level. Fasting serum lipid concentrations were measured weekly. Food intake was assessed weekly by diet diary, 24-h recall, and 7-day surveys of food eaten.

TABLE II. Responses of Lipid and Bile Metabolism in Men[a]

Measurement	Control diet	Oat-bran diet
Serum cholesterol,[b] mg/dl		
Total	257 ± 17	207 ± 12*
LDL	195 ± 16	148 ± 2*
VLDL	31.8 ± 4.2	30.2 ± 6.4
HDL	30.3 ± 1.2	28.9 ± 2.0
Serum triglyceride, mg/dl	159 ± 21	151 ± 31
Fecal bile acid, mg/dl	109 ± 37	180 ± 43
Fuel neutral steroid, mg/dl	719 ± 140	829 ± 91

[a] Values are mean ± SEM, with significant difference indicated: * p vs. control < 0.05.
[b] LDL, low-density lipoprotein; VLDL, very low-density lipoprotein; HDL, high-density lipoprotein.

2.2.2. Results

Body weights and serum triglyceride concentrations did not change significantly during the study; weights averaged 1 lb heavier while on muffins. Dietary cholesterol and fat intakes were higher during both muffin periods than during control periods; egg intake was twofold higher ($p < 0.01$) while on oat bran muffins than during the control period. Wheat bran muffins did not significantly affect serum cholesterol concentrations. However, with oat bran muffin use, serum cholesterol values were significantly lower ($p < 0.001$) at 3, 4, 5, and 6 weeks; during the control period serum cholesterol values averaged 185 ± 7 mg/dl (mean $<$ SEM), while with oat bran muffins, values averaged 164 ± 7 mg/dl. While wheat bran muffins did not affect serum cholesterol values, oat bran muffins lowered serum cholesterol values by 12%.

2.3. Long-Term Effects

The effectiveness and acceptability of high-soluble-fiber diets were assessed in ten hypercholesterolemic men followed for 24–99 weeks (Anderson *et al.*, 1984a). After an initial 1-week control period these men were treated with soluble-fiber-rich diets for 3 weeks on a metabolic ward. Oat bran or bean diets lowered serum total cholesterol and LDL-cholesterol concentrations by 23% (Anderson *et al.*, 1984a). Following discharge from the hospital these men used high-fiber diets, including an average of 41 g of oat bran and 145 g of cooked beans daily. After 24 weeks, serum cholesterol values were 26% lower and LDL-cholesterol values were 24% lower than control values. Four men were followed for 99 weeks; serum cholesterol values were 22% lower and LDL-cholesterol values were 29% lower than control values, while HDL-cholesterol values were 9% higher than control values (Fig. 2). Adherence to diet was rated good to excellent in eight of ten men. This study indicates that soluble-fiber-rich diets are acceptable to selected individuals and maintain significant reductions in serum cholesterol concentrations; oat bran intake appears to sustain a selective reduction in serum LDL-cholesterol while tending to increase HDL-cholesterol concentrations.

3. ANIMAL STUDIES

3.1. Oat Bran Feeding

3.1.1. Experimental Design

Oat bran was fed to rats to determine its effects on serum and liver cholesterol concentrations as well as biliary bile acid and cholesterol concen-

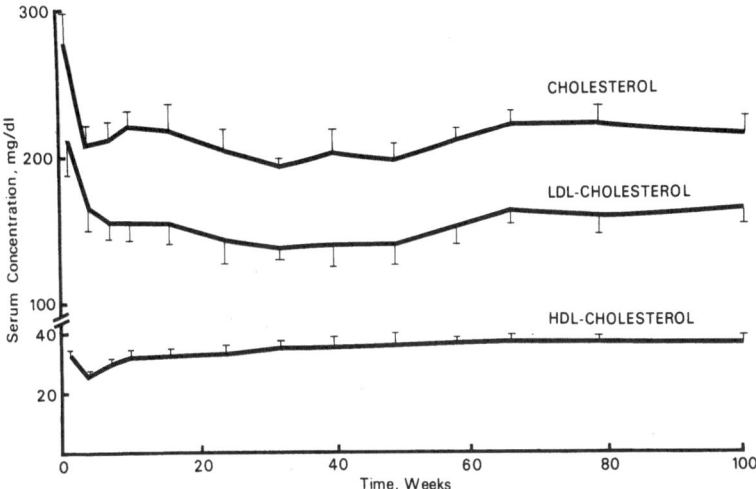

FIGURE 2. Response of serum cholesterol, LDL-, and HDL-cholesterol concentrations of four hypercholesterolemic men to oat bran-supplemented diets for 99 weeks as outpatients.

trations, using previously described approaches (Chen and Anderson, 1979; Chen et al., 1981). Male Sprague-Dawley rats were divided into three groups of ten rats each. Each group received one of three experimental diets for 3 weeks. All diets included the basal diet (Table III). The cellulose diet included the basal diet plus 10% cellulose; the control diet included the basal diet plus 10% cellulose plus 1% cholesterol and 0.2% cholic acid; and the oat bran diet included 10% oat bran fiber plus 1% cholesterol and 0.2% cholic acid.

3.1.2. Results

The oat bran diet was accompanied by significantly lower serum cholesterol concentrations than the control diet (Table IV). Oat bran did not affect serum HDL-cholesterol concentrations. Liver cholesterol concentrations were significantly lower for oat bran- than for control-fed rats. Biliary bile flow, bile acid, and cholesterol concentrations were significantly higher for oat bran-fed rats. These observations are consistent with our human studies, where oat bran intake increased fecal bile acid excretion (Table II).

3.2. Portal Vein Short-Chain Fatty Acids

Short-chain fatty acids (SCFA) are produced in the colon by bacterial fermentation of dietary fiber and other carbohydrates. These SCFAs, in-

TABLE III. Composition of Basal Diet

Ingredient	Amount, g/100 g
Carbohydrate	62.5
Protein	15.0
DL-Methionine	0.3
Fat	6.0
Salt mix	4.0
Vitamin fortification	1.0
Plant fiber	10.0

cluding acetate, propionate, and butyrate, are virtually completely absorbed from the colon (Cummings, 1981; Schmitt et al., 1976). Butyrate is utilized by the colonic endothelium and some appears in the portal vein for uptake by the liver (Cummings, 1981). Propionate is largely extracted from portal venous blood by the liver, while acetate reaches the peripheral circulation and is metabolized by peripheral tissues (Cummings and Branch, this volume, Chapter 10). We have evaluated the potential role of these fiber metabolites on cholesterol homoestasis.

To determine the effects of oat bran feeding on portal vein short-chain fatty acid (SCFA) concentrations, rats were fed a cellulose diet (basal diet with 0.3% cholesterol and 10% cellulose) or an oat bran diet (basal diet with 0.3% cholesterol and 10% oat bran fiber) ad libitum for 3 weeks. Hepatic portal vein samples were analyzed for SCFA. Similar to previous observations (Topping et al., 1982; Storer et al., 1983), serum acetate, butyrate, and propionate concentrations were significantly higher in oat bran-fed rats than in cellulose-fed rats (Table V).

TABLE IV. Cholesterol and Bile Metabolism in Rats[a]

	Normal	Control	Oat bran
Serum total cholesterol, mg/dl	$87 \pm 7*$	$181 \pm 7\dagger$	$123 \pm 7*$
Serum HDL-cholesterol,[a] mg/dl	$43 \pm 2*$	$26 \pm 2\dagger$	$24 \pm 1\dagger$
Liver cholesterol, mg/g liver	$3.1 \pm 0.3*$	$44.3 \pm 2.7\dagger$	$30.0 \pm 1.5\ddagger$
Biliary bile flow, $\mu l/min$ per g liver	$0.97 \pm 0.06*$	$1.24 \pm 0.05\dagger$	$1.58 \pm 0.08\ddagger$
Biliary bile acid, nmol/min per g liver	$23.7 \pm 1.9*$	$30.8 \pm 2.3\dagger$	$45.6 \pm 2.8\ddagger$
Biliary bile cholesterol, nmol/min per g liver	$0.55 \pm 0.06*$	$0.80 \pm 0.06\dagger$	$1.00 \pm 0.06\ddagger$

[a] Values are mean ± SEM for 9–10 rats. Means in the same row with different symbols differ significantly ($p < 0.05$).
[b] HDL, high-density lipoprotein.

TABLE V. SCFA Concentrations in Hepatic Portal Vein of Rats[a]

	Cellulose diet	Oat bran diet
Acetate, μM	1020 ± 44	1346 ± 53*
Butyrate, μM	22 ± 3	71 ± 13*
Propionate, μM	51 ± 3	92 ± 10*

[a] Values are mean ± SEM, with significant difference indicated: * p vs. control < 0.005.

Postmeal portal vein SCFA concentrations were evaluated in another experiment. Rats were randomly assigned to three dietary groups and meal-fed from 8:30 to 10:30 A.M. for 3 weeks. The basal diet (Table III) had no dietary fiber, the control diet with 0.3% cholesterol had no dietary fiber, while the oat bran diet had 10% oat bran fiber with 0.3% cholesterol. Rats were killed at 4, 8, 12, and 24 h after their last meal. Serum propionate concentrations in portal vein were significantly higher in oat bran-fed rats than in control animals (Fig. 3). Propionate concentrations were highest at 4 h and similar at 8 h after meals and returned to baseline by 12 h. These studies indicate that serum propionate concentrations in rats fed oat bran reach peak values in the absorptive period and return to basal values 8–12 h after a meal.

3.3. Hepatic Cholesterol Synthesis

The regulation of hepatic cholesterol synthesis can be assessed in isolated rat hepatocytes (Gibbons and Pullinger, 1979). Using modifications of these techniques, we assessed the effect of propionate on [^{14}C]acetate incorporation into cholesterol of isolated rat hepatocytes. At concentrations as low as

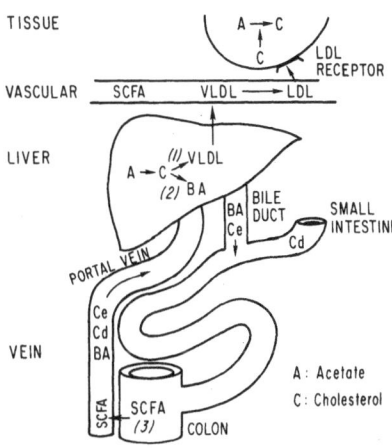

FIGURE 3. Schematic illustration of the regulation of cholesterol metabolism. Abbreviations: A, acetate; C, cholesterol; LDL, low-density lipoprotein; VLDL, very low-density lipoprotein; SCFA, short-chain fatty acids; BA, bile acids; Ce, endogenous cholesterol; Cd, dietary cholesterol.

0.2 mM, propionate significantly inhibited [¹⁴C]acetate incorporation into cholesterol (Fig. 4).

To extend these observations, the effects of propionate feeding on cholesterol homeostasis in rats was evaluated. Rats fed 0.5% sodium propionate for 3 weeks had significantly lower serum and liver cholesterol concentrations than did control animals (Chen and Anderson, 1984). Thus propionate, a metabolic product of fiber fermentation, may mediate some at the cholesterol-lowering effects of soluble fibers.

4. PROPOSED MECHANISMS

Soluble fibers could affect serum cholesterol concentrations by altering cholesterol or bile acid absorption, by altering hepatic production of lipoproteins, by altering peripheral disposal of lipoproteins, or by other actions. Previously, most of the attention has been focused on possible alterations of cholesterol or bile acid absorption or reabsorption (Anderson and Chen, 1979). However, our studies (Anderson *et al.*, 1984b; Chen and Anderson, 1984) suggest that soluble fibers may influence cholesterol metabolism at hepatic or peripheral sites. Figure 5 illustrates some aspects of cholesterol and soluble fiber metabolism.

4.1. Bile Acid Metabolism

Some soluble fibers, such as guar, pectin, and oat bran, increase fecal bile acid excretion, while others, such as gum arabic and beans, do not (Kay

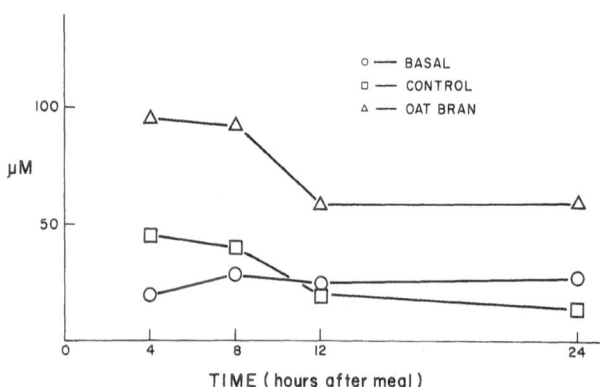

FIGURE 4. Serum propionate concentrations in portal veins of rats fed basal, control, and oat bran diets as described in text.

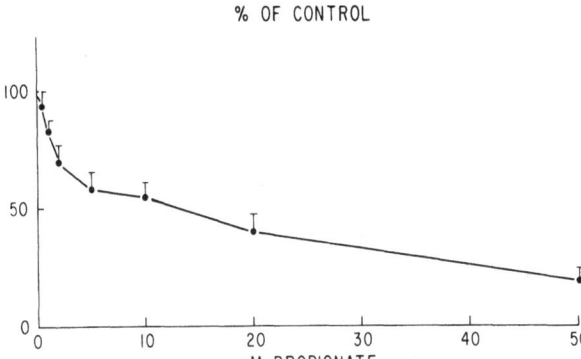

FIGURE 5. Effect of propionate concentration on cholesterol synthesis in isolated rat hepatocytes.

and Truswell, 1977; Anderson *et al.*, 1984b; Anderson and Chen, 1985). Even when soluble fibers increase fecal loss of bile acids, the magnitude of the loss is small compared to that observed with cholestyramine (Moutafes *et al.*, 1977). With oat bran, for example, the fecal bile acid loss is less than twofold greater than on control diets. The liver should easily be able to compensate for these small losses. Dietary fibers may alter the metabolism of bile acids in the gut and change the ratio of primary to secondary bile acids (Story and Thomes, 1982); this could influence hepatic cholesterol or bile acid metabolism. Thus, while alterations in bile acid excretion or metabolism may mediate some of the hypocholesterolemic effects of soluble fibers, other factors probably play a role.

4.2. Hepatic Cholesterol Metabolism

Oat bran, oat gum, guar, pectin, and other soluble fibers lower liver cholesterol concentrations consistently in rats (Chen and Anderson, 1985). Based on the studies outlined above, we postulate the following sequence of events. Oat bran feeding increases bile acid synthesis and secretion. With increased cholesterol entry into the bile acid synthetic pathway, less cholesterol enters the lipoprotein synthetic pathway and less VLDL is available for secretion into the circulation. Soluble fiber-induced increases in portal vein SCFAs, especially propionate, act to decrease hepatic cholesterol synthesis and interfere with usual hepatic compensatory mechanisms. These events result in decreased hepatic cholesterol concentrations and decreased secretion of VLDL-cholesterol.

4.3. Lipoprotein Metabolism

Oat bran feeding rapidly lowers LDL-cholesterol concentrations without altering VLDL-cholesterol concentrations (Fig. 1 and Table II). Since VLDL particles are precursors of LDL particles (Goldstein and Brown, 1982), an increased rate of LDL catabolism might explain these observations. Cholestyramine administration decreases LDL pool size and increases LDL catabolism (Levy and Langer, 1972). Although an increased rate of clearance of LDL has not been demonstrated after oat bran intake, we postulate that oat bran may increase LDL catabolism by the following mechanism. Soluble fibers increase peripheral serum acetate concentrations (Cummings and Branch, this volume, Chapter 10), which may inhibit cholesterol synthesis (Beymen et al., 1982) in peripheral tissues, resulting in an increase in peripheral LDL receptors; this increase would then increase LDL clearance. Although this is hypothetical, our data are consistent with the possibility that oat bran may increase clearance of LDL-cholesterol.

5. CONCLUSIONS

Oat bran has impressive hypocholesterolemic effects, which appear to be mediated by its rich content of water-soluble fiber. Oat bran, 100 g daily, lowers serum cholesterol concentrations of hypercholesterolemic men by 19%; these reductions occur on a metabolic ward where intake of fat and cholesterol are maintained constant over a 21-day period. The LDL-cholesterol concentrations in serum are selectively decreased by oat bran, while HDL-cholesterol concentrations are not affected. Long-term use of oat bran as part of a prudent diet sustains reductions in LDL-cholesterol concentrations for up to 99 weeks, while HDL-cholesterol concentrations increase slowly over this time period.

For healthy college students oat bran muffins lower serum cholesterol concentrations by 12% over a 6-week period. Only 50 g of oat bran daily, about two average muffins, was required to achieve these reductions. Since a 12% reduction in serum cholesterol concentration decreases the estimated risk for amyocardial infarction by 24% (Lipid Research Clinics Program, 1984), oat bran intake may offer a distinct health advantage for selected individuals.

While the hypocholesterolemic effects of oat bran and other sources of soluble fiber are well described, the mechanisms have not been delineated. Some soluble fibers such as oat bran increase fecal bile acid excretion and may influence cholesterol homeostasis in this manner. Oat bran also increases portal vein concentrations of SCFAs such as acetate, propionate, and butyrate. These SCFAs may attenuate hepatic cholesterol synthesis and contribute to the cholesterol-lowering effect of oat bran. Since oat bran intake is accompanied by selective reductions in serum LDL-cholesterol concentrations without alterations in serum VLDL-cholesterol concentrations, it may enhance clearance of LDL-cholesterol. Further studies are required to examine the mechanisms responsible for the important hypocholesterolemic effects of oat bran.

REFERENCES

Anderson, J. W., and Chen. W. L., 1979, Plant fiber: Carbohydrate and lipid metabolism, *Am. J. Clin. Nutr.* **32**:346–363.

Anderson, J. W., and Chen, W. L., 1985, Cholesterol-lowering properties of oat products, in: *Oats* (F. Webster, ed.), in press.

Anderson, J. W., Story, L., Sieling, B., and Chen, W. L., 1984a, Hypocholesterolemic effects of high-fiber diets rich in water-soluble plant fibers, *J. Can. Dietet. Assoc.* **45**:140–149.

Anderson, J. W., Story, L., Sieling, B., Chen, W. L., Petro, M. S., and Story, J., 1984b, Hypocholesterolemic effects of oat-bran or bean intake for hypercholesterolemic men, *Am. J. Clin. Nutr.* **40**:1146–1155.

Aro, A., Uusitupa, M., Voutilainen, E., and Korhonen, T., 1984, Effects of guar gum in male subjects with hypercholesterolemia, *Am. J. Clin. Nutr.* **39**:911–916.

Beymen, A. C., Buechler, K. F., Van der Molen, A. J., and Geelen, M. J. H., 1982, The effects of lactate and acetate on fatty acid and cholesterol biosynthesis by isolated rat hepatocytes, *Int. J. Biochem.* **14**:165–169.

Chen, W. L., and Anderson, J. W., 1979, Effects of plant fiber in decreasing plasma total cholesterol and increasing high density lipoprotein cholesterol, *Proc. Soc. Exp. Biol. Med.* **162**:310–313.

Chen, W. L., Anderson, J. W., and Gould, M. R., 1981, Cholesterol-lowering effects of oat bran and oat gum, *Nutr. Rep. Int.* **24**:1093–1098.

Chen, W. L., Anderson, J. W., and Jennings, D., 1984, Propionate may mediate the hypocholesterolemic effects of certain soluble plant fibers in cholesterol-fed rats, *Proc. Soc. Exp. Biol. Med.* **175**:215–218.

Cummings, J. H., 1981, Short chain fatty acids in the human colon, *Gut* **22**:763–779.

deGroot, A. P., Luyken, R., and Pikaar, N. A., 1963, Cholesterol-lowering effects of rolled oats, *Lancet* **2**:303–304.

Gibbons, G. F., and Pullinger, C. R., 1977, Measurement of the absolute rates of cholesterol biosynthesis in isolated rat liver cells, *Biochem. J.* **162**:321–330.

Gibbons, G. F., and Pullinger, C. R., 1979, Utilization endogenous and exogenous sources substrate for cholesterol bile synthesis by isolated hepatocytes, *Biochem. J.* **177**:255–263.

Goldstein, J. L., and Brown, M. S., 1982, The LDL receptor defect in familial hypercholesterolemia: Implications the pathogenesis and therapy, *Med. Clin. North Am.* **66**:335–362.

Jenkins, D. J. A., Leeds, A. R., Newton, C., and Cummings, J. H., 1975, Effect of pectin, guar gum, and wheat fibre on serum-cholesterol, *Lancet* **2**:1116–1118.

Jenkins, D. J. A., Reynolds, D., Slavin, B., Leeds, A. R., Jenkins, A. R., and Jepson, E. M., 1980, Dietary fiber and blood lipids: Treatment of hypercholesterolemia with guar crispbread, *Am. J. Clin. Nutr.* **33**:575–581.

Judd, P. A., and Truswell, S. A., 1981, The effect of rolled oats on blood lipids and fecal steroid excretion in man, *Am. J. Clin. Nutr.* **34**:2061–2067.

Kay, R. M., and Truswell, A. S., 1977, Effect of citrus pectin on blood lipids and fecal steroid excretion in men, *Am. J. Clin. Nutr.* **30**:171–175.

Kirby, R. W., Anderson, J. W., Sieling, B., Rees, E. D., Chen, W. L., Miller, R. E., and Kay, R. M., 1981, Oat bran intake selectively lowers serum low-density lipoprotein cholesterol concentrations of hypercholesterolemic men, *Am. J. Clin. Nutr.* **34**:824–829.

Levy, R. I., and Langer, T., 1972, Hypolipidemic drugs and lipoprotein metabolism, in: *Drugs Affecting Lipid Metabolism,* Volume 26 (W. L. S. Holms, R. Paoletti, and D. Kritchevsky, eds.), Plenum, New York, pp. 155–163.

Lipid Research Clinics Program, 1984, The lipid research clinic's coronary primary precaution trial results: I. Reduction in incidence of coronary heart disease, *J. Am. Med. Assoc.* **251**:351–358.

Moutafes, C. D., Simmons, L. A., Myant, N. D., Edams, T. W., and Wynn, V., 1977, Effect of cholestyramine of faecal excretion bile acid and neutral steroid in familar hypercholesterolemia, *Atherosclerosis* **26**:329.

Schmitt, M. G., Soegrel, K. H., and Wood, C. M., 1976, Absorption of short chain fatty acids from the human jejunum, *Gastroentology* **70**:211–215.

Storch, K., Anderson, J. W., and Young, V. R., 1984, Oat bran muffins lower serum cholesterol of healthy young people, *Clin. Res.* **32**:740A.

Stores, G. B., Trimble, R. P., Illman, R. J., Snoswell, A. M., and Topping, D. L., 1983, Effects of dietary oat bran and diabetes on plasma volatile fatty acids in the rat, *Nutr. Res.* **3**:519–526.

Story, J. A., and Thomas, J. N., 1982, Modification of bile acid spectrum by dietary fiber, in: *Dietary Fiber in Health and Disease* (G. V. Vahouny and D. Kritchevsky, eds.), Plenum, New York, pp. 193–201.

Topping, D.L., Illman, R. J., Storer, G. B., Timble, R. P., McIntosh, G. H., and Snoswell, A. M., 1982, Oat products and plasma volatile fatty acids in the rat and pig, *Proc. Nutr. Soc. Abstr.* **7**:140.

19

Dietary Fiber and Intestinal Lipoprotein Secretion

KATSUMI IMAIZUMI and MICHIHIRO SUGANO

1. INTRODUCTION

A lowered incidence of coronary artery disease can be attributed in part to a diet characterized by a high fiber content (Anderson *et al.*, 1973; Walker, 1975; Rowell and Burkitt, 1977; Kay *et al.*, 1980). Various human and experimental animal studies on the effects of fiber on lipid metabolism have been principally concerned with the interaction of fiber with lipid components in the intestinal lumen (Eastwood and Boyd, 1967; Eastwood and Hamilton, 1968; Balmer and Zilversmit, 1974; Birkner and Kern, 1974; Kritchevsky and Story, 1974, 1975; Story and Kritchevsky, 1975, 1976; Eastwood and Mowbray, 1976; Eastwood *et al.*, 1976; Vahouny *et al.*, 1980c, 1981) and measurements of serum lipoprotein components (Anderson and Chen, 1979; Kay, 1982). It is also becoming apparent that dietary fiber alters anatomic features of the intestine and the biochemical function of intestinal epithelial cells (Ecknauer *et al.*, 1981; Cassidy *et al.*, 1982; Farness and Schneeman, 1982; Gordon *et al.*, 1983; Gordon and Besch-Williford, 1983), and may affect the regulation of endocrinologic factors (Goulder *et al.*, 1978; Morgan *et al.*, 1979; Jenkins *et al.*, 1980a; Poksay and Schneeman, 1983).

The intestine is now recognized as an organ active in lipoprotein synthesis and as an important source of lipoprotein constituents for serum

KATSUMI IMAIZUMI and MICHIHIRO SUGANO • Laboratory of Nutrition Chemistry, Kyushu University School of Agriculture, Fukuoka 812, Japan.

lipoproteins (Green and Glickman, 1981). Endogenous and exogenous lipids do not accumulate in significant amounts in the intestinal mucosa (Vahouny, 1982) and therefore the absorbed lipids are transported as intestinal lipoproteins. Until now there have been few studies on how dietary fiber affects intestinal lipids and lipoproteins, aside from the studies of Vahouny *et al.* (1978, 1980b). In this chapter, we concentrate on the effects of water-soluble (guar gum) and water-insoluble (cellulose) fibers on the secretion of dietary fats as chylomicrons in rats.

2. SECRETION OF DIETARY LIPIDS INTO MESENTERIC LYMPH

2.1. Overview of Intestinal Lipoprotein Synthesis and Secretion

Several reviews have appeared over the last few years summarizing the current state of knowledge on the composition, synthesis, and secretion of the intestinal lipoproteins and their apoproteins (Friedman and Nylund, 1980; Scanu and Landsberger, 1980; Green and Glickman, 1981). Much of what is known about intestinal lipoprotein formation has resulted from biochemical and electron microscopic studies of triglyceride absorption and chylomicron secretion into lymph.

Chylomicrons are heterogeneous, with a size range from 750 to 6000 Å, and the size is largely determined by the flux of triglyceride through the intestinal cells (Lossow *et al.*, 1969; Fraser, 1970). After fasting, intestinal lymph contains lipid transport particles (280–750 Å) comparable to very low-density lipoproteins (VLDL) of plasma with respect to flotation and composition, except for the absence of apoproteins (Ockner *et al.*, 1968; Glickman and Green, 1977; Imaizumi *et al.*, 1978a), so-called intestinal VLDLs or small chylomicrons (Redgrave and Dunne, 1975). Intestinal VLDL, but not serum VLDL, contains apo A-I. These lipoproteins are biological emulsion droplets composed predominantly of a triglyceride and cholesterol ester core and a phospholipid and protein surface (Miller and Small, 1983a). Cholesterol is partitioned into both surface layer and oil core phases in these particles (Zilversmit, 1965; Miller and Small, 1983b). Although during active fat absorption triglycerides are transported predominantly as large chylomicrons, cholesterol and probably phospholipid are partitioned between large and small chylomicrons (Frazer and Courtice, 1969; Vahouny *et al.*, 1980a). During fat absorption the formation of large lymph particles would allow more triglyceride to be transported, while surface constituents appear to be conserved (Sata *et al.*, 1972; Mjøs *et al.*, 1975).

Using ultrastructural and radioautographic techniques, it has been shown that newly absorbed fatty acids and 2-monoglycerides appear as triglyceride droplets in smooth endoplasmic reticulum in the enterocytes (Strauss, 1966; Sabesin and Frase, 1977). The *de novo* synthesis (Haessler and Isselbacher, 1963) of triglycerides and phospholipids may not be important compared to the monoglyceride pathway (Senior and Isselbacher, 1961; Clark and Hübscher, 1961) and the reacylation of absorbed lysolecithin (Mansbach, 1973) in active chylomicron formation. The protein constituents of chylomicrons are synthesized in the rough endoplasmic reticulum (Hatch *et al.*, 1963; Isselbacher and Budz, 1963; Kessler *et al.*, 1975). Among the apoproteins associated with lymph chylomicrons, apo B, apo A-I, and apo A-IV are synthesized in the intestine in significant amounts, while apo E and apo C are principally of hepatic origin (Wu and Windmueller, 1979; Glickman and Green, 1977; Imaizumi *et al.*, 1978b; Krishnaiah *et al.*, 1980). Recently, Gordon *et al.* (1982a–c, 1984) have shown that apo A-IV, unlike apo A-I, does not contain prosegments, although the primary translation products of human and rat intestinal apo A-I and apo A-IV contain signal peptides (presegments). Human intestinal biopsies show the active synthesis of apo A-II (Rachmilewitz *et al.*, 1978), while this apoprotein is a minor protein in rat chylomicrons (Imaizumi *et al.*, 1978a). Fidge and McCullagh (1981) found a new apoprotein, called apo A-V, in ultracentrifugally isolated lymph chylomicrons, although this protein is easily removed from chylomicrons after gel filtration.

Lipids and proteins are believed to associate in the endoplasmic reticulum; subsequently the lipid droplets accumulate as prechylomicrons in the Golgi apparatus (Redgrave, 1971; Mahley *et al.*, 1971). Discharge of chylomicrons into the intracellular space occurs morphologically by reverse pinocytosis with fusion of Golgi membranes with the basolateral membrane (Strauss, 1966; Sabesin and Frase, 1977). The formation and release of chylomicrons are dependent on protein and phospholipid synthesis, since protein synthesis inhibitors interrupt the release of chylomicrons (Glickman and Kirsch, 1973) and also modify intestinal phospholipid metabolism (O'Doherty *et al.*, 1973).

In addition to chylomicrons, intestinal lymph contains particles corresponding to serum low-density lipoproteins (LDL) and high-density lipoproteins (HDL) (Glickman and Green, 1977; Riley *et al.*, 1980). Krause *et al.* (1981) have shown that intestinal lymph contains predominantly low-molecular weight apo B, which differs immunologically from hepatic apo B (Krishnaiah *et al.*, 1980), in rats treated with ethynyl estradiol, which prevents transfer of plasma apoprotein into lymph (Davis and Roheim, 1978). Lymph HDLs are of diverse morphology, including discs and spheres (Green *et al.*, 1978). A substantial fraction of the lymph apo A-I in fasting rats is shown to be present in lymph HDL (Glickman and Green, 1977; Imaizumi *et al.*, 1978b). Forester *et al.* (1983) have demonstrated that intestine secretes these HDLs directly. The effect of diet on the secretion of lymph LDL and HDL is not well characterized.

2.2 The Effect of Fiber on Dietary Fat Transport

The measurement of the transport rate of mesenteric lymph triglyceride does not address issues of the respective processes of dietary fat handling as described above; rather, it represents the efficiency of the overall processes for fat absorption *in vivo*. To examine *in vivo* the effect of dietary fiber on the transport of dietary fat, we have collected intestinal lymph at selected times after the last meal from meal-fed rats. Dietary and experimental conditions are shown in Fig. 1. As shown in Fig. 1, the concentration of lymph triglycerides increased gradually in guar gum-fed rats and reached a peak value 6 h after feeding. This delay was marked compared to that in rats fed cellulose or fiber-free diets, although cellulose exhibited some delay effect. The concentration of lymph triglycerides decreased most rapidly in rats fed a fiber-free diet. The amount of food ingested and the body weights of rats appeared not to be related to the secretion pattern of lymphatic triglyceride.

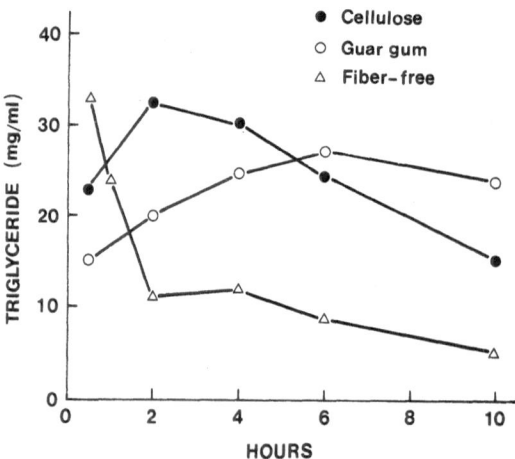

FIGURE 1. Concentration of mesenteric lymph triglycerides at selected times after the last meal. Male Wistar rats, weighing 270–290 g, were trained to meal feed a semipurified diet containing 10% corn oil and cellulose or guar gum (4%), 1 h daily (9–10 A.M.) for 2–3 weeks. Body weights on the experimental day were 279 ± 6 g for guar gum, 246 ± 12 g for cellulose, and 244 ± 9 g for fiber-free diet, respectively. Average food intake per day was 11.7 ± 0.6 g for guar gum, 13 ± 1.5 g for cellulose, and 11.5 ± 1.3 g for fiber-free diet. Mesenteric lymph (approximately 50 μl) was withdrawn by needle directly from the intestinal lymph duct under ether anesthesia. Values are representative of two separate experiments.

When lymph triglyceride is greater than 1.5–3.0 mg/ml, most triglycerides are transported in large chylomicron-sized particles (Redgrave and Dunne, 1975; Imaizumi et al., 1978a). Therefore, the triglycerides in the lymph shown in Fig. 1 are of dietary, not endogenous origin. Taken together, the results suggest that it is likely that ingestion of fiber, especially guar gum, may retard the lymphatic transport of dietary triglycerides as large chylomicrons.

As shown in Fig. 2, lymphatic apo A-I secretion also differed for different dietary fibers. Since fat feeding does not significantly affect the synthetic rate of intestinal apo A-I, but rather increases the secretion rate of apo A-I into mesenteric lymph (Windmueller and Wu, 1981; Bearnot et al., 1982), the results in Fig. 2 may be simply explained as indicating that guar gum in the diet delays the intestinal secretion of apo A-I compared to cellulose. However, since dietary factors, such as the types of protein, also alter the synthetic capacity of intestinal apo A-I, as shown by Tanaka et al. (1983), further study is necessary to determine whether fibers affect apo A-I synthesis in the intestine.

3. THE EFFECT OF FIBER ON MUCOSAL ASPECTS OF CHYLOMICRON SECRETION

Recent work suggests that some of the physiological effects of fiber are not caused simply by intraluminal processes (Cassidy et al., 1982; Vahouny, 1982; Schwartz et al., 1983). Sustained supplementation with fiber alters intestinal surface morphology, the membrane function involved in the transmural transport of nutrients, and biosynthetic events in mucosal cells. In relation to chylomicron formation and secretion, we summarize the effect of fiber on the synthesis of intestinal lipids and changes in villus topographical characteristics as follows.

3.1. Intestinal Lipid Synthesis

Few studies have been carried out to determine the effect of fiber ingestion on intestinal lipid synthesis. The data reported by Schwartz et al. (1983) suggest that ingestion of dietary fiber modifies intestinal cholesterol and phospholipid synthesis. Prolonged pectin (10%) ingestion in rats for 6 weeks decreased the incorporation of [^{14}C]acetate into jejunal and ileal cholesterol in everted intestinal sacs when compared to that in rats maintained on a fiber-free diet. The crypt cells appear to be more responsible for the decreased cholesterol synthesis due to pectin ingestion than the villus cells. Schwartz et al. (1983) also showed that ingestion of a fiber-free diet supplemented with either cellulose or pectin (10 and 5%, respectively) de-

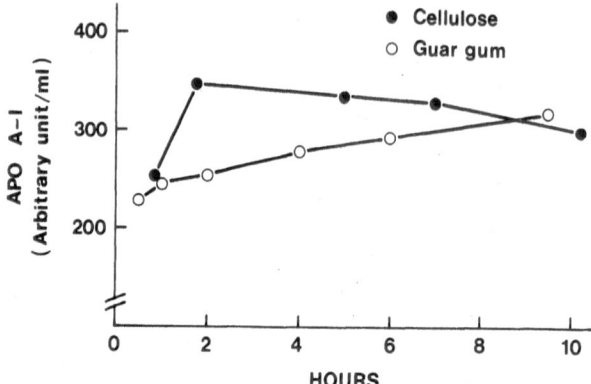

FIGURE 2. Concentration of apo A-I in the mesenteric lymph at selected times after the last meal. Lymph was collected as described in the legend to Fig. 1. Values represent two separate experiments.

creased the incorporation of [^{14}]oleic acid into lecithin in the everted jejunal rings, whereas the incorporation of oleic acid into triglycerides was unaffected by the supplemented fibers. Unfortunately, they failed to show significant differences in the specific activities of lysolecithin acyltransferase (located predominantly in villus cells) and choline phosphotransferase (located predominantly in crypt cells) between the fiber-supplemented and fiber-free groups. Both enzymes are considered to be rate-limiting in the synthesis and resynthesis of endogenous and exogenous lecithin, respectively.

We have examined the effect of the short-term ingestion of fiber on the 3-hydroxy-3-methylglutaryl coenzyme A (HMG-CoA) reductase in intestinal villi and crypts isolated by scraping (Sugano et al., 1982). This enzyme is believed to be rate-limiting for cholesterogenesis in the intestine as well as in the liver (Dietschy and Wilson, 1970). As shown in Table I, dietary cellulose (4%) decreased jejunoileal reductase activities, except in the ileal crypt, as compared to the fiber-free condition. In contrast, when the cellulose content was increased to 20%, the HMG-CoA reductase activity of the villi was elevated slightly, while the crypt activity tended to decrease. Thus, dietary cellulose modified the intercellular distribution of the reductase activity.

The flux of bile acids through the mucosa is a regulatory factor in intestinal cholesterogenesis, since the diversion of bile acids has been shown to stimulate cholesterogenesis, especially synthesis in the ileum (Dietschy, 1968). It has been shown that pectin (Miettinen and Tarpila, 1977; Kay and Truswell, 1977) as well as cellulose (Shurpalekar et al., 1971; Stanley et al., 1973) increase fecal excretion of bile acids. If the alterations in cholesterol metabolism observed with pectin and cellulose are related to the decreased absorption of bile acids due to fecal excretion, ileal cholesterogenesis should increase with fiber supplementation. Hence, it is suggested that cellulose or pectin ingestion may alter intestinal cholesterogenesis by a mechanism other than increased loss of bile acid.

3.2. Intestinal Morphology

Topographic characteristics in the epithelial cell surface have provided useful clues for estimating alterations in the absorptive capacity of dispersed lipid in the intestinal tract. Recently, Cassidy et al. (1982) have shown, by scanning electron microscopy, morphological deviations in the small intestine in rats consuming different sources of dietary fiber (15%). According to Cassidy et al. (1982), feeding of pectin and alfalfa results in characteristic villus cell swelling, loss of microvilli, and distortion and disruption of epithelial cells, while these are not found in rats fed chow, cellulose, or bran. However, it is interesting to note a finding by Gordon et al. (1983) that ingestion of cellulose increases the number of neutrophils, an indicator of some type of inflammatory stimulus, and mitotic figure in the epithelial cells when compared to a fiber-free diet. The most significant connection pointed out by Cassidy et al. (1982) between the morphological and biochemical characteristics appears to be the bile acid-sequestration ability of these fibers rather than lymphatic cholesterol absorption (see Section 3.3). Among the fibers tested, cellulose appears to be the most suppressive for the lymphatic transport of cholesterol (Vahouny et al., 1980b). From these histological observations by Cassidy et al. (1982) and Gordon et al. (1983), it might be expected that cellulose may affect such intracellular activities as assembly and transport of cholesterol as intestinal lipoproteins.

Farness and Schneeman (1982) have reported that the ingestion of pectin increases the length of the small intestine and mucosal weight in rats

TABLE I. HMG-CoA Reductase Activity in Proximal and
Distal Intestine[a]

	Jejunum		Ileum	
Diet	Villi	Crypt	Villi	Crypt
Experiment 1				
Fiber-free	115 ± 6	171 ± 13	36.6 ± 8.5	61.5 ± 3.4
4% Cellulose	$52.7 \pm 2.6^*$	$83.5 \pm 4.7^*$	$14.8 \pm 0.9^*$	68.3 ± 5.1
Experiment 2				
4% Cellulose	74.3 ± 3.3	157 ± 4	18.8 ± 1.0	62.2 ± 2.6
20% Cellulose	$86.8 \pm 2.9^*$	$122 + 8$	$22.0 \pm 0.8^*$	$44.6 \pm 3.1^*$

[a] From Sugano et al. (1982). Rats were fed ad libitum a semipurified diet containing 0, 4, or 20% of cellulose for 6 days. Values (pmol/min per mg protein) are mean $\pm$ SEM for five rats per group. Asterisk indicates significance at $p < 0.05$ from the corresponding group.

relative to a fiber-free diet. Although residual pectin sticks to the mucosa, Brown *et al.* (1979) also showed an increased cell size in rats fed pectin. Longer small intestine and increased cell size are considered to be compensations due to a slowed absorption of nutrients in rats fed gel-forming fibers, such as pectin and guar gum (Farness and Schneeman, 1982). As shown in Table II, the villus size in the lower ileum in guar gum-fed rats is about 30% greater than that for cellulose-fed rats, whereas the corresponding differences in the duodenum and jejunum are not as evident as in the ileum. Decreased cell renewal appeared to be responsible for the increased cell size in the lower ileum of rats fed guar gum, since ingestion of guar gum significantly decreased the incorporation of [³H]thymidine into ileal cells (Imaizumi and Sugano, unpublished observation). Table II also shows that the mucosal weight in rats ingesting guar gum and cellulose tends to be heavier than that in the fiber-free group. Intestinal mucosa from the guar gum group appears to contain more lipids than that from the cellulose group. This finding suggests an interference with intestinal lipid transport in rats fed guar gum. The morphological changes described above will be correlated with the lymphatic secretion of lipids in the next section.

3.3. Secretion Rate of Lymphatic Chylomicrons

In order to circumvent the effects of different rates of gastric emptying and direct interactions of fiber on the test dose of lipids during absorption studies, Vahouny *et al.* (1978, 1980b) fed defined diets containing 15% levels

TABLE II. Villus Size, Mucosal Weight, and Content of Mucosal Lipids in Small Intestine[a]

Diet	Villus size,[b] number of cells per villus			Mucosal weight,[c] g		Total lipids,[d] mg/15 cm length	
	Duodenum	Jejunum	Ileum	Proximal	Distal	Proximal	Distal
Cellulose	85 ± 3	75 ± 3	$41 \pm 2^*$	2.18 ± 0.28	0.43 ± 0.10	$18.3 \pm 2.2^*$	7.0 ± 1.3
Guar gum	89 ± 2	78 ± 2	54 ± 1	2.52 ± 0.31	0.59 ± 0.10	29.5 ± 2.7	13.6 ± 3.6
Fiber-free	ND	ND	ND	1.94 ± 0.20	$0.34 \pm 0.05^*$	ND	ND

[a] Rats were trained on meal feeding. Asterisk indicates significance at $p < 0.05$ from the guar gum group. ND, not determined.
[b] Two hours after the last meal, duodenum (6 cm below pylorus), jejunum (midportion of intestine), and ileum (6 cm above cecum) were examined by microscopy. Villus size was estimated by counting the number of epithelial cells. Villus size is mean ± SEM of cell number for 30 villi from three rats per group (from Imaizumi *et al.*, 1982).
[c] Six hours after the last meal, intestinal mucosa was obtained by scraping the proximal (two-thirds portion below pyrolus) and distal (one-third portion above cecum) intestine. Values are mean ± SEM for six rats per group.
[d] Six hours after the last meal, intestinal mucosa was obtained from the proximal (15 cm below pyrolus) and distal (15 cm above cecum) intestine. Values are mean ± SEM for five rats per group.

of the fiber (wheat bran, alfalfa, yeast cell wall glycan, and pectin) to rats for 5–6 weeks prior to determination of lymphatic absorption of cholesterol and triglyceride. Following catheterization of the thoracic duct, animals were fasted for 24 h prior to receiving a single intraduodenal test meal containing [³H]cholesterol and triolein. The lymph was collected at 4-h intervals during the first 12 h after administration of the test emulsion. Cumulative accumulation of cholesterol and triglyceride in the thoracic lymph appeared to be linear during the first 8 h and declined thereafter. In this experiment they showed that pectin, alfalfa, and cellulose feeding all result in a significant reduction of lymphatic transport of cholesterol and triglyceride compared to the chow-fed control, while wheat bran and yeast glycan appeared to be without effect. The least dramatic result is with a pectin-containing diet.

Although these observations (Vahouny et al., 1978, 1980b) clearly demonstrate that the overall efficiency of the intestinal absorption of triglyceride and cholesterol is modified by the fiber ingested, the capacity to form and secrete chylomicrons in the intestine was not addressed. By using a slightly modified technique as described by Wu et al. (1975), we have measured the effect of fiber (cellulose and guar gum) on the maximum and fractional output rates of test triglyceride and cholesterol into mesenteric lymph in the proximal and distal intestine under the condition where diets do not remain in the lumen. Male Wistar or Sprague-Dawley rats were trained to meal feeding on the diets as described in Fig. 1. Two hours after the last meal, mesenteric lymph duct was cannulated and the infusion tube was placed in either the duodenum or the midportion or lower one-third of the small intestine. After the operation rats were placed in restraining cages and infused through the intestinal cannula with a glucose (10%)–saline (0.9%) solution at a constant rate of 1.9 ml/h. At 21–24 h after the last meal rats were given a fat emulsion (2% triolein, 2% Intralipid–triglyceride, 0.2% egg lecithin, 0.04% cholesterol, and 0.9% NaCl) through the intestinal cannula at a constant rate. After 5 h of the infusion of fat emulsion containing radioactive lipids, the glucose–saline solution or nonradioactive fat emulsion was subsequently infused similarly.

In our first experiment fat emulsion containing [³H]triolein was infused through the duodenum or midportion of the intestine in rats ingesting guar gum and cellulose. As shown in Fig. 3, the proximal output rate of [³H]triglyceride reached a plateau of 50–70% of the infusion rate as early as 3 h after the infusion began. In the distal intestine of rats fed cellulose, the appearance of [³H]triglyceride in the lymph was delayed, reaching a maximum outpute rate at 4 h after emulsion infusion. The maximum output rate of [³H]triolein from the distal intestine was about five times as high in guar gum-fed rats as in cellulose-fed rats (Table III). The maximum output rate from the proximal intestine appears to be higher, but not significantly so, in rats ingesting cellulose compared to guar gum.

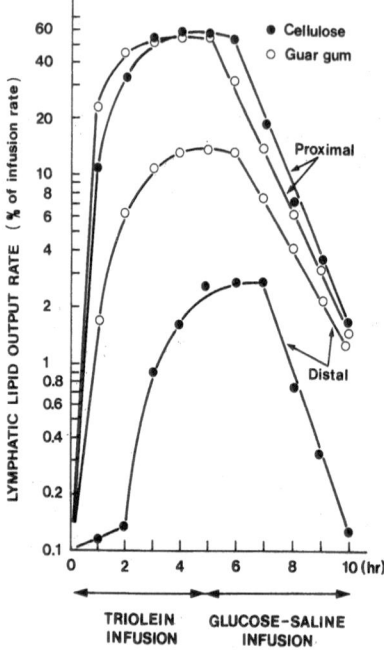

FIGURE 3. Lymphatic output rate of proximally and distally infused [³H]triolein. Male Wistar rats were trained on meal feeding as described in the legend to Fig. 1. Two hours after the last meal, the mesenteric lymph duct was cannulated and the infusion cannula was placed in the proximal (duodenum) or distal (midportion of intestine) positions of intestine under ether anesthesia. After infusion with glucose (10%)-saline (0.9%) solution at the rate of 1.9 ml/h overnight, rats were infused with a fat emulsion containing triolein (2%), Intralipid-triglyceride (2%), egg lecithin (0.2%), cholesterol (0.04%), NaCl (0.9%), and a trace of [³H]triolein. Five hours after the fat infusion, the glucose-saline solution was infused. Each point represents the mean of three or four rats per group. [From Imaizumi et al. (1982).]

Since the decay of [³H]triglyceride output follows first-order kinetics, as shown in Fig. 3, after the infusion was replaced by the fat-free solution, the fractional output rate (0.693/half-time) of lymphatic [³H]triglyceride can be calculated from the linear decay slope by least square fitting. As shown in Table III, guar gum caused a decrease in the fractional output rate of lymphatic [³H]triglyceride from the distal, but not proximal, intestine compared to cellulose ingestion.

In a second experiment fat emulsion containing both [³H]triolein and [¹⁴C]cholesterol was infused into the duodenum or the lower one-third of the small intestine in rats ingesting guar gum, cellulose, or fiber-free diets. The lymphatic output rate of the lipids was measured in terms of large chylomicrons instead of whole lymph. Although the output pattern of [³H]triglyceride in the chylomicrons was essentially similar to that in the first experiment (Fig. 3), the maximum output rate was low (compare Tables III and IV). Since the composition of the infused fat emulsion was identical in the two experiments, the decreased output rate in the second experiment appears to be due to the strain of rats (Wistar and Sprague-Dawley) and also the loss of radioactivity during the preparation of chylomicrons. In the proximal intestine, the maximum output rate of [³H]chylomicrons appeared to be highest in rats ingesting cellulose among the three dietary groups. In the distal intestine, however, the maximum output rate was remarkably low in the cellulose group compared to the guar gum and fiber-free groups. The fractional output rate of [³H]chylomicrons in the proximal intestine was high, although the differences were not significant, in the following order: fiber-free, cellulose, and guar gum. In contrast to the first experiment, the fractional output rate in the distal intestine was lower in the cellulose group than in the guar gum group, which was comparable to the fiber-free group. It seems that the position of infusion cannula may be responsible for the different rates between the two experiments.

The secretion of [¹⁴C]cholesterol in chylomicrons delayed the maximum output rate at 6–8 h after the fat infusion compared to that of [³H]triglyceride. In the proximal intestine guar gum decreased the maximum output rate of [¹⁴C]chylomicrons as in the case of [³H]chylomicrons when compared to the cellulose and fiber-free groups. In the distal intestine the radioactivity of ¹⁴C was not sufficient to be measured accurately. The effect of the fiber on the fractional output rate of [¹⁴C]chylomicrons appeared to be similar to that of [³H]chylomicrons.

Since the lymph flow did not differ significantly among the groups (1.1–1.9 ml/h), the observed differences in the transport of chylomicrons cannot be ascribed to a change in the lymph flow. The results of the two sets of experiments can be summerized in relation to the morphological observations (Section 3.2) as follows:

1. Ingestion of fibers alters the lymphatic transport rate of chylomicrons from the distal as well as proximal intestine. Although two limiting factors, transmural transport of lipids and subsequent assembly to chylomicrons, contribute to the altered lymphatic transport of chylomicrons, the former may be more relevant to the different secretion patterns of chylomicrons between rats ingesting guar gum and those ingesting cellulose.

2. It may not be reasonable to compare the present results on lymphatic

TABLE III. Maximum and Fractional Output Rate of
[³H]Triolein into Mesenteric Lymph[a]

Diet	Maximum output rate, percent of infusion rate	Fractional output rate per hour
Proximal		
Cellulose	65.9 ± 9.1	0.93 ± 0.05
Guar gum	55.6 ± 5.6	0.87 ± 0.15
Distal		
Cellulose	$2.6 \pm 0.1^*$	$1.25 \pm 0.04^*$
Guar gum	13.2 ± 1.8	0.63 ± 0.05

[a]From Imaizumi *et al.* (1982). See legends to Figs. 1 and 3. The fractional output rate was calculated from the linear decay slope. Values are mean $\pm$ SEM for three or four rats per group. Asterisk indicates significance at $p < 0.05$ from the guar gum group.

TABLE IV. Maximum and Fractional Output Rates of [3H]Triolein
and [14C]Cholesterol into Lymphatic Chylomicrons[a]

Diet	Maximum output rate, percent of infusion rate	Fractional output rate per hour
[3H]Triolein		
Proximal		
Cellulose	15.5 ± 0.61*	0.49 ± 0.09
Guar gum	9.4 ± 0.39	0.37 ± 0.01
Fiber-free[b]	12.3 ± 0.25	0.64 ± 0.04
Distal		
Cellulose	0.47 ± 0.07*	0.13 ± 0.03*
Guar gum	1.72 ± 0.26	0.33 ± 0.05
Fiber-free	1.50 ± 0.11	0.45 ± 0.05
[14C]Cholesterol		
Proximal		
Cellulose	15.2 ± 1.02*	0.23 ± 0.01
Guar gum	6.74 ± 0.99	0.16 ± 0.03
Fiber-free[b]	14.2 ± 3.18	0.48 ± 0.17

[a] Fat emulsion containing [3H]triglyceride and [14C]cholesterol was infused through proximal (duodenum) or distal (lower one-third of the small intestine) cannula, respectively. Large chylomicrons were obtained by centrifuging the lymph at 3.2×10^6 g av.-min. Values are mean ± SEM for three rats per group. Asterisk indicates significance at $p < 0.05$ from the guar gum group.
[b] Mean of two separate experiments.

lipid transport with those of Vahouny et al. (1980b), since the experimental conditions differ markedly. Vahouny (1982) suggested that cellulose interferes with the absorption of lipids compared to pectin, a viscous fiber. However, our data suggest that the viscous fiber (guar gum) compared to cellulose may interfere with the intestinal bulk phase diffusion not only of glucose, as suggested by Jenkins et al. (1977, 1978), but also of lipids.

3. Increased cell size in the distal intestine in rats ingesting guar gum may cause the increase in the absorption of triglyceride and cholesterol compared to rats ingesting cellulose. However, increased cell size is not an absolute requisite for the lipid absorption in the lower intestine, since the maximum transport rate of triglyceride was comparable between rats ingesting guar gum and fiber-free diets.

4. It is also emphasized, as suggested by Vahouny (1982) that no single mechanism of action can be assigned to the effect of a given type of dietary fiber on the transport of chylomicrons.

3.4. Chemical Composition of Intestinal Chylomicrons

Analysis of the chemical composition of triglyceride-rich lipoproteins secreted into the mesenteric lymph allows one to some extent to estimate the processing of absorbed lipids in epithelial cells. In this section we describe the effect of dietary fiber on the lipid and apoprotein composition of intestinal chylomicrons.

Mesenteric lymph was collected from rats fed guar gum and cellulose as described in Section 3.3. Table V shows the lipid composition of triglyceride-rich lipoproteins ($d < 1.006$ g/ml) prepared by centrifuging (1×10^8 $\bar{g}$-min) the mesenteric lymph collected overnight from rats trained on meal feeding. The position of the infusion cannula did not affect the lipid composition inasmuch as the lymph was collected overnight. Judging from the high percentage (84–88%) of triglyceride, the collected lymph is considered to contain considerable amounts of diet-derived triglycerides. In general, small chylomicrons (lymph $d < 1.006$ g/ml lipoproteins) contain 70%–75% of triglycerides in the fasting state (Imaizumi et al., 1978a). The average secretion rate of lymphatic triglyceride was higher in the guar gum group than in the cellulose group (23.9 vs. 17.6 mg/h). This result seems to coincide with our suggestion (Section 3.3) that the ingestion of guar gum delays the fat absorption and subsequent lymphatic transport of triglycerides.

The higher ratio of triglyceride to phospholipid in triglyceride-rich lipoproteins observed in rats fed guar gum appears to be the reflection of the delayed fat handling.

TABLE V. Chemical Composition of Triglyceride-Rich
Lipoproteins in Mesenteric Lymph[a]

Diet	Composition, %				
	Cholesterol	Triglyceride (A)	Phospholipid (B)	Protein	A/B
Before fat infusion[b]					
Cellulose	0.8 ± 0.1	83.9 ± 1.8*	12.3 ± 1.8	2.9 ± 0.5	7.7 ± 1.2*
Guar gum	1.2 ± 0.3	88.1 ± 0.6	7.8 ± 0.5	2.9 ± 0.3	11.5 ± 0.7
During fat infusion[c]					
Proximal					
Cellulose	1.1 ± 0.5	83.3 ± 3.8	13.5 ± 3.0	2.2 ± 0.5	7.0 ± 1.9
Guar gum	0.9 ± 0.2	83.8 ± 1.2	13.5 ± 1.2	1.9 ± 0.3	6.3 ± 0.7
Distal					
Cellulose	1.5 ± 0.3	78.8 ± 4.0	16.6 ± 3.9	3.1 ± 0.7	5.4 ± 1.4
Guar gum	1.3 ± 0.2	83.4 ± 1.5	12.7 ± 1.5	2.6 ± 0.8	6.9 ± 0.8

[a] Lymph duct cannulation was performed on rats trained on meal feeding. Values are mean ± SEM for three rats per group. Asterisk indicates significance at $p < 0.05$ from the guar gum group.
[b] Lymph was collected overnight from 10 h after the last meal. The $d < 1.006$ g/ml lipoproteins were obtained by centrifuging the lymph at 1×10^8 $\bar{g}$ min. Since the chemical composition of lymph $d < 1.006$ g/ml lipoproteins was essentially similar when the infusion cannula was put into proximal or distal intestine, these values were combined.
[c] Following overnight infusion of glucose saline, fat emulsion was infused from the proximal or distal intestine. Large chylomicrons were obtained by centrifuging at 3.2×10^6 $\bar{g}$-min the fatty lymph collected during 4–6 h after fat infusion.

During fat infusion through the proximal intestine, the average transport rate of lymphatic triglyceride increased two- to threefold relative to that during the collection of lymph overnight. The chemical composition of large chylomicrons secreted from the proximal intestine was comparable between both dietary groups. This result suggests that the proximal bulk phase diffusion and the subsequent assembly of all the chylomicron components may be interfered with to a similar extent even on feeding guar gum, since guar gum ingestion suppresses the lymphatic transport of chylomicrons, as shown in Section 3.3. In rats ingesting guar gum, the chemical composition of the proximal and distal large chylomicrons were essentially similar. It is therefore suggested that dietary guar gum may not disturb the assembly of chylomicron components in the distal (midportion) intestine, although the export rate to the lymph may be altered.

The apoprotein composition of the $d < 1.006$ g/ml lipoproteins is shown in Fig. 4 and Table VI. In contrast to lipid composition, apoprotein patterns were influenced markedly by the position of the infusion cannula. The relative percentage of apo A-V was 4–6 times higher at the expense of apo A-I and apo C when the infusion cannula was put in the distal intestine. The fiber effect was not evident in the apoprotein composition of $d < 1.006$ g/ml lipoproteins.

With fat infusion, large chylomicrons obtained from the proximal intestine of rats fed fiber were enriched in apo A-IV. Fat ingestion induces apo A-IV mRNA, but not apo A-I mRNA (Gordon, 1982c), and increases a corresponding proportion of apo A-IV in chylomicron apoproteins (Krause *et al.*, 1981). Fiber ingestion appears to have no significant effect on apopro-

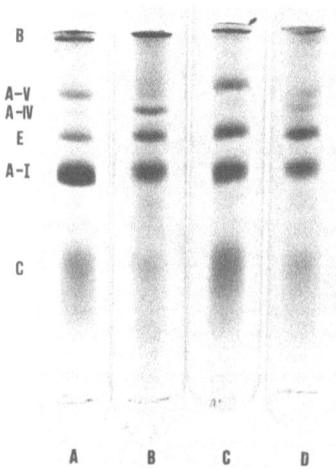

FIGURE 4. Sodium dodecyl sulfate-polyacrylamide gel electrophoretograms of apoproteins of lymph triglyceride-rich lipoproteins. Apoproteins of the triglyceride-rich lipoproteins were separated on polyacrylamide (10%) gel electrophoresis. Glucose-saline was infused into the proximal (A) or distal (C) intestine in the guar gum group. Fat emulsion was infused into the proximal intestine in the guar gum group (B) and into the distal intestine in the cellulose group (D).

TABLE VI. Apolipoprotein Composition of Triglyceride-Rich
Lipoproteins in Mesenteric Lymph[a]

Diet	Composition, %				
	Apo A-V	Apo A-IV	Apo E	Apo A-I	Apo C
Before fat infusion[b]					
Proximal					
Cellulose	3.1 ± 1.9	0.4 ± 0.2	13.8 ± 2.5	38.9 ± 4.7	43.8 ± 5.2
Guar gum	5.8 ± 3.1	1.7 ± 1.0	11.4 ± 2.8	37.1 ± 4.1	44.0 ± 5.2
Distal					
Cellulose	19.4 ± 3.6	3.8 ± 3.0	16.1 ± 3.2	26.8 ± 5.0	34.1 ± 1.9
Guar gum	21.6 ± 3.4	0.6 ± 0.3	21.7 ± 2.6	25.5 ± 3.4	30.6 ± 4.1
During fat infusion[c]					
Proximal					
Cellulose	1.3 ± 0.7	19.7 ± 2.1	14.5 ± 2.7	40.4 ± 3.3	24.1 ± 3.9
Guar gum	2.7 ± 1.6	14.0 ± 1.1	15.1 ± 2.0	36.1 ± 2.9	32.0 ± 3.5
Distal					
Cellulose	5.7 ± 5.0*	2.2 ± 2.0	27.5 ± 2.3	29.2 ± 0.4	35.5 ± 5.5
Guar gum	20.8 ± 1.3	5.8 ± 3.3	21.1 ± 3.8	31.1 ± 4.8	21.3 ± 5.5

[a] See Table V, footnote a.
[b] See Table V, footnote b.
[c] See Table V, footnote c.

tein patterns in the chylomicrons secreted from the proximal intestine. This result is also compatible with our suggestion mentioned above that the assembly of the chylomicron components may not be affected by the kind of fiber. However, the apoprotein composition was altered when fat emulsion was infused through the distal intestine. Ingestion of guar gum significantly increased apo A-V and, to a lesser extent, apo A-IV compared to cellulose ingestion. This phenomenon may be explained as indicating that the synthesis of apo A-IV in the distal intestine may not be sufficient to compensate for an increased absorption of fat. Therefore, apo A-V may have some relevance to the transport of triglyceride-rich lipoproteins in the distal part of the intestine. Although it is not clear whether apo A-V is synthesized in the intestine or originates in the circulation (Fidge and McCullagh, 1981), we have found that [³H]lysine infused through the proximal intestine is incorporated into apo A-V at the level of 4–15% of whole apoproteins (Imaizumi and Sugano, unpublished observations).

In order to correlate the intestinal capacity for secreting chylomicrons or the fractional output rate to the apoproteins, a determination of the synthetic activity of apoproteins is a prerequisite (J. I. Gordon, 1982a–c). In addition, changes in the availability of calcium ion and other ions that may be essential for the release of prechylomicrons (Strauss and Jacob,

1981) should also be considered, since some dietary fibers on occasion inhibit mineral absorption in the small intestine (James *et al.*, 1978).

4. THE EFFECT OF FIBER ON PLASMIC METABOLISM OF CHYLOMICRONS

Long-chain fatty acids absorbed in the intestine are transported to blood serum as chylomicrons. The triglyceride core of the chylomicrons is hydrolyzed by peripheral lipoprotein lipase and the resulting chylomicron remnants are taken up mainly in the liver (Redgrave, 1970; Mjøs *et al.*, 1975). During the metabolism of chylomicrons, the surface components (phospholipid, cholesterol, and apoproteins) are transferred to serum HDL (Tall and Small, 1978). As shown in Fig. 5, metabolism of chylomicron triglyceride appears to be more rapid in rats ingesting cellulose than in rats fed guar gum and fiber-free diets. The decay rate of chylomicron triglyceride in serum is generally determined by the balance between the input from the intestine and the output to the vascular space. The input pattern of the triglyceride is shown in Fig. 1. By comparison of Fig. 1 with Fig. 5, it can be suggested that cellulose ingestion increases plasmic clearance of chylomicrons compared to the case of the fiber-free diet. These data also indicate that guar gum may not disturb specifically a series of plasmic metabolic chains for chylomicrons, such as hydrolysis and uptake, since the plasmic decay is only slightly slower than in the fiber-free group, although the input into the serum compartment appears to be considerably slower. Recently, Mueller *et al.* (1983) have shown, by using rats trained on meal feeding, that the activity of lipoprotein lipase in the adipose tissue is low in cellulose supplementation

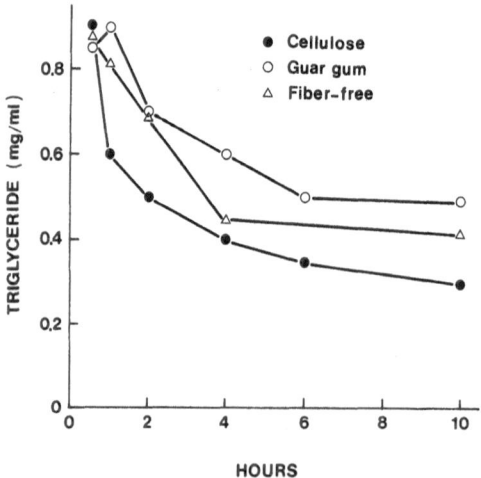

FIGURE 5. Concentration of serum chylomicron triglyceride. Rats were trained on meal feeding as described in the legend to Fig. 1. Values are for one of two separate experiments.

compared to the fiber-free group. Since they measured the lipase activity 24 h after the last meal, when lipoprotein lipase activity in adipose tissue is considerably low due to fasting (Fielding, 1976), it may not be reasonable to apply their finding to our study, where the decay of plasmic chylomicrons was measured within 10 h after the last meal.

An inverse relationship is observed between the decay of plasmic chylomicrons (Fig. 5) and the concentration of serum apo A-I and cholesterol (Fig. 6) in rats fed guar gum, cellulose, and fiber-free diets. The concentration of apo A-I and cholesterol is lower in the guar gum group than in the cellulose and fiber-free groups. These results suggest that the transfer of surface components of chylomicrons to HDL (Tall and Small, 1978) may not be as efficient in rats ingesting guar gum as in rats ingesting cellulose or the fiber-free diet. This phenomenon explains to some extent why ingestion of guar gum decreases serum HDL in man (Jenkins et al., 1980b) and rats (Koo and Stanton, 1981).

5. CONCLUSION

Until now few studies had been performed on how dietary fiber as well as other dietary components affect intestinal lipoprotein formation and secretion. In this chapter we have shown that guar gum exerts a different effect on the intestinal absorption and secretion of dietary fat compared to cellulose in rats. Intestinal activities resulting from fiber ingestion also appear to have a profound effect on the serum lipoprotein metabolism. Thus, the study of fiber should not be restricted to "entrance and exit" phenomena. More detailed biochemical as well as histological study is

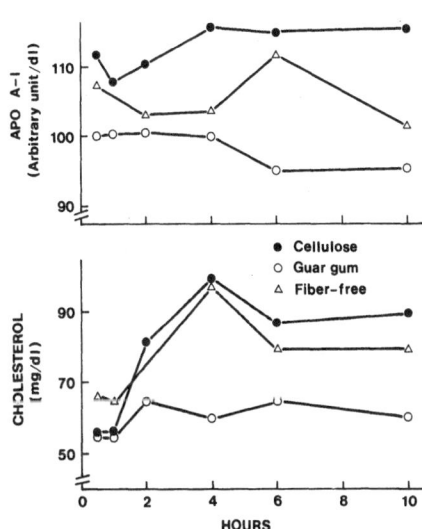

FIGURE 6. Concentration of serum apo A-I and cholesterol. Values are for one of two separate experiments.

definitely necessary to define the underlying mechanism of the altered metabolism of intestinal and serum lipoproteins caused by fibers.

REFERENCES

Anderson, J. W., and Chen, W. J. L., 1979, Plant fiber, carbohydrate and lipid metabolism, *Am. J. Clin. Nutr.* **32:**346–363.

Anderson, J., Grande, F., and Keys, A., 1973, Cholesterol-lowering diets. Experimental trials and literature reviews, *J. Am. Diet. Assoc.* **62:**133–142.

Balmer, J., and Zilversmit, D. B., 1974, Effects of dietary roughage on cholesterol absorption, cholesterol turnover and steroid secretion in the rat, *J. Nutr.* **104:**1319–1328.

Bearnot, H. R., Glickman, R. M., Weinberg, L., Green, P. H. R., and Tall, A. R., 1982, Effect of biliary diversion on rat mesenteric lymph apolipoprotein A-I and high density lipoprotein, *J. Clin. Invest.* **69:**210–217.

Birkner, N. J., and Kern, F., Jr., 1974, *In vitro* adsorption of bile salts to food residues, salicylazosulfapyridine and hemicellulose, *Gastroenterology* **67:**237–244.

Brown, R. C., Kelleher, J., and Losowsky, M. S., 1979, The effect of pectin on the structure and function of the rat small intestine, *Br. J. Nutr.* **42:**357–365.

Cassidy, M. M., Lightfoot, F. G., and Vahouny, G. V., 1982, Morphological aspects of dietary fibers in the intestine, *Adv. Lipid Res.* **19:**203–229.

Clark, B., and Hübscher, G., 1961, Biosynthesis of glycerides in subcellular fractions of intestinal mucosa, *Biochim. Biophys. Acta* **46:**479–494.

Davis, R. A., and Roheim, P. S., 1978, Pharmacologically induced hypolipidemia. The ethinyl estradiol-treated rat, *Atherosclerosis* **30:**293–299.

Dietschy, J. M., 1968, The role of bile salts in controlling the rate of intestinal cholesterogenesis, *J. Clin. Invest.* **47:**286–300.

Dietschy, J. M., and Wilson, J. D., 1970, Regulation of cholesterol metabolism, *N. Engl. J. Med.* **282:**1128–1136.

Eastwood, M. A., and Boyd, G. S., 1967, The distribution of bile salts along the small intestine of rats, *Biochim. Biophys. Acta* **137:**393–396.

Eastwood, M. A., and Hamilton, D., 1968, Studies on the absorption of bile salts to nonabsorbed components of the diet, *Biochim. Biophys. Acta* **152:**165–173.

Eastwood, M. A., and Mowbray, L., 1976, The binding of components of mixed micelles to dietary fiber, *Am. J. Clin. Nutr.* **29:**1461–1467.

Eastwood, M. A., Anderson, R., Michell, W. D., Robertso, J., and Pocock, S., 1976, A method to measure the adsorption of bile salts to vegetable fiber of different water holding capacity, *J. Nutr.* **106:**1429–1432.

Ecknauer, R., Sircar, B., and Johnson, L. R., 1981, Effect of dietary bulk on small intestinal morphology and cell removal in the rat, *Gastroenterology* **81:**781–786.

Farness, P. L., and Schneeman, B. O., 1982, Effects of dietary cellulose, pectin and oat bran on small intestine in the rat, *J. Nutr.* **112:**1315–1319.

Fidge, N. H., and McCullagh, P. J., 1981, Studies on the apoproteins of rat lymph chylomicrons: Characterization and metabolism of a new chylomicron-associated apoprotein, *J. Lipid Res.* **22:**138–146.

Fielding, C. J., 1976, Lipoprotein lipase: Evidence for high- and low-affinity enzyme sites, *Biochemistry* **15:**879–884.

Forester, G. P., Tall, A. R., Bisgaier, C. L., and Glickman, R. M., 1983, Rat intestine secretes spherical high density lipoproteins, *J. Biol. Chem.* **258:**5938–5943.

Fraser, R., 1970, Size and lipid composition of chylomicrons of different svedberg units of flotation, *J. Lipid Res.* **11:**60–65.

Fraser, R., and Courtice, F. C., 1969, The transport of cholesterol in thoracic duct lymph of animals fed cholesterol with varying triglyceride loads, *Aust. J. Exp. Biol. Med. Sci.* **47**:723-732.

Friedman, H. I., and Nylund, B., 1980, Intestinal fat digestion, absorption, and transport. A review, *Am. J. Clin. Nutr.* **33**:1108-1139.

Glickman, R. M., and Green, P. H. R., 1977, The intestine as a source of apolipoprotein A-I, *Proc. Nat. Acad. Sci. USA* **74**:2567-2573.

Glickman, R. M., and Kirsch, K., 1973, Lymph chylomicron formation during the inhibition of protein synthesis. Studies of chylomicron apoproteins, *J. Clin. Invest.* **52**:2910-2920.

Gordon, D. T., and Besch-Williford, C., 1983, Chitin and chitosan: Influence on element absorption in rats, in: *Unconventional Sources of Dietary Fiber,* ACS Symposium Series, no. 214 (I. Furda, ed.), American Chemical Society, Washington, D. C., pp. 155-184.

Gordon, D. T., Besch-Williford, C., and Ellersieck, M. R., 1983, The action of cellulose on the intestinal mucosa and element absorption by the rat, *J. Nutr.* **113**:2545-2556.

Gordon, J. I., Biesgaier, C. L., Sims, H. F., Sachdev, O. P., Glickman, R. M., and Strauss, A. W., 1984, Biosynthesis of human preapolipoprotein A-IV, *J. Biol. Chem.* **259**:468-474.

Gordon, J. I., Smith, D. P., Alpers, D. H., and Strauss, A. W., 1982a, Cloning of a complementary deoxyribonucleic acid encoding a portion of rat intestinal preapolipoprotein A-IV messenger ribonucleic acid, *Biochemistry* **21**:5424-5431.

Gordon, J. I., Smith, D. P., Alpers, D. H., and Strauss, A. W., 1982b, Proteolytic processing of the primary translation product of rat intestinal apolipoprotein A-IV mRNA. Comparison with preproapolipoprotein A-I processing, *J. Biol. Chem.* **257**:8418-8423.

Gordon, J. I., Smith, D. P., Andy, R., Alpers, D. H., Shonfeld, G., and Strauss, A. W., 1982c, The primary translation product of rat intestinal apolipoprotein A-I mRNA is an unusual preprotein, *J. Biol. Chem.* **257**:971-978.

Goulder, T. J., Morgan, L. M., Marks, V., Smythe, T., and Hinks, L., 1978, Effects of guar on metabolic and hormonal responses to meals in normal and diabetic subjects. *Diabetalogia* **14**:235-237.

Green, P. H. R., and Glickman, R. M., 1981, Intestinal lipoprotein metabolism, *J. Lipid Res.* **22**:1153-1173.

Green, P. H. R., Tall, A. R., and Glickman, R. M., 1978, Rat intestine secretes discoid high density lipoprotein, *J. Clin. Invest.* **61**:528-534.

Haessler, H. A., and Isselbacher, K. J., 1963, The metabolism of glycerol by the intestinal mucosa, *Biochim. Biophys. Acta* **73**:427-436.

Hatch, F. T., Hogopian, L. M., Rubenstein, I. J., and Canellos, G. P., 1963, Incorporation of labeled leucine into lipoprotein protein by rat intestinal mucosa, *Circulation* **28**:659.

Imaizumi, K., Fainaru, M., and Havel, R. J., 1978a, Composition of proteins of mesenteric lymph chylomicrons in the rat and alterations produced upon exposure of chylomicrons to blood serum and serum proteins, *J. Lipid Res.* **19**:712-722.

Imaizumi, K., Havel, R. J., Fainaru, M., and Vigne, J.-L., 1978b, Origin and transport of the A-I and arginine-rich apolipoproteins in mesenteric lymph of rats, *J. Lipid Res.* **19**: 1038-1046.

Imaizumi, K., Tominaga, A., Mawatari, K., and Sugano, M., 1982, Effect of cellulose and guar gum on the secretion of mesenteric lymph chylomicrons in meal-fed rats, *Nutr. Rep. Int.* **26**:263-269.

Isselbacher, K. J., and Budz, D. M., 1963, Synthesis of lipoproteins by rat intestinal mucosa, *Nature* **200**:364.

James, W. P. T., Branch, W. J., and Southgate, D. A. T., 1978, Calcium binding by dietary fibre, *Lancet* **i**:638-639.

Jenkins, D. J. A., Leeds, A. R., Bloom, S. R., Sarson, D. L. Albuquerque, R. H., Metz, G. L., and Alberti, K. G. M. M., 1980a, Pectin and post-gastric surgery complications: Normalization of postprandial glucose and endocrine responses, *Gut* **21**:574-579.

Jenkins, D. J. A., Leeds, A. R., Gassull, M. A., Cochet, B., and Alberti, K. G., 1977, Decrease in postprandial insulin and glucose concentrations by guar and pectin, *Ann. Intern. Med.* **86**:20–23.

Jenkins, D. J. A., Reynolds, D., Slavin, B., Leeds, A. R., Jenkins, A. L., and Jepson, E. M., 1980b, Dietary fiber and blood lipids: Treatment of hypercholesterolemia with guar crispbread, *Am. J. Clin. Nutr.* **33**:575–581.

Jenkins, D. J. A., Wolever, T. M. S., Leeds, A. R., Gassull, M. A., Haisman, P., Dilawari, J., Goff, D. V., Metz, G. L., and Alberti, K. G., 1978, Dietary fibers, fiber analogues and glucose tolerance: Importance of viscosity, *Br. Med. J.* **1**:1392–1394.

Kay, R. M., 1982, Dietary fiber, *J. Lipid Res.* **23**:221–242.

Kay, R. M., and Truswell, A. S., 1977, Effect of citrus pectin on blood lipids and fecal steroid excretion in man, *Am. J. Clin. Nutr.* **30**:171–175.

Kay, R. M., Sabry, Z. I., and Csima, A., 1980, Multivariate analysis of diet and serum lipids, *Am. J. Clin. Nutr.* **33**:2566–2572.

Kessler, J. I. P., Narcessian, P., and Mauldin, D. P., 1975, Biosynthesis of lipoproteins by intestinal epithelium. Site of synthesis and sequence of association of lipid, sugar and protein moieties, *Gastroenterology* **68**:1058 (Abstract).

Koo, S. I., and Stanton, P., 1981, Effect of cellulose, pectin and guar gum on the distribution of serum cholesterol among lipoprotein fractions, *Nutr. Rep. Int.* **24**:394–401.

Krause, B. R., Sloop, C. H., Castle, C. K., and Roheim, P. S., 1981, Mesenteric lymph apolipoproteins in control and ethinyl estradiol-treated rats: A model for studying apolipoproteins of intestinal origin, *J. Lipid Res.* **22**:610–619.

Krishnaiah, K. V., Walker, L. F., Borensztajn, J., Shonfeld, G., and Getz, G. S., 1980, Apolipoprotein B variant derived from rat intestine, *Proc. Nat. Acad. Sci. USA* **77**:3806–3810.

Kritchevsky, D., and Story, J. A., 1974, Binding of bile salts *in vitro* by non-nutritive fiber, *J. Nutr.* **104**:458–462.

Kritchevsky, D., and Story, J. A., 1975, *In vitro* binding of bile acids and bile salts, *Am. J. Clin. Nutr.* **28**:305–306.

Lossow, W. J., Lindgren, F. T., Murchio, J. C., Stevens, G. R., and Jensen, L. C., 1969, Particle size and protein content of six fractions of the $S_f > 20$ plasma lipoproteins isolated by density gradient centrifugation, *J. Lipid Res.* **10**:68–76.

Mahley, R. W., Bennet, B. D., Morré, D. J., Gray, M. E., Thistlethwaite, W., and Lequire, V. S., 1971, Lipoproteins associated with Golgi apparatus isolated from epithelial cells of rat small intestine, *Lab. Invest.* **25**:435–444.

Mansbach, C. M., II, 1973, Complex lipid synthesis in hamster intestine, *Biochim. Biophys. Acta* **296**:386–400.

Miettinen, T. A., and Tarpila, S., 1977, Effects of pectin on serum cholesterol, fecal bile acids and biliary lipids in normolipidemic and hyperlipidemic individuals, *Clin. Chim. Acta* **79**:471–477.

Miller, K. W., and Small, D. M., 1983a, Triolein-cholesteryl oleate-cholesterol-lecithin emulsion: Structural models of triglyceride-rich lipoproteins, *Biochemistry* **22**:443–451.

Miller, K. W., and Small, D. M., 1983b, Surface-to-core and interparticle equilibrium distributions of triglyceride-rich lipoprotein lipids, *J. Biol. Chem.* **258**:13772–13784.

Mjøs, O. D., Faergman, O., Hamilton, R. L., and Havel, R. J., 1975, Characterization of remnants produced during the metabolism of triglyceride-rich lipoproteins of blood plasma and intestinal lymph in the rat, *J. Clin. Invest.* **56**:603–615.

Morgan, L. M., Goulder, T. J., Tsiolakis, D., Marks, V., and Alberti, K. G. M. M., 1979, The effect of unabsorbable carbohydrate on gut hormones, *Diabetalogia* **17**:85–89.

Mueller, M. A., Cleary, M. P., and Kritchevsky, D., 1983, Influence of dietary fiber on lipid metabolism in meal-fed rats, *J. Nutr.* **113**:2229–2238.

Ockner, R. K., Block, K. J., and Isselbacher, K. J., 1968, Very low density lipoprotein in intestinal lymph: Evidence for presence of the A protein, *Science* **162**:1285–1286.

O'Doherty, P. J. A., Yousef, I. M., and Kuksis, A., 1973, Effect of puromycin on protein and glycerolipid biosynthesis in isolated mucosal cells, *Arch. Biochem. Biophys.* **156**:586–594.

Poksay, K. S., and Schneeman, B. O., 1983, Pancreatic and intestinal response to dietary guar gum in rats, *J. Nutr.* **113**:1544–1549.

Rachmilewitz, D., Albers, J. J., Saunders, D. R., and Fainaru, M., 1978, Apolipoprotein synthesis by human duodenojejunal mucosa, *Gastroenterology* **75**:667–682.

Redgrave, T. G., 1970, Formation of cholesteryl ester-rich particulate lipid during metabolism of chylomicrons, *J. Clin. Invest.* **49**:465–471.

Redgrave, T. G., 1971, Association of Golgi membranes with lipid droplets (pre-chylomicrons) within intestinal epithelial cells during absorption of fat, *Aust. J. Exp. Biol. Med. Sci.* **49**:209–224.

Redgrave, T. G., and Dunne, K. B., 1975, Chylomicron formation and composition in anesthetized rabbits, *Atherosclerosis* **22**:389–400.

Riley, J. W., Glickman, R. M., Green, P. H. R., and Tall, A. R., 1980, The effect of chronic cholesterol feeding on intestinal lipoproteins in the rat, *J. Lipid Res.* **21**:942–952.

Rowell, H., and Burkitt, D. R., 1977, Dietary fibre and cardiovascular disease, *Artery* **3**:107–119.

Sabesin, S. M., and Frase, S., 1977, Electron microscopic studies of the assembly, intracellular transport, and secretion of chylomicrons by rat intestine, *J. Lipid Res.* **18**:496–511.

Sata, T., Havel, R. J., and Jones, A. L., 1972, Characterization of subfraction of triglyceride-rich lipoproteins separated by gel chromatography from blood plasma of normolipidemic and hyperlipidemic humans, *J. Lipid Res.* **13**:757–767.

Scanu, A. M., and Landsberger, F. R., 1980, Lipoprotein structure, *N. Y. Acad. Sci.* **348**:1–436.

Schwartz, S. E., Starr, C., Bachman, S., and Holtzapple, P. G., 1983, Dietary fiber decreases cholesterol and phospholipid synthesis in rat intestine, *J. Lipid Res.* **24**:746–752.

Senior, J. R., and Isselbacher, K. J., 1961, Formation of higher glycerides from monopalmitin and palmityl CoA by microsomes of rat intestinal mucosa, *Biochem. Biophys. Res. Commun.* **6**:274–278.

Shurpalekar, K. S., Doraiswany, T. R., Sundaravalli, O. E., and Reo, M. N., 1971, Effect of inclusion of cellulose in an atherogenic diet on the blood lipids of children, *Nature* **232**:554 555.

Stanley, M. M., Paul, D., Gacke, D., and Murphy, J., 1973, Effect of cholestyramine, Metamucil and cellulose on fecal bile acid excretion in man, *Gastroenterology* **65**:889.

Story, J. A., and Kritchevsky, D., 1975, Binding of sodium taurocholate by various foodstuffs, *Nutr. Rep. Int.* **11**:161–163.

Story, J. A., and Kritchevsky, D., 1976, Comparison of the binding of various bile acids and bile salts *in vitro* by several types of fiber, *J. Nutr.* **106**:1292–1294.

Strauss, E. S., 1966, Electron microscopic study of intestinal fat absorption, *J. Lipid Res.* **7**:307–323.

Strauss, E. W., and Jacob, J. W., 1981, Some factors affecting the lipid secretory phase of fat absorption by intestine *in vitro* from golden hamster, *J. Lipid Res.* **22**:147–156.

Sugano, M., Fujisaki, Y., Oku, H., and Ide, T., 1982, 3-Hydroxy-3-methylglutaryl coenzyme A reductase activity in the small intestine of rats fed non-purified and semipurified diets, *J. Nutr.* **112**:51–59.

Tall, A. R., and Small, D. M., 1978, Plasma high density lipoproteins, *N. Engl. J. Med.* **299**:1232–1236.

Tanaka, K., Imaizumi, K., and Sugano, M., 1983, Effect of dietary proteins on the intestinal synthesis and transport of cholesterol and apolipoprotein A-I in rats, *J. Nutr.* **113**:1388–1394.

Vahouny, G. V., 1982, Dietary fibers and intestinal absorption of lipids, in: *Dietary Fiber in*

Health and Disease (G. V. Vahouny and D. Kritchevsky, eds.), Plenum, New York, pp. 203–227.

Vahouny, G. V., Blendermann, E. M., Gallo, L. L., and Treadwell, C. R., 1980a, Differential transport of cholesterol and oleic acid in lymph lipoproteins: Sex differences in puromycin sensitivity, *J. Lipid Res.* **21**:415–424.

Vahouny, G. V., Roy, T., Gallo, L. L., Story, J. A., Kritchevsky, D., Cassidy, M., Grund, B. M., and Treadwell, C. R., 1978, Dietary fiber and lymphatic absorption of cholesterol in the rat, *Am. J. Clin. Nutr.* **31**:208–212.

Vahouny, G. V., Timothy, R., Gallo, L. L., Story, J. A., Kritchevsky, D., and Cassidy, M., 1980b, Dietary fibers. III. Effect of chronic intake on cholesterol absorption and metabolism in the rat, *Am. J. Clin. Nutr.* **331**:2182–2191.

Vahouny, G. V., Tombes, R., Cassidy, M. M., Kritchevsky, D., and Gallo, L. L., 1980c, Dietary fibers. V. Binding of bile salts, phospholipids and cholesterol from mixed micelles by bile acid sequestrants and dietary fibers, *Lipids* **15**:1012–1018.

Vahouny, G. V., Tombes, R., Cassidy, M. M. Kritchevsky, D., and Gallo, L. L., 1981, Dietary fibers. VI. Binding of fatty acids and monolein from mixed micelles containing bile salts and lecithin, *Proc. Soc. Exp. Biol. Med.* **166**:12–16.

Walker, A. R. P., 1975, The epidemiological emergency of ischemic arterial disease, *Am. Heart J.* **89**:133–136.

Windmueller, H. G., and Wu, A.-L., 1981, Biosynthesis of plasma apolipoproteins by rat small intestine without dietary or biliary fat, *J. Biol. Chem.* **256**:3012–3016.

Wu, A.-L., and Windmueller, H. G., 1979, Relative contributions by liver and intestine to individual plasma apolipoproteins in the rat, *J. Biol. Chem.* **254**:7316–7322.

Wu, A.-L., Clark, B. S., and Holt, P. R., 1975, Transmucosal triglyceride transport rates in proximal and distal rat intestine *in vivo*, *J. Lipid Res.* **16**:251–257.

Zilversmit, D. G., 1965, The composition and structure of lymph chylomicrons in dog, rat, and man, *J. Clin. Invest.* **44**:1610–1622.

20

Effects of Fiber on Plasma Lipoprotein Composition

BARBARA OLDS SCHNEEMAN and
MICHAEL LEFEVRE

Elevated plasma cholesterol levels have been associated with an increased risk of cardiovascular disease. Because of this association, considerable research effort has been focused on elucidating dietary factors that may be associated with lower plasma cholesterol levels. Reduction of plasma cholesterol by drug intervention has recently been associated with reduced risk of heart disease. Vegetarian diets and diets rich in plant foods relative to animal foods have been associated with lower plasma cholesterol and there is some evidence that vegetarianism may be associated with protection from heart disease (Burr and Sweetnam, 1982; Phillips *et al.*, 1978). Several aspects of a diet rich in plant foods may be protective, including amount and type of fat, protein, and fiber. This chapter will focus on the potential effects of dietary fiber on plasma lipids and lipoproteins.

The ability of several sources of dietary fiber to lower plasma cholesterol level has been demonstrated in both human clinical studies and experimental animal studies. Several recent reviews summarize many of these studies (Anderson and Chen, 1979, 1983; Kritchevsky, 1982; Miettinen, 1983; Story and Kelley, 1982). The percent change in plasma cholesterol due to fiber treatment that was observed in several recent human clinical studies is summarized in Table I. The water-soluble fiber sources appear to be the most effective in lowering plasma cholesterol levels. Oat bran, several gums, legumes, and pectin reduced plasma cholesterol 6–19%. Wheat bran, cellu-

---

BARBARA OLDS SCHNEEMAN and MICHAEL LEFEVRE • Department of Nutrition, University of California, Davis, California 95616.

TABLE I. Effect Of Dietary Fiber On Plasma Cholesterol in Humans[a]

Fiber source (g/day)	Percent of control plasma cholesterol	Subjects		Reference
		Normal	Disorder[b]	
Wheat bran (7–25)	98–106	X	X	Liebman et al. (1983), Kay and Truswell (1977a), Anderson and Chen (1979), Jenkins et al. (1979)
Cellulose (16–27)	104	X		Anderson and Chen (1979), Behall et al. (1984)
Corn bran (26)	97		X	Mahalko et al. (1984)
Soy hulls (21–52)	100–114*	X	X	Mahalko et al. (1984), Schweizer et al. (1983)
Carboxymethylcellulose (19–27)	84*	X		Behall et al. (1984)
Oat bran (27)	87*		X	Kirby et al. (1981), Anderson and Chen (1983)
Apple[c] (20–25)	92*–99	X	X	Gormley et al. (1977), Jenkins et al. (1979)
Vegetables (carrot, cabbage) (20–60)	99–102	X		Jenkins et al. (1979)
Mixed sources (60 g)	97–98	X		Raymond et al. (1977), Ullrich and Albrink (1982)
Gums				
Guar (13–20)	87*	X	X	Jenkins et al. (1979), Jenkins et al. (1980)
Locust bean (10–27)	86*		X	Zavoral et al. (1983ab)
Locust bean (10–27)	86*–90	X		Zavoral et al. (1983ab), Behall et al. (1984)
Gum arabic (25)	94*	X		Ross et al. (1983)
Karaya (19–27)	90*	X		Behall et al. (1984)
Pectin (15–50)	87*	X	X	Miettinen and Tarpila (1977), Kay and Truswell (1977b), Jenkins et al. (1979)
Legumes (30–42)	81*–93*	X	X	Anderson and Chen (1983), Jenkins et al. (1983)

[a] Asterisk indicates that a significant effect of the fiber treatment was reported in the study.
[b] Disorder is some form of hyperlipidemia or diabetes.
[c] Fiber amount unknown.

lose, various vegetables, and soy hulls did not have a hypocholesterolemic effect. Two studies have been reported in which a mixed diet of fiber-rich foods was used to increase fiber intake (Ullrich and Albrink, 1982; Raymond *et al.*, 1977). A significant reduction of plasma cholesterol was not observed in either study; however, the subjects used already had low plasma cholesterol values and further reductions may not have been achievable with the dietary protocols used. The effectiveness of gums, pectin, and other sources of viscous polysaccharides in lowering plasma cholesterol and the lack of response to wheat bran and cellulose have been confirmed by animal experiments as well (Anderson and Chen, 1979, 1983; Elliot *et al.*, 1981; Sarathy and Saraswathi, 1983; Ebihara *et al.*, 1979; Asp *et al.*, 1981, 1983; Chen *et al.*, 1981; Jayakumari and Kurup, 1979; Koo and Stanton, 1981). In addition, chitosan has been reported to be hypocholesterolemic in rats, and soy flour has been reported to elevate serum cholesterol (Sugano *et al.*, 1980; Chang and Johnson, 1977). The response in experimental animals to dietary fibers is usually dependent on the species under examination as well as the hypercholesterolemic nature of the diet. Because of these variables, animal experiments are often difficult to compare.

The cholesterol-lowering ability of these fiber sources frequently appears to be greatest in hyperlipidemic patients. Locust bean gum incorporated into bakery products reduced plasma cholesterol 10–17% in patients with familial hypercholesterolemia and 6–10% in normal subjects (Zavoral *et al.*, 1983a,b). The effectiveness of gums in lowering cholesterol has led to their suggested use as a therapeutic agent in the treatment of hyperlipidemias (Zavoral *et al.*, 1983a,b; Jenkins *et al.*, 1980). The cost and patient acceptability of incorporating a gum into the diet may be better than that associated with use of a drug such as cholestyramine. Use of such fiber-enriched foods may have potential as either a primary treatment or as an enhancement to pharmacological therapy (Zavoral *et al.*, 1983a,b).

Several mechanisms are probably involved in the hypocholesterolemic effects of fiber. The ability of certain fibers to increase the fecal excretion of bile acids may increase the conversion of cholesterol to bile acids and enhance the loss of cholesterol (Kritchevsky 1982; Miettinen and Tarpila, 1977, 1983). In addition, the absorption of cholesterol is reduced by certain fibers (Vahouny *et al.*, 1980, Vahouny, 1982). A third possible mechanism is a delay in the rate and site of lipid absorption from the small intestine. Binding of micellar components and disruption of micelle formation in the small intestine may be involved in the effects of fiber on lipid digestion and absorption.

The distribution of cholesterol in the lipoprotein fractions is a better indication of the associated risk of heart disease (Eder and Gidez, 1982). Table II summarizes studies done in humans in which the effect of fiber on

TABLE II. Lipoprotein Cholesterol Level in Humans Fed Fiber[a]

Fiber Source	Percent of Control		Level in diet g/day	Reference
	HDL-C	LDL-C		
Wheat bran	91	97	20–44	Liebman et al. (1983), Jenkins et al. (1979)
Soy hulls	99–104	99–119	21–52	Schweizer et al. (1983), Mahalko et al. (1984)
Cellulose	100	108*	19–27	Behall et al. (1984)
Carboxymethylcellulose	93	82*	19–27	Behall et al. (1984)
Corn bran	99	97	26	Mahalko et al. (1984)
Oat bran	100	86*	27	Kirby et al. (1981)
Apple	96	NA	20	Jenkins et al. (1979)
Vegetables (carrot, cabbage)	83*–94	NA	20	Jenkins et al. (1979)
Gums				
Guar	95	84*	13–20	Jenkins et al. (1979, 1980)
Locust bean	93	83–90*	10–27	Zavoral et al. (1983ab), Behall et al. (1984)
Karaya	98	90	19–27	Behall et al. (1984)
Pectin	98	NA	31	Jenkins et al. (1979)
Beans	85*	77*	30	Anderson and Chen (1983)
Legumes	108	95	42	Jenkins et al. (1983)

[a]Asterisk indicates that a significant effect of the fiber treatment was reported in the study. NA, Not available.

lipoprotein cholesterol levels were determined. Oat bran, legumes, and gums from guar, locust bean, and karaya were all able to lower the low-density lipoprotein (LDL) cholesterol levels in humans. Oat bran and gums lowered LDL-cholesterol, while high-density lipoprotein (HDL) cholesterol level remained unchanged, supporting the concept that they may be useful therapeutic agents. In the experimental animal studies, results vary based on the hypercholesterolemic nature of the diet. In rats fed cholesterol, oat bran and gums appear to be effective in lowering the concentration of LDL-cholesterol (Anderson and Chen, 1983). Often animal studies have been difficult to interpret because the methods for lipoprotein analysis used were originally developed for human clinical tests and may not be directly applicable to experimental animals. The presentation of data in Table II demonstrates that we have very little information on the effect of dietary fibers on lipoprotein composition and cholesterol distribution. Most of the research has focused only on the HDL and LDL fractions and cholesterol has been the primary component of the lipoprotein measured. Little information is available on the remaining composition of the particles. Given that these studies have demonstrated the potential of oat bran and gums for reducing LDL-cholesterol, information is now needed on the protein and lipid composition of the lipoprotein particles to determine if this reduction can be associated with a reduced atherogenicity of the diet.

The two lipoprotein fractions that have been studied and characterized the most in relation to fiber consumption are LDL and HDL. Elevated LDL particles have been associated with increased risk of cardiovascular disease (Eder and Gidez, 1982). In humans LDL is about 45 to 50% cholesterol, of which about 42% is esterified. Triglycerides contribute 10% and phospholipid comprises about 22%. Protein is about 25% of the particle and over 95% of this protein is the apolipoprotein B (Figure 1). Apo B can be synthesized in the intestine or liver and is recognized by the hepatic and extrahepatic LDL receptor (Brown and Goldstein, 1983; Schonfeld, 1983). Elevated apo B levels have been suggested as a better risk indicator that elevated LDL-cholesterol (Vega et al., 1982). Parallel reduction of both LDL-cholesterol and apo B content would indicate that the number of LDL particles were reduced, which presumably will be associated with reduced atherogenic risk.

HDL particles contain 45–50% protein (Fig. 1). The major apoprotein in HDL is apo A-I, which is the activator of LCAT (Schonfeld, 1983). A recent survey indicated that apo A-I was significantly lower in patients with coronary artery disease and may provide useful information on cardiovascular disease potential, especially in patients who have normal plasma cholesterol levels (Maciejko et al., 1983). The C apoproteins are also associated with HDL particles. The HDL particles exchange the C apoproteins with VLDL particles during alimentary hyperlipemia. These proteins are impor-

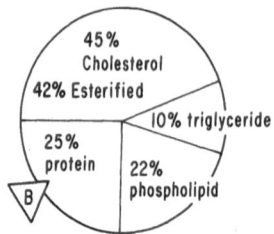

LDL = Low Density Lipoprotein

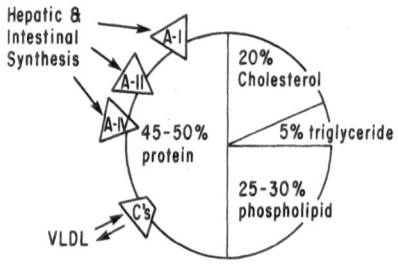

HDL = High Density Lipoprotein

FIGURE 1. Composition of low- and high-density lipoproteins.

tant in regulating triglyceride clearance from the plasma. Small amounts of apoproteins A-II, A-IV, and E are also associated with the HDL fraction; less is known about their function in association with HDL, but they are undoubtedly important in HDL metabolism (Mahley, 1982; DeLamatre *et al.*, 1983; Blum, 1982).

No information is available on the effect of dietary fiber on plasma apoprotein levels in humans. Some information available from vegetarians suggests that alterations in lipoprotein composition can occur in individuals consuming plant foods. Figure 2 shows the cholesterol distribution and apolipoprotein B and A-I patterns in a vegetarian and a nonvegetarian population (Nestel *et al.*, 1981). Total plasma and LDL-cholesterol were reduced in the vegetarian population; HDL-cholesterol levels were similar. Vegetarians have a significantly lower level of LDL-apo B and the plasma level of apo A-I tended to be reduced. A separate study reported similar apoprotein levels and statistically significant reductions in the plasma apo A-I and apo B content of vegetarians in comparison to a nonvegetarian population (Burslem *et al.*, 1978). Kinetic analysis indicates that the flux of apo B-containing particles was significantly reduced in the vegetarians (9.1 vs. 11.8 mg/kg per day.) Although the total flux was reduced, the fractional removal rate was similar between groups (0.025 h^{-1}); hence, the lower LDL-apo B level appears to be the result of reduced synthesis of particles containing apo B. Kinetic analysis indicated that the flux of apo A-I was similar (11.2 mg/kg per day), but the fractional removal rate was increased in vegetarians (0.043 vs. 0.027 h^{-1}), suggesting that the lower plasma A-I in vegetarians was due to a higher rate of clearance of HDL particles. This analytical approach has provided insight into the mechanism by which vegetarian diets may be asociated with protection from cardiovascular disease. Reducing the production of apo B may be associated with less saturation of specific LDL-receptor-mediated clearance (Nestel *et al.*, 1981). The observations sugget that some component of plant diets contributes to the lower apo B and A-I level and the altered turnover; however, it is not clear whether differences in fiber intake or total fat and protein intake are of primary importance.

Some experimental animal data suggest that guar gum may affect plasma apoprotein levels. A preliminary study in our laboratory has indicated that the plasma level of apo B may be reduced by one-third in rats given a guar gum supplement (Schneeman *et al.*, unpublished observations). Imaizumi *et al.* (1982) reported a 25% decrease in serum apo A-I levels when rats were fed guar gum in place of cellulose in the diet. This reduction in the plasma level seemed to be associated with reduced output of the apoprotein and delayed lipid absorption from the intestine during fat absorption. The intestine is known to be a major site of synthesis of apolipoproteins, which are transferred from the intestinal lipoproteins formed during fat absorption to the plasma lipoproteins (Green and Glickman, 1981). The reduction in intestinal synthesis could be associated with the altered rate and site of lipid absorption caused by viscous, water-soluble fibers such as guar gum.

The composition of the HDL fraction isolated from the plasma of rats can be altered by feeding various fiber sources (Schneeman *et al.*, 1984). In an experiment in our laboratory, rats were fed either a basal mixture that contained no fiber or the basal mixture supplemented with either cellulose,

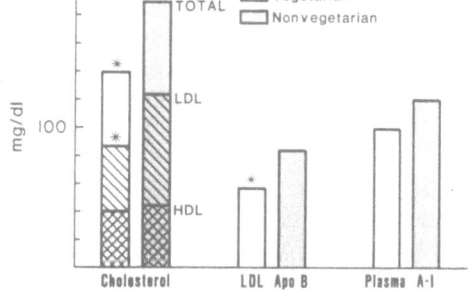

FIGURE 2. Plasma cholesterol, lipoprotein, and apoprotein B and A-I in a vegetarian and a nonvegetarian population. (Adapted from Nestel *et al.*, 1981.)

wheat bran, oat bran, pectin, or guar gum. After 4 weeks, lipoproteins were isolated from the plasma by ultracentrifugation at 100,000 g for 40 h at d 1.216, and the HDL fraction was isolated by gel filtration. The total plasma cholesterol values in these animals tended to be low, probably due to the use of unsaturated fat and cornstarch in the basal diet (Table III). The highest plasma cholesterol value occurred in the wheat bran group, which was significantly higher than the basal or pectin group. HDL cholesterol levels did not differ among the treatments, nor did the concentration of protein measured in the plasma total lipoprotein and HDL fractions (Table III). Figure 3 shows the proportion of apoproteins associated with the HDL fraction based on their separation on sodium dodecylsulfate polyacrylamide gel electrophoresis. The primary differences in apoprotein pattern were noted between the wheat bran group relative to the oat bran and guar gum groups (see Fig. 3; when a significant difference occurred, the parameters are designated by a different letter). The other groups did not differ from these three groups. The wheat bran group has a smaller percentage of apo A-I than either the oat bran or guar gum groups and the proportion of apo E and apo C is larger in this group relative to the guar gum group. Apo E in the HDL fraction of rats has been associated with an increased occurrence of HDL particles that are larger and of lower density (Mahley, 1982). The metabolism of this particle is poorly understood; however, it is known that the apo E can be recognized by LDL-type receptors and it is possible that apo-E-enriched HDL is involved in the transport of cholesterol esters to extrahepatic and hepatic tissue cells with these receptors (Van't Hooft and Havel, 1982). The slight increase of apo E in the HDL fraction can be due to increased synthesis or reduced clearance of the particle; at present nothing is known about the possible effects of dietary fiber on the clearance and synthesis of HDL particles. An understanding of these relationships is necessary to determine the importance of dietary fiber in protecting against heart disease.

TABLE III. Plasma and HDL-Cholesterol and Apolipoprotein Concentration[a]

Diet	Plasma cholesterol,[b] mg/dl	Plasma apoprotein, mg/dl	HDL cholesterol, mg/dl	HDL apoprotein,
Fiber-free	49.0 ± 3.0*	130 ± 8	34.3 ± 5.2	104 ± 6
Cellulose	57.5 ± 4.9*	127 ± 9	33.8 ± 9.2	98 ± 8
Wheat bran	62.7 ± 4.2	118 ± 9	39.1 ± 6.7	99 ± 8
Oat bran	52.6 ± 3.8*	122 ± 11	36.0 ± 5.9	102 ± 10
Pectin	48.1 ± 2.3*	125 ± 6	36.2 ± 4.2	99 ± 7
Guar gum	59.6 ± 3.8*	136 ± 11	34.5 ± 2.7	109 ± 8

[a] From Schneeman et al. (1984).
[b] Values with different symbols differ significantly.

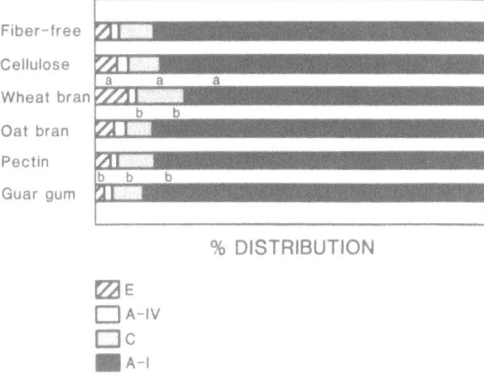

FIGURE 3. Percentage distribution of apoproteins in the HDL fraction of rats fed various sources of dietary fiber. Different letters (a,b) indicate that a significant difference occurred. (Adapted from Schneeman et al., 1984.)

The proportion of C apoproteins was also increased in the HDL fraction of the wheat bran group. These apoproteins are important in the metabolism of triglyceride-rich particles (Schonfeld, 1983). During alimentary lipemia the C apoproteins are transferred to the triglyceride-rich particles, VLDLs and chylomicrons. As the lipid is cleared, these proteins are transferred back to the HDL fraction; hence, an increase in the percent of HDL protein of fasted rats might reflect some shift in the total plasma pool of the C apoproteins. Figure 4 shows the percentages of C apoprotein that are C-II and C-III. C-II apoprotein is an activator of lipoprotein lipase, which is important in the hydrolysis of lipid and clearance of triglyceride-rich particles from the plasma. The C-III apoprotein appears to retard the clearance of these particles by the liver in humans, preventing their premature removal from the plasma (Windler et al., 1980). The ratio of C-II to C-III may provide some indication of clearance relative to inhibition of clearance. In humans a decrease in this ratio in the VLDL fraction has been associated with diets that elevate plasma triglycerides (Kashyap et al., 1982, 1983; Falko et al., 1980). The C-II to C-III ratio in the HDL fraction in these rats, shown inside the bars in Fig. 4, was significantly higher in the guar gum group than in the cellulose or wheat bran groups, suggesting a higher rate of lipolysis and clearance if the pattern reflects the plasma pattern. This result is a preliminary observation and suggests that the pattern of C apoprotein in other lipoprotein fractions, especially VLDL, should be examined. This elevated ratio in the guar gum group could be associated with a reduction in the postprandial hypertriglyceridemia due to a slower rate of lipid absorption in animals fed guar gum (Imaizumi et al., 1982). A reduction in the postprandial hypertriglyceridemia in men receiving a high-fiber diet has been reported (Anderson and Chen, 1979). Consumption of this type of diet or diets rich in water-soluble, viscous fibers might reduce the circulating levels of apo C associated with human VLDL and HDL and raise the ratio of C-II to C-III.

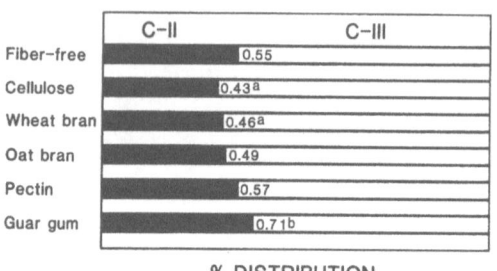

FIGURE 4. Proportion of C-II and C-III of the total apoprotein in the HDL fraction of rats fed various sources of dietary fiber. C-II to C-III ratio is shown inside the bar. Different letters (a,b) indicate that a significant difference occurred. (Adapted from Schneeman et al., 1984.)

Research in humans and in experimental animals has pointed to the potential of dietary fibers, especially the water-soluble, viscous polysaccharides, in lowering plasma cholesterol and LDL-cholesterol. These reductions could be associated with reduced risk of cardiovascular disease, especially in hyperlipidemic individuals. Future research must determine the changes in protein and lipid composition and the changes in particle size associated with these reductions as well as determine the mechanisms for the alterations in plasma lipoproteins. This research approach is needed to evaluate the usefulness of dietary fiber as a therapeutic agent in the treatment of hyperlipidemias and as a protective factor in the diet to reduce the risk of cardiovascular disease.

ACKNOWLEDGMENTS.   This work has been supported in part by NIH AM 20446 and by a grant from American Heart Association, California Affiliate.

REFERENCES

Anderson, J. W., and Chen, W. L., 1979, Plant fiber. Carbohydrate and lipid metabolism, *Am. J. Clin. Nutr.* **32:**346–363.

Anderson, J. W., and Chen, W. L., 1983, Legumes and their soluble fiber: Effect on cholesterol-rich lipoproteins, in: *Unconventional Sources of Dietary Fiber*, ACS Symposium Series, no. 214 (I.Furda, ed.) American Chemical Society, Washington, D.C., pp. 49–59.

Asp, N. G., Bauer, H. G., Nilsson-Ehle, P., Nyman, M., and Oste, R., 1981, Wheat bran increases high-density lipoproteins in the rat, *Br. J. Nutr.* **46:**385–393.

Behall, K. M., Lee, K. H., Mosher, P. B., 1984, Blood lipids and lipoproteins in adult men fed four refined fibers, *Am. J. Clin. Nutr.* **39:**209–214.

Blum, C. B., 1983, Dynamics of apolipoprotein E metabolism in humans, *J. Lipid Res.* **23:** 1308–1316.

Brown, M. S., and Goldstein, J. L., 1983, Lipoprotein receptors in the liver: Control signals for plasma cholesterol traffic, *J. Clin. Invest.* **72:**743–747.

Burr, M. L., and Sweetnam, P. M., 1982, Vegetarianism, dietary fiber, and mortality, *Am. J. Clin. Nutr.* **36:**873–877.

Burslem, J., Schonfeld, G., Howald, M. A., Weidman, S. W., and Miller, J. P., 1978, Plasma apoprotein and lipoprotein lipid levels in vegetarians, *Metabolism* **27:**711–719.

Chang, M. L., and Johnson, M. A., 1977, Influence of dietary fiber (from soybean flour) on lipid metabolism in rats, *Nutr. Rep. Int.* **16**:573-577.

Chen, W. L., Anderson, J. W., and Gould, M. R., 1981, Effects of oat bran and pectin on lipid metabolism of cholesterol-fed rats, *Nutr. Rep. Int.* **24**:1093-1098.

DeLamatre, J. G., Hoffmeire, C. A., Lacko, A. G., Roheim, P. S., 1983, Distribution of apoprotein A-IV between the lipoprotein and the lipoprotein-free fractions of rat plasma: possible role of lecithin: cholesterol acyltransferase, *J. Lipid Res.* **24**:1578-1585.

Ebihara, K., Kiriyama, S., and Manabe, M., 1979, Cholesterol-lowering activity of various natural pectins and synthetic pectin-derivatives with different physico-chemical properties, *Nutr. Rep. Int.* **20**:519-526.

Eder, H. A., and Gidez, L. I., 1982. The clinical significance of the plasma high density lipoproteins, *Med. Clin. North Am.* **66**:431-440.

Elliot, J., Mulvihill, E., Duncan, C., Forsythe, R., and Kritchevsky, D., 1981, Effects of tomato pomace and mixed-vegetable pomace on serum and liver cholesterol in rats, *J. Nutr.* **111**:2203-2211.

Falko, J. M., Schonfeld, G., Witztum, J. T., Kolar, J. B., and Salmon, P., 1980, Effects of short-term high carbohydrate, fat-free diet on plasma level of apo C-II and apo C-III and on the apo C subspecies in human plasma lipoproteins, *Metabolism* **29**:654-661.

Gormley, T. R., Kevany, J., Egan, J. P., and McFarlane, R., 1977, Effect of apples on serum cholesterol in humans, *Ir. J. Food Sci. Technol.* **1**:117-128.

Green, P. H. R., and Glickman, R. M., 1981, Intestinal lipoprotein metabolism, *J. Lipid Res.* **22**:1153-1173.

Imaizumi, K., Tominaga, A., Mawatari, K., and Sugano, M., 1982, Effect of cellulose and guar gum on the secretion of mesenteric lymph chylomicrons in meal-fed rats, *Nutr. Rep. Int.* **26**:263-269.

Jayakumari, N., and Kurup, P. A., 1979, Dietary fiber and cholesterol metabolism in rats fed a high cholesterol diet, *Atherosclerosis* **33**:41-47.

Jenkins, D. J. A., Reynolds, D., Leeds, A. R., Waller, A. L., and Cummings, J. H., 1979, Hypocholesterolemic action of dietary fiber unrelated to fecal bulking effect, *Am. J. Clin. Nutr.* **32**:2430-2435.

Jenkins, D. J. A., Reynolds, D., Slavin, B., Leeds, A. R., Jenkins, A. L., and Jepson, E. M., 1980, Dietary fiber and blood lipids: Treatment of hypercholesterolemia with guar crispread, *Am. J. Clin. Nutr.* **33**:575-581.

Jenkins, D. J. A., Wong, G. S., Patten, R., Bird, J., Hall, M., Buckley, G. C., McGuire, V., Reichert, R., and Little, J. A., 1983, Leguminous seeds in the dietary management of hyperlipidemia, *Am. J. Clin. Nutr.* **38**:567-573.

Kashyap, M. L., Barnhart, R. L., and Srivastava, L. S., 1982, Effects of dietary carbohydrate and fat on plasma lipoproteins and apolipoproteins C-II and C-III in healthy men, *J. Lipid. Res.* **23**:877-886.

Kashyap, M. L., Barnhart, R. L., and Srivastava, L. S., 1983, Alimentary lipemia: Plasma high-density lipoproteins and apolipoproteins C-II and C-III in healthy subject, *Am. J. Clin. Nutr.* **37**:233-234.

Kay, R. M., and Truswell, A. S., 1977a, The effect of wheat fibre on plasma lipids and fecal steroid excretion in man, *Br. J. Nutr.* **37**:227-235.

Kay, R. M., and Truswell, A. S., 1977b, Effect of citrus pectin on blood lipids and fecal steroid excretion in man, *Am. J. Clin. Nutr.* **30**:171-175.

Kirby, R. W., Anderson, J. W., Sieling, B., Rees, E. D., Chen, W. L., Miller, R. F., and Kay, R. M., 1981, Oat-bran intake selectively lowers low-density lipoprotein cholesterol concentrations of hypercholesterolemic men, *Am. J. Clin. Nutr.* **34**:824-829.

Koo, S. I., and Stanton, P., 1981, Effects of cellulose, pectin and guar gum on the distribution of serum cholesterol among lipoprotein fractions, *Nutr. Rep. Int.* **24**:395-401.

Kritchevsky, D., 1982, Fiber and Lipids, in: *Dietary Fibers in Health and Disease*, (G. V. Vahouny and D. Kritchevsky, eds.), Plenum, New York, pp. 187–192.

Liebman, M., Smith, M. C., Iverson, J., Thye, F. W., Hinkle, D. E., Herbert, W. G., Ritchey, S. J., and Driskell, J. A., 1983, Effects of coarse wheat bran fiber and exercise on plasma lipids and lipoproteins in moderately overweight men, *Am. J. Clin. Nutr.* **36**:71–81.

Maciejko, J. J., Holmes, D. R., Kottke, B. A., Zinsmeister, A. R., Dinh, D. M., and Mao, S. J. T., 1983, Apolipoprotein A-I as a marker of angiographically assessed coronary-artery disease, *N. Engl. J. Med.* **309**:385–389.

Mahalko, J. R., Sandstead, H. H., Johnson, L. K., Inman, L. F., Milne, D. B., Warner, R. C., and Haunz, E. A., 1984, Effect of consuming fiber from corn bean, soy hulls, or apple powder on glucose tolerance and plasma lipids in type II diabetes, *Am. J. Clin. Nutr.* **39**:25–34.

Mahley, R. W., 1982, Atherogenic hyperlipoproteinemia, *Med. Clin. North Am.* **66**:375–402.

Miettinen, T. A., 1983, Effects of dietary fibre on cholesterol metabolism in man, in: *Bulletin 20, Fibre in Human and Animal Nutrition* (G. Wallace and L. Bell, eds.), The Royal Society of New Zealand, pp. 173–177.

Miettinen, T. A., and Tarpila, S., 1977, Effect of pectin on serum cholesterol, fecal bile acids and biliary lipids in normolipidemic and hyperlipidemic individuals, *Clin. Chim. Acta* **79**:471–477.

Nestel, P. J., Billington, T., and Smith, B., 1981, Low density and high density lipoprotein kinetics and sterol balance in vegetarians, *Metabolism* **30**:941–945.

Phillips, R. L., Lemon, F. R., Beeson, W. L., and Kuzma, J. W., 1978, Coronary heart disease mortality among Seventh-day Adventists with differing dietary habits: A preliminary report, *Am. J. Clin. Nutr.* **31**:191–198.

Raymond, T. L., Connor, W. E., Lin, D. S., Warner, S., Frey, M. M., and Connor, S. L., 1977, The interaction of dietary fibers and cholesterol upon the plasma lipids and lipoproteins, sterol balance, and bowel function in human subjects, *J. Clin. Invest.* **60**:1429–1437.

Ross, A. H. M., Eastwood, M. A., Anderson, J. R., and Anderson, D. M. W., 1983, A study of the effects of dietary gum arabic in humans, *Am. J. Clin. Nutr.* **37**:368–375.

Sarathy, R., and Saraswathi, G., 1983, Effect of tender bean pods *(cyamopsis tetragonoloba)* on cholesterol levels in rats, *Am. J. Clin. Nutr.* **38**:295–299.

Schneeman, B. O., Cimmarusti, J., Cohen, W., Downes, L., and Lefevre, M., 1984, Composition of high density lipoproteins in rats, *J. Nutr.*, **114**:1320–1326.

Schonfeld, G., 1983, Disorders of lipid transport—Update 1983, *Progr. Cardiovasc. Dis.* **26**:89–108.

Schweizer, T. F., Bekhechi, A. K., Koellreutter, B., Riemann, S., Pometta, D., and Bron, B. A., 1983, Metabolic effects of dietary fiber from dehulled soybeans in humans, *Am. J. Clin. Nutr.* **38**:1–11.

Story, J. A., and Kelley, M. J., 1982, Dietary fiber and lipoproteins, in: *Dietary Fiber in Health and Disease* (G. V. Vahouny and D. Kritchevsky, eds.), Plenum, New York, pp. 229–236.

Sugano, M., Fujikawa, T., Hiratsuji, Y., Nakashima, K., Fukuda, N., and Hasegawa, Y., 1980, A novel use of chitosan as a hypocholesterolemic agent in rats, *Am. J. Clin. Nutr.* **33**:787–793.

Ullrich, I. H., and Albrink, M. J., 1982, Lack of effect of dietary fiber on serum lipids, glucose, and insulin in healthy young men fed high starch diets, *Am. J. Clin. Nutr.* **36**:1–9.

Vahouny, G. V., 1982, Dietary fibers and intestinal absorption of lipids, in: *Dietary Fiber in Health and Disease* (G. V. Vahouny and D. Kritchevsky, eds.), Plenum, New York, pp. 203–227.

Vahouny, G. V., Roy, T., Gallo, L. L., Story, J. A., Kritchevsky, D., and Cassidy, M. M., 1980, Dietary fibers. III. Effects of chronic intake on cholesterol absorption and metabolism in the rat, *Am. J. Clin. Nutr.* **33**:2182–2191.

Van't Hooft, F., and Havel, R. J., 1982, Metabolism of apolipoprotein E in plasma high density lipoproteins from normal and cholesterol-fed rats, *J. Biol. Chem.* **257**:10996–11001.

Vega, G. L., Grosezek, E., Wolf, R., and Grundy, S. M., 1982, Influence of polyunsaturated fats on composition of plasma lipoproteins and apolipoproteins, *J. Lipid Res.* **23**:811–811.

Windler, E., Chao, Y. S., and Havel, R. J., 1980, Determination of hepatic uptake of triglyceride-rich lipoproteins and their remnants in the rat, *J. Biol. Chem.* **255**:5475–5480.

Zavoral, J. H., Hannan, P., Fields, D. J., Hanson, M. N., Frantz, I. D., Kuba, K. Elmer, P., and Jacobs, Jr., D. R., 1983a, The hypolipidemic effects of locust bean gum food products in familial hypercholesterolemic adults and children, *Am. J. Clin. Nutr.* **38**:285–294.

Zavoral, J. H., Hannan, P., Smith, C. M., Hedlund, B. E., Hanson, M. N., Fields, D., Kuba, K., Frantz, I., and Jacobs, Jr., D. R., 1983b, Locust bean gum in food products fed to familial hypercholesterolemic families and a type II patient, in: *Unconventional Sources of Dietary Fiber,* ACS Symposium Series, no. 214 (Furda, I., ed.), American Chemical Society, Washington, D. C., pp. 77–92.

21

Dietary Fiber, Sucrose, and Serum Lipids

MARGARET J. ALBRINK and IRMA H. ULLRICH

1. INTRODUCTION

The best known effects of diet on serum cholesterol were elaborated during a series of experiments on adult men carried out by Keys and others during the 1960s (Keys *et al.*, 1965; Anderson *et al.*, 1973). The conclusions reached from these experiments were that saturated fat was the most powerful cholesterol-raising dietary component, dietary cholesterol having a small additional effect, and polyunsaturated fat having a cholesterol-lowering effect about half as effective as the cholesterol-raising effect of saturated fat. Pectin, certain vegetables, and plant sterols were also found to have a cholesterol-lowering effect. Most of these studies were carried out using diets of usual Western composition, i.e., moderately high in saturated fat and cholesterol. The amount and type of carbohydrate was found to have little or no effect. When an effect was found, sucrose and other sugars had a cholesterol-raising effect compared to starch. By and large, the type of carbohydrate was thought to be of little significance compared to the large effect of type of fat (McGandy *et al.*, 1967). So strong is this impression that in many studies the type of carbohydrate is not even stated.

Epidemiologic evidence that dietary fiber might protect against atherosclerosis (Trowell, 1972) led to the hypothesis that dietary fiber as a component of complex carbohydrates might have a cholesterol-lowering effect. A number of studies have now reported a cholesterol-lowering effect of dietary fiber, either as part of normal foods or added to low-fiber diets (reviewed by

MARGARET J. ALBRINK and IRMA H. ULLRICH • Department of Medicine, West Virginia University School of Medicine, Morgantown, West Virginia 26506.

Kay, 1982). However, such a cholesterol-lowering effect of fiber is far from universally found. Where a cholesterol-lowering effect has been found the fiber has usually been added to diets relatively high in fat (reviewed by Kelsay, 1978).

In very low-fat diets, such as those recommended for maximal cholesterol-lowering effect (Connor and Connor, 1982), the powerful effect of type of fat on cholesterol is removed and the effect of nonfat components of the diet may thus become more important. Differences between types of carbohydrate may be more clearly manifest in such low-fat diets. The effects on serum cholesterol of dietary components likely to be present in high concentrations in high-carbohydrate diets are thus of particular interest: fiber, sucrose and other sugars, and starch.

It is the purpose of the present chapter to report the effects on serum cholesterol of dietary fiber and of certain sugars when fed as constituents of very low-fat diets. Diets of varying types of carbohydrate will be compared with each other and with high-fat "usual Western" diets. In these studies it becomes evident that dietary fiber has little effect on serum cholesterol in high-starch, high-carbohydrate diets, while sucrose compared to starch has a cholesterol-raising effect.

2. EXPERIMENTS WITH VERY LOW-FAT DIETS

2.1. Interaction of Sucrose and Fiber

The effects of varying amounts of sucrose and of fiber in very low-fat diets was assessed in diets consisting of 15% calories from protein, 15% from fat, and 70% from carbohydrate (Albrink and Ullrich, 1984). Twenty-four young men were divided into four groups of six each. Each group was assigned to one of four very low-fat diets, in which sucrose constituted 0, 18, 36, or 52% of calories. At each level of sucrose, the diet was fed in both low- and high-fiber form for 10 days each. The diets were composed of normal foods. Dietary fiber, measured as neutral detergent fiber (Van Soest and Robertson, 1976), comprised 15 g daily for the low-fiber diets and 68 g in the high-fiber diets, except for the 52% sucrose diet, in which, in order to accommodate the high amount of sucrose, it was necessary to eliminate some of the high-fiber foods, with the result that the fiber content of the 52% high-fiber diet was 34 g daily. The nonsucrose carbohydrate foods were chiefly starchy vegetables and fruit. In order to maintain the subjects' usual dietary cholesterol intake of about 500 mg daily, two eggs daily were included in all diets. Dietary history revealed that the subjects' usual diets consisted of 16% calories from protein, 39% from fat, 40% from carbohydrate, and 5% from alcohol, with 450 mg cholesterol daily.

The subjects' triglyceride concentrations after the 0 and 18% sucrose diets were not different from those during their usual diets, and fiber had no effect. There was, however, an increase in triglycerides with the 36 and 52% sucrose diets, and fiber appeared to protect partially against this increase (Ullrich and Albrink, 1980) for the 36% but not the 52% sucrose diet, suggesting that 68 g but not 34 g fiber daily was sufficient to protect against the triglyceride-raising effect of sucrose. A blunting of the insulin response to a representative high-fiber meal was also seen for the 36% carbohydrate diet (Ullrich and Albrink, 1980).

Of particular interest to us was the serum cholesterol response to the diets. The cholesterol decreased by 15 and 14% when the men changed from their usual high-fat diets to the 0 and 18% sucrose diets, but by only 3 and 6% during the 36 and 52% sucrose diets (not significant). Dietary fiber was without effect at any level of sucrose. Sucrose in the amount of 36% or more of calories thus nearly eradicated the cholesterol-lowering effect of removing fat from the diet, and sucrose in these amounts had an effect on serum cholesterol about equal to the effect of their usual intake of saturated fat, which sucrose replaced.

2.2. Effect of High- and Low-Fiber Starches

In another short-term study, two diets composed of starchy foods, one high and one low in fiber, were consumed by seven young men for 4 days. The usual cholesterol intake was maintained by inclusion of two eggs daily. The serum cholesterol declined equally with both diets from that observed during their usual high-fat diets (Ullrich and Albrink, 1982). Thus, as in the experiment outlined above in Section 2.1, dietary fiber did not modify the cholesterol-lowering effect of the change from a high-fat to a very low-fat diet. The cholesterol-lowering effect took place despite the maintenance of usual cholesterol intake. We concluded from these results that dietary fiber, while it prevented carbohydrate-induced lipemia, had no further cholesterol-lowering effect than the powerful effect of substituting starch for fat in the diet.

These findings prompted us to ask several questions about the effects of diet on serum cholesterol during very low-fat diets. Was the sucrose effect shared by other sugars, such as glucose, or was it peculiar to sucrose and other fructose-containing sugars or fructose itself? Did the fact that dietary cholesterol was maintained at relatively high levels have anything to do with the hypercholesterolemic effect of sucrose compared to starch in these very high-carbohydrate diets? Was sufficient fiber given to evoke a cholesterol-lowering effect, or to have any physiological effect?

2.3. Effect of Glucose

In an earlier study (Albrink et al., 1979) we noted the effect on serum cholesterol of two very high-carbohydrate diets, 70% of calories, in one of which glucose in liquid formula form constituted 50% of calories, lactose constituting the remainder of the carbohydrate, with the other diet was composed of high-fiber starchy foods. Seven healthy young adults consumed both diets, in random order, for 7 days. Unlike the sucrose diets, the cholesterol content of these diets was very low, only slightly more than 100 mg daily. Upon changing from their usual high-fat diets, the serum cholesterol in the subjects decreased after 1 week of both the high-fiber diet and the liquid glucose diet, only slightly more so for the high-fiber diet (23% vs 16% below baseline). Thus, when the dietary carbohydrate was glucose, the cholesterol-raising effect seen with sucrose did not occur.

An identical high-glucose, low-cholesterol liquid formula diet was also consumed by ten middle-aged, nondiabetic, normotriglyceridemic men for 1 week, preceded by 3 days of a 300-g carbohydrate diet of usual Western high cholesterol and fat content. As was the case with the young adults, the cholesterol decreased 14% following the high-glucose diet (Albrink *et al.*, 1984a).

These diets were low in cholesterol, while the sucrose diets were high in cholesterol. It is possible that the combination of cholesterol and sucrose accounted for the cholesterol-raising effect of sucrose compared to equally high-cholesterol starchy diets.

2.4. Glucose versus Fructose

While we have not compared high- and low-cholesterol intake in high-sucrose diets, we have compared high-fructose with high-glucose diets, both low in cholesterol (Albrink *et al.*, 1984a). For these diets, two liquid formula diets were consumed, one the same as the high-glucose diet described in Section 2.3, the other similar except that fructose rather than glucose constituted 50% of the calories. The diets were consumed for 1 week by four normoglyceridemic men and one hypertriglyceridemic man. The serum cholesterol was 14% higher for the fructose than the glucose diet. Thus high-cholesterol intake is not necessary for the cholesterol-raising effect of fructose compared to starch or glucose. Since fructose is thought to be the cholesterol-raising component of sucrose, it seems likely that high intake of cholesterol is not necessary for a cholesterol-raising effect of sucrose.

2.5. Effect of Low- and High-Fiber Diets on Fecal Steroids

The lack of fiber effect on serum cholesterol does not mean that the fiber had no effect on steroid metabolism. Fecal fiber and steroid results were available for two of the above studies: the low- and high-fiber starchy foods (Ullrich *et al.*, 1981), in which fiber constituted 21 or 58 g daily, and in 52% sucrose low- and high-fiber studies (Albrink, *et al.*, 1984b), in which fiber constituted 5 and 34 g fiber daily. The concentration of all fiber elements in the stool virtually doubled during the high-fiber compared to the low-fiber diets. The fiber was measured by the method of Van Soest and Robertson (1976). In both high-fiber diets there was a decrease in concentration of secondary bile acids, and thus an increase in the relative prominence of primary bile acids.

3. DISCUSSION

The studies outlined indicate a strong cholesterol-lowering effect of dietary starch and a cholesterol-raising effect of sucrose but not glucose. Fiber appeared to have no effect on cholesterol beyond the effect of the starch of which it was a part. On the other hand, fiber appeared to protect against carbohydrate-induced lipemia and hyperinsulinemia. The possible mechanisms of sucrose, starch, and fiber will be examined in an attempt to explain the strong sucrose and starch effect and lack of fiber effect on cholesterol, and the diminution of carbohydrate-induced rise in triglycerides by fiber in these studies.

3.1. Effect of Sucrose and Fiber on Serum Tryglycerides

The mechanism and degree of carbohydrate-induced lipemia have been debated since the first description of the phenomenon by Ahrens *et al.* (1961). It is thought that dietary glucose is incorporated into liver triglycerides under the influence of insulin (Liu *et al.*, 1983). Our finding that dietary fiber protected against carbohydrate-induced lipemia and blunted the insulin response to a representative meal supports the hypothesis that insulin response to a diet determines the triglyceride-raising potential of the diet (Liu *et al.*, 1983).

3.2. Effect of Diet on Serum Cholesterol

Anderson *et al.* (1973) stated that sucrose, in mixed-carbohydrate diets high in fat, was not found to raise plasma cholesterol concentration. In our very high-carbohydrate diets we found that sucrose did have a cholesterol-raising effect, and fiber had no effect. In order to explain these discrepancies, it is necessary to review several aspects of the regulation of serum cholesterol.

3.2.1. Effect of Sucrose, Glucose, and Starch on Serum Cholesterol

Consistent with our findings, a number of studies have demonstrated, in addition to a rise in triglycerides, an increase in serum cholesterol concentration with very high carbohydrates when sucrose compared to starch is the chief source of carbohydrate (Keys *et al.*, 1960; Groen *et al.*, 1966; Macdonald and Braethwaite 1964). On the other hand, when glucose was the chief source of carbohydrate in such very high-carbohydrate diets, while triglycerides increased as they did with sucrose, cholesterol usually decreased (Beveridge *et al.*, 1964; Schreibman and Ahrens, 1976). In a few studies sucrose and glucose have been compared in the same paper, and sucrose found to be hypercholesterolemic compared to glucose (Winitz, 1964; Kaufman *et al.*, 1966). Others, however, found no difference between glucose and sucrose regarding their effect on serum cholesterol (Macdonald, 1966; Anderson *et al.*, 1963).

In diets high in polyunsaturated fats and moderately high in carbohydrate there was no difference between the effects of sucrose and dextrins on cholesterol (Richardson *et al.*, 1980; Hayford *et al.*, 1979). The amount of sugars could have been too small, although in carefully controlled high-fat diets Hallfrisch *et al.*, (1983) demonstrated a cholesterol-raising effect of only 7.5% of calories as fructose. The effect of amount and type of dietary fat may be all-important in determining the difference, if any, between sucrose (or fructose) and glucose on serum cholesterol. The above negative studies could have been due to a high content of polyunsaturated fat. Relatively small increases in the ratio of polyunsaturated to saturated fatty acids in the diet may have a definite cholesterol-lowering effect (Jackson *et al.*, 1984).

In higher fat diets a cholesterol-raising effect of sucrose has also been found (Antar and Ohlson, 1965; McGandy *et al.*, 1966). In more recent studies a cholesterol-raising effect of 30% of calories from sucrose vs. 30% from starch in diets containing 15, 42, and 43% of calories from protein, fat, and carbohydrate and 562 mg cholesterol has been reported (Reiser *et al.*, 1979). A similar cholesterol-raising effect was found from as little as 7% of calories from fructose (Hallfrisch *et al.*, 1983).

Not all investigators have found sucrose to be hypercholesterolemic compared to starch or equicholesterolemic compared to usual high-fat diets as we did. Grande *et al.* (1974), making modest substitutions of sucrose for starch, to the extent of about 16% of calories, found no difference in the effect on cholesterol. Dunnigan *et al.* (1970) also found no difference. Negative studies may be the result of the large influence of type of fat in high-fat diets. In moderate- or high-fat diets the sucrose effect is abolished by polyunsaturated fat and exaggerated by saturated fat (Antar *et al.*, 1970) and possibly by dietary cholesterol. The powerful cholesterol-raising effect of saturated fat and cholesterol-lowering effect of polyunsaturated fat (Anderson et al., 1973) may obliterate the effect of type of carbohydrate in diets rather high in fat.

The amount of sucrose may be critical, large amounts being necesary to show a cholesterol-raising effect except under the most carefully controlled conditions, such as those of Hallfrisch et al. (1983). Thus we found no effect of 18% sucrose calories compared to starch on cholesterol. When similar small substitutions were made there was no difference between sucrose and starch (Anderson et al., 1963; Grande et al., 1974), although in older men replacement of sucrose by legumes lowered cholesterol (Grande et al., 1965). They attributed the difference to the older age of the subjects.

The reason for the differing effect of sucrose and starch on serum cholesterol is unknown. Portman (1962) was the first to report a cholesterol-lowering effect of starch compared to sucrose and other sugars. He attributed the starch effect to the impaired reabsorption of bile acids secondary to the greater residue in the gut of rats fed high-starch diets. The interruption of the return of bile acids to the liver resulted in increased secretion and turnover of bile acids, the ultimate effect being a reduction in serum cholesterol concentration. When sucrose replaced starch, bile acids were efficiently reabsorbed, resulting in decreased turnover of bile acids with resultant decreased degradation and excretion of cholesterol and finally in higher serum cholesterol levels.

Goldstein et al. (1983) hypothesize that dietary factors that lead to increased hepatic cholesterol content cause downregulation of the hepatic LDL receptor, which in turn results in increased concentration of circulating cholesterol, which has thus escaped clearing. It is possible that sucrose feeding, by stimulating hepatic (MacDonald and Roberts, 1965) and/or intestinal (Holt et al., 1979) cholesterogenesis, could lead to increased hepatic cholesterol concentration with subsequent downregulation of the LDL receptor and resulting increased circulating cholesterol. In such an event the VLDL remnants resulting from carbohydrate-induced lipemia, instead of being promptly removed by the liver via specific receptors, would be converted into LDL, thus raising the serum cholesterol.

Early work by Kritchevsky (1978) and Grande et al. (1965) suggested that some factor in certain natural foods protected against hypercholesterolemia. Dietary fiber has since been shown to be one such factor. Kelsay (1978) reviewed the subject and concluded that fiber would be most hypocholesterolemic in high-fat diets. More recent studies show that fibers most consistently causing a reduction of cholesterol or low-density cholesterol are guars, pectins, gums, and oat bran (Behall et al., 1984; Jenkins et al., 1980, 1983; Zavoral et al., 1983; Kirby et al., 1981). On the other hand, a variety of fibers added to usual diets had little effect (Mahalko *et al.*, 1984; Tsai *et al.*, 1983). In none of the above studies was the dietary fat as low as in our studies.

Dietary fiber may act in a manner similar to cholestyramine: binding of bile acids with subsequent stimulation of conversion of cholesterol to bile acids and their excretion in the bile. The consequent decrease in hepatic cholesterol would lead to an increase in hepatic LDL receptors, with consequent facilitated removal of circulating cholesterol by the liver (Shepherd *et al.*, 1980). Starch was hypothesized by Portman (1962) to bind bile acids in a similar manner. Thus, fiber might act in the same way as starch. A maximal cholesterol-lowering effect of the large amounts of starch in our studies might preclude any additional cholesterol-lowering effect of fiber. A weak additional bile acid binding effect of fiber could easily be compensated for by increased cholesterol synthesis (Maranhão and Quintão, 1983). Even with the powerful bile acid binding capacity of cholestyramine it is often necessary to add an agent that inhibits cholesterol synthesis in order to realize a cholesterol-lowering effect of cholestyramine (Mabuchi *et al.*, 1983).

The possible reasons for our lack of effect of dietary fiber on serum cholesterol are many, but it seems most likely that in very high-carbohydrate diets with high starch content the effect of starch is so great that fiber as no additional effect. An alternative explanation is that the effect on cholesterol metabolism, such as seen in our fecal steroid studies (Ullrich *et al.*, 1981), is easily overcome by increased cholesterol synthesis. We found an increase in primary at the expense of secondary fecal bile acids during high-fiber diets, even though we found no cholesterol-lowering effect. This is the change usually reported when a cholesterol-lowering effect is found upon feeding high-fiber diets (Kay 1982).

SUMMARY AND CONCLUSIONS

In very-high carbohydrate diets the powerful influence of amount and type of dietary fat on serum lipids is removed, and the effect of nonfat components of the diet becomes more important. The present chapter has reviewed the short-term influence of various very high-carbohydrate diets on serum cholesterol concentrations. Of particular interest to us were the components likely to be prominent in high-carbohydrate diets; fiber, sucrose, and other sugar.

In 70% carbohydrate diets, when sugars constituted 36% or more of calories, triglycerides increased in all cases and fiber protected partially against this change. When the sugar was sucrose, cholesterol was higher than with diets devoid of sugar or with diets in which glucose was the sugar. Fructose was more hypercholesterolemic than glucose. At a lower content of sucrose (less than 18% of calories) no effect on serum cholesterol or triglycerides was seen.

Dietary fiber had no effect on serum cholesterol regardless of the presence or absence of sucrose in the diet. Nonetheless, the high-fiber diets caused an increases in fecal primary bile acids at the expense of secondary bile acids, a change usually associated with increased excretion of cholesterol in the bile. An effect of fiber in removing cholesterol from the body was probably counteracted by increased cholesterol synthesis.

We conclude that dietary fiber has little effect on serum cholesterol in very high-carbohydrate diets, but that type and amount of sugar have large effects.

ACKNOWLEDGMENTS.   This work was supported in part by Research Career Award 5K6HL00486, NHLBI (M. J. A.), and by a grant from the Sugar Association (SA-3-099/78).

REFERENCES

Aherns, E. H., Jr., Hirsch, J., Oette, K., Farquhar, J. W., and Stein, Y., 1961, Carbohydrate-induced and fat-induced lipemia, *Trans. Assoc. Am. Physicians* **74**:124–146.

Albrink, M. J., and Ullrich, I. H., 1985, Interactions of dietary fiber and sucrose on serumm lipids, cholesterol and high density lipoprotein cholesterol in healthy young men fed high carbohydrate diets, (submitted for publication).

Albrink, M. J., Newman, T. and Davidson, P. C., 1979, Effect of high- and low-fiber diets on plasma lipids and insulin, *Am. J. Clin. Nutr.* **32**:1486–1491.

Albrink, M. J., Harper, L., and Davidson, P. C., 1985a, Curtailment of carbohydrate-induced lipemia by impaired glucose tolerance, (submitted for publication).

Albrink, M. J., Ullrich, I. H., Beamer, K., Reid, R., and Watne, R., 1985b, Response of fecal fiber and steroid to high fiber high sucrose diets, (submitted for publication).

Anderson, J. T., Grande, F., Matsumoto, V., and Keys, A., 1963, Glucose, sucrose and lactose in the diet and blood lipids in man, *J. Nutr.* **79**:349–359.

Anderson, J. T., Grande, F., and Keys, A., 1973, Cholesterol-lowering diets. *J. Am. Diet. Assoc.* **62**:133–142.

Antar, M. A., and Ohlson, M. A., 1965, Effect of simple and complex carbohydrates upon total lipids, non-phospholipids, and different fractions of phospholipids of serum in young men and women, *J. Nutr.* **75**:329–337.

Antar, M. A., Little, J. A., Lucas, C., Buckley, G. C., and Csima, A., 1970, Interrelationship between the kinds of dietary carbohydrate and fat in hyperlipoproteinemic patients. Part 3. Synergistic effect of sucrose and animal fat on serum lipids, *Atherosclerosis* **11**:191–201.

Behall, K. M., Lee, K. H., and Moser, P. B., 1984, Blood lipids and lipoproteins in adult men fed four refined fibers, *Am. J. Clin. Nutr.* **39**:209–214.

Beveridge, J. M. R., Jagannathan, S. N., and Connell, W. F., 1964, The effect of the type and amount of dietary fat on the level of plasma triglycerides in human subjects in the post-absorptive state, *Can. J. Biochem.* **42**:999–1003.

Connor, W. E., and Connor, S. L., 1982, The dietary treatment of hyperlipidemia. Rationale, technique and efficacy, *Med. Clin. North Am.* **66**:485–518.

Dunnigan, M. G., Fyfe, T., McKiddle, M. T., and Crosbie, C. M., 1970, The effects of isocaloric exchange of dietary starch and sucrose on glucose tolerance, plasma insulin and serum lipids in man, *Clin. Sci.* **38**:1–9.

Goldstein, J. L., Kita, T., and Brown, M. S., 1983, Defective lipoprotein receptors and atherosclerosis. Lessons from an animal counterpart of familial hypercholesterolemia, *N. Engl. J. Med.* **309**:288–296.

Grande, F., Anderson, J. T., and Keys, A., 1965, Effect of carbohydrates of leguminous seeds, wheat and potatoes on serum cholesterol concentration in man, *J. Nutr.* **86**:313–317.

Grande, F., Anderson, J. T., and Keys, A., 1974, Sucrose and various carbohydrate-containing foods and serum lipids in man, *Am. J. Clin. Nutr.* **27**:1043–1051.

Groen, J. J., Balogh, M., Yaron, E., and Cohen, A. M., 1966, Effect of interchanging bread and sucrose as main source of carbohydrate in a low fat diet on the serum cholesterol levels of healthy volunteer subjects, *Am. J. Clin. Nutr.* **19**:46–58.

Hallfrisch, J., Reiser, S., and Prather, E. S., 1983, Blood lipid distribution of hyperinsulinemic men consuming three leves of fructose, *Am. J. Clin. Nutr.* **37**:740–748.

Hayford, J. T., Danney, M. M., Wiebe, D., Roberts, S., and Thompson, R. G., 1979, *Am. J. Clin. Nutr.* **32**:1670–1678.

Holt, P. R., Dominquez, A. A., and Kwartler, J., 1979, Effect of sucrose feeding upon intestinal and hepatic lipid synthesis, *Am. J. Clin. Nutr.* **32**:1792–1798.

Jackson, R. L., Kashyap, M. L., Barnhard, R. L., Allen, C., Hogg, E., and Glueck, C. J., 1984, Influence of polyunsaturated and saturated fats on plasma lipids and lipoproteins in man, *Am. J. Clin. Nutr.* **39**:589–597.

Jenkins, D. J. A., Reynolds, D., Slavin, B., Leeds, A. R., Jenkins, A. L., and Jepson, E. W., 1980, Dietary fiber and blood lipids: Treatment of hypercholesterolemia with guar crispbread, *Am. J. Clin. Nutr.* **33**:575–581.

Jenkins, D. J. A., Wong, G. S., Patten, R., Bird, J., Hall, M., Buckley, G. C., McGuire, V., Reichert, R., and Little, J. A., 1983, Leguminous seeds in the dietary management of hypercholesterolemia, *J. Am. Clin. Nutr.* **38**:567–573.

Kaufman, N. A., Poznanski, R., Blondheim, S. H., and Stein, V., 1966, Changes in serum lipid levels of hyperlipemic patients following the feeding of starch, sucrose and glucose, *Am. J. Clin. Nutr.* **18**:261–269.

Kay, R. M., 1982, Dietary fiber, *J. Lipid Res.* **23**:221–242.

Kelsay, J. L., 1978, A review of research on effects of fiber intake in man, *Am. J. Clin. Nutr.* **31**:142–159.

Keys, A., Anderson, J. T., and Grande, F., 1965, Serum cholesterol response to changes in the diet. II. Effect of cholesterol in the diet, *Metabolism* **14**:759–765.

Keys, A., Anderson, J. T., and Grande, F., 1966, Diet-type (fats constant) and blood lipids in man, *J. Nutr.* **70**:257–266.

Kirby, R. W., Anderson, J. W., Sieling, B., Rees, E. D., Chen, W.-J. L., Miller, R. E., and Kay, R. M., 1981, Oat-bran intake selectively lowers serum low-density lipoprotein cholesterol concentrations of hypercholeterolemic men, *Am. J. Clin. Nutr.* **34**:824–829.

Kritchevsky, D., 1978, Effect of dietary fiber on lipid metabolism and atherosclerosis, in: *International Conference on Atherosclerosis* (L. A. Carlson, ed.), Raven, New York, 1978, pp. 160–172.

Liu, G. C., Coulston, A. M., and Reaven, G. M., 1983. Effect of high-carbohydrate low-fat diets on plasma glucose, insulin and lipid responses in hypertriglyceridemic humans, *Metabolism* **32**:750–753.

Mabuchi, H., Sakai, T., Sakai, Y., Yoshimura, A., Watanabe, A., Wakasugi, T., Koizumi, J., Takeda, R., 1983, Reduction of serum cholesterol in heterozygous patients with familial hypercholesterolemia. Additive effects of compactin and cholestyramine, *N. Engl. J. Med.* **308**:609–613.

MacDonald, I., 1966, Influence of fructose and glucose on serum lipid levels in men and pre and post-menopausal women, *Am. J. Clin. Nutr.* **18**:369–372.

MacDonald, I., and Braethwaite, D. M., 1964, The influence of dietary carbohydrates on the lipid pattern in serum and in adipose tissue, *Clin. Sci.* **27**:23–30.

MacDonald, I., and Roberts, J. B., 1965, The incorporation of various C14 dietary carbohydrates into serum and liver lipids, *Metabolism* **14**:991–999.

Mahalko, J. R., Sandstead, H. H., Johnson, L. K., Inman, L. F., Milne, D. B., Warner, R. C., and Haunz, E. A., 1984, Effect of consuming fiber from corn bran, soy hulls, or apple powder on glucose tolerance and plasma lipids in type II diabetes, *Am. J. Clin. Nutr.* **39**:25–34.

Maranhão, R. C., and Quintão, E. C. R., 1983, Long term steroid metabolism balance studies in subjects on cholesterol-free and cholesterol-rich diets: Comparison between normal and hypercholesterolemic individuals, *J. Lipid Res.* **24**:167–173.

McGandy, R. B., Hegsted, D. M., Myers, M. L., and Stare, F. J., 1966, Dietary carbohydrate and serum cholesterol levels in man, *Am. J. Clin. Nutr.* **18**:237–242.

McGandy, R. B., Hegsted, D. M., and Stare, F. J., 1967, Dietary fats, carbohydrates and atherosclerotic vascular disease, *N. Engl. J. Med.* **277**:186–192, 242–247.

Portman, O. W., 1962, Importance of diet, species, and intestinal flora in bile acid metabolism, *Fed. Proc. Fed. Am. Soc. Exp. Biol.* **21**:896–902.

Reiser, S., Hallfrisch, J., Michaelis, O. E., IV, Lazar, F. L., Martin, R. E., and Prather, E. S., 1979, Isocaloric exchange of dietary starch and sucrose in humans. I. Effect on levels of fasting blood lipids, *Am. J. Clin. Nutr.* **32**:1659–1668.

Richardson, D. P., Scrimshaw, N. S., and Young, V. R., 1980, The effect of dietary sucrose on protein utilization in healthy young men, *Am. J. Clin. Nutr.* **33**:264–272.

Schreibman, P. H., and Ahrens, E. J., Jr., 1976, Sterol balance in hyperlipidemic patients after dietary exchange of carbohydrate for fat, *J. Lipid Res.* **17**:97–106.

Shepherd, J., Packard, C. J., Bicker, S., Lawrie, T. D. V., and Morgan, H. G., 1980, Cholestyramine promotes receptor-mediated low-density-lipoprotein catabolism, *N. Engl. J. Med.* **302**:1219–1222.

Trowell, H., 1972, Ischemic heart disease and dietary fiber, *Am. J. Clin. Nutr.* **25**:926–932.

Tsai, A. C., Mott, E. L., Owen, G. M., Bennick, M. R., Lo, G. S., and Steinke, F. H., 1983, Effects of soy polysaccharide on gastrointestinal functions, nutrient balance, steroid excretions, glucose tolerance, serum lipids, and other parameters in humans, *Am. J. Clin. Nutr.* **38**:504–511.

Ullrich, I. H., and Albrink, M. J., 1980, Dietary fiber protects against sucrose-induced-hypertriglyceridemia, *Clin. Res.* **28**:816A.

Ullrich, I. H., and Albrink, M. J., 1982, Lack of effect of dietary fiber on serum lipids, glucose tolerance and insulin in healthy young men fed high starch diets, *Am. J. Clin. Nutr.* **36**:1–9.

Ullrich, I. H., Lai, H.-Y., Vona, L., Reid, R. L., and Albrink, M. J., 1981, Alterations of fecal steroid composition induced by changes in dietary fiber consumption, *Am. J. Clin. Nutr.* **34**:2054–2060.

Van Soest, P. J., and Robertson, J. B., 1976, Chemical and physical properties of dietary fiber, presented at Miles Symposium on Dietary Fiber, Nutrition Society of Canada, Rexdale, Ontario.

Winitz, M., 1964, Effect of dietary carbohydrate on serum cholesterol levels, *Arch. Biochem.* **108**:576–579.

Zavoral, J. H., Hannan, P., Stat, M., Fields, D. J., Hanson, M. N., Frantz, I. D., Kuba, K., Elmer, P., and Jacobs, D. R., 1983, The hypolipidemic effect of locust bean gum food products in familial hypercholesterolemic adults and children, *Am. J. Clin. Nutr.* **38**:285–294.

22

Dietary Fiber and Weight Management

ANTHONY R. LEEDS and
PATRICIA A. JUDD

1. INTRODUCTION

That dietary fiber may have important effects in the genesis and management of obesity has been considered possible since the "dietary fiber hypothesis" was first proposed (Heaton, 1973; Trowell, 1975). Despite intense public interest in a potential beneficial effect for fiber, as demonstrated by the enormous popularity of some high-fiber diet books, such as the *F-Plan Diet* (Eyton, 1982), very few attempts have been made to test this idea. Since dietary fiber is a complex mixture of materials, which may have different effects depending on its chemical structure and physical relationships to adjacent materials (i.e., its physical form), it is an oversimplication of the problem to ask the question: Does dietary fiber help the obese to lose weight? Even if one particular study were able to provide a scientifically acceptable affirmative answer to the question, it would not follow that this could be translated into an effective message for the obese and overweight public, since the factors operating to facilitate or prevent success in the most frequent weight management situations (overweight or moderately obese individuals seeking advice from nonmedical sources such as slimming clubs) would not be the same as were operating in the experimental situation.

ANTHONY R. LEEDS • Department of Nutrition, Queen Elizabeth College, University of London, London W8 7AH, and Department of General Medicine and Endocrinology, Central Middlesex Hospital, London NW10 7NS, United Kingdom   PATRICIA A. JUDD • Department of Nutrition, Queen Elizabeth College, University of London, London W8 7AH, United Kingdom.

Successful weight reduction usually involves a reduction of oral energy input and many of the techniques developed to facilitate weight reduction, such as wiring of the jaws, are simply aids to achieve compliance with the prescribed energy-reduced diet. Other techniques, such as the use of some anorectic drugs, may involve direct effects on metabolic processes as well as facilitation of compliance. Thus, a useful initial question is: Can dietary fiber components and high-fiber diets have specific effects in obesity, or, if they have any effect at all, are they simply another aid to compliance with the energy-reduced diet? Figure 1 illustrates some possible effects of dietary fiber on energy balance. Before being eaten, fiber may by its very presence influence the physical properties of a food so as to affect the ease with which the food can be eaten (Heaton, 1980), and may, but not necessarily, be related to energy density, a sufficient lowering of which may reduce total energy intake. After being eaten, effects of fiber on gastric distension and emptying, small intestinal distension and motility, nutrient absorption rates, and fluxes of energy to the liver may provide neurological signals, as well as hormonal signals, to control the rate of energy intake. The effects of fiber on the gut have been discussed by Read (this volume, Chapter 7). Fiber also alters the palatability of food, and it is now recognized that designing satiety studies to examine effects of fiber are difficult, because unless food items or diets are equally palatable, differences in satiety scores may be due to differences of palatability rather than fiber content (Spitzer and Rodin, 1981).

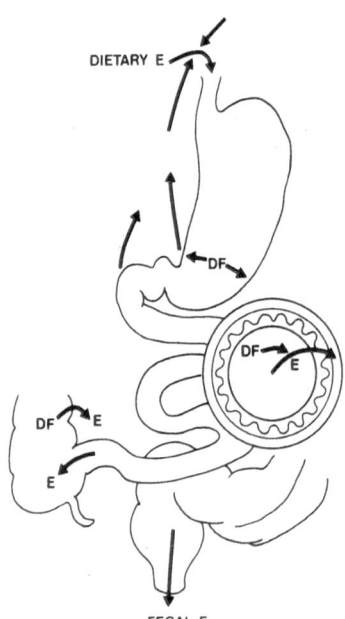

FIGURE 1. Sites of action of dietary fiber in the gut related to energy balance. E, energy; DF, dietary fiber. (Reproduced with permission.)

Fiber may also have an effect on the rate and completeness of energy absorption (Fig. 1), and some of the metabolic effects of fiber may have beneficial effects beyond controlling satiety.

2. MECHANISMS OF ACTION

2.1. Satiety

Satiety is listed here in order to provide a complete list, but has been reviewed elsewhere (Heaton, 1980).

2.2. Absorption of Energy

Cummings and Branch (this volume, Chapter 10) have presented some of the evidence showing that fecal energy may be increased under some circumstances. McCance and Widdowson (1947) showed that the digestibility of energy and protein was lower in six subjects when 90% extraction wheat flour was substituted for 80% extraction flour. Southgate and Durnin (1970) demonstrated in 49 subjects in four groups that increasing unavailable carbohydrate (dietary fiber) increased fecal energy losses and in most cases fecal nitrogen and fat losses. Increasing fiber intake by a factor of 2–3 reduced apparent digestibility of energy by about 2% from about 95%. Significant increases of fecal energy loss have been shown by Farrell et al. (1978) and Kelsay et al. (1978) in well-controlled studies. Fecal energy was approximately doubled in both studies and digestibility reduced by 2% in Farrell's study and 4% in Kelsay's study. Reductions of energy digestibility of only 2% may seem insignificant, but in absolute terms the additional energy losses may represent 50–100 kcal/day. If such changes persisted, they might be important, but it is possible that man may adapt to high-fiber diets to become more efficient with regard to energy absorption. It is not possible from the work referred to above to determine whether any adaptation occurred. The study periods were 11 days (McCance and Widdowson, 1947), 7 days after 5-day run-ins (Southgate and Durnin, 1970), 26 days (Kelsay et al., 1978), and 24 days (Farrell et al., 1978). Recalculation of data reported in a study by Judd (1982) suggest the possibility of improvement of the efficiency of energy absorption with time. Nine young people were studied for 42 days, during which time weighed diet records were kept; dietary fiber intakes were calculated from these records (Fig. 2). The normal diet was taken during the first 7 days, then barley bread and barley were substituted for wheat bread in the diets, building up the amount of barley during days 8–14. After day 28 the subjects reverted to the normal wheat-based diets. Three-day duplicate food collections and 3-day fecal collections were made

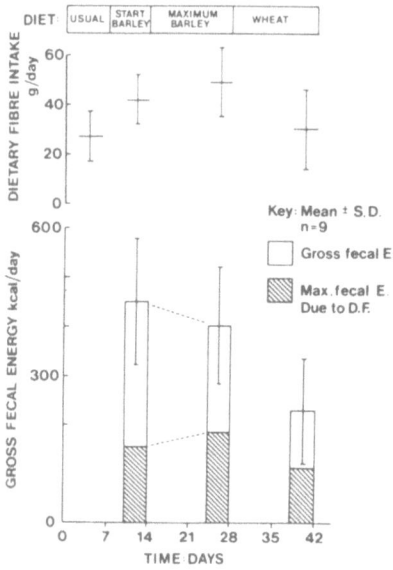

FIGURE 2. Dietary fiber intake (calculated) and gross fecal energy (measured) in nine subjects. Values are mean ± SD. Hatching on the columns represents the calculated maximum contribution to gross fecal energy that could be contributed to dietary fiber in the feces. [Data derived from Judd (1982), reproduced with permission.]

at the end of the "start-barley" period, the end of the maximum barley period, and the end of the wheat period. Bomb calorimetry of food and feces gave data from which apparent digestibility of energy could be calculated: this was 82 ± 7% after the maximum barley diet and 90 ± 4% after the wheat diet (Table I). The mean gross fecal energy was 448 ± 130 kcal/day after 1 week of barley and 402 ± 117 kcal/day (mean ± SD) after a further 14 days of barley at a higher intake level. Since the calculated dietary fiber intake was higher from day 14 to day 28 of the study, it follows that if there were to be no fecal degradation of dietary fiber at either time, then fecal energy from other sources has fallen more than total gross fecal energy (Fig. 2). Clearly there would have been some degradation of dietary fiber and the loss of energy from this source may have been different on the two occasions; however, the calculated gross fecal energy less the maximum possible contribution to fecal energy due to dietary fiber (assuming the calculated figures to reflect the true values) fell from 289 ± 114 after the "start–barley" period to 217 ± 111 kcal/day (mean ± SD) after the "maximum-barley" period; individual changes are illustrated in Fig. 3. These calculated figures do nothing more than suggest the possibility that there could be an adaptation of fecal energy loss. Fecal energy losses of the order of magnitude described above are sometimes dismissed as being of no consequence; if evidence for increased efficiency of energy absorption after adaptation to a high-fiber diet could be obtained, this view would be supported.

TABLE I. Apparent Digestibilities of Dry Matter, Nitrogen, Fat and Energy in Nine Subjects after High-Barley and Wheat-Based Diets[a]

	Barley	Wheat
Dry matter digestibility, %	78 ± 6	89 ± 5
Energy digestibility, %	82 ± 7	90 ± 4
Nitrogen digestibility, %	89 ± 4	95 ± 3
Fat digestibility, %	92 ± 5	95 ± 5

[a] From Judd (1982). Values are mean ± SEM.

Another important consideration is that if energy balance were to be persistently altered by high-fiber diets, weight changes would not necessarily follow. It is possible that downward adjustment of basal metabolic rate (BMR), perhaps as a consequence of thyroid hormone level changes, might occur. Certainly large reductions of energy intake may reduce BMR (Garrow, 1981); whether persistent increased fecal energy loss would do the same is uncertain.

2.3. Metabolic Effects

Some types of dietary fiber modify the absorption of carbohydrate, resulting in a flattening of postprandial glucose and insulin responses (Jenkins et al., 1978). Rebound hypoglycemia, which may induce hunger and commencement of feeding, may not occur after high-fiber meals. Rebound hypoglycemia can certainly be prevented by the use of pectin in the dumping syndrome, where hypoglycemia may be severe (Leeds et al., 1981). Persistently low insulin responses to meals may result in changes in receptor numbers or function on peripheral tissues, reflected in an increased sensitivity to insulin, which would be a beneficial change in obese patients with hyperinsulinism. Gastrointestinal hormone levels in blood may be reduced by fiber (Morgan et al., 1979); thus, lower glucose-dependent insulinotropic polypeptide (GIP) levels may mediate the reduced insulin responses and possibly modify upper gut motility.

Reduction of LDL-cholesterol by some types of fiber (Smith and Holm, 1982), while not relevant to body weight management, may be a beneficial effect in some patients.

3. EFFECTS ON WEIGHT LOSS

In Chapter 23 of this volume Anderson describes the beneficial effects of high-carbohydrate, high-fiber diets, including marked weight losses in some cases. High-fiber breads have been demonstrated to facilitate weight

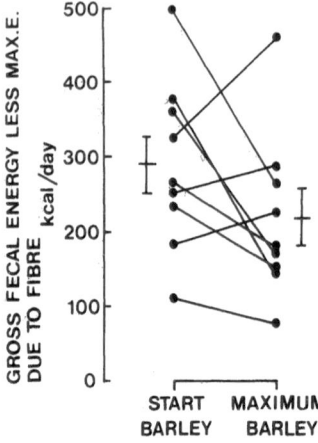

FIGURE 3. Calculated gross fecal energy less maximum energy derived from dietary fiber. Values for individual subjects. [Data derived from Judd (1982), reproduced with permission.]

loss in association with an energy-restricted diet (Michelsen *et al.*, 1979) and fiber components such as guar gum have also been demonstrated to cause weight loss (Tuomilehto *et al.*, 1980; Krotkiewski, 1984). In Krotkiewski's study nine obese women were given 20 g guar gum granules before two main meals daily for 8 weeks and were specifically asked not to make dietary changes. Mean (± SEM) body weight fell from 95.6 ± 3.1 to 91.3 ± 2.1 kg and body fat from 46.1 ± 2.9 to 43.6 ± 2.8 kg, while dietary records suggested no change in intake. In a second study (Krotkiewski, 1984) guar gum was taken for 1 week followed by wheat bran taken for 1 week, then gum for 1 week, and so on, alternating weekly for 10 weeks, by 21 obese patients whose initial mean (± SEM) weight was 92.5 ± 4.2 kg and final weight was 85.4 ± 3.7 kg. Mean (± SEM) weekly weight loss was 0.94 ± 0.2 kg when guar was taken and 0.64 ± 0.1 kg when wheat bran was taken. The patients had been advised to maintain habitual dietary intake, but it is not clear whether they did so.

Some of the difficulties encountered in fiber and obesity studies concern the preparation of satisfactory placebo preparations. For a mixed barley-bran and pectin fiber tablet a suitable placebo has been made and two studies have been undertaken. In a study by S. Rössner (personal communication) there was no significant difference in weight loss between the study groups in patients intensively managed in hospital practice and prescribed an 1100-kcal diet. By contrast, a study by Ryttig (personal communication) where 90 women, more than 115% of their ideal body weight were prescribed a 1200-kcal diet in a slimming clinic and also given fiber tablets or placebo, the mean weight loss in the fiber tablet group was 6.3 kg and in the placebo group 4.2 kg over an 11-week period. Dietary data were collected, but were not able to indicate clearly whether energy intakes had been lower in the fiber tablet group than in the placebo group. These two studies, possibly the first to use acceptable placebos, suggest that fiber preparations (and it is also just possible high-fiber diets as well) may be more effective in situations where the conscious effort to reduce food intake is not very strong: they may be aids to compliance with the prescribed energy-reduced diet. It follows from this that it is possible that fiber preparations, and possibly high-fiber diets, may be more effective in situations where the intensity of management effort is not great and where therefore the compliance with the dietary prescription may not be so good. Thus it would be reasonable to expect that fiber preparations and possibly diets would be more effective when applied in slimming clubs than in hospital clinics, where intensity of effort may be expected to be high. The greater proportion of overweight and moderately obese patients seek advice from nonmedical sources and these include slimming clubs. It follows that research studies undertaken in such clubs may give results of more practical relevance than studies undertaken in hospital environments.

4. CONCLUSION

The evidence suggests that the most important effect of fiber related to obesity is its role in modifying energy intake. If energy intake reduction in obese patients can be achieved by other means, fiber may have little additional effect, but if energy intake reduction has been insufficient, fiber may facilitate further reduction. This idea needs to be tested in well-controlled studies.

ACKNOWLEDGMENTS. We are grateful to Sue Elliott, Mike Ethrington, and J. Glass for preparing the artwork, plates, and typescript, respectively.

REFERENCES

Eyton, A., 1982, The F-Plan Diet, Penguin, Harmondsworth, Middlesex, England.
Farrell, D. J., Girle, L., and Arthur, J., 1978, Effects of dietary fibre on the apparent digestibility of major food components and on blood lipids in men, Aust. J. Exp. Biol. Med. Sci. 56:469–479.
Garrow, J. S., 1981, The physics and physiology of obesity, in: Treat Obesity Seriously: A Clinical Manual, Churchill Livingstone, Edinburgh, pp. 18–60.
Heaton, K. W., 1973, Food fibre as an obstacle to energy intake, Lancet 2:1418–1421.
Heaton, K. W., 1980, Food intake regulation and fiber, in: Medical Aspects of Dietary Fiber (G. A. Spiller and R. M. Kay, eds.), Plenum, New York, pp. 223–238.
Jenkins, D. J. A., Wolever, T. M. S., Leeds, A. R., Gassull, M. A., Haisman, P., Diliwari, J., Goff, D. V., Metz, G. L., and Alberti, K. G. M. M., 1978, Dietary fibres, fibre analogues and glucose tolerance, importance of viscosity, Br. Med. J. 1:1392–1394.

Judd, P. A., 1982, The effects of high intakes of barley on gastrointestinal function and apparent digestibilities of dry matter, nitrogen and fat in human volunteers, *J. Plant Foods* 4:79-88.

Kelsay, J. L., Behall, K. M., and Prather, E. S., 1978, Effect of fiber from fruits and vegetables on metabolic responses of human subjects. I. Bowel transit time, number of defecations, fecal weight, urinary excretions of energy and nitrogen and apparent digestibilities of energy, nitrogen, and fat, *Am. J. Clin. Nutr.* 31:1149-1153.

Krotkiewski, M., 1984, Effect of guar gum on body-weight, hunger ratings and metabolism in obese subjects, *Br. J. Nutr.* 52:97-105.

Leeds, A. R., Ralphs, D. N. L., Ebied, F., Metz, G., and Dilawari, J. B., 1981, Pectin and the dumping syndrome: Reduction of symptoms and plasma volume changes, *Lancet* 1:1075-1078.

McCance, R. A., and Widdowson, E. M., 1947, The digestibility of English and Canadian wheats with special reference to the digestibility of protein by man, *J. Hyg.* 45:59-64.

Michelsen, O., Makdani, D. P., Cotton, R. H., Titcomb, S. T., Colmey, J. C., and Gatty, R., 1979, Effects of a high fiber bread on weight loss in college-age males, *Am. J. Clin Nutr.* 32:1703-1709.

Morgan, L. M., Goulder, I. J., Tsiolakis, D., Marks, V., and Alberti, K. G. M. M., 1979, The effect of unabsorbable carbohydrate on gut hormones, *Diabetologia* 17:85-89.

Smith, U., and Holm, G., 1982, Effect of a modified guar gum preparation on glucose and lipid levels in diabetics and healthy volunteers, *Atherosclerosis* 45:1-10.

Southgate, D. A. T., and Durnin, J. V. G. A., 1970, Calorie conversion factors. An experimental reassessment of the factors used in the calculation of the energy value of human diets, *Br. J. Nutr.* 24:517-535.

Spitzer, L., and Rodin, J., 1981, Human eating behaviour: A critical review of studies in normal weight and overweight individuals, *Appetite* 2:293-329.

Trowell, H., 1975, Diabetes mellitus and obesity, in: *Refined Carbohydrate Foods and Disease. Some Implications of Dietary Fibre* (D. P. Burkitt and H. C. Trowell, eds.), Academic, London, pp. 227-249.

Tuomilehto, J., Vontilainen, E., Huttunen, J., Vinni, S., and Homan, K., 1980, Effect of guar gum on body weight and serum lipids in hypercholesterolemic females, *Acta Med. Scand.* 208:45-48.

23

Dietary Fiber in Nutrition Management of Diabetes

JAMES W. ANDERSON

1. INTRODUCTION

Dietary fiber intake benefits individuals with a wide variety of metabolic conditions or gastrointestinal disorders. In the past decade the advantages of generous fiber intakes have been reported for persons with diabetes (Anderson, 1979; Anderson and Chen, 1979; Anderson and Ward, 1979; Jenkins *et al.*, 1982), hypercholesterolemia (Anderson *et al.*, 1984), hypertriglyceridemia (Anderson, 1980), obesity (Anderson *et al.*, 1980a), or hypertension (Anderson, 1983). Individuals with high levels of dietary fiber intake are less likely to develop coronary heart disease (Morris *et al.*, 1977; Kromhout *et al.*, 1982; Liu *et al.*, 1982) or colon cancer (Bingham *et al.*, 1979) than their neighbors with low-fiber intakes. The role of dietary fiber in the prevention (Trowell, 1975) and management of diabetes (Anderson, 1979, Anderson and Chen, 1979; Anderson and Ward, 1979) has been studied extensively. This review will examine the effects of dietary fiber intake on glucose and lipid metabolism of lean diabetic individuals.

Interactions between fiber intake and diabetes have been examined in three major ways. First, meal studies have incorporated various types of fiber into test meals and examined the postprandial responses of blood glucose and hormone concentrations. Second, fiber-supplement studies have evaluated the short-term and long-term impact of fiber supplements on glycemic control, insulin requirements, and blood lipid concentrations of diabetic subjects. Third, high-fiber diets have been fed to diabetic subjects

JAMES W. ANDERSON • Medical Service, Veterans Administration Medical Center, and Department of Medicine, University of Kentucky College of Medicine, Lexington, Kentucky 40511.

for short-term and long-term periods to assess their effects on glycemic control, insulin requirements, and blood lipid concentrations. Before discussing proposed mechanisms to explain the actions of fiber, studies using these three approaches will be summarized.

2. MEAL STUDIES

Jenkins *et al.* (1976, 1977, 1979a,b), in a series of innovative studies, reported that incorporating purified fibers into meals reduced the blood glucose response to meals. They documented that water-soluble fibers such as guar or pectin decrease the postprandial glycemic response to mixed meals or oral ᵍlucose loads. When guar, for example, was included with the morning meal, postmeal blood glucose values were significantly lower than after similar meals without guar. These observations have important implications for the management of individuals with diabetes.

The pioneering studies of Jenkins *et al.* (1976, 1977, 1979a,b) were confirmed by many other groups (Monnier *et al.*, 1978; Morgan *et al.*, 1979). These studies documented that water-soluble fibers such as guar and pectin decrease postprandial glycemic responses to meals, while water-insoluble fibers such as cellulose or wheat bran do not exert these effects. From most effective to least effective these fibers can be rated as follows: guar, pectin, cellulose, wheat bran. Figure 1 illustrates these comparisons. The metabolic effects of soluble fibers with respect to glucose metabolism clearly differ from the effects of water-insoluble fibers.

Hormone responses to meals or oral glucose administration also are influenced by fiber intake. Jenkins *et al.* (1976) first documented clearly that serum insulin responses to fiber-containing meals were lower than observed after meals without fiber supplements. These early studies suggested that fiber intake somehow increased peripheral sensitivity to insulin, since oral

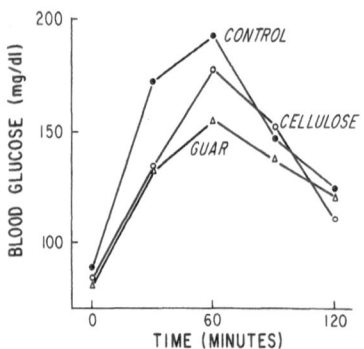

FIGURE 1. Glycemic response of subjects with impaired glucose tolerance to oral administration of glucose, glucose and guar, or glucose and cellulose. [Modified from the data of Monnier *et al.* (1978) and Jenkins *et al.* (1976).]

glucose loads were metabolized with substantially lower peripheral insulin concentrations.

Responses of gut hormones and other pancreatic hormones also are affected by fiber supplements. Serum concentrations of gastric inhibitory polypeptide (GIP), vasoactive inhibitory polypeptide (VIP), and gut glucagon are lower after high-fiber meals than after low-fiber meals (Morgan *et al.*, 1979). Serum pancreatic glucagon cencentrations also are lower with high-fiber diets than with low-fiber diets (Miranda and Horwitz, 1978). Since glucagon and some gut hormones have hepatic effects that oppose those of insulin, lower serum concentrations of these hormones may enhance insulin effects on the liver and perhaps on peripheral tissues.

3. FIBER SUPPLEMENTS

3.1 Glycemic Effects

Jenkins *et al.* (1978, 1979a,b, 1980) developed guar supplements to evaluate the long-term effects of fiber supplements for diabetic individuals. Compared to values with control diets, guar supplements were associated with better glycemic control, lower insulin requirements, and lower serum cholesterol concentrations.

Fiber supplements usually improve glycemic control, lower insulin or oral agent requirements, and lower serum cholesterol concentrations. Table I summarizes the responses reported for 24 groups of subjects given fiber-supplemented diets for 1–52 weeks. A total of 347 diabetic subjects were treated for an average of 10 weeks. Improved glycemic control, judged by lower plasma glucose concentrations, less glycosuria, or decreased insulin requirements, was noted by 22 of 24 groups (92%).

Two groups (Botha *et al.*, 1981; Cohen *et al.*, 1980) reported that fiber-supplemented diets offered no advantages for their patients. Many individuals do not tolerate fiber supplements well (Aro *et al.*, 1981; Carroll *et al.*, 1981; Christiansen *et al.*, 1980; Cohen *et al.*, 1980; Johansen, 1981; U. Smith and Holm, 1982). While a soluble fiber supplement usually improve glucose metabolism of diabetic subjects, it frequently produces nausea, vomiting, or other gastrointestinal side effects (Anderson, 1979; Anderson and Chen, 1979; Anderson and Ward, 1979). This remains the major limitation to the wider use of fiber supplements for type II diabetic subjects. Palatable preparations of guar or other soluble fiber supplements may offer major advantages for the nutrition management of obese type II diabetic subjects.

The guar crispbread preparation developed by Jenkins *et al.* (1978, 1980) was well tolerated by their English diabetic subjects and effectively improved glycemic control. We were able to use this guar crispbread prepa-

TABLE I. Response of Diabetic Subjects to Fiber-Supplemented Diets

Reference	Number of subjects	Type of fiber	Duration of study, days	Response of Blood			Weight change
				Glucose	Cholesterol	Triglyceride	
Aro et al. (1981)	9	Guar	91	Improved	Lower	Unchanged	None
Bosello et al. (1980)	38	Wheat bran	30	Improved	Lower	Lower	—
Botha et al. (1981)	10	Guar	91	Unchanged	Lower	—	—
Carroll et al. (1981)	6	Guar	28	Improved	Lower	—	—
Cohen et al. (1980)	22	Guar or wheat bran	91	Unchanged	—	—	None
Dobson et al. (1981)	9	Guar or wheat bran	91	Improved	Lower	—	Lower
Doi et al. (1979)	13	Glucomannan	90	Improved	Lower	—	—
Fagerberg (1982)	40	Psylium	122	Improved	Lower	Unchanged	—
Jenkins et al. (1978)	6	Guar	56	Improved	—	—	—
Jenkins et al. (1979a)	9	Guar	84–140	Improved	Lower	—	—
Jenkins et al. (1980)	11	Guar	183–365	Improved	Lower	—	—
Johansen (1981)	10	Guar	28	Improved	Lower	—	—
Koepp and Hegewisch (1981)	10	Guar	28	Improved	—	—	None
Kuhl et al. (1983)	12	Guar	7	Improved	—	—	—
Kyllastinen and Lahikainen (1981)	14	Guar	61	Improved	Lower	—	—
Mayne et al. (1982)	12	Apple fiber	49	Improved	Lower	Unchanged	—
Miranda and Horwitz (1978)	8	Cellulose	10	Improved	—	—	Unchanged
Monnier et al. (1981)	17	Wheat bran	10–15	Improved	—	—	—
Nugren et al. (1980)	14	Wheat bran	14–28	Improved	—	—	—
Ray et al. (1983)	12	Guar or wheat bran	61	Improved	Lower	Unchanged	—
C. J. Smith et al. (1982b)	17	Guar	7–21	Improved	Lower	Unchanged	Lower
U. Smith et al. (1982a)	18	Guar	7–14	Improved	—	—	—
Stokholm et al. (1981)	10	Guar	7	Improved	—	—	Lower

ration for several subjects. The crispbread or Melba toast-like preparation is not widely used in our area. Nevertheless, most subjects found it acceptable. Two subjects, however, developed nausea and vomiting after several days on the guar preparation, requiring it to be discontinued (J. W. Anderson, unpublished observations). After examining a number of guar preparations, we find that the Glucotard® formulation (Boehringer Mannheim, Mannheim, West Germany) has the greatest potential for patient acceptance; however, it is not available in the U.S.

3.2 Lipid Effects

Soluble fiber supplements also lower serum cholesterol concentrations. Table I illustrates that hypocholesterolemic effects were reported in 13 or 14 studies (93%). These supplements usually did not lower serum triglyceride concentrations. As discussed elsewhere (Chen and Anderson, this volume, Chapter 18), foods rich in water-soluble fiber, such as oat or bean products, have specific hypocholesterolemic effects but do not lower serum triglyceride values significantly. On the other hand, wheat bran (Heaton and Pomare, 1974; Bosello *et al.*, 1980) or a mixture of different fibers may have hypotriglyceridemic effects (Anderson, 1980; Anderson *et al.*, 1980b).

4. HIGH-FIBER DIETS

4.1 High-Carbohydrate/Fiber Diet Studies

In 1974 we developed high-carbohydrate/fiber (HCF) diets for the management of lean diabetic individuals (Kiehm *et al.*, 1976). Intensive nutrition managment with HCF diets lowers insulin requirements of lean individuals with either type I or type II diabetes (Anderson and Ward, 1978, 1979; Anderson, 1979; Anderson and Chen, 1979; Anderson *et al.*, 1980a,b). HCF diets also lower fasting serum cholesterol and triglyceride concentrations significantly.

4.1.1. Composition of High-Fiber Diets

HCF diets differ from traditional diets used to treat diabetes in several regards; Table II highlights some of these differences. HCF diets are higher in complex carbohydrate and fiber and lower in fat and cholesterol than traditional diets. All diets consist of commonly available foods, and purified fibers such as guar have not been included. HCF diets have been used only for intensive management in the hospital; because they provide only 30–45 g (1–1.5 oz.) of meat daily we did not consider them practical for home use.

High-fiber maintenance (HFM) diets were developed for long-term management at home (Table II).

4.1.2. Responses of Type I Diabetic Individuals

Lean diabetic adults consistently benefit from HCF diets. Table III summarizes the responses of 25 individuals with insulin-dependent (IDDM or type I) diabetes and 25 individuals with non-insulin-dependent (NIDDM or type II) diabetes. In both groups HCF diets significantly lowered insulin requirements, fasting plasma glucose, and cholesterol concentrations.

Insulin requirements for type I diabetic individuals decrease rapidly with HCF diets (Fig. 2). Eight subjects were maintained for 1 week on a metabolic ward with control diets and then were switched to weight-maintaining HCF diets for an average of 3 weeks. Subjects maintained consistent exercise patterns throughout the study and weight changes were minimal. With HCF diets for these individuals, insulin requirements dropped to 40% of initial values and remained at this level for the rest of the hospital stay. Most individuals used similar insulin doses after discharge from the hospital if they followed the HFM diet.

For type I diabetic subjects HCF diets not only lower insulin requirements, but also improve glycemic control and reduce the frequency of insulin reactions. For 25 lean type I individuals, HCF diets lowered insulin requirements by approximately 40% (range of 15–77%). Fasting plasma glucose values averaged 30 mg/dl lower on HCF diets despite lower insulin doses.

TABLE II. Comparison of American Diabetes Association (ADA),
Induction High-Carbohydrate, High-Fiber (HCF), and
High-Fiber Maintenance (HFM) Diets[a]

	ADA		HCF		HFM	
Carbohydrate, total, g/day	215	(43%)	350	(70%)	281	(57%)
Complex	108		255		191	
Simple	107		95		94	
Protein, g/day	100	(20%)	100	(20%)	100	(20%)
Fat, total, g/day	82	(37%)	22	(10%)	51	(23%)
Saturated	28		5		12	
Monounsaturated	42		6		25	
Polyunsaturated	10		8		12	
Cholesterol, mg/day	450		50		180	
Dietary fiber, total, g/day	15		65		50	
Insoluble	11		51		37	
Soluble	4		14		13	

[a]Values are for 2000-kcal diets. Parentheses refer to percent of energy. ADA, American Diabetes Association.

TABLE III. Response of Insulin-Dependent (Type I) and
Non-Insulin-Dependent (Type II) Diabetic Men to High-
Carbohydrate, High-Fiber (HCF) Diets[a]

Measurement	Type I		Type II	
	Control	HCF	Control	HCF
Number of subjects	25	—	25	—
Insulin dose, U/day	32 ± 4	20 ± 4	19 ± 1	1 ± 1
Fasting serum values, mg/dl				
Glucose	186 ± 12	156 ± 12	161 ± 11	135 ± 7
Cholesterol	200 ± 8	139 ± 6	194 ± 15	149 ± 8
Triglycerides	111 ± 12	105 ± 12	116 ± 9	111 ± 11
Body weight, lb	148 ± 7	147 ± 7	152 ± 5	150 ± 4

[a] Subjects ate control diets for 1 week and then HCF diets for about 3 weeks on a metabolic research ward. Values are mean ± SEM.

HCF diets lowered serum cholesterol concentrations by 30%. HCF diets did not induce hypertriglyceridemia in these subjects and average triglyceride values were similar on control and HCF diets.

4.1.3. Responses of Type II Diabetic Individuals

Insulin can usually be discontinued when lean type II individuals are treated intensively with HCF diets. Figure 2 shows the time course for eight subjects. The response time to HCF diets was quite variable. In some instances insulin could be discontinued by 10 days after starting HCF diets, whereas other patients required more than 5 weeks of intensive treatment before insulin could be discontinued.

HCF diet therapy has required us to change the classification of some lean individuals from type I to type II diabetes. One man was admitted to the metabolic ward taking 35 units of insulin daily with a 21-year history of diabetes. With the HCF diet his insulin requirements dropped to 8 units/day in 3 weeks and he discontinued insulin using the HFM diet after 8 weeks at home. For the next 3 years this lean individual had good glycemic control with the HFM diet without insulin or oral hypoglycemic agents.

Glycemic control and serum lipids improve with HCF diets (Table III). These diets allowed us to discontinue insulin therapy for 24 of 25 lean type II men. With insulin doses averaging only 3% of doses with control diets, fasting plasma glucose values were 26 mg/dl lower with HCF diets. Serum cholesterol concentrations were 24% lower on HCF than control diets, but fasting serum triglyceride values were similar.

Long-term responses to HFM diets are summarized in Table IV and elsewhere (Anderson and Ward, 1978; Anderson, 1982; Story et al., 1985).

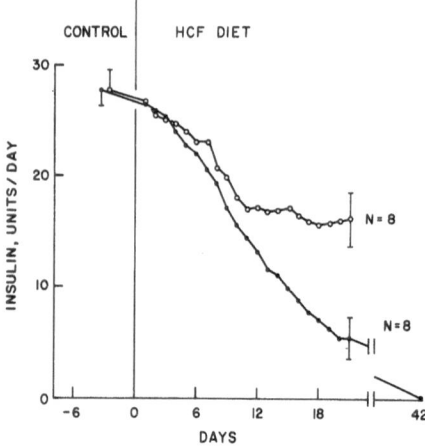

FIGURE 2. Insulin responses of subjects with (O) insulin-dependent (type I) and (●) non-insulin-dependent (type II) diabetes to high-carbohydrate, high-fiber (HCF) diets.

When lean individuals closely adhere to HFM diets they maintain the improvements achieved with the hospital HCF diet. Insulin requirements, glycemic control, and serum lipids are well maintained by HFM diets for up to 10 years of followup.

4.2. High-Fiber Diets

Since 1976 approximately 30 full-length studies of high-fiber diets for diabetic subjects have been reported in peer-reviewed, English language journals. Table IV summarizes the responses of 415 diabetic subjects given high-fiber diets for a minimum of 10 days; two studies of shorter duration (Burke *et al.*, 1982; Hoffman *et al.*, 1982) are not included. Most of these investigators have used high-fiber, high-carbohydrate diets, but four groups examined the influence of high-fiber standard carbohydrate diets, These studies included insulin-dependent diabetic subjects (four studies), non-insulin-dependent diabetic subjects (eight studies), and both types of individuals (12 studies). The reported glycemic and lipid responses will be reviewed.

4.2.1. Glycemic Responses

Average glycemic control, estimated by average blood glucose values, glycosuria, or insulin requirements, improved in 21 of 23 studies (91%). The acceptability of high-fiber diets is reflected by the 42-day median and 194-day average duration of these studies. The two groups reporting that fiber intake had no appreciable effect included a study of poorly controlled children treated for 14 days (Lindsay *et al.*, 1984) and the study using moderate-fiber, low-carbohydrate diets (Manhire *et al.*, 1981). Thus, 15 different groups have tested high-fiber diets for diabetic subjects and 13

TABLE IV. Response of Diabetic Subjects to High-Fiber Diets

Reference	Number of subjects	Type of diet[a]	Duration of study, days	Response of Blood			Weight change
				Glucose	Cholesterol	Triglyceride	
Anderson and Ward (1978)	10	HFHC	183–1095	Improved	Lower	Lower	None
Anderson et al. (1979a)	20	HFHC	16	Improved	Lower	Lower	Unchanged
Anderson et al. (1980a)	21	HFHC	12–42	Improved	Lower	Lower	Lower
Anderson et al. (1980b)	11	HFHC	18–26	Improved	Lower	Lower	Unchanged
Barnard et al. (1982)	60	HFHC	26	Improved	Lower	Lower	Lower
Barnard et al. (1983)	69	HFHC	730–1095	Improved	Lower	Lower	Lower
Hjollund et al. (1983)	9	HFHC	21	Improved	Lower	Unchanged	Unchanged
Karlstrom et al. (1984)	14	HF	21	Improved	Unchanged	Unchanged	Unchanged
Kay et al. (1981)	5	HF	14	Improved	–	–	Unchanged
Kiehm et al. (1976)	13	HFHC	14–28	Improved	Lower	Lower	Lower
Kinmonth et al. (1982)	10	HF	42	Improved	–	–	–
Lindsay et al. (1984)	12	HFHC	14	Unchanged	–	–	Unchanged
Manhire et al. (1981)	16	MFLC	42	Unchanged	Unchanged	–	–
Ney et al. (1982)	20	HFHC	28–210	Improved	–	–	Increased
Pedersen et al. (1982)	40	HFHC	28	Improved	Lower	Unchanged	–
Riccardi et al. (1984)	14	HFHC	10	Improved	Lower	Lower	Increased
Rivellese et al. (1980)	8	HFHC	10	Improved	Lower	Lower	–
Rosman et al. (1983)	10	HF	91	Improved	–	Lower	–
H. C. Simpson et al.(1981)	27	HFHC	42	Improved	Lower	–	Unchanged
H. C. Simpson et al. (1982)	10	HFHC	42	Improved	Unchanged	Unchanged	Unchanged
R. W. Simpson et al. (1979a)	14	HFHC	42	Improved	Lower	Unchanged	–
R. W. Simpson et al. (1979b)	11	HFHC	42	Improved	Lower	–	–
Taskinen et al. (1983)	21	HFHC	42	Improved	Lower	Unchanged	–

[a] HFHC, high-fiber, high-carbohydrate; HF, high-fiber; MFLC, moderate-fiber, low-carbohydrate.

report benefits. High-fiber diets offer benefits for insulin-dependent as well as non-insulin-dependent diabetic individuals.

4.2.2. Lipid Responses

High-fiber, high-carbohydrate diets lower serum cholesterol and triglyceride concentrations (Anderson *et al.*, 1980a). Table IV summarizes the responses reported in 18 studies. High-fiber diets lowered serum cholesterol concentrations in 15 of 18 studies (83%). Serum cholesterol reductions of 10–20% were common. Similarly, these diets lowered fasting serum triglycerides in 10 of 16 studies (63%). The long-term triglyceride responses that we observe are representative of the type of response that can be expected. Thus, high-fiber diets lower both serum cholesterol and triglyceride concentrations significantly.

4.2.3. Other Effects

High-carbohydrate, high-fiber diets offer other benefits for diabetic individuals. In addition to improving glycemic control and lowering serum lipids, these diets also assist in weight control and lower blood pressure. The utility of high-fiber, low-energy-dense foods as part of a weight-reduction and maintenance program is reviewed elsewhere (Anderson, 1981; Duncan *et al.*, 1983). These diets lower blood pressure of our patients by 10% during their hospital stay (Anderson, 1983). Others also document the beneficial effects of fiber intake on blood pressure (Dobson *et al.*, 1983; Barnard *et al.*, 1983; Rouse *et al.*, 1983).

5. MECHANISMS

5.1. Insulin Secretion

High-carbohydrate diets improve glucose metabolism without increasing insulin secretion (Anderson, 1982). In non-diabetic as well as non-insulin-dependent diabetic subjects these diets lower fasting serum insulin concentrations and peripheral serum insulin responses to oral glucose administration.

Recently we (Fukagawa *et al.*, 1984) assessed the effects of HCF diets (Table II) on insulin sensitivity of six healthy young college students. After 3 weeks with these diets fasting serum insulin concentrations were significantly lower than with their usual diets. These lower insulin concentrations were associated with twofold increases in estimated sensitivity to insulin.

Urinary C-peptide excretion was used to evaluate endogenous insulin secretion in non-insulin-dependent diabetic subjects treated with HCF diets. As noted above, these diets usually allowed us to discontinue use of insulin therapy for these patients. The C-peptide excretion was similar with control diets and insulin therapy to values with HCF diets and no insulin therapy (Whitley and Anderson, unpublished observations). Thus, our data suggest that reductions in insulin requirements with HCF diets are related to improved peripheral sensitivity to insulin and that these diets do not stimulate the secretion of increased amounts of endogenous insulin.

5.2. Insulin Receptors

Insulin binding to tissue receptors plays a vital role in insulin action. The number of insulin receptors and their affinity for insulin may influence the changes in insulin sensitivity associated with high-fiber diets. By 1976 we noted that HCF diets increased insulin receptor number for circulating monocytes (Anderson, 1979).

Increased insulin binding to circulating monocytes has subsequently been noted by several investigators (Pedersen et al., 1982; Ward et al., 1982) with high-fiber diets. These observations confirm studies in animals that high-carbohydrate diets increase the number of insulin receptors for various tissues (Sun et al., 1977). Increased binding of insulin to receptors of peripheral tissues may contribute to the enhanced insulin sensitivity associated with high-fiber diets.

5.3. Insulin Sensitivity

Until recently sensitivity to insulin was difficult to assess. The euglycemic insulin clamp technique (DeFronzo et al., 1979) provides an estimate of insulin sensitivity and has been widely used (Rowe et al., 1983; Fink et al., 1982; Rizza et al., 1982). We have used this technique to estimate the impact of HCF diets on healthy subjects and insulin-dependent diabetic subjects.

To further evaluate HCF diets for healthy individuals, we recruited six male college students. On their usual diet we performed a baseline euglycemic insulin clamp study. They then ate weight-maintaining HCF diets (Table II) for 3 weeks and the second clamp study was performed. They resumed their usual diet for 4–8 weeks and the last clamp study was completed. During each clamp study plasma glucose concentrations were maintained at approximately 100 mg/dl throughout the study. Insulin was infused at a rate of $10\mu U/M^2$ per min for 3 h.

HCF diets produced a twofold increase in glucose use during the euglycemic insulin clamp study (Fig. 3). With their usual diets, glucose use during the 3-h clamp study averaged 1.8 mg/kg per min; with the HCF diet,

GLUCOSE USE (mg/kg/min)

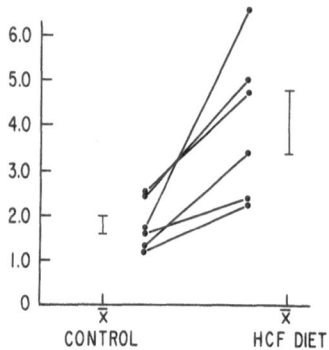

FIGURE 3. Glucose utilization by healthy young men on control or high-carbohydrate, high-fiber (HCF) diets as measured by the euglycemic insulin clamp technique.

glucose use averaged 3.7 mg/kg per min ($p < 0.001$ vs. control). Thus, HCF diets were accompanied by a twofold increase in apparent insulin sensitivity for these healthy subjects.

Similar studies were performed for a 58-year-old, insulin-dependent diabetic subject. On a metabolic ward he was fed an HCF diet for 4 weeks. After a clamp study he was discharged and used his customary diet for 5 weeks. He then was readmitted to the metabolic ward and fed a high-protein, low-carbohydrate diet (Anderson, 1983) for 4 weeks. Euglycemic insulin clamp studies were performed at the completion of each diet. With the high-protein diet, glucose use averaged 1.0 mg/kg per min (Fig. 4) while glucose use was 1.8 mg/kg per min with the HCF diet ($p < 0.001$ vs. high-protein diet). Thus, for this insulin-dependent subject, an HCF diet was accompanied by an 80% increase in apparent insulin sensitivity.

Intracellular changes responsible for these changes in insulin sensitivity are discussed elsewhere (Hjollund et al., 1983). Increasing carbohydrate

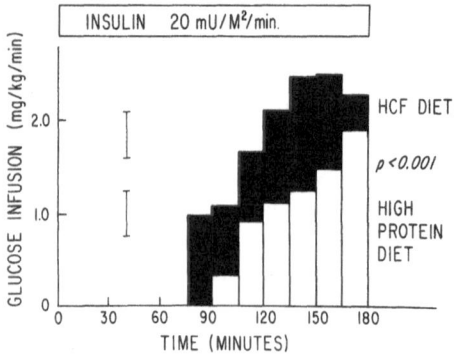

FIGURE 4. Glucose utilization of an insulin-dependent (type I) diabetic man to high-carbohydrate, high-fiber (HCF) and high-protein, low-carbohydrate diets as measured by the euglycemic insulin clamp technique.

intake enhances intracellular capacities to use glucose. Glycolytic rates are increased, as are activities of key glycolytic enzymes; hepatic gluconeogenesis is suppressed, as are activities of key gluconeogenic enzymes; glycogen synthetic rates are increased, as are glycogen concentrations of several tissues. All of these processes facilitate glucose use and act to lower the plasma glucose concentration.

Fiber intake may enhance tissue sensitivity to insulin, in part through its short-chain fatty acid metabolic products. Our studies (Anderson and Bridges, 1984) indicate that propionate stimulates rates of glycolysis in isolated rat hepatocytes and inhibits rates of gluconeogenesis. We suggest that some of the favorable effects of fiber intake on glucose metabolism may be mediated by these metabolic products.

6. CONCLUSIONS

High-fiber diets produce distinct benefits for persons with diabetes. Increased intake of dietary fiber improves glycemic control and lowers insulin requirements. Diets generous in both complex carbohydrate and fiber and restricted in fat are expecially advantageous. For adults with insulin-dependent (type I) diabetes HCF (high-carbohydrate, high-fiber) diets lower insulin requirements by an average of 40%; for lean adults with non-insulin-dependent (type II) diabetes HCF diets lower insulin needs by 80–100% and allow insulin to be discontinued in approximately 90% of individuals.

Generous intakes of dietary fiber also lower serum cholesterol, triglycerides, and blood pressure. HCF diets, for example, lower serum cholesterol an average of 30% and triglycerides 15%. Soluble fibers from oat products or beans selectively lower atherogenic low-density lipoprotein cholesterol and raise protective high-density lipoprotein cholesterol. Generous intakes of fiber can lower blood pressure by 10%.

Mechanisms responsible for the beneficial effects of fiber are not fully defined. Fiber intake slows the digestion and absorption of carbohydrates and reduces their glycemic effects. Fiber also enhances peripheral sensitivity to insulin; insulin binding to circulating monocytes is greater with high-fiber diets than with low-fiber intakes.

Peripheral sensitivity to insulin increases with HCF diets. When healthy college students used them for 3 weeks, glucose use during an euglycemic clamp study doubled. An insulin-dependent diabetic adult man also used twice as much glucose during the insulin clamp study on the HCF diet than on a high-fat, low-carbohydrate diet.

A prudent diet, with 55–60% of energy from carbohydrate, 15–20% from protein, and less than 30% from fat, and less than 300 mg/day of cholesterol and generous in dietary fiber, provides distinct health advantages. Most persons with diabetes would benefit from a nutrition plan restricted in fat and cholesterol and plenteous with complex carbohydrate and fiber.

REFERENCES

Anderson, J. W., 1979, High carbohydrate, high fiber diets for patients with diabetes, in: *Treatment of Early Diabetes* (R. A. Camerini-Davalos and B. Hanover, eds.), Plenum, New York, pp. 263–273.

Anderson, J. W., 1980, High fiber diets in diabetes and hypertriglyceridemia, *Can. Med. Assoc. J.* **123**:975–979.

Anderson, J. W., 1981, Plant fiber treatment for metabolic diseases, *Spec. Top. Endocrinol. Metab.* **2**:1–42.

Anderson, J. W., 1982, High carbohydrate diet effects on glucose and triglyceride metabolism of normal and diabetic men, in: *Metabolic Effects of Utilizable Dietary Carbohydrate* (S. Reiser, ed.), Marcel Dekker, New York, pp. 285–313.

Anderson, J. W., 1983, Plant fiber and blood pressure, *Ann. Intern. Med.* **98**:842–846.

Anderson, J. W., and Bridges, S. R., 1984, Short-chain fatty acids affect glucose metabolism in isolated rat hepatocytes, *Proc. Soc. Exp. Biol. Med.*, **177**:372–376.

Anderson, J. W., and Ward, K., 1978, Long term effects of high carbohydrate, high fiber diets on glucose and lipid metabolism: A preliminary report on patients with diabetes, *Diabetes Care* **1**:77–82.

Anderson, J. W., and Chen, W. L., 1979, Plant fiber: Carbohydrate and lipid metabolism, *Am. J. Clin. Nutr.* **32**:346–363.

Anderson, J. W., Chen, W. J. L., and Sieling, B., 1980b, Hypolipidemic effects of high carbohydrate, high fiber diets, *Metabolism* **29**:551–558.

Anderson, J. W., Ferguson, S. K., Karounos, D., O'Malley, L., Sieling, B., and Chen, W. L., 1980a, Mineral and vitamin status on high fiber diets: Long term studies of diabetic patients, *Diabetes Care* **3**:38–40.

Anderson, J. W., Story, L., Sieling, B., Chen, W. L., Petro, M. S., and Story, J., 1984, Hypocholesterolemic effects of oat-bran or bean intake for hypercholesterolemic men, *Am. J. Clin. Nutr.* **40**:1146–1155.

Anderson, J. W., and Ward, K., 1978, Long term effects of high carbohydrate, high fiber diets on glucose and lipid metabolism: A preliminary report on patients with diabetes, *Diabetes Care* **1**:77–82.

Anderson, J. W., and Ward, K., 1979, High carbohydrate, high fiber diets for isulin-treated men with diabetes mellitus, *Am. J. Clin. Nutr.* **32**:2312–2321.

Aro, A., Uusitupa, M., Voitilanen, E., Hersio, K., Korhonen, T., and Siitonen, O., 1981, Improved diabetic control and hypocholesterolemic effect induced by long term dietary supplementation with guar gum in type II (noninsulin-dependent) diabetes, *Diabetologia* **21**:29–33.

Barnard, R. J., Lattimore, L., Holley, R. G., Cherny, S., and Pritikin, N., 1982, Response of noninsulin dependent diabetic patients to an intensive program of diet and exercising, *Diabetes Care* **5**:370–374.

Barnard, R. J., Massey, M. R., Cherny, S., O'Brien, L. T., and Pritikin, N., 1983, Long term use of a high complex carbohydrate, high fiber, low fat diet and exercise in the treatment of NIDDM patients, *Diabetes Care* **6**:268–273.

Bingham, S., Williams, D. R. R., Cole, T. J., and James, W. P. T., 1979, Dietary fiber and regional large bowel cancer mortality in Britain, *Br. J. Cancer* **40**:456–463.

Bosello, O., Ostuzzi, R., Armellini, F., Miccolo, R., and Scuro, L. A., 1980, Glucose tolerance and blood lipids in bran fed patients with impaired glucose tolerance, *Diabetes Care* 3:46–49.

Botha, A. P. J., Steyn, A. F., Esteruysen, A. J., and Slabbert, M., 1981, Glycosylated hemoglobin, blood glucose and serum cholesterol levels in diabetics treated with guar gum, *S. Afr. Med. J.* 59:333–334.

Burke, B. J., Hartog, M., Heaton, K. W., and Hooper, S., 1982, Assessment of the metabolic effects of dietary carbohydrate and fibre by measuring urinary excretion of C-peptide, *Hum. Nutr. Clin. Nutr.* 36C:373–380.

Carroll, D. G., Dykes, V., and Hodgson, W., 1981, Guar gum is not a panacea in diabetes management, *N. Z. Med. J.* 93:292.

Christiansen, J. S., Bonnevie-Neilsen, V., Svendsen, P. A., Ronn, B., and Nerup, J., 1980, Effect of guar gum on 24-hour insulin requirements of insulin-dependent diabetic subjects as assessed by artificial pancreas, *Diabetes Care* 3:659–662.

Cohen, M., Leong, V. W., Salmon, E., and Martin, F. I. R., 1980, Role of guar and dietary fibre in the management of diabetes mellitus, *Med. J. Aust.* 1:59–61.

DeFronzo, R. A., Tobin, J. D., and Andres, R., 1979, Glucose clamp technique: A method of quantifying insulin secretion and resistance, *Am. J. Physiol.* 237:E214–223.

Dobson, P. M., Stocks, J., Holdsworth, G., and Galton, D. J., 1981, High fibre and low fat diets in diabetes mellitus, *Br. J. Nutr.* 46:289–294.

Dobson, P. M., Pacy, P. J., Beevers, M., Bal, P., Fletcher, R. F., and Taylor, K. G., 1983, The effects of a high fibre, low fat and low sodium dietary regime in diabetic hypertensive patients of different ethnic groups, *Postgrad. Med. J.* 59:641–644.

Doi, K., Matsuura, Kawara, A., and Baba, S., 1979, Treatment of diabetes with glucomannan (Konjac Mannan), *Lancet* 1:987–988.

Duncan, K. H., Bacon, J. A., and Weinsier, R. L., 1983, The effects of high and low energy density diets on satiety, energy intake and eating time of obese and non-obese subjects, *Am. J. Clin. Nutr.* 37:763–767.

Fagerberg, S. E., 1982, The effects of bulk laxative (Metamucil) on fasting blood glucose, serum lipids, and other variables in constipated patients with noninsulin dependent adult diabetes, *Curr. Therapeut. Res.* 31:166–172.

Fink, R. I., Kolterman, O. G., Griffin, J., and Olefsky, J. M., 1983, Mechanisms of insulin resistance in aging, *J. Clin. Invest.* 71:1523–1535.

Fukagawa, N. K., Minaker, K. L., Hageman, G., Young, V. R., and Anderson, J. W., 1984, High carbohydrate, high fiber diets increase peripheral insulin sensitivity of healthy young men, *Clin. Res.* 32:796A.

Heaton, K. L., and Pomare, E. W., 1974, Effect of bran on blood lipids and calcium, *Lancet* 1:49–51.

Hjollund, E., Pedersen, O., Richelsen, B., Beck-Nielsen, H., and Sorensen, N., 1983, Increased insulin binding to adipocytes and monocytes and increased insulin sensitivity of glucose transport and metabolism in adipocytes from noninsulin dependent diabetics after a low fat/high starch/high fiber diet, *Metabolism* 32:1067–1075.

Hoffman, C. R., Fineberg, S. E., Howey, D. C., Clark, C. M., and Pronsky, Z., 1982, Short term effects of a high fiber, high carbohydrate diet in very obese diabetic individuals, *Diabetes Care* 5:506.

Jenkins, D. J. A., Goff, D. V., Leeds, A. R., Alberti, K. G. M. M., Wolever, T. M. S., Gassull, M. A., and Hockaday, T. D. R., 1976, Unabsorbable carbohydrates and diabetes: Decreased postprandial hyperglycemia, *Lancet* 2:172 174.

Jenkins, D. J. A., Wolever, T. M. S., Hockaday, T. D. R., Leeds A. R., Howarth, R., Bacon, S., Apling, E. C., and Dilawari, J., 1977, Treatment of diabetes with guar gum. Reduction of urine glucose loss in diabetics, *Lancet* 2:779–780.

Jenkins, D. J. A., Wolever, T. M. S., Nineham, R., Metz, G. L., Bacon, S., and Hockaday, T. D. R., 1978, Guar crispbread in the diabetic diet, *Br. Med. J.* **2:**1744–1746.

Jenkins, D. J. A., Wolever, T. M. S., Nineham, R., Bacon, S., Smith, R., and Hockaday, T. D. R., 1979a, Dietary fiber and diabetic therapy: A progressive effect with time, *Adv. Exp. Med. Biol.* **119:**275–279.

Jenkins, D. J. A., Hockaday, T. D. R., Wolever, T. M. S., Nineham, R., Goff, D. V., Haisman, P., Charnock, R., Taylor, R. H., and Bacon, S., 1979b, Dietary fibre and ketone bodies: Reduced urinary 3-hydroxy-butyrate excretion in diabetes on guar, *Br. Med. J.* **2:**1555.

Jenkins, D. J. A., Wolever, T. M. S., Bacon, S., Nineham, R., Lees, R., Rowden, R., Love, M., and Hockaday, T. D. R., 1980, Diabetic diets: High carbohydrate combined with high fiber, *Am. J. Clin. Nutr.* **33:**1729–1733.

Jenkins, D. J. A., Taylor, R. H., and Wolever, T. M. S., 1982, The diabetic diet, dietary carbohydrate and differences in digestibility, *Diabetologia* **23:**477–484.

Johansen, K., 1981, Decreased urinary glucose excretion and plasma cholesterol levels in non-insulin dependent diabetic patients with guar, *Diabete Metab.* **7:**87–90.

Karlstrom, B., Vessby, B., Asp, N.-G., Boberg, M., Gustafsson, I.-B., Lithell, H., and Werner, I., 1984, Effects of an increased content of cereal fibre in the diet of type II (non-insulin dependent) diabetic patients, *Diabetologia* **26:**272–277.

Kay, R. M., Grobin, W., and Track, N. S., 1981, Diets rich in natural fibre improve carbohydrate tolerance in maturity onset, non-insulin dependent diabetics, *Diabetologia* **20:**18–21.

Kiehm. T. G., Anderson, J. W., and Ward, K., 1976, Beneficial effects of a high carbohydrate, high fiber diet on hyperglycemic diabetic men, *Am. J. Clin. Nutr.* **29:**895–899.

Kinmonth, A. L., Angus, R. H., Jenkins, P. A., Smith, M. A., and Baum, J. D., 1982, Whole foods and increased dietary fibre improve blood glucose control in diabetic children, *Arch. Dis. Child.* **57:**187–194.

Koepp, P., and Hegewisch, S., 1981, Effect of guar on plasma viscosity and related parameters in diabetic children, *Eur. J. Pediatr.* **137:**31–33.

Kromhout, O., Bosschieter, E. B., and deLezenne Coulander, C., 1982, Dietary fiber and 10-year mortality from coronary heart disease, cancer and all causes, *Lancet* **2:**518–522.

Kuhl, C., Molsted-Pederson, L., and Hornnes, P. J., 1983, Guar gum and glycemic control of pregnant insulin-dependent diabetic patients, *Diabetes Care* **6:**152–154.

Kyllastinen, M., and Lahilainen, T., 1981, Long term dietary supplementation with a fiber product (guar gum) in elderly diabetics, *Curr. Ther. Res.* **30:**872.

Lindsay, A. N., Hardy, S., Jarrett, L., and Rallison, M. L., 1984, High carbohydrate, high fiber diet in children with type I diabetes, *Diabetes Care* **7:**63–67.

Liu, K., Stamler, J., Trevisan, M., and Moss, D., 1982, Dietary lipids, sugar, fiber, and mortality from coronary heart disease, *Atherosclerosis* **2:**221–227.

Manhire, A., Henry, C. L., Hartog, M., and Heaton, K. W., 1981, Unrefined carbohydrate and dietary fibre in the treatment of diabetes mellitus, *J. Hum. Nutr.* **35:**99–101.

Mayne, P. D., McGill, A. R., Gormley, T. R., Tomkin, G. H., Julian, T. R., and O'Moore, R. R., 1982, The effect of apple fibre on diabetic control and plasma lipids, *Ir. J. Med. Sci.* **151:**36–41.

Miranda, P. M., and Horwitz, D. L., 1978, High fiber diets in the treatment of diabetes mellitus, *Ann. Intern. Med.* **88:**482–486.

Monnier, L., Pham, T. C., Aquirre, L., Orsetti, A., and Mirouze, J., 1978, Influence of indigestible fibers on glucose tolerance, *Diabetes Care* **1:**83–88.

Monnier, L. H., Blotman, M. J., Colette, C., Monnier, M. P., and Mirouze, J., 1981, Effect of dietary fibre supplements in stable and labile insulin dependent diabetics, *Diabetologia* **20:**12–17.

Morgan, L. M., Goulder, T. J., Tsiolakis, D., Marks, V., and Alberti, K. G. M. M., 1979, The effect of unabsorbable carbohydrate on gut hormones, *Diabetologia* **17:**85–89.

Morris, J. N., Marr, J. W., and Clayton, D. G., 1977, Diet and heart; A postscript, *Br. Med. J.* 2:1307–1314.

Ney, D., Hollingsworth, D. R., and Cousins, L., 1982, Decreased insulin requirement and improved control of diabetes in pregnant women given a high carbohydrate, high fiber, low fat diet, *Diabetes Care* 5:529.

Nugren, C., Berglund, O., Hallmans, G., Lithner, F., and Taljehahl, I. B., 1980, The effect of a high-bran diet on diabetes in mice and humans, *Acta Endocrinol.* 94 (S237):66.

Pedersen, O., Hjollund, E., Lindkov, H. O., Helms, P., Sorensen, N. S., and Ditzel, J., 1982, Increased insulin receptor binding to monocytes from insulin dependent diabetic patients after a low fat, high starch, high fiber diet, *Diabetes Care* 5:284–291.

Ray, T. K., Mansell, K. M., Knight, L. C., Malmud, L. S., and Owen, O. E., 1983, Long term effects of dietary fiber on glucose tolerance and gastric emptying in noninsulin dependent diabetic patients, *Am. J. Clin. Nutr.* 37:376–381.

Riccardi, G., Rivellese, A., Pacioni, D., Genevese, S., Mastranzo, P., and Mancini, M., 1984, Separate influence of dietary carbohydrate and fibre on the metabolic control of diabetes, *Diabetologia* 26:116–121.

Rivellese, A., Riccardi, G., Giacco, A., Pacioni, D., Genovese, S., Mattiole, P. L., and Mancini, M., 1980, Effect of dietary fibre on glucose control and serum lipoproteins in diabetic patients, *Lancet* 2:447–449.

Rizza, R. A., Mandarino, L. J., and Gerich, J. E., 1982, Cortisol induced insulin resistance in man, *J. Clin. Endocrinol. Metab.* 54:131–138.

Rosman, M. S., Smith, C. J., and Jackson, W. P. U., 1983, The effect of long term high fiber diets in diabetic outpatients, *S. Afr. Med. J.* 63:310–313.

Rouse, I. L., Beilin, L. J., Armstrong, B. K., and Vandongen, R., 1983, Blood pressure lowering effect of a vegetarian diet, *Lancet* 1:5–9.

Rowe, J. W., Minaker, K. L., Pallotta, J. A., and Flier, J. S., 1983, Characterization of the insulin resistance of aging, *J. Clin. Invest.* 71:1581–1587.

Simpson, H. C. R., Simpson, R. W., Lousley, S., Carter, R. D., Geekie, M., Hockaday, T. D. R., and Mann, J. I., 1981, A high carbohydrate leguminous fibre diet improves all aspects of diabetic control, *Lancet* 1:1–5.

Simpson, H. C., Mann, J. I., Chakrabarti, R., Imeson, J. D., Stirling, Y., Tozer, M., Woolf, L., and Meade, T. W., 1982, Effect of high fibre diet on haemostatic variables in diabetes, *Br. Med. J.* 284:1608.

Simpson, R. W., Mann, J. I., Eaton, J., Moore, R. A., Carter, R. D., and Hockaday, T. D. R., 1979a, Improved glucose control in maturity onset diabetes treated with high carbohydrate, modified fat diet, *Br. Med. J.* 1:1753–1756.

Simpson, R. W., Mann, J. I., Eaton, J., Carter, R. D., and Hockaday, T. D. R., 1979, High carbohydrate diets and insulin dependent diabetes, *Br. Med. J.* 2 :523 –525.

Smith, C. J., Rosman, M. S., Levitt, N. S., and Jackson, W. P. U., 1982, Guar biscuits in the diabetic diet, *S. Afr. Med. J.* 61 :196 –198.

Smith, U., and Holm, G., 1982, Effect of a modified guar gum preparation on glucose and lipid levels in diabetics and healthy volunteers, *Atherosclerosis* 45:1–10.

Stokholm, K. H., Laurtsen, H. B., and Larsen, S., 1981, Reduced glysuria during guar gum supplementation in noninsulin dependent diabetes, *Dan. Med. Bull.* 28:41–42.

Story, L., Anderson, J. W., Chen, W. J. L., Karounos, D., and Jefferson, B., 1985, Adherence to high carbohydrate, high fiber diets: Long term studies of nonobese diabetic men, *J. Am. Diet. Assoc.*, (in press).

Sun, J. V , Tepperman, H. M., and Tepperman, J., 1977, A comparison of insulin binding by liver plasma membranes of rats fed a high glucose diet or a high fat diet, *J. Lipid Res.* 18:533–539.

Taskinen, M., Nikkila, E. A., and Allus, A., 1983, Serum lipids and lipoproteins in insulin dependent diabetic subjects during high carbohydrate, high fiber diet, *Diabetes Care* 6:224–230.

Trowell, H. C., 1975, Dietary fiber hypothesis of the etiology of diabetes mellitus, *Diabetes* 24:762–765.

Ward, G. M., Simpson, R. W., Simpson, H. C. R., Naylor, B. A., Mann, J. I., Turner, R. C., 1982, Insulin receptor binding increased by high carbohydrate low fat diet in noninsulin dependent diabetics, *Eur. J. Clin. Invest.* 12:93–96.

24

Update on Fiber and Mineral Availability

JUNE L. KELSAY

1. INTRODUCTION

Due to the binding capabilities of fiber, there has been much concern about the effect of high-fiber diets on nutrient availability, particularly of minerals. Studies on effects of fiber on mineral and vitamin bioavailability were reviewed previously (Kelsay, 1981, 1982). Although there were some reports that high-fiber diets adversely affected mineral balances, the subject remains controversial. This chapter will deal with recent studies on fiber and mineral availability, with particular emphasis on other factors that may complicate the interpretation of results.

2. *IN VITRO* STUDIES ON MINERAL BINDING

Several *in vitro* studies have been conducted on factors affecting mineral binding by fiber. Iron binding has been most frequently investigated. Studies have involved fiber from wheat, maize, and pinto beans, and purified fibers such as hemicellulose, lignin, cellulose, and pectin. The solubilities of minerals in cereals of different phytate content were also determined.

Reinhold *et al.* (1981) found that the amount of iron bound by neutral detergent fiber (NDF) (cellulose, hemicellulose, and lignin) from wheat or maize depended upon iron concentration, pH, quantity of fiber, the presence of inhibitors, and quantities of inhibitors. Iron binding by fiber was strongly

JUNE L. KELSAY • Carbohydrate Nutrition Laboratory, U. S. Department of Agriculture Agricultural Research Service, Beltsville, Maryland 20705.

inhibited by citrate, EDTA, ascorbate, and phytate. Cysteine and hydrazine sulfate were also inhibitory. However, in a later study using rat intestinal segments, Reinhold *et al.* (1982) reported that ascorbate, citrate, cysteine, or phytate did not inhibit binding of iron by fiber.

Kojima *et al.* (1981) examined the solubilization of iron from cooked pinto beans. They also found that citrate, EDTA, ascorbate, cysteine, and a number of other agents inhibited iron binding *in vitro*. The effects of ascorbate and citrate were additive, but effect of ascorbate with other agents was not. Tea decreased iron solubility, and whole spinach suspension and the insoluble spinach residue removed iron from solution that was previously solubilized from beans. Both tea and spinach contain oxalic acid, which might account for some of the binding; however, oxalate alone had little effect. Tea also contains tannic acid, which can bind divalent cations.

Fernandez and Phillips (1982) studied interactions among individual fiber components, inorganic iron, and substances known to chelate iron. Lignin and hemicellulose (from psyllium mucilage) bound iron in ranges that might be found in physiological circumstances; cellulose and pectin were less effective. Binding increased as pH was increased to 6.8. Citrate and EDTA had inhibitory effects on the binding of iron to lignin and cellulose; fructose, cysteine, and ascorbate did not.

Leigh and Miller (1983) measured iron binding by isolated wheat bran fiber in the presence of iron ligands. Iron binding was inhibited by EDTA, lactobionate, citrate, nitrilotriacetic acid, and ascorbate. When iron was added to a meal of beef, bread, green beans, and milk, availability was not affected by fiber, citrate, and ascorbate, but was enhanced by nitrilotriacetic acid and EDTA. When iron was added to a semisynthetic meal, fiber, ascorbate, citrate, nitrilotriacetic acid, and EDTA increased iron availability.

A further complicating factor in cereals is phytate. Lyon (1984) studied the solubility of calcium, magnesium, zinc, and copper in cereal products containing different levels of phytate. The minerals were released from cereals by extraction with HCl. The addition of sodium bicarbonate to pH 7.0 resulted in various degrees of precipitation of the different minerals. Precipitation was greatest for zinc in high-phytate cereals and least for calcium in low-phytate cereals. Extracted copper was not precipitated. The addition of EDTA and citrate prevented precipitation.

These *in vitro* studies show that although fiber may bind minerals, a number of agents in foods and in the digestive tract may affect the amount of binding. It is different to compare results of the above studies, due to differences in experimental conditions. However, in general, *in vitro* iron binding was inhibited by citrate, EDTA, and ascorbate. Effects of different substances on binding become increasingly unpredictable as more variables are introduced. Tea and spinach contain substances that increased iron binding by insoluble bean residue. Phytate inhibited binding of iron in one study, but appeared to increase binding of calcium, magnesium, and zinc in another. Different fibers vary in their capacity to bind minerals. It is difficult to separate the capabilities of the different fibers, because the fibers occur together in most foods. In one study of purified fibers, cellulose and pectin did not bind as much iron as did lignin and hemicellulose.

3. MINERAL AVAILABILITY FROM TEST MEALS

It has been reported that absorption of iron as measured by serum iron or by whole body counter was less in human subjects given whole meal (whole wheat) flour in place of white flour (Vellar *et al.*, 1968; Elwood *et al.*, 1970; Dobbs and Baird, 1977) and when bran was added to rolls (Bjorn-Rasmussen, 1974).

Sandstrom *et al.* (1980), using ^{65}Zn and whole body counting, measured zinc absorption in humans fed meals based on bread. A lower amount of zinc was absorbed from white bread than from an equal amount of whole meal bread; however, the zinc content of the white bread was lower. When $ZnCl_2$ was added to the breads so that they contained equal amounts of zinc, the amount of absorption was higher from the white than from the whole meal bread. The addition of milk, eggs, beef, or cheese to whole meal bread resulted in improved zinc absorption. A significant positive correlation was found between zinc absorption and the protein content of the meals.

In a subsequent study of zinc absorption as affected by protein source, Sandstrom and Cederblad (1980) substituted defatted soy flour for 25% of the protein in chicken in meals given to human subjects. Neither the zinc content of the meal nor the amount of zinc absorption was influenced. Soy flour in a beef meal resulted in a decrease in zinc content and also a lower zinc absorption than from beef alone. The absorption of zinc from a soybean meal was not different from that when an animal protein meal with the same zinc content was fed. Zinc absorption was lower when the calcium content of a soybean meal was increased by the addition of milk.

When evaluating results of studies in which test meals were fed, it is necessary to consider carefully the relative amounts of fiber, phytate, protein, and other nutrients, as well as levels of the mineral being investigated. Both the whole meal bread and soybeans fed in the above studies contain fiber and phytate.

Test meals will give information on the effects of other nutrients or other agents on the availability of a mineral from that particular meal, but they do not give the total picture of bodily retention for a day or a longer period of time. The total daily intake of the nutrient being studied and that of other interacting agents are of the utmost importance.

4. FIBER INTAKES

One of the problems in evaluating studies on the effects of fiber is that it is difficult to compare levels of fiber intake among studies. The crude fiber (CF) values give only an indication of relative fiber levels, since much of the fiber is destroyed in the analysis. The Southgate method for total dietary fiber (DF), which includes soluble fibers, gives higher values for fiber than does the NDF method, except for cereals. Because of this discrepancy in values obtained by the different methods, it is difficult to make recommendations about levels of fiber intake.

Hardinge *et al.* (1958) reported crude fiber intakes of vegetarians and nonvegetarians (Table I). These values are higher than those reported in later studies, but they do indicate that the fiber intake of vegetarians is higher than that for nonvegetarians. Reported crude fiber intakes in the later studies (Table I) range from 2.8 to 4.8 g/day for nonvegetarians and from 6.2 to 8.9 g/day for vegetarians. Dietary fiber intakes range from 13.4 to 20.2 g/day for nonvegetarians and from 30.9 to 33.2 g/day for vegetarians. Marlett and Bokram (1981) found higher crude fiber and dietary fiber intakes for males than for females.

In a study conducted in our laboratory, 29 subjects collected food in amounts equivalent to that eaten during 1 week for each of the four seasons. We calculated crude fiber intakes and determined NDF intakes for these 4

TABLE I. Calculated Crude Fiber and Dietary Fiber Intakes

Reference	Subjects	Crude fiber g/day	Dietary fiber g/day
Hardinge *et al.* (1958)	Fifteen male nonvegetarians	10.7	—
	Fifteen male lacto-ovovegetarians	16.3	—
	Fourteen male pure vegetarians	23.9	—
	Fifteen female nonvegetarians	8.4	—
	Fifteen female lacto-ovovegetarians	12.6	—
	Eleven female pure vegetarians	20.7	—
Dorfman *et al.* (1976)	Seven males and 14 females	2.8	—
Bingham *et al.* (1979)	Sixty-three males and females	—	19.9
King *et al.* (1981)	Five vegetarians	6.2	—
	Pregnant women:		
	Nine vegetarians	8.9	—
	Six nonvegetarians	4.8	—
Marlett and Bokram (1981)	Fifty-seven males	4.8	19.9
	One hundred forty-three females	3.8	13.4
Anderson *et al.* (1981)	Forty-nine female vegetarians	—	30.9
Gibson *et al.* (1983)	Thirty-six vegetarians	—	33.2
	Thirty nonvegetarians	—	20.2

weeks. Mean intakes were higher for the males than for the females, but the difference was not statistically significant, due to the large variation in intakes for both sexes. Although the crude fiber values are comparable to those reported from other studies, the NDF values of 9.5 g/day for 13 males and 7.7 g/day for 16 females are about half the calculated dietary fiber intakes reported by Marlett and Bokram (1981) (Table I).

5. MINERAL STATUS OF VEGETARIANS

Because it is generally believed that vegetarians have a higher fiber intake than nonvegetarians, studies have been conducted measuring the mineral status of vegetarians (Table II).

Anderson et al. (1981) investigated the iron and zinc status of 56 vegetarian women (mean age, 53 years). Mean dietary fiber, iron, and zinc intakes were 30.9 g, 12.5 mg, and 9.2 mg, respectively, as calculated from 3-day diet records. Mean hemoglobin, serum transferrin saturation, and serum and hair zinc were within the normal ranges for these parameters. These findings suggest that the iron and zinc status of these women was not adversely affected by the high intakes of fiber and phytate, and that increased absorption of dietary iron and zinc may have resulted as an adaptation to the vegetarian diet.

TABLE II. Trace Element Status of Vegetarians

Reference	Subjects	Intake	Finding
Anderson et al. (1981)	Fifty-six vegetarians, mean age, 53 years	12.5 mg Fe, 9.2 mg Zn	Mean hemoglobin, serum transferrin saturation, and serum and hair Zn within normal range
Gibson et al. (1983)	Thirty-six vegetarians, mean age, 69 years	2.1 mg Cu, 4.4 mg Mn, 113 μg Se	Copper and Se status of the two groups comparable; hair Mn levels higher in vegetarians
	Thirty nonvegetarians, mean age, 60 years	1.6 mg Cu, 2.6 mg Mn, 109 μg Se	
King et al. (1981)	Five vegetarians Pregnant women:	6.4 mg Zn	Plasma, urinary, and hair Zn similar for vegetarian
	Nine vegetarians	12.3 mg Zn	and nonvegetarian pregnant
	Six nonvegetarians	14.4 mg Zn	women; plasma Zn levels higher in nonpregnant vegetarians

Gibson *et al.* (1983) conducted further studies on vegetarians in which they were compared with nonvegetarians. They determined trace metal status of 36 vegetarian women (mean age, 69 years) and 30 women consuming mixed diets (mean age, 60 years). Three-day diet records were kept and blood and hair samples were taken. The vegetarians had higher intakes of dietary fiber, copper, and manganese than did the women consuming mixed diets. Dried legumes, nuts, and soya products contributed more to energy, copper, manganese, and selenium intakes for vegetarians than for nonvegetarians. Serum copper levels for the vegetarians were within the normal range for persons consuming mixed diets. Hair copper and selenium levels were comparable for the two groups of women. However, hair manganese levels were higher in the vegetarians, probably due to the higher manganese intakes. The authors pointed out that calculated dietary trace element intake data are probably limited in accuracy due to lack of available data. The use of hair for assessment of trace element status is controversial. However, the copper and selenium status of the vegetarians appears to be comparable to that of nonvegetarians, and the manganese status better, in spite of the higher intake of fiber.

King *et al.* (1981) evaluated the zinc status of 12 pregnant vegetarian women, six pregnant nonvegetarian women, and five nonpregnant vegetarian women. Crude fiber intake calculated from 3-day diet records was 8.9 g for nine pregnant vegetarians and 4.8 g for six pregnant nonvegetarians, and values were not significantly different. Calculated zinc intakes for the two groups were also comparable. Plasma, urinary, and hair zinc levels were similar for the two groups of pregnant women. Even though the dietary levels of zinc for the nonpregnant vegetarian women were lower than for the other two groups, plasma zinc levels were about 20% higher than in the pregnant women. The lacto-ovovegetarian diet did not appear to affect zinc status in the pregnant women.

From these studies, it appears that if vegetarians have a decreased availability of minerals due to high fiber and/or phytate intakes, they are able to adjust to the situation and maintain mineral status comparable to that of nonvegetarians.

6. CONSUMPTION OF VEGETARIAN DIETS BY NONVEGETARIANS

Nonvegetarians, who may not consume as much fiber as vegetarians, may respond with decreased mineral utilization to a vegetarian diet. Two studies have been conducted on nonvegetarians consuming vegetarian diets.

Freeland-Graves *et al.* (1981) measured plasma and saliva zinc levels of 12 nonvegetarian women (20–29 years of age) who consumed a lacto-ovovegetarian diet for 22 days. The diet contained 7.8 g of crude fiber and 15.3 mg of zinc per day. Zinc levels of salivary sediment (consisting primarily of epithelial cells) significantly decreased as compared to initial values. Zinc levels of plasma or whole mixed saliva were not affected by the diet. Significantly greater plasma zinc uptake and an increase in the area under the zinc tolerance curve after an oral load of zinc were found after consumption of the vegetarian diet as determined in five of the subjects. The authors concluded that these results indicate that the vegetarian diet adversely affected zinc status in nonvegetarian women.

Kies *et al.* (1983) reported zinc balances of 12 vegetarians and 12 omnivores consuming controlled vegetarian diets. Fecal zinc excretion and zinc balances of subjects indicated better utilization of zinc from vegetarian diets by practicing vegetarians than by omnivores consuming vegetarian diets. The authors stated that the zinc intakes of the omnivores may have been greater prior to the study and that they may have been adjusting also to a lower level of zinc intake as well as to a higher fiber diet.

Feeding nonvegetarians a vegetarian diet will likely result in an increase in fiber intake. However, it may also involve differences in nutrient intakes. A knowledge of previous nutrient intakes of the subjects and a sufficient length of time on the new diet to adjust to differences in nutrient intakes are important.

7. MINERAL BALANCE STUDIES

A few controlled diet balance studies have been carried out in recent years, which provide additional information on the effects of fiber on mineral balances.

Rao and Rao (1980) determined mineral balances of six young men from a low socioeconomic group in India who were working as gardeners. Diets were formulated on the basis of prevailing dietary practices of low- and very low-income groups in four regions of India. The diets were largely lactovegetarian diets; however, two diets contained eggs and two contained fish. In addition, a diet containing fish, a diet containing legumes, and a diet containing mutton were fed. The diets were consumed for 11 days each, with the first 7 days serving as a stabilization period, and collections were made during the last 4 days. Mean analyzed dietary fiber intakes ranged from 48.0 to 81.6 g/day. Mean balances were positive for chromium, copper, and manganese. The chromium intake values were high, and urinary values extremely high. Zinc balance was negative on the very low-income diet of Maharashtra, and magnesium balances were negative on both the low- and very low-income diets of the same region. The absorption of magnesium from the regional diets was negatively correlated with the fiber content of the diets. The diets provided 2700 kcal and 60 g protein per day. The men weighed from 39.9 to 49.5 kg, and this caloric intake seems high for them. This caloric intake is also probably higher than the usual intake for low-income groups in India. Possibly the mean positive balances on so many of the diets were due to increased food intake during the study; however, no weight changes were reported.

Van Dokkum et al. (1982) compared effects of white bread and coarse-bran bread diets on mineral balances. Twelve men consumed the white bread diet (9 g NDF) and a medium-fiber coarse-bran bread diet (22 g NDF). Four of the men then consumed a high-fiber coarse-bran bread diet (35 g NDF), a medium-fiber fine-bran diet (22 g NDF), or a whole meal bread diet (22 g NDF). Twenty-day balances were determined on each diet. Increasing the fiber from 9 to 22 g NDF as coarse bran resulted in increased mineral intake and increased fecal excretion, but no difference in retention. On 35 g NDF, mean iron balance was negative and significantly lower than on the 22 g NDF diet. Although fecal amounts of all other minerals except calcium significantly increased, balances were not significantly different. Balances were negative for calcium, magnesium, iron, and zinc on the highest fiber diet. There was no apparent effect of bran particle size on mineral balances. The whole meal bread diet resulted in higher balances of magnesium and copper. The authors concluded that although on the 35 g NDF diet the mineral intakes were increased, this diet might not be advisable, since there were so many negative mineral balances.

Tsai et al. (1983) fed a basal diet containing 2.8 g crude fiber or the same diet with 25 g soy polysaccharide to 14 subjects for 17-day periods. The soy polysaccharide contained 60% total dietary fiber or 30% NDF. Feces were collected for 4 days, beginning with day 10 of each period. Fecal excretions of calcium, phosphorus, iron, magnesium, zinc, and copper were not significantly different on the two diets.

Morris and Ellis (1983) determined zinc balances of ten men fed diets containing whole bran muffins or dephytinized bran muffins. All subjects consumed both diets for 15 days each. The diets contained 16 g NDF and 17 mg zinc per day. Phytic acid intake was 2.0 and 0.2 g/day on the whole bran and dephytinized bran diets, respectively. Zinc balances for the last 10 days on each diet were positive and not significantly different.

We previously reported negative balances of calcium, magnesium, zinc, and copper for subjects consuming a diet containing approximately 24 g NDF per day in fruits and vegetables (Kelsay et al., 1970a,b). There was some question about the possible effect of oxalic acid from spinach in this diet, particularly on calcium balance (Kelsay et al., 1981). Therefore, we investigated further the effect of spinach and fiber on mineral balances (Kelsay and Prather, 1983).

Twelve men consumed the following diets for 4 weeks each: (1) low-fiber (5 g NDF) diet with spinach; (2) higher fiber (27 g NDF) diet containing fruits and vegetables with spinach; and (3) higher fiber diet in which cauliflower, which is low in oxalic acid content, replaced the spinach. The mean intake of spinach in diets 1 and 2 was 110 g every other day. During week 4, the mean calcium balance was negative and significantly lower on the higher fiber diet with spinach than on the low-fiber diet with spinach. Mean magnesium and zinc balances were negative and significantly lower on the higher fiber diet with spinach than on the low-fiber diet containing spinach or the higher fiber diet containing cauliflower. Mean copper balance was significantly lower on the higher fiber diet containing cauliflower than on the low-fiber diet with spinach. Although the mineral balances on the higher fiber diet with spinach were not significantly lower than on the other diets during week 3, we feel that these differences during week 4 are real and important. This is the second study in which we have found negative mineral balances during the fourth week on a diet containing fruits and vegetables and including spinach. Results of this study suggest that oxalic acid in combination with fiber adversely affects balances of some minerals. The response appears to be time-related, and may be only transient.

Preliminary results of a study by Behall et al. (1983) indicate that the addition of 19.5 g cellulose, sodium carboxymethylcellulose, locust bean gum, or karaya to a 2600-kcal diet containing 6.3 g NDF did not significantly alter balances of zinc, copper, calcium, iron, and magnesium.

Prather et al. (1984) determined mineral balances of 20 men and 33 women during the sixth week on a diet containing 35% of the kcal from complex carbohydrates. The NDF intakes ranged from 22 g/1500 kcal to 58 g/3900 kcal. Preliminary determinations indicated that there were negative balances of some minerals when these high levels of NDF were consumed.

Results of the balance studies reviewed here and of others previously reported indicate that intakes of about 25 g NDF/day may be consumed without adverse effects on mineral balances. Higher levels of fiber intake, however, may not be advisable. The added effects of other mineral binders such as phytic acid and oxalic acid will complicate interpretation of results and also must be considered.

8. SUMMARY AND CONCLUSIONS

Although it has been shown that fibers will bind to minerals in vitro, many agents in food and in the digestive tract will affect this binding. Some agents may inhibit binding, whereas others will enhance binding.

In studies with test meals it was shown that the amount of protein and calcium in the meal could affect zinc absorption. Intakes of nutrients for the whole day or several days will determine total utilization.

It is difficult to make recommendations about levels of fiber intake due to the discrepancy of fiber values obtained with different methodologies.

Calculated fiber intakes of vegetarians appear to be higher than for nonvegetarians. There are indications that the mineral status of vegetarians is comparable to that of nonvegetarians. If there is a decreased availability of minerals due to the high-fiber diets of vegetarians, they seem to be able to adjust to it.

The mineral status of nonvegetarians consuming a vegetarian diet may not be as good as that of vegetarians, because of the unaccustomed increase in fiber intake.

The effect of fiber on mineral balances continues to be a controversial issue. Carefully controlled balance studies with higher levels of fiber intake are needed. Time of adjustment to a change in diet must be sufficient to eliminate effects of a former diet. Other factors that affect mineral availability should be considered in planning experimental diets.

REFERENCES

Anderson, B. M., Gibson, R. S., and Sabry, J. H., 1981, The iron and zinc status of long-term vegetarian women, *Am. J. Clin. Nutr.* **34:**1042–1048.

Behall, K. M., Lee, K., Wilson, A., and Prather, E. S., 1983, Effect of purified fibers added to a basic diet on apparent mineral balance of male subjects, *Fed. Proc. Fed. Am. Soc. Exp. Biol.* **42:**1063.

Bingham, S., Cummings, J. H., and McNeil, N. I., 1979, Intakes and sources of dietary fiber in the British population, *Am. J. Clin. Nutr.* **32:**1313–1319.

Bjorn-Rasmussen, E., 1974, Iron absorption from wheat bread. Influence of various amounts of bran, *Nutr. Metab.* **16:**101–110.

Dobbs, R. J., and Baird, I. M., 1977, Effect of wholemeal and white bread on iron absorption in normal people, *Br. Med. J.* **2:**1641–1642.

Dorfman, S. H., Ali, M., and Floch, M. H., 1976, Low fiber content of Connecticut diets, *Am. J. Clin. Nutr.* **29:**87–89.

Elwood, P. C., Benjamin, I. T., Fry, F. A., Eakins, J. D., Brown, D. A., DeKock, P. C., and Shah, J. U., 1970, Absorption of iron from chapatti made from wheat flour, *Am. J. Clin. Nutr.* **23:**1267–1271.

Fernandez, R., and Phillips, S. F., 1982, Components of fiber bind iron *in vitro, Am. J. Clin. Nutr.* **35:**100–106.

Freeland-Graves, J. H., Ebangit, M. L., and Hendrikson, P. J., 1980, Alterations in zinc absorption and salivary sediment zinc after a lacto-ovo-vegetarian diet, *Am. J. Clin. Nutr.* **33:**1757–1766.

Gibson, R. S., Anderson, B. M., and Sabry, J. H., 1983, The trace metal status of a group of post-menopausal women vegetarians, *J. Am. Diet. Assoc.* **82:**246–250.

Hardinge, M. G., Chambers, A. C., Crooks, H., and Stare, F. J., 1958, Nutritional studies of vegetarians. III. Dietary levels of fiber, *Am. J. Clin, Nutr.* **6:**523–525.

Kelsay, J. L., 1981, Effect of diet fiber level on bowel function and trace mineral balances of human subjects, *Cereal Chem.* **58:**2–5.

Kelsay, J. L., 1982, Effects of fiber on mineral and vitamin bioavailability, in: *Dietary Fiber* in *Health and Disease* (G. V. Vahouny and D. Kritchevsky, eds.), Plenum, New York, pp. 91–103.

Kelsay, J. L., and Prather, E. S., 1983, Mineral balances of human subjects consuming spinach in a low-fiber diet and in a diet containing fruits and vegetables, *Am. J. Clin. Nutr.* **38:**12–19.

Kelsay, J. L., Behall, K. M., and Prather, E. S., 1979a, Effect of fiber from fruits and vegetables on metabolic responses of human subjects. II. Calcium, magnesium, iron, and silicon balances, *Am. J. Clin. Nutr.* **32:**1876–1880.

Kelsay, J. L., Behall, K. M., and Prather, E. S., 1979a, Effect of fiber from fruits and vegetables on metabolic responses of human subjects. III. Zinc, copper, and phosphorus balances, *Am. J. Clin. Nutr.* *32:*2307–2311.

Kelsay, J. L., Clark, W. M., Herbst, B. J., and Prather, E. S., 1981, Nutrient utilization by human subjects consuming fruits and vegetables as sources of fiber, *J. Agric. Food Chem.* **29:**461–465.

Kies, C., Young, E., and McEndree, L., 1983, Zinc bioavailability from vegetarian diets. Influence of dietary fiber, ascorbic acid, and past dietary practices, in: *Nutritional Bioavailability of Zinc* (G. E. Inglett, ed.), ACS Symposium Series, no. 210, American Chemical Society, Washington, D.C., pp. 115–126.

King, J. C., Stein, T., and Doyle, M., 1981, Effect of vegetarianism on the zinc status of pregnant women, *Am. J. Clin. Nutr.* **34:**1049–1055.

Kojima, N., Wallace, D., and Bates, G. W., 1981, The effect of chemical agents, beverages, and spinach on the *in vitro* solubilization of iron from cooked pinto beans, *Am. J. Clin. Nutr.* **34:**1392–1401.

Leigh, M. J., and Miller, D. D., 1983, Effects of pH and chelating agents on iron binding by dietary fiber: Implications for iron availability, *Am. J. Clin. Nutr.* **38:**202–213.

Lyon, D. B., 1984, Studies on the solubility of Ca, Mg, Zn and Cu in cereal products, *Am. J. Clin. Nutr.* **39:**190–195.

Marlett, J. A., and Bokram, R. L., 1981, Relationship between calculated dietary and crude fiber intakes of 200 college students, *Am. J. Clin. Nutr.* **34:**335–342.

Morris, E. R., and Ellis, R., 1983, Dietary phytate/zinc molar ratio and zinc balance in humans, in: *Nutritional Bioavailability of Zinc* (G. E. Inglett, ed.). ACS Symposium Series no. 210, American Chemical Society, Washington, D.C., pp. 159–172.

Prather, E. S., Wilson, A., Reiser, S., Carafelli, C., and Hallfrisch, J., 1984, Mineral balances of men and premenopausal and postmenopausal women consuming a high complex carbohydrate diet, *Fed. Proc. Fed. Am. Soc. Exp. Biol.* **43:**615.

Rao, C. N., and Rao, B. S. N., 1980, Absorption and retention of magnesium and some trace elements by man from typical Indian diets, *Nutr. Metab.* **24:**244–254.

Reinhold, J. G. Garcia, L. J. S., and Garzon, P., 1981, Binding of iron by fiber of wheat and maize, *Am. J. Clin. Nutr.* **34:**1384–1391.

Reinhold, J. G., Garcia, L. P. M., Arias-Amado, L., and Garzon, P., 1982, Dietary fiber–iron interactions: Fiber-modified uptakes of iron by segments of rat intestine, in: *Dietary Fiber in Health and Disease* (G. V. Vahouny and D. Kritchevsky, eds.), Plenum, New York, pp. 117–132.

Sandstrom, B., and Cederblad, A., 1980, Zinc absorption from composite meals. 2. Influence of the main protein source, *Am. J. Clin. Nutr.* **33:**1778–1783.

Sandstrom, B., Arvidsson, B., Cederblad, A., and Bjorn-Rasmussen, E., 1980, Zinc absorption from composite meals. 1. The significance of wheat extraction rate, zinc, calcium, and protein content in meals based on bread, *Am. J. Clin. Nutr.* **33:**739–745.

Tsai, A. C., Mott, E. L., Owen, G. M., Bennick, M. R., Lo, G. S., and Steinke, F. H., 1983, Effects of soy polysaccharide on gastrointestinal functions, nutrient balance, steroid excretions, glucose tolerance, serum lipids, and other parameters in humans, *Am. J. Clin. Nutr.* **38:**504–511.

Van Dokkum, W., Wesstra, A., and Schippers, F. A., 1982, Physiological effects of fibre-rich types of bread. I. The effect of dietary fibre from bread on the mineral balance of young men, *Br. J. Nutr.* **47**:451–460.

Vellar, O. D., Borchgrevink, C., and Natvig, H., 1968, Iron fortified bread. Absorption and utilization studies, *Acta Med. Scand.* **183**:251–256.

25

Role of Dietary Fiber in Geriatric Nutrition: A Review

R. ALI, G. M. OWEN, and
L. M. SCHANBACHER

1. INTRODUCTION

Demographic evidence and statistical data support the fact that the population in the developed countries is growing older. The decline in birth rate and increased life expectancy both contributed to this phenomenon, which, by all indications, should continue well beyond the year 2000. Studies on population dynamics show that in 1976, the segment of world population over 65 years of age was 6%, while in the U. S. and Europe this age group represented 10 and 14%, respectively (Metropolitan Life Foundation, 1982; Young, 1983; Russell, 1983). It is estimated that by the year 2025 the population over the age of 65 in the U. S. will quadruple from the current 26 million to well over 100 million and that the "very old" population (85 years of age and older) will reach 6.7 million (Hayflick, 1974; Shank, 1976; Butler and McGuire, 1982). It is of interest to note that the "senior-boom" predicted for the first quarter of the 21st century correlates in time to the "baby-boom" witnessed in the early 1960s.

All these predictions, however, represent extrapolations from current population dynamics; these dynamics reflect the state of our knowledge of the aging phenomenon at the organic and cellular levels, which can be described as scanty at best. It is conceivable, therefore, that these statistics

R. ALI, G. M. OWEN, and L. M. SCHANBACHER • Nutritional Research and Development, Bristol-Myers International Division, New York, New York 10154.

could be dramatically changed, both quantitatively and qualitatively, if our understanding of the causes of aging advances faster than the biological clock that controls the life span of man.

This review is an attempt to examine the role of dietary fiber in nutrition of the elderly, arbitrarily defined as those who are 65 years of age and older. Given the current state of knowledge on the nutritional requirements of this age group and the present understanding of the role of fiber in the diet, one can appreciate the challenge of objectively reviewing the subject. Nonetheless, if the only contribution of the review is to draw the attention of health professionals to the serious gaps in our knowledge on the nutritional needs of the elderly, who represent the fastest growing segment in our society, it is a cause worth every effort.

Although there is no absolute requirement for dietary fiber, it is well established that physiological dependence on fiber in the diet does exist, at least in a segment of the population, to modulate gut function and manage constipation (Dwyer, 1983). As various systems begin to slow down with age under the control of a preset genetic code, promotion of regularity takes on added significance in the geriatric population, judging from the rate of usage of laxatives by this age group. General nutritional concerns may arise as a result of potentially higher than average intake of dietary fiber or chronic use of laxatives in the presence of marginal intake of some essential nutrients. Age-related changes in the gut may influence digestion and absorption of nutrients and could lead to nutritional deficiencies.

2. NUTRITIONAL STATUS OF THE ELDERLY

The relation between nutrition and aging has been recently reviewed (Munro, 1981; Bowman and Rosenberg, 1982; Roe, 1983). Using two-thirds of the recommended daily allowances (RDAs) (Food and Nutrition Board, 1980) as the standard and comparing it to the survey data from the National Institute of Health at the Aging Center in Baltimore (McGandy et al., 1966), the Health and Nutrition Examination Survey of National Center for Health and Statistics (1979), and the Oregon study reported by Yearick et al. (1980), one may conclude that there are some general areas of concern with implications for the nutrition and health of the elderly.

First, the RDAs may have overestimated the need for energy, calcium, iron, vitamin A, and certain B vitamins reported low in the diet of the elderly population (O'Hanlon and Kohlrs, 1978; Rivlin, 1981; Bowman and Rosenberg, 1982; Young, 1983). Second, the elderly may indeed be receiving less than their optimal dietary allowances from those nutrients (Eckstein, 1983). Third, anthropometric measures and dietary methods used in assessing the nutritional status of the young adult may not be suitable tools for evaluating nutritional intake and requirements of the older adult population (Bowman and Rosenberg, 1982; Russell, 1983).

Resolutions to these concerns have not been reached, and several approaches were suggested by Russell (1983). He emphasized the need to establish dietary, anthropometric, and biochemical standards that are specific for assessing the nutritional status of the elderly; with such standards, it is possible to balance their nutrition and improve their state of health. It may be necessary to adjust the RDAs for each added decade of life above 50 years of age and to correlate them with a new and dynamic set of anthropometric measures that are representative of the changes in the human body associated with growing older.

3. AGING OF THE GASTROINTESTINAL TRACT AND THE IMPLICATION FOR NUTRITION

A number of age-related physiological and biochemical changes in the gastrointestinal tract can influence nutritional needs, alter dietary intake and utilization of the nutrients, and compromise the overall health status of the elderly (Butler and McGuire, 1982). The prevalence of gastrointestinal (GI) symptoms and diseases increases with age. In patients over 70 years of age, carcinoma of the stomach or large bowel, peptic ulcer disease, and intestinal obstruction due to hernias and colonic diverticular disease account for the major portion of the 20% of all deaths attributable to GI disease. Such disorders in the older patient require the same modalities of management, including the attempts to maintain caloric and nitrogen balance, as in younger individuals (Taylor, 1983).

Various oral and esophageal functions as well as gastric emptying should be examined in older subjects who present difficulties in eating. Adequate dentition and appropriate swallowing should be checked in individuals who have difficulties in consuming bulky or high-fiber diets that require proper chewing to facilitate the ease of delivery of food to the stomach.

After digested food reaches the stomach, it must be properly mixed and liquified by the effective action of retrograde gastric contractal activity and digestion with acidified gastric juices. It has been suspected for many years that changes in the gastric mucosa related to age lead to altered secretory function. Baron, 1963, using a modified version of the Kay's augmentation histamine test, found that both basal and maximal gastric acid secretion declined with age and that acid secretion was less for females than for males. Evidence reveals an increasing tendency to achlorhydria with advancing age. It appears that this tendency is associated with atrophic changes in the gastric mucosa. Diminished maximal secretory function of the remaining cells also contributes to the tendency for a lower acid secretory function in the aged.

The incidence of gastritis in the elderly is not well documented. However, it is generally recognized that acute gastritis, chronic atrophic gastritis, and chronic hypertrophic gastritis increase in incidence in the elderly and may be the cause of dyspeptic symptoms in patients with normal barium X-ray examination. Reported changes in gastric function may indirectly affect the nutritional status of the elderly by influencing food selection and intake.

Other age-related changes occur in both the small intestine and large bowel. Noticeable alterations that tend to decrease functional absorptive capacity are seen by flattening of the fingerlike villi, which appear borader, and a reduction in villus height (Chacko *et al.*, 1969; Webster and Leeming, 1975) accompanied by a decrease in the total cellular population of the gut mucosa.

Changes in pancreatic digestive enzyme secretion occur, which reflect alterations in the total functional capacity of the pancreas in older individuals. Structural changes such as proliferation of duct cell and an overall ductual system hyperplasia may displace acinar cellular mass and contribute to the decreased secretory capacity (Keel and Sandin, 1973).

Functional changes related to reduced pancreatic lipase excretion in the elderly have been reported (Necheles *et al.*, 1942; Becker *et al.*, 1950; Garcia *et al.*, 1955; Bartos and Groh, 1969). Inappropriate digestion of fat can result in lower bowel distress associated with an increase in flatulence, acute bouts of abdominal cramps, and pain and diarrhea. Care must be taken to assess the total digestive and secretory capacity of the small bowel as it relates to these aging processes to be certain that appropriate types and quantities of essential nutrients are provided in the diet.

4. DIETARY FIBER AND ITS NUTRITIONAL IMPLICATION FOR THE ELDERLY

The effect of dietary fiber on the digestion and utilization of nutrients has been recently reviewed (Ali *et al.*, 1981, 1982; Vahouny, 1981; Staub and Ali, 1982). Southgate and Durnin (1970) and Southgate (1973) found a positive correlation between transit time and digestibility of cellulose. Older subjects, both men and women, consistently show a higher percent apparent digestibility of cellulose and pentosan at low and high fiber intake than younger subjects (Figures 1 and 2). No difference was noted in apparent digestibility of protein, energy, and fat between young and older subjects (Figs. 3–5). Southgate speculated that increased bulk in the diet could decrease transit time and therefore allow less residence of digesta in the gut

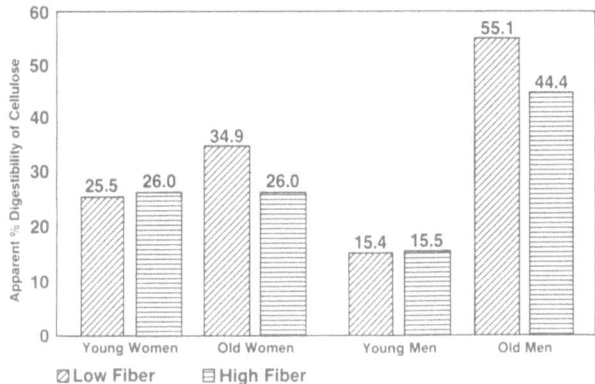

FIGURE 1. The effect of the level of dietary fiber intake on the apparent digestibility of cellulose. (Adapted from Southgate and Durnin, 1970.)

to permit optimal digestion and absorption of nutrients; alternatively, availability for absorption of the products of digestion may be impaired as a result of the water-binding capacity of dietary fiber in the intestinal lumen. Unfortunately, few data are available to support these speculations (Garrison *et al.*, 1978; Slavin and Marlett, 1980).

Certain unabsorbable plant polysaccharides may reduce postprandial hyperglycemia. Attention must be given to the possibility that such complex

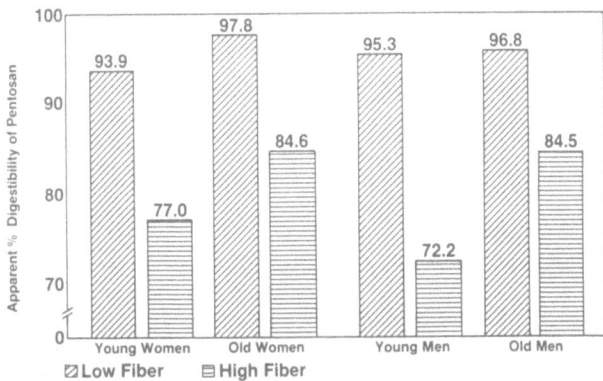

FIGURE 2. The effect of the level of dietary fiber on the apparent digestibility of pentosan. (Adapted from Southgate and Durnin, 1970.)

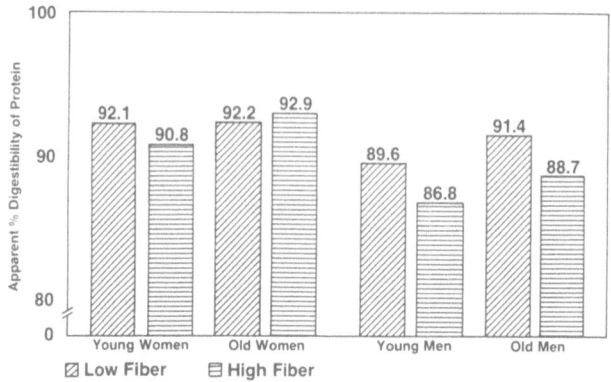

FIGURE 3. The effect of the level of dietary fiber on the apparent digestibility of protein. (Adapted from Southgate and Durnin, 1970.)

carbohydrate substances as guar gum may exert undesirable effects on other components of the diet, e.g., fat, while apparently benefiting patients with regard to carbohydrate metabolism (Jenkins *et al.*, 1978). Tsai *et al.* (1983) were not able to determine that soy polysaccharide exerted any undesirable effects on nutrient balances, including fat and minerals, at least in young adults studied over a relatively short period of time.

Dietary fiber alters fat absorption to some extent, depending upon the fiber components examined. Pectin, 15 g/day, can double fecal fat excretion

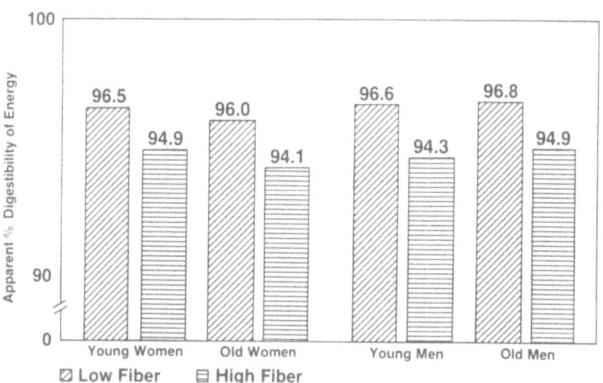

FIGURE 4. The effect of the level of dietary fiber on the apparent digestibility of energy. (Adapted from Southgate and Durnin, 1970.)

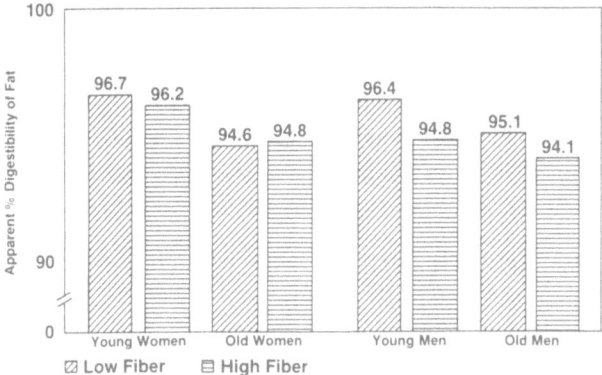

FIGURE 5. The effect of the level of dietary fiber on the apparent digestibility of fat. (Adapted from Southgate and Durnin, 1970.)

(Kay and Truswell, 1977). Wheat bran, 25–30 g/day, increased fecal fat and fatty acid excretion in healthy medical students (Cummings *et al.*, 1976). Similarly, fecal nitrogen increases when dietary fiber is increased. This may result from the presence of undigested protein complexes, increase in endogenous nitrogen excretion, or increase in fecal microorganisms.

A number of studies have been undertaken to look at the effect of dietary fiber on mineral absorption. Most attention has been focused on calcium, phosphorus, and iron, although increasing attention is being given to zinc, copper, and other trace metals. The association of calcium malabsorption with whole-grain products was initially reported by McCance and Widdowson (1942) and McCance and Walsham (1948) and examined further by Rheinhold *et al.* (1976). Fiber itself, independent of the presence of phytate, may exert some effects on calcium and magnesium absorption in metabolism.

Persson *et al.* (1976) found some decrease in serum calcium levels in elderly patients whose diets were supplemented with 10 or 20 g wheat bran daily for 6 weeks.

Rheinhold *et al.* (1975) showed that zinc binds quite strongly to low-phytate wheat bran. Removal of phytate from bran or whole meal (whole wheat) bread or the addition of calcium to the preparations seemed to increase zinc binding, *in vitro*.

Sandstead *et al.* (1978) showed that wheat bran (26 g/day) added to an average diet of the sort consumed by many American men appeared to decrease retention of zinc in four of five volunteer study subjects. In contrast, added corn bran had no effects on zinc retention and neither wheat nor corn appeared to have adverse effects on retention of iron or copper.

In the gut, interaction of cell wall materials with the process of mineral absorption represents a possible disadvantage of high-fiber diets, particularly when diets are supplemented with high-fiber preparations. One area where caution would seem to be needed is in supplementing the diets of older persons with whole wheat products to improve bowel habits when their dietary intakes of iron and calcium may be marginal (Cummings, 1978).

5. MEDICAL AND CLINICAL IMPLICATIONS OF DIETARY FIBER FOR THE ELDERLY

The aging process involves physiological changes that alter nutrient requirements, but is often accompanied by changes in total food intake and selection that run counter to the evolving age-related change in demand (Young and Solomons, 1983). While long-term dietary habits have implications in the development of various medical disorders or conditions, attention here is focused on the medical implications of the ingestion of dietary fiber by older persons.

5.1. Diverticular Disease

The incidence of diverticular disease in both the duodenum and the colon increases with age. Manousos *et al.* (1967) and Parks (1969) have shown that both the incidence and time of onset of symptoms of this disease increase almost threefold from age 40 (18%) to 80 years (32%). This condition appears to result in changes in muscular tone and lack of coordination of aboral propulsive movement of gut contents. Thus, intraluminal pressure increases, creating regional high-pressure zones that produce outpocketing of the aged intestinal wall (Hughes, 1969). Effective treatment to reduce the pain and normalize muscular tone with a return toward more effective aboral motility functions includes the use of high-residue dietary fiber sources. Recent experimental evidence in rabbits suggest that maintaining a low-residue diet or switching from a high- to a low-residue diet drastically increases the occurrence of diverticula (Hodgson, 1972). Adding wheat bran and psyllium seed husks to the diet in moderate or prescribed amounts appears to be common practice and somewhat effective in helping to regain more normal gut functions. More objective studies are needed to better define the appropriate sources and levels of dietary fiber that are useful in the management of this age-related disease.

5.2. Constipation

Constipation has different meanings for different individuals. Most persons consider constipation to be an abnormally low frequency of defecation, but difficulty of expulsion is second as a complaint; hard consistency of the stool is another way of characterizing constipation (Devroede, 1978). It is difficult to study the effects of various fibers on bowel habits, because all diets have a substantial placebo effect. This has been demonstrated in studies of patients with irritable bowel syndrome and patients with diverticular disease, where the placebo effect was equal to or greater than the treatment effect (Soltoft *et al.*, 1976).

Contributory causes of constipation in adults include low-fiber diet, irregular bowel habits, debility, use of narcotic analgesics, and obstruction. Fecal water and fecal weight and volume may be reduced if a diet low in fiber is regularly consumed. If a person has pain on defecation because of an anal fissure or hemorrhoids, normal urges to defecate may be suppressed. For example, ingestion of food or beverage is usually associated with a gastro-colic reflex that initiates mass movement of the colon content. Sudden changes in bowel habits leading to constipation should prompt medical attention, because obstructive constipation normally results from cancer of the colon or rectum.

Increasing the amount of fiber in the diet increases the stool bulk and increases intestinal muscle tone, which can help control constipation. Addition of fiber to the diet of individuals with either acute or chronic constipation helps to restore more normal fecal excretion patterns and regularity. Both a bulking capacity and a water-holding activity of these fibers are thought to contribute to a more coordinated intestinal proportion of content and delivery of feces through the large bowel. An increase in dietary fiber can be best achieved by inclusion of whole grain cereal brans or muffins and encouraging consumption of bran-containing breakfast cereals daily. Increased intake of vegetables may be acceptable to some elderly persons, but others may complain of the increased bulk of the diet (Mendeloff, 1978). Sudden increases in the fiber content of the diet of elderly persons are generally not well tolerated. They may complain of excess gas, abdominal bloating, and loose bowel movements.

It is recommended that the successful use of selected dietary fiber sources for this indication can be achieved with increasing amounts until effective relief is obtained. Obstruction of the intestine or large bowel can occur if older subjects do not consume adequate volumes of water while receiving a high-fiber diet.

5.3. Laxatives

It is worth noting that about half of the elderly persons in the U. S. use laxatives occasionally or regularly (Fingl and Freston, 1979). Reasons for the use of laxatives are: (1) simple constipation, reflecting (a) low-fiber intake or (b) use of constipating drugs; (2) medical conditions that make defection difficult and/or painful; and (3) habit. Among the laxatives used are bulk formulations including methylcellulose, cereal brans, and psyllium seeds. Bulk-forming laxative agents taken before food can reduce appetite because the user has a "full feeling." This may be more true among elderly persons than among young adults. Smith *et al.* (1980) showed in animal studies that bulk-forming laxatives such as psyllium seeds reduce the absorption of dietary minerals, including calcium, magnesium, and zinc. Hemicellulose from cereal brans as well as fruits and vegetables containing pectin and lignin also act by increasing intestinal motility. Electrolyte fluxes in the intestine may also be altered by substances that promote intestinal motility. Dietary fiber sources that have some effect on intestinal transport do not exert significantly change intestinal absorption except by absorption of micronutrients such as trace elements in the intestinal lumen (Rheinhold *et al.*, 1976).

It is clear that attention must be given to the use of various laxative agents by elderly persons, whether or not dietary recommendations with respect to fiber intake are to be made.

5.4. Cardiovascular Disease

Work in the field of cardiovascular disease is focused to a large extent on cholesterol metabolism with respect to its synthesis, absorption, and degradation. Degradation of cholesterol proceeds to neutral steroids via microbiological hydrogenation to coprostanol and further oxidation of this compound, or to bile acid formation, which involves a combination of enzymatic and microbial steps. Since fiber appears to affect the spectrum of metabolites of cholesterol found in feces, more data on the effects of fiber on intestinal microflora are needed.

In vitro experiments have shown that different types of fiber exhibit varying affinities for bile acids and bile salts. In fact, the same material will bind different bile acids and salts to different extents.

While it has been shown among Seventh-Day Adventists (SDA) that vegetarian/nonvegetarian status was strongly related to the risk of coronary heart disease (CHD) in males below age 65 years, there was no relation between dietary habits and risk of CHD deaths among males over age 65 or among females of any age (Phillips *et al.*, 1978). It was postulated that reduced CHD risk among younger SDA males might reflect lower intake of total fat or saturated fat or higher intake of dietary fiber. Failure to see diet-related differences in SDA males above age 65 years may reflect shifts in diet by individuals who develop risk factors for CHD or who have initial manifestations of CHD.

It seems unlikely that diet (vegetarian vs. nonvegetarian) or relative levels of fat or saturated fat in a diet of persons 70 years of age or older will have any measurable effects on the evolution of coronary heart disease or other cardiovascular disorders.

5.5. Diabetes Mellitus

The elderly individual is less able to tolerate glucose than is the younger person. Reduction in tolerance is a metabolic change that becomes progressively more evident throughout life, but varies widely among different individuals (Andres and Topin, 1977).

Diabetes mellitus in elderly persons is most commonly of the maturity-onset type. Etiologic factors in the development of maturity-onset diabetes include obesity and declining glucose tolerance associated with the aging process. Even though pancreatic production of insulin may be impaired, most elderly patients with maturity-onset diabetes do not require insulin. Weight reduction may be necessary to improve glucose tolerance. Other facets of nutritional and dietary management of diabetes are control of hyperlipidemia and maintenance of blood sugars to avoid hyperglycemia or/and hypoglycemia. Modifications in the diet that can be recommended include reduced intake of simple carbohydrate, and increased intake of complex carbohydrates from cereal foods and tuberous vegetables to supply about 60% of total daily energy requirements. It is questionable that the fiber content of this diet has any special role, but instead the benefit comes from a decrease in simple carbohydrate intake (Simpson *et al.*, 1979). It must be recognized that older persons may have difficulty consuming this bulkier diet, and compliance with its use may be poor among the elderly unaccustomed to consuming relatively bulky diets.

5.6. Fiber and Drugs

Although there are several changes in the structure and function of the GI tract that occur during aging and could affect rate and quantity of drug absorption, no significant change in drug absorption attributable to aging has been identified (Vestal, 1980). Nonnutrient components of the diet, including specific forms of dietary fiber, e.g., pectin, may adsorb drugs, producing a transient or net reduction in drug absorption. Delayed absorption of common drugs can occur when the drug is taken at the same time as food or within 1–2 h after food has been consumed.

Slower gastric emptying time may promote absorption of drugs. Either the delay in stomach emptying permits more drug to be dissolved in the stomach before it passes into the duodenum to be absorbed or more drug may be absorbed when it slowly reaches the absorption sites in the small intestine (Welling, 1977). Dietary fiber in the stomach is retained longer than are fluid or semifluid components. The rate at which a drug leaves the stomach depends on whether it is absorbed to dietary fiber or suspended or dissolved in fluid components.

6. SUMMARY AND CONCLUSIONS

Health implications of dietary fiber take an added significance in geriatric nutrition because of limited knowledge of age-related changes in the gut and possible modifying effects of dietary fiber on nutrient digestion and absorption (Table I).

It appears that susceptibility to constipation, hemorrhoids, diverticular disease, and irritable bowel symptoms are reduced when daily intake of dietary fiber, from a variety of sources, is maintained between 20 and 25 g. Although dietary fiber may protect from development of colon cancer, the evidence is indirect and inconclusive. There is no evidence for a direct protective effect of levels of fiber intake against atherosclerosis. Most types of dietary fiber do not directly influence plasma lipid or glucose levels, although some types will reduce postprandial hyperglycemia.

The question of essential mineral deficiency resulting from high fiber intake and reduced mineral absorption has been partially examined, but research in this area is needed to further our knowledge in nutrition and health of the elderly.

TABLE I. Age-Related Changes in Gut Function versus Physiological Action of Dietary Fiber in the Gut[a]

Gastrointestinal function	Age-related change	Dietary fiber-related modification	Type of fiber
Mastication	↓	↑	Polysaccharides, lignins
Gastric emptying	?	↓	Pectin, mucilages
Gastric acid secretion	↓	?	Pectin, mucilages
Small intestinal absorption	?	?	Pectin, mucilages
Mouth-to-colon transit time	↑	↓	Pectin, mucilages, polysaccharides
Mouth-to-rectum transit time	↑	↓	Polysaccharides, lignin
Bacterial metabolism (colon)	↑	↑	Polysaccharides, lignins, mucilages, pectin
Water absorption (colon)	?	↓	Polysaccharides, lignins
Intraluminal pressure	?	↓	Polysaccharides, mucilages, pectin
Fecal minerals	?	↑	Acidic polysaccharides
Fecal electrolytes	?	↑	Polysaccharides, lignin
Fecal Steroids	?	↑	Lignins
Fecal weight	?	↑	Polysaccharides, lignins, mucilages, pectin

[a] Adapted from Eastwood and Kay (1979).

It is questionable whether elderly persons should implement major changes in dietary habits. They may find changes difficult to accept on the one hand and it may be questioned whether assumed benefits can be documented on the other hand. Some attention must be given to the total diet consumed by the elderly person and the levels of nutrients provided by the diet. Emphasis should be placed on eating a variety of foods in moderation. The health care advisor must be aware of drugs being taken and the use of laxatives and intake of vitamin/mineral supplements to be certain that energy, protein, and essential micronutrient needs are being met.

ACKNOWLEDGMENTS. The authors wish to acknowledge C. M. Dominguez for her editorial assistance and D. R. Brudno for the preparation of the manuscript.

REFERENCES

Ali, R., Staub, H., Coccodrilli, H. G., Jr., and Schanbacher, L., 1981, Nutritional significance of dietary fiber: Effect on nutrient bioavailability and selected gastrointestinal functions, *J. Agric. Food Chem.* **29**:465–472.

Ali, R., Staub, H., Leveille, G. A., and Boyle, P. C., 1982, Dietary fiber and obesity. A Review, in: *Dietary Fiber in Health and Disease* (G. V. Vahouny and D. Kritchevsky, eds.), Plenum, New York, pp. 139–144.

Andres, R., and Topin, J. D., 1977, Endocrine systems, in: *Handbook of Biology of Aging* (C. E. Finch and L. Hayflick, eds.), Van Nostrand Reinhold, New York, pp. 357–378.

Baron, J. H., 1963, An assessment of the augmented histamine test in the diagnosis of peptic ulcer, *Gut* **4**:243–253.

Bartos, V., and Groh, J., 1969, The effect of repeated stimulation of the pancreas on pancreatic secretion in young and aged men, *Gerontol. Clin.* **II**:56–62.

Becker, G. H., Meyer, J., and Necheles, H., 1950, Fat absorption in young and old age, *Gastroenterology* **14**:80–92.

Bowman, B. ., and Rosenberg, I. H., 1982, Assessment of the nutritional status of the elderly, *Am. J. Clin. Nutr.* **35**:1142–1151.

Butler, R. N., and McGuire, E. A. H., 1982, Evidence relating selected vitamins and minerals to health and disease in the elderly population in the United States, Forward, *Am. J. Clin. Nutr.* **36**:977–978.

Chacko, C. J. G., Paulson, K. A., Mathan, V. I., and Baker, S. J., 1969, The villus architecture of the small intestine in the tropics—A necropsy study, *J. Pathol. Bacteriol.* **98**:146–151.

Cummings, J. H., 1978, Nutritional implications of dietary fiber, *Am. J. Clin. Nutr.* **31**:521–529.

Cummings, J. H., Hill, M. J., Jenkins, D. J. A., Pearson, J. R., and Wiggins, H. S., 1976, Changes in fecal composition and colonic function due to serial fiber, *Am. J. Clin. Nutr.* **29**:1468–1471.

Devroede, G., 1978, Dietary fiber, bowel habits, and colonic function, *Am. J. Clin. Nutr.* **31**: 5157–5160.

Dwyer, J., 1983, Vegetarian and other alternative dietary practices, in: *Manual of Clinical Nutrition* (D. M. Paige, ed.), Nutrition Publication, Pleasantville, New Jersey, pp. 42.1–42.23.

Eastwood, M. A., and Kay, R. M., 1979, A hypothesis for the action of dietary fiber along the gastrointestinal tract, *Am. J. Clin. Nutr.* **32**:364–367.

Eckstein, D., 1983, Nutritional care of the elderly, *Clin. Nutr. (Manual Clin. Nutr. Suppl.)* **2**(6):19–23.

Fingl, E., and Freston, J. W., 1979, Antidiarrheal agents and laxatives: Changing concepts, *Clin. Gastroenterol.* **8:**161-86.

Food and Nutrition Board, 1980, *Recommended Dietary Allowances,* 9th ed., National Academy of Science, National Research Council, Washington, D.C.

Garcia, P., Roderick, C., and Swanson, P., 1955, The relation of age to fat absorption in adult women with observations on concentration of serum cholesterol, *J. Nutr.* **55:**601-609.

Garrison, M. V., Reel, R. L., Fawley, P., and Breidenstem, C. P., 1978, Comparative digestibility of acid detergent fiber by laboratory albino and wild polynesian rats, *J. Nutr.* **108:**191-195.

Hayflick, L., 1974, On mortality and immortality, *Executive Health* **X**(4).

Hodgson, W. J. B., 1972, An interim report on the production of colonic diverticula in the rabbit, *Gut* **13:**302-304.

Hughes, L. W., 1969, *Postmortem* survey of diverticular disease, *Gut* **10:**336-351.

Jenkins, D. D. A., Wolever, T. M. S., and Nineham, R., 1978, Guar crispbread in the diabetic diet, *Br. Med. J.* **2:**1744-1746.

Kay, R. M., and Truswell, S., 1977, Effect of citrus pectin on blood lipids and fecal steroids secretion in man, *Am. J. Clin. Nutr.* **30:**171-175.

Keel, L., and Sandin, B., 1973, Changes in pancreatic morphology associated with aging, *Gut* **14:**962-970.

Manousos, O. N., Truelove, S. C., and Lumsden, K., 1967, Transit times of food in patients with diverticulosis or irritable colon syndrome and normal subjects, *Br. Med. J.* **iii:** 760-762.

McCance, R. A., and Walsham, C. M., 1948, The digestion and absorption of the calories, protein, purines, fat and calcium in whole meal wheat bread, *Br. J. Nutr.* **2:**26-28.

McCance, R. A., and Widdowson, E. M., 1942, Mineral metabolism of healthy adults on white and brown bread dietaries, *J. Physiol.* **101:**44-46.

McGandy, R. B., Barrows, C. H., Spanias, A., Meredith, A., Stone, J. L., and Norris, A. H., 1966, Nutrient intakes and energy expenditure in men of different ages, *J. Gerontol.* **21:** 581-587.

Mendeloff, A. I., 1978, Fiber and gastrointestinal tract: Summary and recommendations workshop III, *Am. J. Clin. Nutr.* **31:**5145-5147.

Metropolitan Life Foundation, 1982, Continued increase in elderly population, *Stat. Bull. Metrop. Life Insur. Co.* **63**(3):6-10.

Munro, H. M., 1981, Nutrition and aging, *Br. Med. Bull.* **37:**83.

National Center for Health and Statistics, 1979, Dietary Intake Source Data, United States, 1971-1974, DHEW Publ. no., PHS 79-1221, National Center for Health Statistics, Hyattsville, Maryland.

Necheles, H., Plotke, F., and Meyer, J., 1942, Studies in old age V. active pancreatic secretion in the aged, *Am. J. Dig. Dis.* **9:**157-159.

O'Hanlon, P., and Kohlrs, M. B., 1978, Dietary studies of older Americans, *Am. J. Clin. Nutr.* **31:**1257-1269.

Parks, T. G., 1969, Natural history of diverticular disease of the colon. A review of 521 cases, *Br. Med. J.* **4:**639-642.

Persson, I., Raby, K., Font-Bech, P., and Jensen, E., 1976, Effective prolonged bran administration on serum levels of cholesterol, ionised calcium and iron in the elderly, *J. Am. Gerontol. Soc.* **24:**334-339.

Phillips, B. L., Lemmon, F. R., Beeson, W. L., and Kuzma, J. W., 1978, Coronary heart disease mortality among Seventh Day Adventists with differing dietary habits: A preliminary report, *Am. J. Clin. Nutr.* **31:**5191-5198.

Rheinhold, J. G., Ismael-Beigi, F., and Faradji, B., 1975, Fiber vs. phytate as determinants of the availability of calcium, zinc and iron of bread stuffs, *Nutr. Rep. Int.* **12:**75-78.

Rheinhold, J. G., Faradji, B., Abadi, P., and Ismael-Beigi, F., 1976, Decreased absorption of calcium, magnesium, zinc and phosphorus by humans due to increased fiber and phosphorus consumption as wheat bread, *J. Nutr.* **106:**493-503.

Rivlin, R. S., 1981, Nutrition and aging: Some unanswered questions, *Am. J. Med.* **71**:337.

Roe, D. A., 1983, The nutritional status of the elderly, in: *Geriatric Nutrition,* Prentice Hall, Englewood Cliffs, New Jersey, pp. 56–63.

Russell, R. M., 1983, Evaluating the nutritional status of the elderly, *Clin. Nutr. (Manual Clin. Nutr. Suppl.)* **2**(6):4–8.

Sandstead, H. H., Monoz, J. M., Jacob, R. A., Kleveay, L. M., Reck, S. M. J., Logan, G. M., Dinzis, F. R., Inglell, G. E., Shuey, W. C., 1978, Influence of dietary fiber on trace element balance, *Am. J. Clin. Nutr.* **31**:5180–5184.

Shank, R. E., 1976, *Nutrition, Longevity, and Aging,* Academic, New York, pp.

Simpson, R. W., Mann, J. J., Eaton, J., Moore, R. A., Carter, R., and Hockaday, T. D. R., 1979, Improved glucose control in maturity-onset diabetes treated with high carbohydrate modified fat diet, *Br. Med. J.* **1**:1753–1756.

Slavin, J. L., and Marlett, J. A., 1980, Effect of refined cellulose on apparent energy, fat and nitrogen digestibilities, *J. Nutr.* **110**:2020–2026.

Smith, R. G., Rowe, M. J., Smith, A. N., Eastwood, M. A., Drummond, E., and Brydon, W. G., 1980, A study of bulking agents in elderly patients, *Age Aging* **9**:267–271.

Soltoft, J., Krag, B., Goodman-Hoyer, E., Kristensen, E., and Wulff, H. R., 1976, A double-blind trial of the effect of wheat bran on symptoms of irritable bowel syndrome, *Lancet* **1**:270–271.

Southgate, D. A. T., 1973, Fiber and other unavailable carbohydrates and their effect on the energy value of the diet, *Proc. Nutr. Soc.* **1973**:131–136.

Southgate, D. A. T., and Durnin, J. V. G. A., 1970, Calorie conversion factors. An experimental reassessment of the factors used in the calculation of the energy value of human diets, *Br. J. Nutr.* **24**:517–535.

Staub, H., and Ali, R., 1982, Nutritional and physiological values of gums, in: *Food Hydrocolloids* (M. Glicksman, ed.), CRC, Boca Raton, Florida, pp. 101–121.

Taylor, K. B., 1983, Gastroenterology, in: *Nutritional Support of Medical Practice, 2nd Edition* (H. E. Schneider, C. E. Anderson and D. B. Coursin, eds.), Lippincott, New York, pp. 352–367.

Tsai, A. C., Mott, E. L., Owen, G. M., Bennick, M. R., Lo, G. S., and Steinke, F. H., 1983, Effects of soy polysaccharide on gastrointestinal functions, nutrient balance, steroid excretion, glucose tolerance, serum lipids and other parameters in humans, *Am. J. Clin. Nutr.* **38**:504–511.

Vahouny, G. V., 1981, Conclusions and recommendations of the symposium on "Dietary Fibers in Health and Disease," *Am. J. Clin. Nutr.* **35**:152–156.

Vestal, R. E., 1980, Methodological problems associated with studies of drug metabolism in the elderly, in: *First World Conference on Clinical Pharmacology and Therapeutics* (P. Turner, ed.), MacMillan, London, pp. 110–116.

Webster, S. G. P., and Leeming, J. T., 1975, The appearance of the small bowel mucosa in old age, *Age Aging* **4**:168–174.

Welling, P. G., 1977, Influence of food and diet on gastrointestinal absorption: A review, *J. Pharmacokinet. Biopharmaceut.* **5**:291–331.

Yearick, E. S., Wang, M. L., and Pisias, S. J., 1980, Nutritional status of the elderly: Dietary and biochemical findings, *J. Gerontol.* **35**:663–671.

Young, E. A., 1983, Nutrition, aging and the aged, *Med. Clin. North Am.* **67**(2):295.

Young, V. R., and Solomons, N. W., 1983, Nonnutrient factors in metabolism, in: *Manual of Clinical Nutrition* (D. M. Paige, ed.), Nutrition Publication, Pleasantville, New Jersey, pp. 3.1–3.11.

26

Constipation in Pregnancy Treated with Dumovital Fiber Tablets

ERIK GREGERSEN

More than 25% of all pregnant women in Denmark use some kind of laxative because of constipation. Instead of using special laxatives, we have been using Dumovital fiber tablets to treat and prevent constipation in pregnancy.

In a combined city/rural district in Denmark, 1128 pregnant women were consecutively asked to participate in the investigation in the period February 1980–August 1981. The investigation was performed as a double blind investigation with Dumovital fiber tablets and placebo. The fiber tablets had a fiber content of 0.27 g, with 80% fibers from grain and 20% from citrus. The dietary fiber content was 44%, whereas the placebo tablets contained 6% dietary fiber.

A total of 250 patients started the treatment, and 140 finished the investigation. Of those, 121 filled in the schedules correctly (Table I). No significant difference was found between the two groups. A total of 110 patients stopped treatment after shorter or longer time (Table II); there was no significant difference between the groups. The investigation was conducted during approximately weeks 20 and 36 of pregnancy, which was the period between the first and second control in the outpatient clinic of the department. The patients daily filled in a schedule with questions concerning intake of food, medicine, and laxatives and questions concerning defecation. No resorption studies were performed.

ERIK GREGERSEN • Department of Gynecology and Obstetrics, Sct. Maria Hospital, 7100 Vejle, Denmark.

TABLE I. Number of Patients Completing Treatment

	Fiber tablet	Placebo	Total
Correctly filled in schedules	64	57	121
Patients without control period	5	4	9
Patients using too few tablets	5	5	10
Total completed	74	66	140

The results were collected in 2-week periods. The first 2 weeks were a controlled period without treatment; the treatment started with three tablets daily the first week, six tablets daily next week, and nine tablets daily during the remaining 12 weeks of treatment. A total of about 2.5 g of fiber was given daily. The cautious beginning was chosen because of the possibility of colic and flatulence at the start of treatment. Based on other investigations, nine tablets were estimated to be a suitable daily dose. The patients were recommended to drink water with the tablets and were also informed that the effect of the tablets was like that of fiber-rich food. If medicine or laxatives were used, this was registered in the schedules. Since fiber tablets may be used in the treatment of overweight, the weight gain during pregnancy was also registered.

There was a significant increase in bowel movements in both groups, with a significantly higher increase in the fiber tablet group. There was no significant difference between the two groups in the period without treatment (Fig. 1).

TABLE II. Period of Treatment

	Number of patients		Total
	Fiber tablet	Placebo	
Period of treatment			
About 1 month	27	15	42
About 2 months	22	20	42
About 3 months	10	16	26
Number of patients not completing treatment	59	51	110
Number of patients completing treatment (see Table I)	74	66	140
Total	133	117	250

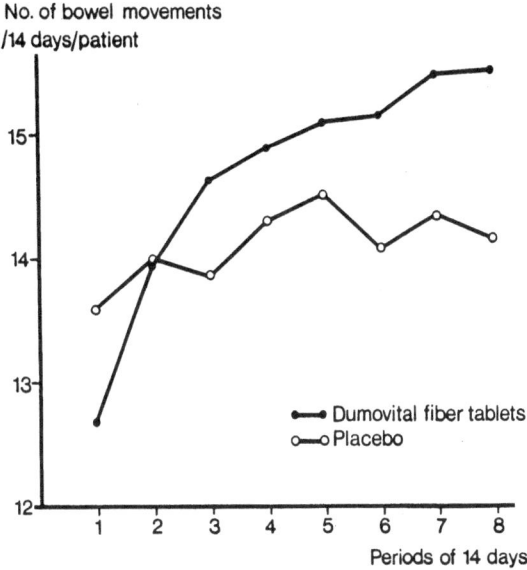

FIGURE 1. Number of bowel movements.

The number of "constipations" shows a significant fall in both groups (Fig. 2), most pronounced in the fiber tablet group, but the difference is not significant.

The reasons for stopping treatment are shown in Table III. A total of 22 out of 51 (43.1%) in the placebo group and nine out of 59 (14.1%) in the fiber tablet group stopped treatment because of lack of effect. The difference is statistically significant. The other reasons for stopping treatment did not show any significant difference between the groups.

There was no statistically significant difference in weight gain or in birth weight in the two groups (Table IV).

The frequency of complications at delivery showed no significant differences, and there were no differences in diagnoses or number of caesarean sections between the two groups (Table V). No deaths occurred.

The increased number of bowel movements during treatment may be troublesome in some patients, and some patients stopped treatment because of diarrhea. Ten patients who completed treatment (five in each group) had taken fewer tablets than planned because the effect was found to be sufficient with those fewer tablets (Table I). Thus the number of tablets necessary probably varies with the individual.

The effect in the placebo group may be explained by the significantly larger number of patients in this group stopping treatment because of lack of

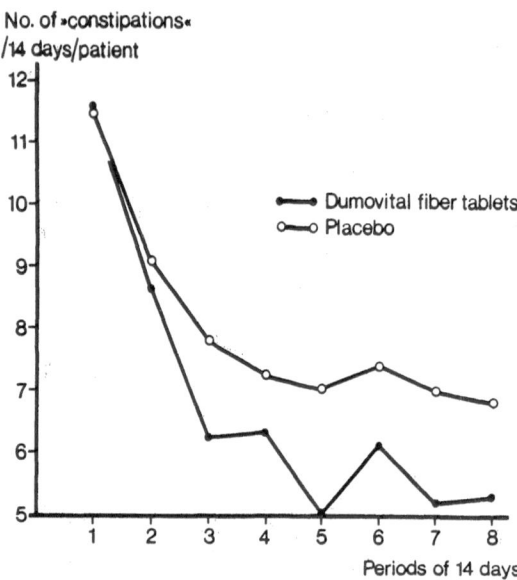

FIGURE 2. Number of constipations (formed stools and/or missing bowel movements).

effect. This was most pronounced in those patients who stopped treatment after a short time. Patients in the fiber tablet group who stopped treatment after a short time had an almost too good effect of the treatment (Fig. 3).

Since there is a small content of fiber in the placebo tablets, this might partly explain the expected placebo effect. The increased intake of water and the information of the effect of fiber-rich food also might have been of some importance.

The patients were not informed of the possible use of fiber tablets in order to lose weight. No differences in weight gain were found between the two groups.

The conclusion is that treatment with fiber tablets increases the number of bowel movements and thus reduces the tendency toward constipation in pregnancy.

SUMMARY

In a randomized double blind investigation of the effect of Dumovital fiber tablets on constipation in pregnancy 121 women were treated with nine

TABLE III. Reasons for Stopping Treatment

	Fiber tablet	Placebo	Total
Number of tablets unacceptably high	6	2	8
Lack of effect	9	22	31
Lack of control period and insufficiently filled in schedules	14	10	24
Colic/diarrhea	8	2	10
Premature labor/abortion	2	2	4
Unexplained	20	13	33
Total	59	51	110

TABLE IV. Weight of Mother and Child

	Fiber tablet	Placebo
Number	63[a]	57
Average weight increase of pregnant patients, kg	7.48	7.24
Average birth weight, kg	3.400	3.410

[a] One patient could not be found because of emigration.

TABLE V. Complications in Pregnancy and at Delivery[a]

	Fiber tablet	Placebo
Contractions absent or reduced	14	10
Fetopelvic disproportion	5 (4)	3 (1)
Threatening death of the child	2	5
Dysfunction of the placenta	0	3 (1)
Toxemia	0	3 (1)
Breech presentation and other abnormal presentations	6 (6)	1 (1)
Total	27 (10)	25 (4)

[a] Parentheses indicate number of caesarean sections.

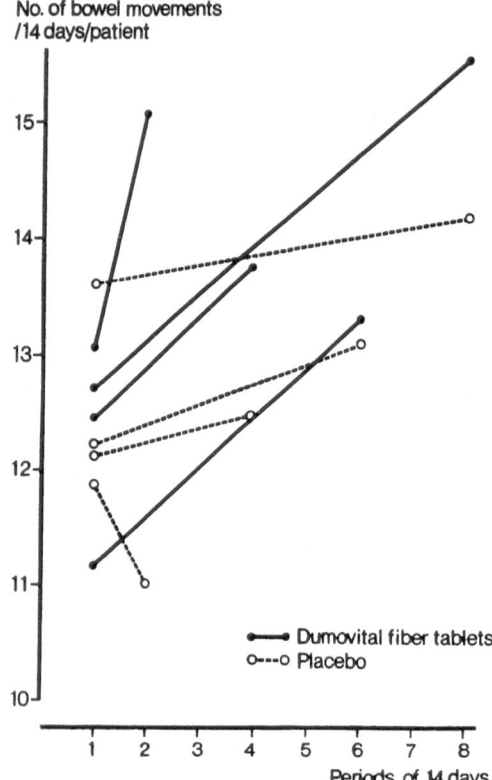

FIGURE 3. Number of bowel movements for those who stopped treatment.

tablets daily (2.5 g) in the period between weeks 20 and 36 of pregnancy after a control period of 2 weeks. The treatment group consisted of 46 patients, the placebo group of 57. A statistically significant increase in number of bowel movements was found in the fiber tablet group compared with the placebo group.

27

Fiber and Duodenal Ulcer

ANDREAS RYDNING and ARNOLD BERSTAD

1. INTRODUCTION

In spite of the widespread use of diets in patients with duodenal ulcer disease, our knowledge of the therapeutic effect of such diets is rather limited. Dietary treatment is based on the belief that small, bland meals might reduce the secretion of acid and pepsin, buffer the acid secreted into the stomach, reduce the gastric motor activity, and maintain the resistance of the gastric mucosa (Roth, 1966). The clinical value of this traditional low-fiber diet has never been documented (Doll *et al.*, 1956). It has been suggested that the refinement of staple carbohydrate foods may be the major etiologic factor accounting for the rising incidence of duodenal ulcer in Western countries during the present century (Cleave, 1962, 1974). In the last few years, therefore, there has been an increasing interest in the study of the possible relationship between the diet and the development of duodenal ulcer as well as the possible therapeutic effect of a staple, high-fiber diet (Malhotra, 1978; Rydning *et al.*, 1982).

2. PREVIOUS STUDIES

2.1. Effects on Gastric Function

Tovey (1974) found that wheat or rice bran and certain unrefined grains do have a greater buffer capacity than do refined carbohydrate foods such as polished rice and white flour. According to Tovey (1974), the staple foods were strong antral stimulants, resulting in an increased output of acid into

ANDREAS RYDNING and ARNOLD BERSTAD • Department of Medicine, Lovisenberg Hospital, Oslo 4, Norway.

the stomach. Only when the buffering effects exceed the stimulus to greater acid output will there be a fall in acid concentration. In practice, however, the quantity of buffer consumed in staple food diets would not reach this level (Tovey, 1974). Lennard-Jones et al. (1968) compared meals with a high and low protein content and found that the acidity of the gastric contents tended to be lowered for a longer period of time after a high-protein meal. However, in the experiments performed there was little difference in protein content between white and whole meal (whole wheat) bread. It is therefore not known which constituents of the high-protein meal may cause this effect; one possibility could be in difference in fiber contents.

Tovey (1974) did not find that bran and unrefined grains inhibited pepsin activity in vitro.

Distension of the stomach will increase acid output. Calloway et al. (1982) found that patients with duodenal ulcer had a rate of spontaneous swallowing four times greater than in the control group. If large quantities of air are swallowed, bloating and distension will result. A diet high in fiber, which shortens the total gut transit time, may enable air to pass more rapidly through the intestines and therefore cause less distension and acid output.

Several studies show a delayed gastric emptying after meals containing large doses of guar gum or pectin. Lawaetz et al. (1983) gave 10.5 g pectin in glucose solution to four patients with dumping symptoms and two healthy volunteers. While the initial fraction emptied from the stomach in dumping patients was reduced, pectin had no effect on gastric emptying in two healthy volunteers. Holt et al. (1979) studied gastric emptying in eight volunteers and gave 400 ml orange juice containing 16 g guar gum and 10 g pectin. Gastric emptying was slowed down after addition of gel fiber. In a chronic experiment, several subjects receiving a low-fiber diet containing 3 g total dietary fiber per day were given an isocaloric diet supplemented with 20 g apple pectin per day for 4 weeks (Schwartz et al., 1982). Gastric emptying half-time was prolonged approximately twofold and returned to normal 3 weeks after discontinuing the pectin supplementation. In all these studies on gastric emptying, large and unphysiological doses of gel fiber were used. Grimes and Goddard (1977) reported that liquid left the stomach significantly more rapidly with white bread than with whole meal bread. Since the difference in protein content was rather small and hardly can explain the differences in results, one may again ask if the differences seen can be explained by differences in fiber content.

Both through geographic surveys as well as through experimental work on animal models, Tovey et al. (1975) found that there is strong evidence that a liposoluble factor is present in wheat bran and certain other high-fiber foods that protects against duodenal ulceration. Since there are areas in the world with a high incidence of duodenal ulcer in the presence of a high dietary intake of fiber in the population (Tovey and Tunstall, 1975; Tovey, 1979), it has been postulated by Jayaraj *et al.* (1976) that there may be a protective factor affecting mucosal resistance in some high-fiber foods but not in others.

2.2. Effects in Ulcer Patients

Several studies have been published comparing a bland, fiber-poor diet to a normal diet (Doll *et al.*, 1956; Truelove, 1960; Buchman *et al.*, 1969). No difference between the dietary groups was found with regard to symptoms and ulcer healing.

Nafstad *et al.* (1967), Nafstad and Tollersrud (1967), and Nafstad (1967) have reviewed some of the nutritional factors of pathogenic importance in the development of gastric ulcers in swine. In a series of experiments they showed that pigs kept on a diet consisting of casein, sugar, potato starch, and unsaturated fatty acids developed gastric ulcers at high incidence. Inclusion of soybean meal in the ration markedly reduced the number of ulcers. A coarsely ground soybean meal gave better protection against development of ulcers than a finely ground one with smaller particle size and lower content of crude fibers (Baustad and Nafstad, 1969). A diet including 5 or 10% meal of coarsely ground barley straw offered full protection against the development of gastric ulcers. The finely ground straw gave no protection as compared to the basal ration.

Malhotra (1978) found that the relapse rate for duodenal ulcer was significantly lower in patients eating unrefined wheat compared to their previous rice diet. He attributes the effect of a staple high-fiber diet to the increased mastication required, which is associated with an increase in saliva, lower stomach acidity, and reduced bile output. Malhotra *et al.* (1965) made the interesting discovery that in cases where saliva was withheld from food entering the stomach, the gastric juice was almost devoid of mucus. Furthermore, a high concentration of mucus was found in the gastric juice when the food eaten required thorough mastication compared to food swallowed without the same need for masticaiton.

3. STUDIES IN THIS LABORATORY

3.1. Prophylactic Effect of a High-Fiber Diet

Rydning *et al.* (1982) carried out a duodenal ulcer relapse study in which 73 patients with a recently healed duodenal ulcer were randomly allocated to a diet high or low in fiber. The two groups were comparable with respect to smoking and previous treatment given (placebo, antacids,

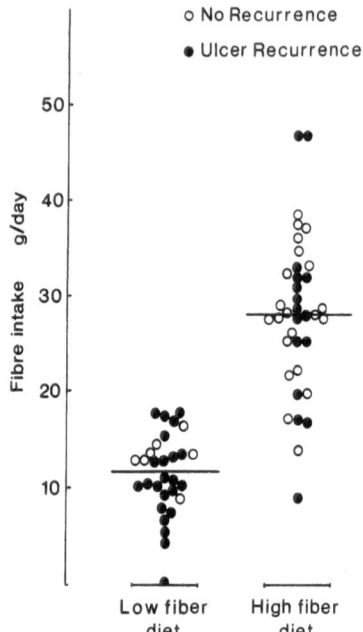

FIGURE 1. Individual dietary fiber intake (g/day) in patients on a low- and a high-fiber diet (median values marked with lines). (From Rydning *et al.*, 1982.)

ranitidine). Ulcer recurrence was studied for a period of 6 months. Patients on a high-fiber diet were asked to eat bread rich in fiber as well as additional sources of fiber, such as porridge made from unrefined flour, vegetables, and fruit. The patients on the low-fiber diet were asked to eat white bread and avoid or reduce other sources of fiber mentioned. The food eaten was recorded daily for 1 week every month during the 6-month follow-up period. The total dietary fiber intake was recorded from a table published by South-

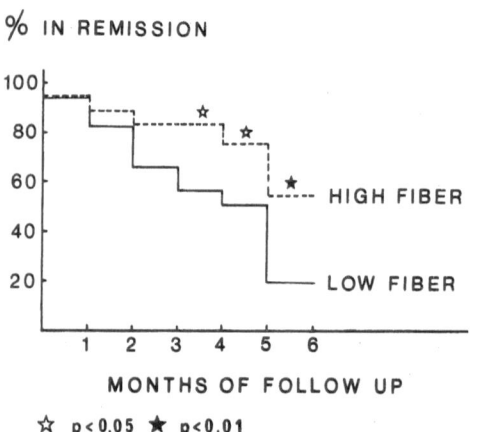

FIGURE 2. Percentage of duodenal ulcer patients in remission during the 6-month follow-up period on a high- or low-fiber diet. (From Rydning *et al.*, 1982.)

gate *et al.* (1976). The median fiber intake in the patients' pretreatment food was 16.2 g/day. During the trial the high-fiber group increased their fiber intake to a median of 28.2 g/day (range 8.9–46.7 g/day, $p < 0.001$), while the low-fiber group decreased their median uptake to 11.4 g/day (range 0–17.7 g/day, $p < 0.001$) (Fig. 1).

During the 6-month follow-up period, ulcer recurrence was found in 28 (80%) of the 35 patients in the group on a low-fiber diet, compared to 17 (45%) of the 38 patients in the group on a high-fiber diet ($p < 0.01$) (Fig. 2). Ulcer recurrence was more frequent in smokers than in nonsmokers ($p < 0.01$). The high-fiber diet was of benefit to both smokers and nonsmokers and the observed differences in ulcer recurrence rate cannot be explained by differences in smoking habits. In conclusion, a diet rich in fiber may protect against relapse of duodenal ulceration. Recurrent ulcers were found at all levels of fiber intake and there was no "dose–response" relationship. One cannot be certain that the fiber itself actually exerts the beneficial effect, and it may be that a diet poor in fiber is unfavorable rather than that a high-fiber diet is of benefit.

3.2. Healing Effect of a High-Fiber Diet

Whether a high-fiber diet would be beneficial in patients with active duodenal ulceration is not known. We have therefore started a clinical trial to investigate the effect of a high-fiber diet compared to a low-fiber diet in patients with duodenal ulceration. The patients are also given antacid tablets, four Link® tablets (Apothekernes Laboratorium, Norway) per day containing a codried gel of aluminum hydroxide and magnesium carbonate and with a neutralizing capacity of 20 mmol HCl per tablet. So far 60 patients out of a total of 80 have been included. Our preliminary data show that there is a higher healing rate in the high- compared to the low-fiber group, but this difference is not statistically significant.

3.3. Mechanisms of Action

3.3.1. *In vitro* Studies

The experiments were carried out with a fiber-enriched wheat bran product, Fiberform® (Tricum AB, Höganäs, Sweden), consisting of 78% fiber (w/w), 7% protein (w/w), and 8% lipid-soluble material (w/w) as well as 0.57 mg phytic acid/g, and a gel-forming fiber product, Guarem® (Orion Corp., Remeda Pharmaceutical, Kuopio, Finland), a guar gum. The fiber products were added to gastric juice.

3.3.1a. Effects on Acidity. A small increase in pH and a slight reduction in titratable hydrogen ion concentration were seen in the gastric juice with

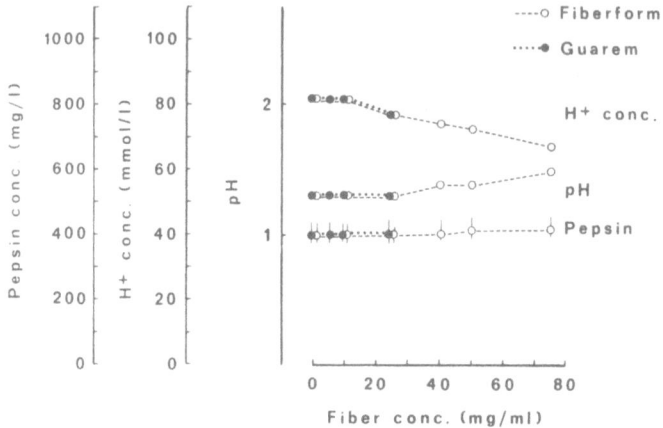

FIGURE 3. The effect of increasing fiber concentration on pH, titratable acid (hydrogen ion concentration), and pepsin concentration in gastric juice. (From Rydning and Berstad, 1984.)

higher amounts of fiber-enriched wheat bran added (Fig. 3). Titratable hydrogen ion concentration was not influenced by guar gum in the concentrations that were possible to test.

3.3.1b. Effects on Pepsin. Pepsin in gastric juice was not influenced by either of the fiber products tested (Fig. 3).

3.3.1c. Effects on Bile Acids. Both fiber products bound bile acids (Fig. 4). The amount of fiber bound by fiber-enriched wheat bran was almost linearly related to the amount added. Guar gum bound less bile acid per unit

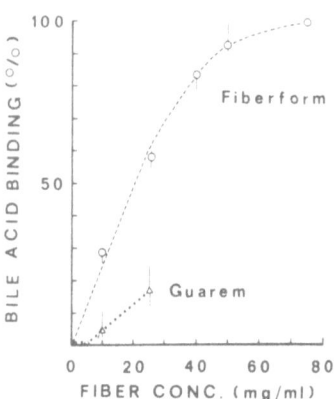

FIGURE 4. The effect of increasing fiber concentration on binding of bile acid (median values). (From Rydning and Berstad, 1984.)

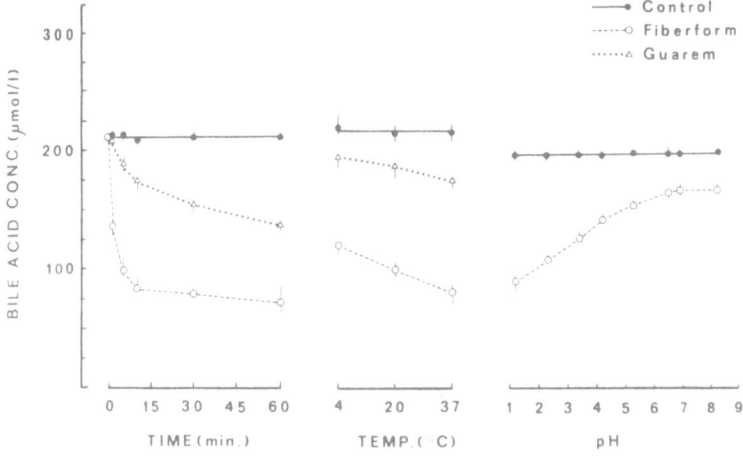

FIGURE 5. The influence of time, temperature, and pH on the bile acid binding by fiber (From Rydning and Berstad, 1984.)

weight than the fiber-enriched wheat bran product. The binding was rapid with both types of fiber and influenced by time, temperature, and pH of the incubation mixture, as shown in Fig. 5. Both fiber products bound more bile acids at 37°C than at 4°C. The amount of bile acid bound by the fiber-enriched wheat bran was pronounced at low pH, i.e., at pH 1.0–3.0 (Fig. 5). Due to gel formation it was impossible to obtain a reproducible pH curve for guar gum.

Fiber-enriched wheat bran was added to 40 samples of gastric juice obtained in 20 consecutive patients examined with a routine pentagastrin test for various reasons. Bile acid concentrations were reduced in all but four samples, which did not contain any bile acid. In the basal samples the bile acid concentrations were reduced from 97 μmol/liter (median value; range 7–4846 μmol/liter) to 55 μmol/liter (range 0–4343 μmol/liter) and in the stimulated samples from 28 μmol/liter (range 0–1171 μmol/liter) to 8 μmol/liter (range 0–839 μmol/liter) (Fig. 6). The binding varied with pH and bile acid concentration. The percent bile acid bound was higher at low than at high pH and the absolute amount of bile acids bound increased with increasing bile acid concentration (Fig. 7). There was no correlation between pH and bile acid concentration before addition of fiber-enriched wheat bran. The bile acid was partly reversed by alkalization (Florèn and Nilsson, 1982; Rydning and Berstad, 1984) and by adding a 6 M urea (Florèn and Nilsson, 1982). The binding is a combination of hydrophobic and hydrophilic interactions (Florèn and Nilsson, 1982).

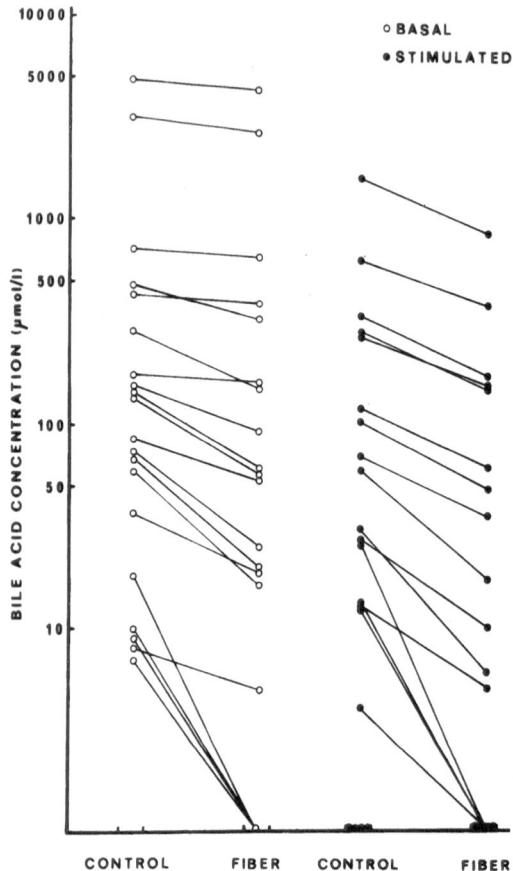

FIGURE 6. The effect of fiber-enriched wheat bran on bile acid concentration in 40 gastric juice samples obtained from 20 consecutive patients admitted for routine pentagastrin test (20 samples collected under basal conditions and 20 after pentagastrin stimulation). The pH range was 1.2–7.1 for the basal samples and 1.0–1.4 for the stimulated samples. A total of 125 mg Fiberform® was added to 5 ml gastric juice and incubated 10 min at 37°C. (From Rydning and Berstad, 1984.)

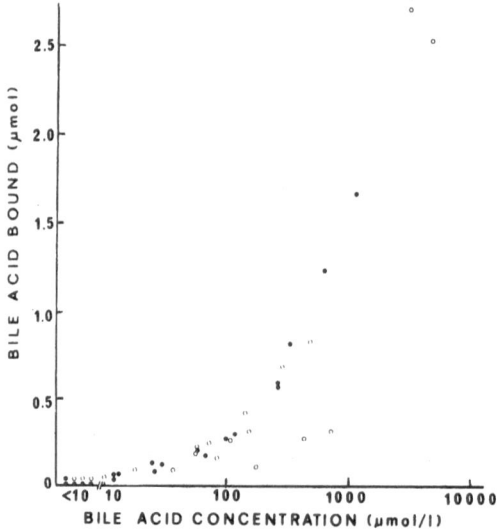

FIGURE 7. The influence of bile acid concentration on bile acid binding by fiber-enriched wheat bran. (O): Basal samples. (●): Stimulated samples. (From Rydning and Berstad, 1984.)

3.3.2. *In Vivo* Studies

The effects of fiber-enriched wheat bran and guar gum on postprandial intragastric juice acidity, pepsin, and bile acid concentrations were studied in ten healthy volunteers. On three different occasions they were given a meal consisting of wheatmeal (whole wheat) porridge and juice alone or with either 10.5 g Fiberform® or 5 g Guarem® added to the porridge. The meals were given in random order. After 12 h fasting, a nasogastric tube was inserted and placed in the most dependent part of the stomach by fluoroscopic control. After emptying the stomach, 5-ml aliquots of gastric content were withdrawn at 10-min intervals for 4 h and 50 min. The contents of available carbohydrates, protein, and fat as well as the caloric value of the meals were almost identical (Rydning *et al.*, 1984).

3.3.2a. Effects on Acidity. Following the porridge containing Fiberform®, the pH rose to a significantly lower peak value (pH 4) than after the control meal, but the elevation lasted significantly longer (Fig. 8) (approximately 30 min longer). With guar gum the pH curve was significantly different from the control, reaching a lower peak value and shortening the acid-neutralizing effect of the meal (pH elevation lasted approximately 20 min shorter than without fiber). The acid rebound effect was apparently of the same magnitude with all three types of meals (Fig. 9). The change in profile of the postprandial intragastric pH curve is probably not due to the neutralizing effect of fiber-enriched wheat bran, since *in vitro* this is modest

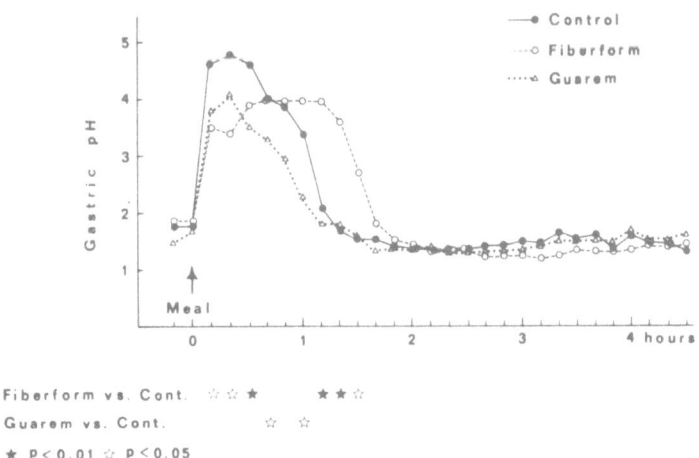

FIGURE 8. The effect of three different meals on intragastric pH (median values) in ten healthy volunteers. Meals consist of (1) wheatmeal porridge with juice (control), (2) meal 1 + 10.5 g fiber-enriched wheat bran, Fiberform®, and (3) meal 1 + 5 g guar gum, Guarem®. (From Rydning *et al.*, 1985.)

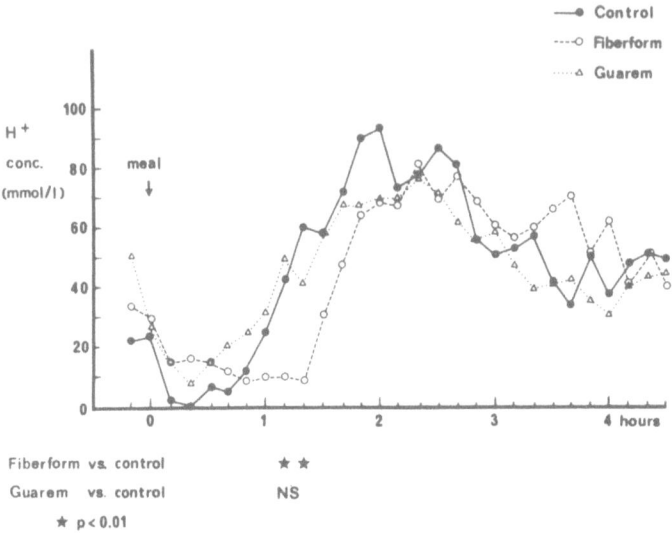

FIGURE 9. The effect of three different meals (see Fig. 8) on intragastric hydrogen ion concentration (median values) in ten healthy volunteers. (From Rydning *et al.*)

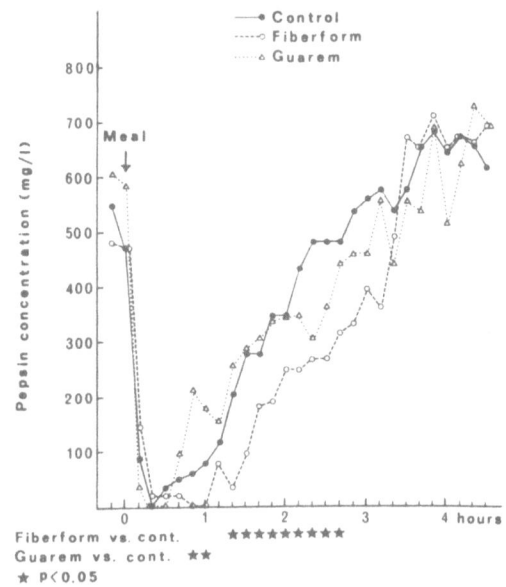

FIGURE 10. The effect of three different meals (see Fig. 8) on intragastric pepsin concentration (median values) in ten healthy volunteers. (From Rydning *et al.*)

Fiberform® neutralizes approximately 2.1 mmol acid). The mechanism for this effect is not known.

3.3.2b. Effects on Pepsin. Fiberform® significantly prolonged the meal-induced decrease in pepsin concentration for a considerable time (significant for 90 min) (Fig. 10). The reason for this reduction in pepsin concentration *in vivo* is not known, since pepsin is not inhibited by fiber *in vitro*. If Fiberform® in some way increases the amount of fluid present within the stomach, a reduction in pepsin concentration due to dilution could occur. Another theoretical but less likely explanation for the reduced pepsin concentration could be a fiber-induced inhibition of pepsin secretion. With Guarem® only small differences compared to the control was seen.

3.3.2c. Effects on Bile Acids. Both meals containing additional fiber lowered bile acid concentrations significantly for a considerable period of time (60–140 min) as compared to the meal poor in fiber (Fig. 11). Mean bile acid concentration during the whole postprandial period ($4\frac{1}{2}$ h) were significantly lower with both fiber-enriched wheat bran (74 μmol/liter) ($p < 0.01$) and guar gum (82.5 μmol/liter) ($p < 0.05$) compared to the control experiments (165 μmol/liter) (Fig. 12). These findings are of potential clinical significance and may be important where regurgitated bile is thought to cause mucosal damage (Kalima, 1982; Rhodes *et al.*, 1969).

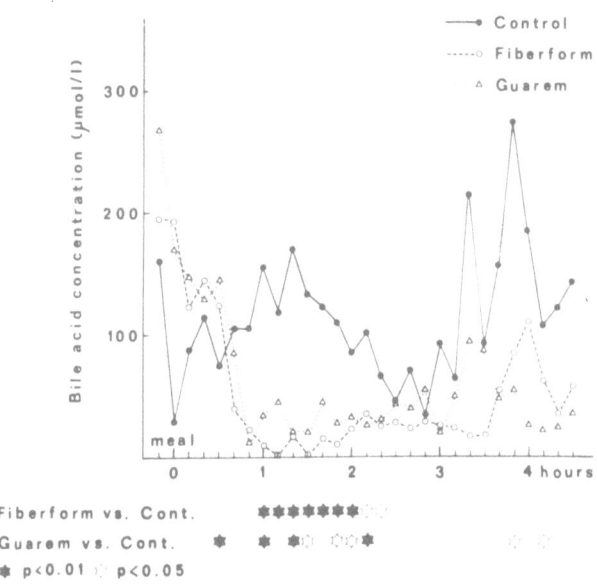

FIGURE 11. The effect of three different meals (see Fig. 8) on bile acid concentration (median values) in ten healthy volunteers. (From Rydning *et al.*,1985.)

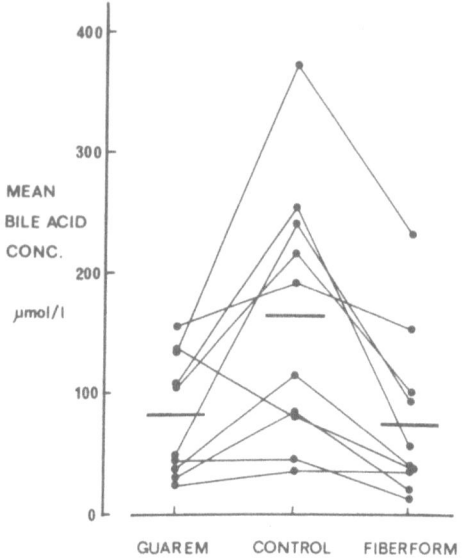

FIGURE 12. Mean bile acid concentration in ten healthy volunteers during the whole 4½-h test period after ingestion of a meal without fiber (control); a meal with 5 g guar gum, Guarem®; or a meal with 10.5 g fiber-enriched wheat bran, Fiberform®, added. Individual values are connected with a line. Mean values for each group are shown with horizontal lines.

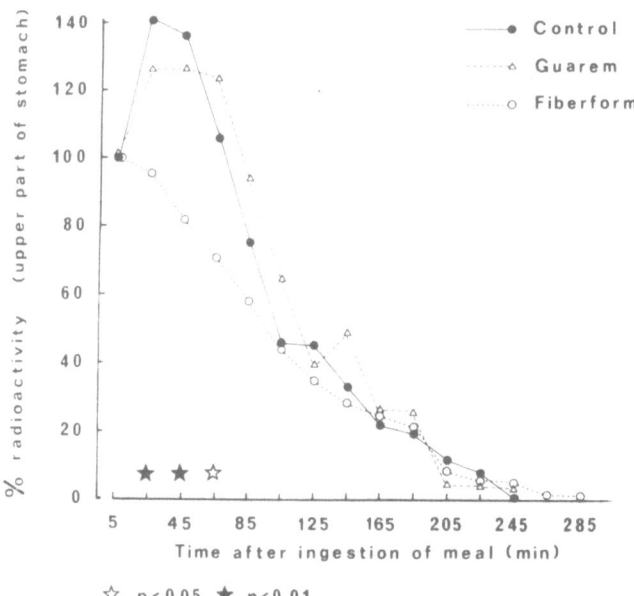

FIGURE 13. The effect of guar gum, Guarem®, 5 g, and fiber-enriched wheat bran, Fiberform®, 10.5 g, on gastric emptying of an isotope-labeled meal as measured by a simple Pitman localization monitor placed over the upper part of the stomach. Mean values in ten healthy volunteers.

3.4. The Influence of Fiber on Gastric Emptying

The effect of 10.5 g Fiberform® and 5 g Guarem® on gastric emptying
has been studied both by a simple isotope detector placed over the upper
part of the abdomen and by gamma camera. The fiber preparations were
added to wheatmeal porridge containing ^{99}Tc-DTPA (diethylenetriamine
pentaacetic acid). Ten healthy volunteers were tested with the simple fundus
isotope detector and eight volunteers were tested with the gamma camera.
With the simple upper abdominal isotope detector an elevation in isotope
activity was seen 25 min postprandially (Fig. 13) for the porridge alone and
for the meal containing guar gum. This difference in isotope activity between
the three meals was not seen with the gamma camera. We therefore think
that the difference in results seen with the simple registration method is due
to differences in distribution of the meals within the stomach in such a way
that the control and Guarem®-containing meals accumulate in the fundic
part of the stomach during the first 60 min after meal ingestion. Neither the
simple isotope registration method nor the gamma camera (Fig. 14) showed
any differences in total gastric emptying time among the three meals given.
The reason we did not confirm previous findings of a prolonged gastric
emptying time using gel fiber may be due to the fact that we employed
smaller and more physiological doses of gel fiber than had been tested
previously.

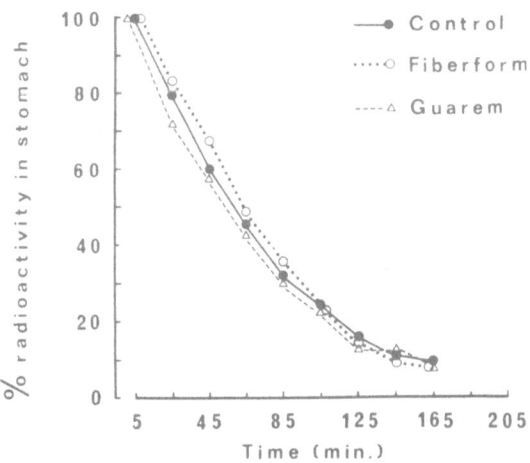

FIGURE 14. The effect of guar gum, Guarem®, 5 g, and fiber-enriched wheat bran,
Fiberform®, 10.5 g, on gastric emptying of an isotope-labeled meal in eight healthy
volunteers using the gamma camera (mean values). No significant differences are seen
among meals.

Having seen that fiber-enriched wheat bran significantly prolonged postprandial pH elevation and reduced pepsin concentrations while there was very little influence on these parameters *in vitro,* we wanted to see if the effect of gastric emptying could explain this discrepency between *in vivo* and *in vitro* results. The conclusion from this study is that fiber in the doses used does not influence gastric emptying and consequently the results cannot explain our previous findings. Whether the observed effect of Fiberform® on the distribution of the meal within the stomach may have any bearing on our previous results is not known.

4. CONCLUSION

A diet rich in fiber has been of value in the prevention of duodenal ulceration. Such a diet is not significantly better than a diet poor in fiber in the treatment of active ulcers. Fiber-enriched wheat bran and guar gum bind bile acids effectively both *in vitro* and *in vivo. In vivo,* fiber-enriched wheat bran reduced postprandial pepsin concentrations for a considerable period of time and the profile of the postprandial pH curve was changed to a lower peak value but showed a longer lasting pH elevation. The mechanisms for the effects on pepsin and acidity *in vivo* are not known. The applied doses of fiber did not affect the gastric emptying of the wheatmeal porridge in healthy volunteers. In addition to the effects on acid and pepsin, the pronounced binding of bile acids by both fiber products may be of clinical importance in conditions where regurgitated bile is thought to cause mucosal damage (Kalima, 1982; Rhodes *et al.,* 1969).

REFERENCES

Baustad, B., and Nafstad, I., 1969, Gastric ulcers in swine. 4. Effects of dietary particle size and crude fiber contents on ulceration, *Pathol. Vet.* **6:**546–556.

Buchman, E., Kaung, D. T., Dolan, K., and Nash Knapp, R., 1969, Unrestricted diet in the treatment of duodenal ulcer, *Gastroenterology* **56:**1016–1020.

Calloway, S. P., Fonagby, P., and Pounder, R. F., 1982, Frequency of swallowing in duodenal ulceration and hiatus hernia, *Br. Med. J.* **285:**23–24.

Cleave, T. L., 1962, *Peptic Ulcer,* Wright, Bristol.

Cleave, T. L., 1974, *The Saccharine Disease,* Wright, Bristol.

Doll, R., Friedlander, P., and Pygott, F., 1956, Dietetic treatment of peptic ulcer, *Lancet* **1:**5–9.

Florèn, C. H., and Nilsson, Å., 1982, Binding of bile salts to fibre-enriched wheat bran, *Clin. Nutr.* **36C:**381–389.

Grimes, D. S., and Goddard, J., 1977, Gastric emptying of wholemeal and white bread, *Gut* **18:**725–729.

Holt, S., Heading, R. C., Carter, D. C., Prescott, L. F., and Tothill, P., 1979, Effect of gel fibre on gastric emptying and absorption of glucose and paracetamol, *Lancet* **1:**636–639.

Jayaraj, A. P., Tovey, F. I., and Clark, C. G., 1976, The possibility of dietary protective factors in duodenal ulcer. II. An investigation into the effect of prefeeding with different diets and of instillation of foodstuffs into the stomach on the incidence of ulcers in pylorus-ligated rats, *Postgrad. Med. J.* **52**:645–650.

Kalima, T. V., 1982, Reflux gastritis unrelated to gastric surgery, in: Non-Ulcer Dyspepsia (A. Walan, ed.), *Scand. J. Gastroenterol.* **17** (suppl. 79):66–71.

Lawaetz, O, Blackburn, A. M., Bloom, S. R., Aritas, Y. and Ralphs, D. N. L., 1983, Effect of pectin on gastric emptying and gut hormone release in the dumping syndrome, *Scand. J. Gastroenterol.* **18**:327–336.

Lennard-Jones, J. E., Fletcher, J., and Shaw, D. G., 1968, Effect of different foods on the acidity of the gastric contents in patients with duodenal ulcer, *Gut* **9**:177–182.

Malhotra, S. L., 1978, A comparison of unrefined wheat and rice diets in the management of duodenal ulcer, *Postgrad. Med. J.* **54**:6–9.

Malhotra, S. L., Saigal, O. N., and Mody, G. D., 1965, Role of saliva in the aetiology of peptic ulcer, *Brit. Med. J.* **1**:1220–1222.

Nafstad, I., 1967, Gastric ulcers in swine. 1. Effect of dietary protein, dietary fat and vitamin E on ulcer development, *Pathol. Vet.* **4**:1–14.

Nafstad, I., and Trollersrud, S., 1967, Gastric ulcers in swine. 2. Effects of high fat diets and vitamin E on ulcer development, *Pathol. Vet.* **4**:15–22.

Nafstad, I., Tollersrud, S., and Baustad, B., 1967, Gastric ulcers in swine. 3. Effect of different proteins and fats on their development, *Pathol. Vet.* **4**:23–30.

Rhodes, J., Barnardo, D. E., Phillips, S. F., Rovelstad, R. A., and Hofmann, A. F., 1969, Increased reflux of bile into the stomach in patients with gastric ulcer, *Gastroenterology* **57**:241–252.

Roth, J. L. A., 1966, The ulcer patient should watch his diet, in: *Controversy in internal Medicine* (F. J. Ingelfinger, A. S. Relman, and M. Finland, eds.), W. B. Saunders, Philadelphia, pp. 161–170.

Rydning, A., and Berstad, A., 1984 Infuence of fiber on acidity, pepsin and bile acids in human gastric juice *in vitro, Scand. J. Gastroenterol.* **19**:953–959.

Rydning, A., Berstad, A., Aadland, E, and Ødegaard, B., 1982, Prophylactic effect of dietary fibre in duodenal ulcer disease, *Lancet* **2**:736–738.

Rydning, A., Nesland, A., and Berstad, A., 1984, Influence of fiber on postprandial intragastric juice acidity, pepsin and bile acids in healthy subjects, *Scand. J. Gastroenterol.* **19**:1039–1044.

Schwartz, S. E., Levine, R. A., Singh, A., Scheidecker, J. R., and Track, N. S., 1982, Sustained pectin ingestion delays gastric emptying, *Gastroenterology* **83**:812–817.

Southgate, D. A. T., Bailey, B., Collinson, E., Walker, A. F., 1976, A guide to calculating intakes of dietary fibre, *J. Hum. Nutr.* **30**:303–313.

Tovey, F. I., 1974, Aetiology of duodenal ulcer: An investigation into the buffering action and effect on pepsin of bran and unrefined carbohydrate foods, *Postgrad. Med. J.* **50**:683–688.

Tovey, F. I., 1979, Peptic ulcer in India and Bangladesh, *Gut* **20**:329–347.

Tovey, F. I., and Tunstall, M., 1975, Duodenal ulcer in black populations in Africa south of the Sahara, *Gut* **16**:564–576.

Tovey, F. I., Jayaraj, A. P., and Clark, C. G., 1975, The possibility of dietary protective factors in duodenal ulcer, *Postgrad. Med. J.* **51**:366–372.

Truelove, S. C., 1960, Stilbestrol, phenobarbitone, and diet in chronic duodenal ulcer, *Br. Med. J.* **2**:559–566.

28

Gallstones

K. W. HEATON

1. INTRODUCTION

Cholelithiasis is one of the commonest diseases of the Western world, affecting 30–60% of women and half that number of men during their lifetime (Heaton, 1981). About three-quarters of these gallstones are composed mainly of crystalline cholesterol, as the monohydrate (Sutor and Wooley, 1971). The fundamental biochemical abnormality leading to the precipitation of cholesterol from bile is the secretion of bile supersaturated with cholesterol, that is, bile containing more cholesterol than can be solubilized by the detergent system in bile, consisting of mixed micelles of bile acids and lecithin (Bouchier, 1983). It has been known for some years that many people have supersaturated bile but remain free of gallstones, suggesting that bile needs to contain nucleating factors in order for crystallization to occur. Now it appears that the gallbladder bile of patients with gallstones does contain a potent nucleating factor (Burnstein *et al.*, 1983) and that this substance (or substances) is absent from nongallstone patients, however supersaturated their bile (Kesäniemi and Grundy, 1983). Antinucleating factors may well be important, too, and there is evidence that apoproteins A-I and A-II may have this property (LaRusso, 1984). Research in this field is very active and major advances in understanding the pathogenesis of gallstones can be expected in the next few years.

Research into preventable, etiologic factors is also active. In particular, large ultrasonographic surveys of gallstone prevalence and associated risk factors including diet are being carried out in Rome, Sirmione (near Milan), Copenhagen, and Oxford. Data from these are not available at this time

K. W. HEATON • Department of Medicine, University of Bristol, and Bristol Royal Infirmary, Bristol BS2 8HW, United Kingdom.

(April 1984) but are expected soon. In the meantime, valuable information is emerging from a large and well-conducted case–control study from Adelaide. This is the first case–control study of gallstone patients that satisfies the criteria of modern epidemiology. It will be extensively quoted in this chapter. The other major source of information on dietary factors in gallstones is experimental studies, which have usually involved chemical analysis of gallbladder bile to determine its degree of saturation with cholesterol.

The role of diet in gallstones will be discovered only by combining information from all sources, epidemiologic and experimental, since no method of study is without limitations. For example, a case–control study may fail to identify a real dietary influence if the threshold intake at which this influence works is exceeded by nearly all the controls as well as the cases. Conversely, an experimental study may fail to register a real effect of a dietary factor if this factor operates slowly and the experiment is of short duration.

The role of diet in gallstones has been extensively reviewed (Heaton, 1984a), including a consideration of dietary fat and cholesterol as well as of dietary fiber and fiber-depleted foods. The present chapter will be concerned only with the last two factors, but this is not a major limitation, since the roles of fat and cholesterol are far from certain. Concerning dietary fiber, this chapter is based on the view that, to be logical, any discussion of the role of fiber must include a consideration of fiber-depleted foods (Cleave, 1974; Trowell *et al.*, 1985). These include sugars, especially sucrose. Thus the two questions to be answered are: (1) Do fiber-depleted foods, including sucrose, favor the formation of gallstones? (2) Does dietary fiber and/or a fiber-rich diet protect against gallstones? On present evidence the best answer to both questions is "Probably yes."

2. EXCESSIVE ENERGY INTAKE

There are strong arguments for the view that the regular consumption of fiber-depleted foods inflates the intake of energy above that obtained from "natural," whole or fiber-rich foods (Heaton, 1973, 1980). Indeed, when volunteers ate *ad libitum* of, alternately, fiber-rich and fiber-depleted foods, their mean energy intake was 28% higher on the fiber-depleted diet (Thornton *et al.*, 1983). This diet was rich in sucrose as well as poor in fiber and it seems to have been its sucrose content that was chiefly responsible for the energy difference, since, in a subsequent study comparing an *ad libitum* sucrose-rich diet with an *ad libitum* sucrose-poor one, the fiber intakes being similar, the same workers found a very similar difference in energy intake, namely 25% higher on the sucrose-rich diet (Werner *et al.*, 1984).

If it is accepted that consuming sucrose *per se* inflates energy intake, then any evidence that in sucrose-consuming communities, high-energy intake, or established obesity, increases the risk of gallstones can be logically taken as one piece of evidence that consuming sucrose increases the risk of gallstones.

The evidence linking gallstones with obesity is overwhelming and will not be rehearsed here. The association is believed to be explained by the fact that obese people almost invariably have gallbladder bile that is supersaturated with cholesterol during the overnight fast (Bennion and Grundy, 1978). Obese people have not necessarily eaten more than nonobese people, but their energy intake has undeniably been excessive for them.

Does increasing energy intake increase a person's chance of gallstones irrespective of obesity? The evidence is conflicting. In the study of sucrose-rich and sucrose-poor diets mentioned above (Werner *et al.*, 1984) there was no difference in the cholesterol saturation of gallbladder bile after 6 weeks on the two regimes, which suggests that, in the short term, a 25% increase in energy does not increase the risk of gallstones. On the other hand, in the Adelaide case–control study a habitually high-energy intake increased the relative risk of gallstones in young and middle-aged women and in young men, but not in older subjects of both sexes (Scragg *et al.*, 1984a). Thus, a high-energy intake may be lithogenic only if it is prolonged. The variations in susceptibility to high-energy intake with age and sex reported by Scragg *et al.* (1984a) have not been noted in earlier case–control studies, probably because they were all too small. The variations may help to explain the inconsistent results of earlier studies.

3. HYPERINSULINISM

Test meals of fiber-depleted sugars generally evoke greater insulin responses than meals of fiber-rich foods, including whole fruit (Haber *et al.*, 1977; Albrink *et al.*, 1979; Bolton *et al.*, 1981). On sucrose-rich diets some individuals develop high fasting plasma insulin levels (Reiser *et al.*, 1981). Disrupting the fibrous architecture of rice by grinding it into flour greatly increases its insulinogenicity (O'Dea *et al.*, 1980). For all these reasons, in a discussion of fiber and gallstones it is pertinent to ask if increased secretion of insulin increases the risk of gallstones.

The Adelaide case–control study is the only adequate epidemiologic study that has investigated the fasting plasma insulin levels of gallstone patients (Scragg *et al.*, 1984b). An elevation of 10 μU/ml in fasting plasma insulin increased the relative risk of gallstones by 1.9 in females and 2.1 in males (95% confidence limits 1.1–3.0 and 1.1–4.2, respectively). This finding was independent of obesity and of dietary intake.

This novel and important finding has a possible biochemical explanation. *In vitro,* insulin increases the activity in rat liver of the rate-limiting enzyme for cholesterol synthesis, β-hydroxymethyl-β-glutaryl CoA reductase (Neprokoeff *et al.,* 1974). Patients with cholesterol gallstones may have raised activity of this enzyme in their liver and most of them secrete excessive amounts of cholesterol into their bile (Bouchier, 1983). However, Thornton *et al.* (1980) found no correlation between the cholesterol saturation index of bile and the fasting or oral-glucose-stimulated levels of plasma insulin in 25 nonobese middle-aged women.

4. SUCROSE

That sucrose *could be* an etiologic factor in gallstones is suggested by the links already mentioned between gallstones and surplus energy intake and between gallstones and hyperinsulinism. Another suggestive link is the effect of sucrose upon *blood lipids.* It is well known that fasting plasma triglyceride concentrations rise with increased carbohydrate intake (Lewis, 1976) and especially with sucrose (Reiser *et al.,* 1978). In the study of Werner *et al.* (1984) plasma triglycerides were 0.98 mmol/liter on a sucrose intake of 16 g/day and 1.33 mmol/liter on an intake of 112 g/day. Hypertriglyceridemia is associated with a high incidence of cholesterol gallstones and with supersaturated gallbladder bile (Ahlberg *et al.,* 1979, 1980). Even in normolipidemic subjects there is a correlation between the plasma triglyceride concentration and the cholesterol saturation index of bile (Thornton *et al.,* 1981). In the Adelaide case–control study a 0.5 mmol/liter rise in the plasma triglyceride concentration doubled the relative risk of gallstones (Scragg *et al.,* 1984b).

Plasma high-density lipoprotein (HDL) cholesterol provides yet another possible link between sucrose and gallstones. Werner *et al.* (1984) found plasma HDL-cholesterol to be 9% lower on their high-sugar diet, an effect of sucrose reported previously only with excessively high intakes (Yudkin *et al.,* 1980). This is relevant because there is an inverse relationship between plasma HDL-cholesterol and the cholesterol saturation index of bile (Thornton *et al.,* 1981) and because people with low levels of HDL-cholesterol have an increased risk of gallstones (Petitti *et al.,* 1981; Scragg *et al.,* 1984b).

Direct evidence that sucrose promotes gallstones is scanty. Over 2- to 6-week periods the level of sucrose in the diet does not seem to affect the cholesterol saturation of gallbladder bile (Cahlin *et al.,* 1973; Andersén and Hellström, 1980; Werner *et al.,* 1984). However, these experimental periods may be too short if sucrose operates by promoting obesity or through some other slowly developing metabolic abnormality. The best direct evidence comes from the Adelaide case–control study (Scragg *et al.,* 1984a). These workers looked at total sugar intake, which consists mainly of refined sucrose in most people, and at sugar in drinks and sweets, which is all refined and is a large proportion of refined sugar intake. As shown in Table I, total sugar intakes were considerably higher in gallstone patients of both sexes under the age of 50, but were not significantly different over this age. On the other hand, sugar in drinks and sweets was higher in all groups of gallstone patients except older men. These findings with regard to sugar were the biggest and most consistent differences in any nutrient in the Adelaide study.

5. PROTECTIVE EFFECT OF DIETARY FIBER

The evidence that a high intake of dietary fiber protects against gallstones is of four kinds:

1. Low prevalence of the disease in groups eating a high-fiber diet.
2. Protection of laboratory animals against gallstones by fiber or fiber-rich foods.
3. Beneficial effect on human bile of a fiber-rich diet.
4. Beneficial effect on human bile of wheat bran.

5.1. Low Prevalence of Gallstones in Populations Eating a High-Fiber Diet

Accurate data on gallstone prevalence and dietary fiber intake are not available for a sufficient number of populations to enable mathematical relationships to be calculated. However, it is reasonably well substantiated that gallstones are rare throughout sub-Saharal Africa (Brett and Barker, 1976; Hcaton, 1981) and it is highly likely that in these regions dietary fiber intakes are very high, as judged by stool weights (Burkitt et al., 1972) and by limited dietary surveys (Bingham and Cummings, 1980).

Vegetarians eat about twice as much dietary fiber as the general population (Gear et al., 1979) and an ultrasonographic survey of vegetarians in Oxford has shown them to have half the expected prevalence of gallstones (Pixley et al., 1985). Vegetarians also have a reduced incidence of diverticular disease of the colon (Gear et al., 1979), a disease widely ascribed to a low-fiber intake and clearly associated with gallstones (Capron et al., 1981).

It must of course be admitted that there are other differences in lifestyle and diet between Africans and Westerners and between vegetarians and meat-eaters, but the data given above at least make it unlikely that there is *no* connection between gallstones and dietary fiber intake.

It is possible that a very high fiber intake protects against the lithogenic effect of obesity. Two rural Third-World communities have been studied in which the women tend to be obese and yet appear to escape gallstones,

TABLE I. Daily Intake of Sugars and Dietary Fiber in Patients with Gallstones and Matched Community Controls—The Adelaide Case-Control Study[a]

	Females				Males			
	Age <50		Age >50		Age <50		Age >50	
	Cases	Controls	Cases	Controls	Cases	Controls	Cases	Controls
Sugars, total, g	147 ± 7***	113 ± 4	128 ± 8	126 ± 7	160 ± 15*	121 ± 10	135 ± 12	153 ± 10
Sugars, drinks and sweets, g	53 ± 4***	28 ± 3	36 ± 4**	23 ± 2	58 ± 5*	40 ± 7	46 ± 6	40 ± 5
Dietary fiber, g	19.2 ± 0.8	17.7 ± 0.7	18.1 ± 0.9	21.9 ± 1.2	17.4 ± 2.1	18.3 ± 1.6	18.5 ± 2.2	22.6 ± 1.9

[a]From Scragg et al. (1984a). Significance: * $p < 0.05$, ** $p < 0.01$, *** $p < 0.001$.

namely a village in Zimbabwe and one of the Tongan islands in the South Pacific. In both places, samples of gallbladder bile have been obtained by duodenal intubation from obese women and, on analysis, the samples have been surprisingly unsaturated with cholesterol (Heaton *et al.*, 1977; Stace *et al.*, 1981). In both places the inhabitants ingest very large amounts of fiber—from maize in Zimbabwe and from fruit in Tonga.

5.2. Protection of Laboratory Animals by Fiber or Fiber-Rich Foods

No experiments have been reported that were designed to test the hypothesis that fiber-depleted diets favor gallstone formation. However, many lithogenic dietary regimes have been described and, while the diets vary widely, they have one feature in common—they are all described as semisynthetic or semipurified (Heaton, 1975). What these vague terms actually mean is that the carbohydrate component of the diet is always fiber-depleted. Usually it is glucose or sucrose, but sometimes it is cooked starch. Sometimes these diets are described as deficient in essential fatty acids (EFA), and there are biochemical arguments linking EFA deficiency with lithogenic bile (Hikasa *et al.*, 1969). However, several observations suggest that the lithogenicity of these diets is due, at least in part, to their lack of fiber. In the hamster, the diet loses its lithogenic action if it is supplemented with bulking agents such as agar, carboxymethylcellulose, and psyllium hydrocolloid, or even if the animal is allowed to eat the straw laid on the floor of its cage (Hikasa *et al.*, 1969; van der Linden and Bergman, 1977). Adding pure lignin to hamsters' diet also reduces the number that develop gallstones (Rotstein *et al.*, 1981). In the rabbit, preformed stones dissolve rapidly if fiber-rich chow is reintroduced (Borgman and Haselden, 1968). The Kyoto group summed up a decade of research into diet-induced cholesterol gallstones in hamsters by identifying "three major factors: (1) an excessive intake of purified and highly absorbable carbohydrate, such as sugar, (2) a large intake of animal fats . . . , and (3) a small intake of indigestible, less absorbable and unpurified carbohydrate and vegetable fibers containing a lot of residue" (Tanimura *et al.*, 1978).

5.3. Beneficial Effect on Human Bile of a Fiber-Rich Diet

The only report of the reaction of human bile to a diet naturally rich in dietary fiber is that of our group (Thornton *et al.*, 1983). Thirteen women with asymptomatic, radiolucent gallstones were studied after 6 weeks on a diet containing frequently consumed amounts of refined sugar and fiber-depleted starchy foods and again, in random order, after 6 weeks on a diet devoid of these products but with free access to all full-fiber or unrefined foods. The intake of dietary fiber averaged 13 and 27 g/day, respectively. The cholesterol saturation index of gallbladder bile aspirated from the duodenum averaged 1.50 on the fiber-depleted diet and 1.20 on the full-fiber diet (Fig. 1). The index was lower on the full-fiber diet in all but one subject (who was atypical in gaining weight on this diet due to overindulgence in nuts!). We wondered if the beneficial effect of the full-fiber diet was due to its containing only 6 g/day refined sugars compared with 106 g/day on the fiber-depleted diet, but in a subsequent, similarly designed study we found no difference in bile composition on sucrose intakes of 16 and 112 g/day when fiber intake was held practically constant (Werner *et al.*, 1984). The full-fiber diet provided significantly more of various vitamins and minerals (Heaton *et al.*, 1983), but bile is not known to be affected by these substances. One is forced to conclude, therefore, that it is the higher fiber content of this diet that explains its beneficial effect on bile. However, the mode of action is obscure. It does not appear to be the same as the bran effect, since the bile acid composition of bile was only altered minimally.

5.4. Beneficial Effect on Human Bile of Wheat Bran

Pomare *et al.* (1976) in Bristol reported that, when ten women with radiolucent gallstones added raw bran 33 g/day to their diet for 4–6 weeks,

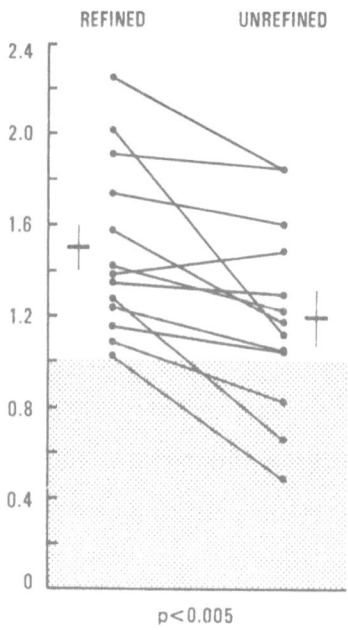

FIGURE 1. Cholesterol saturation index of bile in 13 women after 6 weeks on a refined, fiber-depleted diet and after 6 weeks on an unrefined, fiber-rich diet. (Thornton *et al.*, 1983.)

the cholesterol saturation index of their bile fell from 1.49 to 1.29 ($p < 0.005$). Two years later three further studies were reported that essentially confirmed our findings, although none of the studies followed the same design. In one study the nine subjects had radiolucent gallstones but were given bran cereal (i.e., cooked bran) in the large dose of 50 g daily; the saturation index fell in all, on average, from 1.43 to 0.76 (McDougall *et al.*, 1978). In another study, the subjects did take raw bran 30 g/day but they did not have gallstones (Watts *et al.*, 1978). Nevertheless, duodenal bile was initially supersaturated in five of the subjects (all women) and in all five the saturation index fell, on average, from 1.36 to 0.94. In six subjects with initially unsaturated bile, bran had no effect. In the third study, the subjects were asked to eat 25 g raw bran daily for a year. They did not have gallstones, but had diverticular disease of the colon with diarrhea and high bile acid excretion, so it is questionable how relevant the findings are (Tarpila *et al.*, 1978). Bile was analyzed in only five subjects. The authors stated that bile saturation did not change overall, but they gave no data and, in the discussion, mention that "initially supersaturated bile tended to become less saturated." The lack of effect of bran on bile saturation in healthy young subjects with initially unsaturated bile has been documented by ourselves (Wicks *et al.*, 1978) and by Huijbregts *et al.* (1980). This is perhaps, to be expected, since feeding bran is not giving a drug but is replacing in the diet something that is deficient in most Westerners. Bran can only be expected to improve a situation when this has become abnormal. The published evidence strongly suggests that bran usually does improve the cholesterol saturation of bile when this is initially high.

5.5. Mode of Action of Bran

Unfortunately, there are no reports of the effect of bran on the secretion of cholesterol into bile (a difficult phenomenon to study). However, it is likely that bran acts by reducing this, since the other possible explanation for reduced cholesterol saturation, expansion of the bile acid pool, has been disproved (Pomare *et al.*, 1976; McDougall *et al.*, 1978). One possible explanation of reduced cholesterol secretion, namely loss of weight, can be ruled out. Weight loss has not accompanied bran feeding in any study.

The most plausible mechanism is via alteration of bile acid metabolism and specifically by reduction of the circulating pool of deoxycholic acid (DCA). Bran was first shown to deplete the bile acid pool of deoxycholic acid by Pomare and Heaton (1973) and this has been confirmed in several later studies (Pomare *et al.*, 1976; Wicks *et al.*, 1978; McDougall *et al.*, 1978; Tarpila *et al.*, 1978), although in the study of Watts *et al.* (1978), the percent DCA fell only in the three subjects with initially high levels. Similarly, there was no fall in young Dutchmen who started with initially low levels, probably because they were already eating a high-fiber diet (Huijbregts *et al.*, 1980). The message seems again to be that bran is effective only when there already is an abnormal situation. It may be abnormal to have too much bile acid in circulation that has been dehydroxylated by intestinal bacteria. DCA is derived from cholic acid by 7α-dehydroxylation, a transformation carried out in the colon by anaerobic bacteria.

The idea that bran improves the cholesterol saturation of bile by reducing the input of DCA into the circulating pool is plausible and attractive for several reasons.

1. When the bile acid composition of bile has been compared in patients with cholesterol gallstones and in healthy controls the patients have usually been found to have an increased percentage of DCA (Heaton, 1985).

2. In two large series of gallstone patients the percent DCA has been found to correlate significantly with the cholesterol saturation index (van der Linden and Bergman, 1977; Hofmann *et al.*, 1982).

3. Feeding DCA in physiological doses, 100–150 mg/day, to normal subjects increases the cholesterol content of their bile (Low-Beer and Pomare, 1975). Larger doses, such as 750–1000 mg/day, usually do not have this effect [Ahlberg *et al.* (1977), LaRusso *et al.* (1977), Carulli *et al.* (1980); but Ponz de Leon *et al.* (1983) disagree], probably because at this dosage DCA has toxic effects on the small intestine and reduces cholesterol absorption.

4. When cholic acid, the precursor of DCA, is fed to volunteers, some of them convert it rapidly to DCA and expand their DCA pool; such people have a rise in the cholesterol saturation of their bile (Carulli *et al.*, 1981).

5. Besides bran, five other measures lower the DCA content of bile and all five also reduce the cholesterol saturation of bile. These measures are treatment with ampicillin (Carulli *et al.*, 1981); treatment with metronidazole (Low-Beer and Nutter, 1978); treatment with lactulose, which, like dietary fiber, enters the colon and is fermented there to short-chain fatty acids, acid pH inhibiting bacterial 7α-dehydroxylase (Thornton and Heaton, 1981); oral administration of *Streptococcus faecium,* which presumably acts by displacing the normal anaerobic bacteria (Salvioli *et al.*, 1982); and thyroxine treatment of hypothyroidism, which possibly acts by speeding up colonic transit (Angelin *et al.*, 1983). The unanimity with which these diverse measures affect two aspects of bile is remarkable and suggests the two are linked.

Why should an increased proportion of DCA in bile favor more saturated bile? There are two possible explanations. First, being the most detergent of the bile acids, DCA leaches out more cholesterol from the liver cell as it crosses it on its way from the portal blood to the bile (Carulli *et al.*, 1984). Second, DCA tends to displace chenodeoxycholic acid, another dihydroxy bile acid, but a primary one made by the liver, from the bile (either by competing with it for intestinal absorption or by suppressing its synthesis) [for original references see Heaton (1985)], and this removes an agent that is known to lower cholesterol secretion. Whatever the mode of action of deoxycholic acid, bran may act by reducing it.

Bran could reduce the amount of circulating DCA in two ways. First, it provides solid matter in the cecum to which DCA would tend to adsorb (Eastwood and Hamilton, 1968), thus preventing its absorption. Second, up to 50% of bran is metabolized by colonic bacteria to short-chain fatty acids. These would tend to lower the pH in the cecum. Acid pH would tend to reduce the absorption of DCA because DCA precipitates at acid pH and is rendered unavailable for absorption. Furthermore, at pH < 6.0 the bacterial 7α-dehydroxylase that generates DCA from cholic acid becomes inactive (MacDonald et al., 1978). The mode of action of bran has not been studied, due to the inaccessibility of the cecum. However, the fact that it takes as long as 6 weeks for the effect of bran on biliary DCA to become apparent suggests an effect on bacterial metabolism rather than a direct physical action (Wicks et al., 1978).

Curiously, there are no reports of the effects on human bile of other fiber concentrates or of fiber components, but it is likely that different fiber sources will have different effects, as they do on plasma cholesterol.

The effect of bran on bile composition raises the possibility that the formation or recurrence of gallstones could be prevented by enriching the diet with bran. However, this is yet to be demonstrated. It is likely that other dietary measures will be necessary as well, including sucrose restriction, and weight reduction in overweight patients.

6. CONTRARY EVIDENCE

In the Adelaide case–control study there was no significant difference in mean fiber intake between gallstone patients and controls of either sex or at age <50 or ≥50 (Scragg et al., 1984a). However, on multivariate analysis, the direction of the regression coefficients shows that, for both sexes, fiber intake was negatively associated with gallstone risk. In any case, the possibility exists that to be strongly protective, fiber intake must be higher than that achieved by any of the citizens of Adelaide.

According to a preliminary report (Pomare, 1983), Tongan islanders have a higher percentage of deoxycholic acid in their bile acid pools than New Zealand Tongans despite having a much higher intake of dietary fiber (estimated as 71 g/day) and despite having unsaturated bile (Stace et al., 1981). There is an obvious discrepancy between these findings and the results of work with bran. However, Tongans do not eat wheat fiber and it may be that the fiber in roots and tubers on which they subsist has a different effect on bile acid metabolism to that of bran. Similarly, the obese village women of Zimbabwe had Western levels of deoxycholate in their bile despite having unsaturated bile (Heaton *et al.*, 1977) and despite eating large amounts of maize. Again, perhaps maize fiber and wheat fiber have different effects on bile acid metabolism.

7. SUMMARY AND CONCLUSIONS

Fiber-depleted sugars favor the secretion of bile supersaturated with cholesterol and hence gallstones by inflating energy intake and promoting obesity. Sugars also tend to raise fasting plasma insulin and triglycerides and to depress plasma HDL-cholesterol, and all three of these metabolic changes are associated with an increased risk of gallstones.

The protective effect of dietary fiber is attested to by (1) the low prevalence of gallstones in populations eating a high-fiber diet, (2) protection of laboratory animals against gallstones by fiber or fiber-rich foods, (3) a beneficial effect on human bile of a fiber-rich diet, and (4) a beneficial effect on human bile of wheat bran. Bran appears to work by reducing the input of deoxycholic acid from the colon, but the mode of action of a fiber-rich diet is unknown.

A unifying scheme to show the likely links between fiber-depleted foods and cholesterol gallstones is shown in Fig. 2.

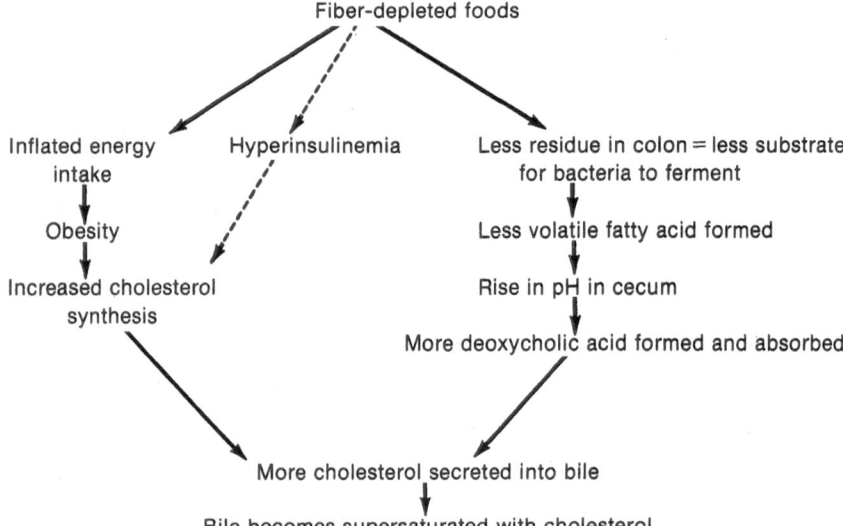

FIGURE 2. Connection between fiber-depleted foods and cholesterol gallstones.

REFERENCES

Ahlberg, J., Angelin, B., Einarsson, K., Hellström, K., and Leijd, B., 1977, Influence of deoxycholic acid on biliary lipids in man, *Clin. Sci. Mol. Med.* **53**:249–256.

Ahlberg, J., Angelin, B., Einarsson, K., Hellström, K., and Leijd, B., 1979, Prevalence of gallbladder disease in hyperlipoproteinemia, *Dig. Dis. Sci.* **24**:459–464.

Ahlberg, J., Angelin, B., Einarsson, K., Hellström, K., and Leijd, B., 1980, Biliary lipid composition in normo- and hyperlipoproteinemia, *Gastroenterology* **79**:90–94.

Albrink, M. J., Newman, T., and Davidson, P. C., 1979, Effect of high- and low-fiber diets on plasma lipids and insulin, *Am. J. Clin. Nutr.* **32**:1486–1491.

Andersén, E., and Hellström, K., 1980, Influence of fat-rich versus carbohydrate-rich diets on bile acid kinetics, biliary lipids, and net steroid balance in hyperlipidemic subjects, *Metabolism* **29**:400–409.

Angelin, B., Einarsson, K., and Leijd, B., 1983, Bile acid metabolism in hypothyroid subjects: Response to substitution therapy, *Eur. J. Clin. Invest.* **13**:99–106.

Bennion, L. J., and Grundy, S. M., 1978, Risk factors for the development of cholelithiasis in man, *N. Engl. J. Med.* **299**:1161–1167, 1221–1227.

Bingham, S., and Cummings, J. H., 1980, Sources and intakes of dietary fiber in man, in: *Medical Aspects of Dietary Fiber* (G. A. Spiller and R. M. Kay, eds.), Plenum, New York, pp. 261–284.

Bolton, R. P., Heaton, K. W., and Burroughs, L. F., 1981, The role of dietary fiber in satiety, glucose, and insulin: Studies with fruit and fruit juice, *Am. J. Clin. Nutr.* **34**:211–217.

Borgman, R. F., and Haselden, F. H., 1968, Cholelithiasis in rabbits: Effects of diet upon formation and dissolution of gallstones, *Am. J. Vet. Res.* **29**:1287–1292.

Bouchier, I. A. D., 1983, Biochemistry of gallstone formation, *Clin. Gastroenterol.* **12**:25–48.

Brett, M., and Barker, D. J. P., 1976, The world distribution of gallstones, *Int. J. Epidemiol.* **5**:335–341.

Burkitt, D. P., Walker, A. R. P., and Painter, N. S., 1972, Effect of dietary fibre on stools and transit-times, and its role in the causation of disease, *Lancet* **ii**:1408–1412.

Burnstein, M. J., Ilson, R. G., Petrunka, C. N., Taylor, R. D., and Strasberg, S. M., 1983, Evidence for a potent nucleating factor in the gallbladder bile of patients with cholesterol gallstones, *Gastroenterology* **85**:801–807.

Cahlin, E., Jönsson, J. Nilsson, S., and Scherstén, T., 1973, Biliary lipid composition in normolipidemic and prebeta hyperlipoproteinemic gallstone patients. Influence of sucrose feeding of the patients on the biliary lipid composition, *Scand. J. Gastroenterol.* **8**:449–456.

Capron, J.-P., Piperaud, R., Dupas, J.-L., Delamarre, J., and Lorriaux, A., 1981, Evidence for an association between cholelithiasis and diverticular disease of the colon: A case-controlled study, *Dig. Dis. Sci.* **26**:523–527.

Carulli, N., Ponz de Leon, M., Zironi, F., Iori, R., and Loria, P., 1980, Bile acid feeding and hepatic sterol metabolism: Effect of deoxycholic acid, *Gastroenterology* **79**:637–641.

Carulli, N., Ponz de Leon, M., Loria, P., Iori, R., Rosi, A., and Romani, M., 1981, Effect of the selective expansion of the cholic acid pool on bile lipid composition: Possible mechanism of bile acid induced biliary cholesterol desaturation, *Gastroenterology* **81**:539–546.

Carulli, N., Loria, P., Bertolotti, M., Ponz de Leon, M., Menozzi, D., Medici, G., and Piccagli, I., 1984, Effects of acute changes of bile acid pool composition on biliary lipid secretion, *J. Clin. Invest.* **74**:614–624.

Cleave, T. L., 1974, *The Saccharine Disease,* Wright, Bristol.

Eastwood, M. A., and Hamilton, D., 1968, Studies on the adsorption of bile salts to non-absorbed components of diet, *Biochim. Biophys. Acta* **152**:165–173.

Gear, J. S. S., Ware, A., Fursdon, P., Mann, J. I., Nolan, D. J., Brodribb, A. J. M., and Vessey, M. P., 1979, Symptomless diverticular disease and intake of dietary fibre, *Lancet* **i**:511–514.

Haber, G. B., Heaton, K. W., Murphy, D., and Burroughs, L., 1977, Depletion and disruption of dietary fibre. Effects on satiety, plasma-glucose, and serum-insulin, *Lancet* ii:679-682.

Heaton, K. W., 1973, Food fibre as an obstacle to energy intake, *Lancet* ii:1418-1421.

Heaton, K. W., 1975, Gallstones and cholecystitis, in: *Refined Carbohydrate Foods and Disease. Some Implications of Dietary Fibre* (D. P. Burkitt and H. C. Trowell, eds.), Academic, London, pp. 173-194.

Heaton, K. W., 1980, Food intake regulation and fiber, in: *Medical Aspects of Dietary Fiber* (G. A. Spiller and R. M. Kay, eds.), Plenum, New York, pp. 223-238.

Heaton, K., 1981, Gallstones, in: *Western Diseases: Their Emergence and Prevention* (H. C. Trowell and D. P. Burkitt, eds.), Arnold, London, pp. 47-59.

Heaton, K. W., 1984, The role of diet in the aetiology of cholelithiasis, *Rev. Clin. Nutr.* **53:** 549-560.

Heaton, K. W., 1985, Bile salts, in: *Liver and Biliary Disease,* 2nd ed., (R. Wright, K. G. M. M. Alberti, S. Karran, and G. H. Millward-Sadler, eds.), Saunders, London.

Heaton, K. W., Wicks, A. C. B., and Yeates, J., 1977, Bile composition in relation to race and diet: Studies in Rhodesian Africans and in British subjects, in: *Bile Acid Metabolism in Health and Disease* (G. Paumgartner and A. Stiehl, eds.), MTP, Lancaster, England, pp. 197-202.

Heaton, K. W., Emmett, P. M., Henry, C. L., Thornton, J. R., Manhire, A., and Hartog, M., 1983, Not just fibre—The nutritional consequences of refined carbohydrate foods, *Hum. Nutr. Clin. Nutr.* **37C:**31-35.

Hikasa, Y., Matsuda, S., Nagase, M., Yoshinaga, M., Tobe, T., Maruyama, I., Shioda, R., Tanimura, H., Muraoka, R., Muroya, H., and Togo, M., 1969, Initiating factors of gallstones, especially cholesterol stones (III), *Arch. Jpn. Chir.* **38:**107-124.

Hofmann, A. F., Grundy, S. M., Lachin, J. M., Lan, S.-P., Baum, R. A., Hanson, R. F., Hersh, T., Hightower, N. C., Marks, J. W., Mekhjian, H., Shaefer, R. A., Soloway, R. D., Thistle, J. L., Thomas, F. B., and Tyor, M. P., 1982, Pre-treatment biliary lipid composition in white patients with radiolucent gallstones in the National Co-operative Gallstone Study, *Gastroenterology* **83:**738-752.

Huijbregts, A. W. M., van Berge-Henegouwen, G. P., Hectors, M. P. C., van Schaik, A., and van der Werf, S. D. J., 1980, Effects of a standardised wheat bran preparation on biliary lipid composition and bile acid metabolism in young healthy males, *Eur. J. Clin. Invest.* **10:**451-458.

Kesäniemi, Y. A., and Grundy, S. M., 1983, Clofibrate, caloric restriction, supersaturation of bile and cholesterol crystals, *Scand. J. Gastroenterol.* **18:**897-902.

LaRusso, N. F., 1984, Apoproteins in bile: Apo A inhibits nucleation, Paper read at 8th International Bile Acid Meeting, Cortina d'Ampezzo, March 1984.

LaRusso, N. F., Szczepanik, P. A., and Hofmann, A. F., 1977, Effect of deoxycholic acid ingestion on bile acid metabolism and biliary lipid secretion in normal subjects, *Gastroenterology* **72:**132-140.

Lewis, B., 1976, Influence of diet, energy balance and hormones on serum lipids, in: *The Hyperlipidaemias. Clinical and Laboratory Practice,* Blackwell, Oxford, pp. 131-180.

Low-Beer, T. S., and Nutter, S., 1978, Colonic bacterial activity, biliary cholesterol saturation, and pathogenesis of gallstones, *Lancet* ii:1063-1065.

Low-Beer, T. S., and Pomare, E. W., 1975, Can colonic bacterial metabolites predispose to cholesterol gallstones? *Br. Med. J.* **1:**438-440.

MacDonald, I. A., Singh, G., Mahony, D. E., and Meier, C. E., 1978, Effect of pH on bile salt degradation by mixed fecal cultures, *Steroids* **32:**245-256.

McDougall, R. M., Yakymyshyn, L., Walker, K., and Thurston, O. G., 1978, The effect of wheat bran on serum lipoproteins and biliary lipids, *Can. J. Surg.* **21:**433-435.

Neprokoeff, C. M., Lakshmanan, M. R., Ness, G. C., Dugan, R. E., and Porter, J. W., 1974,

Regulation of the diurnal rhythm of rat liver β-hydroxy-β-methylglutaryl coenzyme A reductase activity by insulin, glucagon, cyclic AMP, and hydrocortisone, *Arch. Biochem. Biophys.* **160**:387–393.

O'Dea, K., Nestel, P. J., and Antonoff, L., 1980, Physical factors influencing postprandial glucose and insulin responses to starch, *Am. J. Clin. Nutr.* **33**:760–765.

Petitti, D. B., Friedman, G. D., and Klatsky, A. L., 1981, Association of a history of gallbladder disease with a reduced concentration of high-density-lipoprotein cholesterol, *N. Engl. J. Med.* **304**:1396–1398.

Pixley, F., Wilson, D., McPherson, K., and Mann, J., 1985, Effect of vegetarianism on development of gallstones in women, *Br. Med. J.*, **291**:11–12.

Pomare, E. W., 1983, Fibre and bile acid metabolism, in: *Fibre in Human and Animal Nutrition* (G. Wallace and L. Bell, eds.), Royal Society of New Zealand Bulletin 20, pp. 179–182.

Pomare, E. W., and Heaton, K. W., 1973, Alteration of bile salt metabolism by dietary fibre (bran), *Br. Med. J.* **4**:262–264.

Pomare, E. W., Heaton, K. W., Low-Beer, T. S., and Espiner, H. J., 1976, The effect of wheat bran upon bile salt metabolism and upon the lipid composition of bile in gallstone patients, *Am. J. Dig. Dis.* **21**:521–526.

Ponz de Leon, M., Carulli, N., Iori, R., Loria, P., and Romani, M., 1983, Regulation of cholesterol absorption by bile acids: Role of deoxycholic and cholic acid pool expansion on dietary cholesterol absorption, *Ital. J. Gastroenterol.* **15**:86–93.

Reiser, S., Hallfrisch, J., Michaelis, O. E., Lazar, F. L., Martin, R. E., and Prather, E. S., 1978, Isocaloric exchange of dietary starch and sucrose in humans. I. Effects on levels of fasting lipids, *Am. J. Clin. Nutr.* **32**:1659–1669.

Reiser, S., Bohn, E., Hallfrisch, J., Michaelis, O. E., Keeney, M., and Prather, E. S., 1981, Serum insulin and glucose in hyperinsulinemic subjects fed three different levels of sucrose, *Am. J. Clin. Nutr.* **34**:2348–2358.

Rotstein, O. D., Kay, R. M., Wayman, M., and Strasberg, S. M., 1981, Prevention of cholesterol gallstones by lignin and lactulose in the hamster, *Gastroenterology* **81**:1098–1103.

Salvioli, G., Salati, R., Bondi, M., Fratalocchi, A., Sala, B. M., and Gibertini, A., 1982, Bile acid transformation by the intestinal flora and cholesterol saturation in bile, Effects of *Streptococcus faecium* administration, *Digestion* **23**:80–88.

Scragg, R. K. R., Calvert, G. D., and Oliver, J. R., 1984b, Plasma lipids and insulin in gallstone disease, *Br. Med. J.* **289**:521–525.

Scragg, R. K. R., McMichael, A. J., and Baghurst, P. A., 1984a, Diet, alcohol, and relative weight in gallstone disease: A case–control study, *Br. Med. J.* **288**:1113–1119.

Stace, N. H., Pomare, E. W., Peters, S., Thomas, L., and Fisher, A., 1981, Biliary lipids and dietary intakes (including dietary fiber) in four different female populations, *Gastroenterology* **80**:1291.

Sutor, D. J., and Wooley, S. E., 1971, A statistical survey of the composition of gallstones in eight countries, *Gut* **12**:55–64.

Tanimura, H., Shioda, R., Nagase, M., Tafenaka, M., Kobayashi, N., Setoyama, M., Kamato, T., Mukaihara, S., Maruyama, K., Kato, H., Miki, K., and Hikasa, Y., 1978, Initiating factors in formation of cholesterol gallstones, *Arch. Jpn. Chir.* **47**:427–445.

Tarpila, S., Miettinen, T. A., and Metsäranta, L., 1978, Effects of bran on serum cholesterol, faecal mass, fat, bile acids and neutral sterols, and biliary lipids in patients with diverticular disease of the colon, *Gut* **19**:137–145.

Thornton, J. R., and Heaton, K. W., 1981, Do colonic bacteria contribute to cholesterol gallstone formation? Effects of lactulose on bile, *Br. Med. J.* **282**:1018–1020.

Thornton, J. R., Heaton, K. W., and MacFarlane, D. G., 1980, Plasma lipids, insulin and gallstone risk, *Clin. Sci.* **59**:9p.

Thornton, J. R., Heaton, K. W., and Macfarlane, D. G., 1981, A relation between high-density-lipoprotein cholesterol and bile cholesterol saturation, *Br. Med. J.* **283**:1352–1354.

Thornton, J. R., Emmett, P. M., and Heaton, K. W., 1983, Diet and gall stones: Effects of refined and unrefined carbohydrate diets on bile cholesterol saturation and bile acid metabolism, *Gut* **24**:2–6.

Trowell, H. C., Burkitt, D. P., and Heaton, K. W., 1985, *Dietary Fibre, Fibre-Depleted Foods and Disease,* Academic, London.

Van der Linden, W., and Bergman, F., 1977, Formation and dissolution of gallstones in experimental animals, *Int. Rev. Exp. Pathol.* **17**:173–233.

Watts, J. McK., Jablonski, P., and Toouli, J., 1978, The effect of added bran to the diet on the saturation of bile in people without gallstones, *Am. J. Surg.* **135**:321–324.

Werner, D., Emmett, P. M., and Heaton, K. W., 1984, The effects of dietary sucrose on factors influencing cholesterol gallstone formation, *Gut* **25**:269–274.

Wicks, A. C. B., Yeates, J., and Heaton, K. W., 1978, Bran and bile: Time-course of changes in normal young men given a standard dose, *Scand. J. Gastroenterol.* **13**:289–292.

Yudkin, J., Kang, S. S., and Bruckdorfer, K. R., 1980, Effects of high dietary sugar, *Br. Med. J.* **281**:1396.

29

Fiber and Cancer

DAVID KRITCHEVSKY

Dietary fiber, hypothetically, can protect against intestinal cancer in several ways. It can lessen the probability of contact between a potential carcinogen and intestinal mucosa by its role as a diluent of intestinal contents and by reducing intestinal transit time. Dietary fiber can also influence bacterial conversion of precursors of carcinogens by the same mechanisms.

Epidemiologic evidence concerning the role of fiber in carcinogenesis dates to the studies of Stocks and Karns (1933) in England, who found a negative correlation between the incidence of colon cancer and the ingestion of whole meal (whole wheat) bread, vegetables, and milk. In India, Paymaster *et al.* (1968) found a negative correlation between colon cancer incidence and a vegetarian lifestyle and the intake of dairy foods. Studies based on examination of data from the Food and Agricultural Organization have suggested a weakly protective effect of cereals and pulses (Irving and Drasar, 1973; Howell, 1975); no effect of fiber (Armstrong and Doll, 1975); or suggestions of complex intradietary effects (Liu *et al.*, 1970; McMichael *et al.*, 1980). One study in which dietary fiber intake was actually assessed found that the difference between the high colon cancer incidence in Copenhagen, Denmark and the low incidence in Kuopio, Finland was correlated with the high intakes of fiber and milk in the Finnish cohort (IARC, 1977). Bingham *et al.* (1979) studied the relationship between regional large bowel cancer mortality and dietary fiber in England. They found negative correlations with pentose intake (g/day) and vegetable (excluding potatoes) intake (oz./week). No correlations were found between standardized death rates (per 100,000) and total dietary fiber (g/day), fat intake (g/day), or beef consumption (oz./week). This study was the first to suggest a protective role for specific fiber

DAVID KRITCHEVSKY • The Wistar Institute of Anatomy and Biology, Philadelphia, Pennsylvania 19104.

components rather than for fiber *per se*. Variables with which death rates were significantly correlated are presented in Table I. Case-control studies (Bjelke, 1974; Modan *et al.*, 1975) generally support the hypothesis that dietary fiber protects against colon cancer (Burkitt, 1974), but the findings are not uniform (Higginson, 1966; Wynder and Shigematsu, 1967). Clearly, more data are needed on the role of dietary fiber in general and more importantly on the effects of specific fiber components.

The literature on the effects of dietary fibers on colon carcinogenesis in rats does not yield simple or consistent correlations. Variations in basal diet, rat strain, carcinogen, and type and amount of fiber complicate analysis.

There are several studies in Fisher 344 rats (Table II). Cellulose (20–40%) did not protect against azoxymethane (AOM)-induced colon carcinogenesis in male rats (Ward *et al.*, 1973), but Konjac mannan (5%) protected male rats against dimethylhydrazine (DMH)-induced tumors (Mizutani and Mitsuoka, 1983). Male Fisher rats were fed a semipurified diet containing 15% cellulose, hemicellulose, or lignin and were given DMH by gavage (Kritchevsky, Weber, and Klurfeld, unpublished observations). Tumor incidence (%) was: cellulose, 100; hemicellulose, 50; and lignin, 70. The results are detailed in Table III. Female Fisher rats were fed diets containing 15% alfalfa, bran, or pectin and given subcutaneous injection of AOM or intrarectal instillation of methylnitrosourea (MNU). Alfalfa did not affect AOM-induced carcinogenesis, but bran and pectin showed a protective effect. These two fibers were ineffective against MNU, but alfalfa enhanced carcinogenesis (Watanabe *et al.*, 1979) (Table IV). It has been suggested (Kritchevsky, 1983) that the different effects may have been due to the bile acid-binding properties of the various fibers (Kritchevsky and Story, 1974; Story and Kritchevsky, 1976) taken together with the observation (Cassidy *et al.*, 1980, 1981) that the disruption of mucosal integrity by various fibers is correlated with their capacity to bind bile acids.

Male Wistar rats are protected from DMH-induced colon cancer by cellulose (4.5% added to a semipurified diet) (Freeman *et al.*, 1978), but the

TABLE I. Correlation of Dietary Variables with Death Rates from Colon Cancer in England[a]

Variable	r
Pentose	−0.960
All vegetables (excluding potatoes)	−0.940
Fresh green vegetables	−0.861
Vitamin C	−0.842
Lignin	−0.826

[a] After Bingham *et al.* (1979).

TABLE II. Influence of Fiber on Experimental Colon Cancer
in Fisher Rats[a]

Sex	Diet	Fiber (%)	Carcinogen	Effect	Reference
Male	SP	Cellulose (20–40)	AOM (sc)	None	Ward et al. (1973)
Male	C	Konjac mannan (5)	DMH (ip)	Protect	Mizutani and Mitsuoka (1983)
Male	SP	Cellulose (15)	DMH (f)	None	Kritchevsky, Weber, and
		Hemicellulose (15)		Protect	Klurfeld, unpublished results
		Lignin (15)		Protect	
Female	SP	Alfalfa (15)	AOM (sc)	None	Watanabe et al. (1979)
		Bran (15)		Protect	
		Pectin (15)		Protect	
Female	SP	Alfalfa (15)	MNU (ir)	Enhance	Watanabe et al. (1979)
		Bran (15)		None	
		Pectin (15)		None	

[a] SP, semipurified; C, chow; AOM, azoxymethane; DMH, dimethylhydrazine; MNU, methylnitrosourea; sc, subcutaneous; ip, intraperitoneal; f, fed; ir, intrarectal.

TABLE III. Influence of Fiber (15%) on 1,2-Dimethylhydrazine-Induced
Colon Carcinogenesis in Male Fisher Rats[a]

| | Fiber | | |
	Cellulose	Hemicellulose	Lignin
Tumor incidence			
Number	23/23	12/24	16/23
Incidence	100	50	70
Tumors/tumor-bearing rat	4.3 ± 0.5	1.9 ± 0.3	2.8 ± 0.3
Carcinomas, %	47	41	43

[a] After Kritchevsky et al. (1985).

TABLE IV. Influence of Fiber (15%), Carcinogen, and Mode of
Administration on Experimental Colon Cancer in
Female Fisher Rats[a]

| | AOM (sc) | | MNU (ir) | |
Fiber	Incidence, %	Tumors/rat	Incidence, %	Tumors/rat
Control	57	0.8	69	1.0
Alfalfa	53	0.7	83	2.3
Bran	33	0.4	60	0.8
Pectin	10	0.1	59	1.0

[a] After Watanabe et al. (1979). AOM (sc), azoxymethane (subcutaneous); MNU (ir), methylnitrosourea (intrarectal).

TABLE V. Influence of Fiber on Experimental Colon Cancer in
Sprague-Dawley Rats[a]

Sex	Diet	Fiber (%)	Carcinogen	Effect	Reference
Male	SP	Bran (20)	DMH (f)	Protect	Wilson *et al.* (1977)
Male	C	Bran (20)	DMH (f)	Protect	Barbolt and Abraham (1978)
Male	SP	Bran (20)	DMH (sc)	None	Bauer *et al.* (1979)
		Carrot (20)		Enhance	
		Pectin (6.5)		Enhance	
Male	C	Bran (20)	DMH (f)	Protect	Barbolt and Abraham (1980)
Female	C	Bran (20)	DMH (f)	None	Barbolt and Abraham (1980)

[a]See footnote to Table III for explanation of abbreviations.

course of colon carcinogenesis is unaffected in female Wistar rats fed bran (20% added to commercial ration) (Cruse *et al.*, 1978).

Experiments using Sprague-Dawley rats (Table V) have shown similar disparities. Bran (20%) added to a semipurified (Wilson *et al.*, 1977) or a commercial (Barbolt and Abraham, 1978) diet protects against colon cancer induced by feeding DMH. However, when the DMH is given by subcutaneous injection, bran (20% in a semipurified diet) is without effect and carrot (20%) and pectin (6.5%) enhance carcinogenesis (Bauer *et al.*, 1979). Bran (20% added to commercial ration) protects male Sprague-Dawley rats against colon cancer induced by feeding DMH, but has no effect in female Sprague-Dawley rats (Barbolt and Abraham, 1980).

The foregoing suggests a number of variables that have to be examined and their effects delineated. First would be the need for more studies of various fibers in order to ascertain if specific types of fiber (e.g., pentose-rich) are more closely correlated with protective effects. In animals we must have more data on the effects of mode of carcinogen administration and a greater uniformity in diet (e.g., semipurified rather than commercial). The findings that male and female rats react differently to the same fiber and carcinogen suggest a need for investigation into reasons for the sex difference. These studies could also provide important insights into possible hormonal influences. Finally, intradietary effects (fiber vs. fat, protein, or carbohydrate) must also be assessed. Eventually, the precise role of dietary fiber effects in colon carcinogenesis will emerge.

REFERENCES

Armstrong, B., and Doll, R., 1975, Environmental factors with cancer incidences and mortality in different countries with special references to dietary practices, *Int. J. Cancer* **15**:617–631.

Barbolt, T. A., and Abraham, R., 1978, The effect of bran in dimethylhydrazine-induced colon carcinogenesis in the rat, *Proc. Soc. Exp. Biol. Med.* **157**:656–659.

Barbolt, T. A., and Abraham, R., 1980, Dose-response, sex differences and the effect of bran in dimethylhydrazine-induced intestinal carcinogenesis in rats, *Toxicol. Appl. Pharmacol.* **55:**417–422.

Bauer, H. G., Asp, N. G., Oste, R., Dahlquist, A., and Fredlund, P. E., 1979, Effect of dietary fiber on the induction of colorectal tumors and glucuronidase activity in the rat, *Cancer Res.* **39:**3752–3756.

Bingham, S., Williams, D. R. R., Cole, T. J., and James, W. P. T., 1979, Dietary fibre and regional large-bowel cancer mortality in Britain, *Br. J. Cancer* **40:**456–463.

Bjelke, E., 1974, Epidemiological studies of cancer of the stomach, colon and rectum; with special emphasis on the role of diet, *Scand. J. Gastroenterol.* (Suppl.9):1–235.

Burkitt, D. P., 1974, Epidemiology of cancer of the colon and rectum, *Cancer* **28:**3–13.

Cassidy, M. M., Lightfoot, F. G., Grau, L. E., Roy, T., Kritchevsky, D., and Vahouny, G. V., 1980, Effect of bile salt-binding resins on morphology of the rat jejunum and colon: A scanning electron microscope study, *Dig. Dis. Sci.* **25:**609–612.

Cassidy, M. M., Lightfoot, F. G., Grau, L. E., Story, J. A., Kritchevsky, D., and Vahouny, G. V., 1981, Effect of chronic intake of dietary fiber on the ultrastructural topography of rat jejunum and colon: A scanning microscope study, *Am. J. Clin. Nutr.* **34:**218–228.

Cruse, J. P., Lewin, M. R., and Clark, C. G., 1978, Failure of bran to protect against experimental colon cancer in rats, *Lancet* **2:**1278–1280.

Freeman, H. J., Spiller, G. A., and Kim, Y. S., 1978, A double-blind study on the effect of purified cellulose dietary fiber on 1,2-dimethylhydrazine-induced rat colonic neoplasia, *Cancer Res.* **38:**2912–2917.

Higginson, J., 1966, Etiological factors in gastro-intestinal cancer in man, *J. Nat. Cancer Inst.* **37:**527–545.

Howell, M. A., 1975, Diet as an etiological factor in the development of cancers of the colon and rectum, *J. Chronic Dis.* **28:**67–80.

International Agency for Research on Cancer, 1977, Dietary fibre, transit time, faecal bacteria, steroids and colon cancer in two Scandinavian populations, *Lancet* **2:**207–211.

Irving, D., and Drasar, B. S., 1973, Fibre and cancer of the colon, *Br. J. Cancer* **28:**462–463.

Kritchevsky, D., 1983, Fiber, steroids and cancer, *Cancer Res.* **43:**2491S–2495S.

Kritchevsky, D., Weber, M. M., and Klurfeld, D. M., 1984, Unpublished observation.

Kritchevsky, D., and Story, J. A., 1974, Binding of bile salts *in vitro* by nonnutritive fiber, *J. Nutr.* **104:**458–462.

Liu, K., Moss, D., Persky, V., Stamler, J., Garsiole, D., and Saltero, I., 1979, Dietary cholesterol, fat and fibre and colon-cancer mortality: An analysis of international data, *Lancet* **2:**782–785.

McMichael, A. J., McCall, M. G., Hartshorne, J. M., and Woodings, T. L., 1980, Patterns of gastrointestinal cancer in European immigrants to Australia: The role of dietary change, *Int. J. Cancer* **25:**431–437.

Mizutani, T., and Mitsuoka, T., 1983, Effect of Konjac mannan on 1,2-dimethylhydrazine-induced intestinal carcinogenesis in Fischer 344 rats, *Cancer Lett.* **19:**1–6.

Modan, B., Barell, V., Lubin, F., Modan, M., Greenberg, R. A., and Graham, S., 1975, Low fiber intake as an etiologic factor in cancer of the colon, *J. Nat. Cancer Inst.* **55:**15–18.

Paymaster, J. C., Sanghvi, L. D., and Gangodharan, P., 1968, Cancer in the gastrointestinal tract in Western India, *Cancer* **21:**279–288.

Stocks, P., and Karns, M. K., 1933, A cooperative study of the habits, homelife, dietary and family histories of 450 cancer patients and an equal number of control patients, *Ann. Eugen. (London)* **5:**237–280.

Story, J. A., and Kritchevsky, D., 1976, Comparison of the binding of various bile acids and bile salts *in vitro* by several types of fiber, *J. Nutr.* **106:**1292–1294.

Ward, H. M., Yamamoto, R. S., and Weisburger, J. H., 1973, Cellulose dietary bulk and azoxymethane-induced intestinal cancer, *J. Nat. Cancer Inst.* **57**:713–715.

Watanabe, K., Reddy, B. S., Weisburger, J. H., and Kritchevsky, D., 1979, Effect of dietary alfalfa, pectin and wheat bran on azoxymethane or methylnitrosourea-induced colon carcinogenesis in F344 rats, *J. Nat. Cancer Inst.* **63**:141–145.

Wilson, R. B., Hutcheson, D. P., and Widemann, L., 1977, Dimethylhydrazine-induced colon tumors in rats fed diets containing beef fat or corn oil with and without wheat bran, *Am. J. Clin. Nutr.* **30**:176–181.

Wynder, E. L., and Shigematsu, T., 1967, Environmental factors of cancer of the colon and rectum, *Cancer* **20**:1520–1561.

30

Diet and Mammary Carcinogenesis

K. K. CARROLL

1. INTRODUCTION

Examination of epidemiologic data has shown that breast cancer incidence and mortality are positively correlated with a number of dietary parameters, including dietary fat, animal protein, and caloric intake (Carroll and Khor, 1975; National Research Council, 1982). Of these dietary variables, fat has received by far the most attention. The main reason for this is the consistency with which high-fat diets increase the yield of mammary tumors in experimental animals compared to low-fat diets (Carroll and Khor, 1975; National Research Council, 1982; Carroll, 1983). The experimental evidence with respect to dietary fat appears to be much stronger than that for the other dietary variables. Although dietary fiber may help to protect against colorectal cancer (National Research Council, 1982), there are no indications that it has any protective effect in breast cancer.

The ultimate aim of both the epidemiologic and experimental studies is to obtain information that can be used to reduce the high death rate from breast cancer, which has been the single more common cause of cancer deaths among women of the U. S. and Canada in recent years (Wynder *et al.*, 1981; Carroll, 1982). Thus, the evidence linking dietary fat to breast cancer and also to some other types of cancer has led to an interim dietary recommendation that fat intake be reduced to 30% of calories from the present level of approximately 40% (National Research Council, 1982; Palmer and Bakshi, 1983). Since dietary changes of this magnitude have significant

K. K. CARROLL • Department of Biochemistry, University of Western Ontario, London, Ontario N6A 5C1, Canada.

implications for the food industry (Council for Agricultural Science and Technology, 1982), it is important to examine carefully the evidence on which such a recommendation is based.

2. EPIDEMIOLOGIC EVIDENCE

The positive correlation between cancer and dietary fat is more evident in international comparisons as opposed to within-country or case–control studies (Palmer and Bakshi, 1983). There are a number of reasons for this. Differences in dietary fat intake and in breast cancer incidence and mortality are generally greater between countries than within countries (Hems, 1980), so that any correlations are more likely to be apparent in comparing results from different countries. It is probably also easier to see correlations when larger population groups are being compared, since this will tend to minimize effects of genetic variations in the populations.

Studies on migrating populations have shown that when people move from one country to another, their experience of cancer incidence and mortality changes over a period of time from that of their home country to that of their newly adopted country (Gori, 1978). This is best documented by studies on Japanese emigrants to the U. S., but it has also been observed in other migrating populations (Gori, 1978; Adelstein et al., 1979).

Evidence such as this has given rise to the concept that environmental factors are of major importance in carcinogenesis. This does not, however, mean that genetic factors are unimportant. It is well recognized, for example, that women having close relatives with breast cancer are at greater risk of developing it themselves than women in the population at large (Kelsey, 1979). It seems possible that if genetic susceptibility to breast cancer could be quantitated, a plot of the relative risk of different individuals in a population might resemble a standard distribution curve (Fig. 1a). This does not mean that any given individual would necessarily remain in the same part of the curve throughout her life, since somatic mutations could affect susceptibility.

Under a particular set of environmental conditions, one might predict that all individuals with risk greater than that represented by the line marked Environment A would develop breast cancer (Fig. 1a). Under a different set of conditions, breast cancer would develop in all those with risk greater than the line designated Environment B. There would thus be many individuals in the population who would not develop breast cancer under either of these environmental conditions. The conditions would nevertheless play an important role in overall cancer incidence and mortality by influencing whether or not cancer developed in the individuals at high risk.

In comparing two different populations, it cannot be assumed that their genetic susceptibility to cancer will have the same distribution in each case,

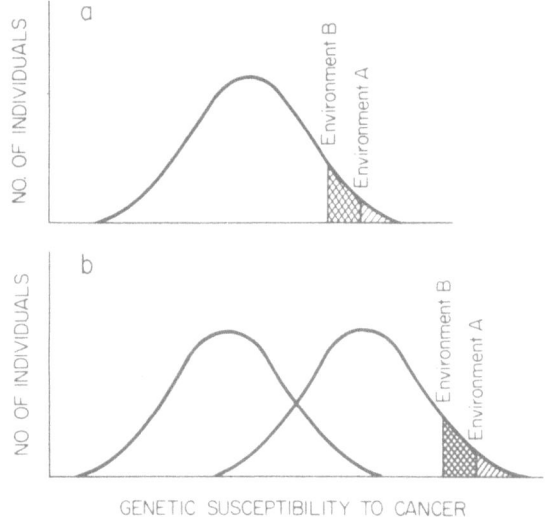

FIGURE 1. (a) Hypothetical variation in the risk of developing breast cancer in a large population of women. It is suggested that because of differences in genetic susceptibility, fewer women would develop breast cancer in Environment A compared to Environment B. (b) Men may also vary in their genetic susceptibility to breast cancer, as indicated by the distribution curve on the left. However, because men are normally much less susceptible than women, few if any men would develop breast cancer in either Environment A or Environment B.

and the smaller the population, the more variable will be the distribution. It is therefore likely to be more difficult to dissociate environmental effects from genetic effects in smaller populations.

An extreme example of the predominance of genetic effects is represented by populations of men and women, who differ markedly in their susceptibility to breast cancer (Kelsey, 1979), so that varying the environmental conditions could influence the incidence of breast cancer in women and not in men (Fig. 1b). There are, however, circumstances in which a substantial number of men can develop breast cancer. This has been reported, for example, in Egypt, where bilharziasis may lead to hyperestrogenism with gynecomastia and increased incidence of breast cancer (El-Gazayerli and Abdel-Aziz, 1963).

Aside from the considerations discussed above, caution must be exercised in interpreting the results of epidemiologic studies. Mortality and morbidity records are often incomplete, and there are many difficulties associated with the estimation of dietary intake of different populations. In spite of this, it seems clear that in a country such as Japan, breast cancer mortality and dietary fat intake are both much lower than in North America and Western Europe. From epidemiologic data alone, however, it is difficult to establish causative relationships. Evidence from studies with experimental animals has therefore been of particular importance in developing the idea that high-fat diets increase the risk of breast cancer. Thus, this evidence should also be scrutinized carefully in order to assess its relevance to human populations.

3. EXPERIMENTAL EVIDENCE

In human populations, the incidence of breast cancer increases with age, and differences in breast cancer mortality between countries with high-fat diets and those with low-fat diets are more pronounced after the menopause (de Waard, 1969). In contrast, most of the experimental studies have been done in relatively young animals, using carcinogens to produce substantial numbers of tumors over a rather short period of time. In some of the early studies by Tannenbaum on spontaneous tumors in mice (Tannenbaum, 1942; Silverstone and Tannenbaum, 1950) the experiments extended over most of the life span, but it seems desirable to carry out further studies on the effects of dietary fat on the development of mammary tumors in older animals. Preliminary results of some of our long-term experiments suggest that dietary fat may have little effect when animals are older (Kalamegham and Carroll, 1984), and this should be explored more fully.

Many of the experiments to date have involved diets containing individual fats or simple mixtures of one or two fats. Such experiments are useful for obtaining information on the effects of different types of dietary fat, but do not reflect human experience. The fat in human diets comes from a variety of different sources and it is desirable to have more information about the effects of such mixtures on mammary tumorigenesis in experimental animals.

If the mechanisms by which dietary fat affects tumorigenesis in animals can be elucidated, it may be possible to apply this knowledge for prevention and treatment of breast cancer in human populations. The evidence indicates that effects of dietary fat on mammary carcinogenesis in animals are exerted largely at the promotional stage, but the exact mechanism is still unclear.

Mammary carcinogenesis as well as normal development of the gland is obviously dependent on the hormonal milieu and it is reasonable to think that this may be affected by dietary fat. Although various workers have studied effects of dietary fat on circulating levels of hormones and on hormone receptors in tissues, there is no consensus on the importance of hormonal alterations as a mechanism of action of dietary fat (Welsch and Aylsworth, 1983; Dao and Chan, 1983).

Of the various other mechanisms that have been proposed (Carroll *et al.*, 1981), the suggestion that prostaglandins may be involved appears to be one of the most promising. It is known that polyunsaturated fats promote mammary carcinogenesis in rats more effectively than saturated fats (Carroll and Khor, 1975) and this difference seems to be related to a requirement for essential fatty acids (Carroll *et al.*, 1981). These serve as precursors of prostaglandins, which can act as promoters of carcinogenesis (Levine, 1981). Other studies have shown that the promoting effect of dietary fat can be prevented by treatment with the prostaglandin synthesis inhibitor indomethacin (Carter *et al.*, 1983; Abraham and Hillyard, 1983).

4. FUTURE PROSPECTS

There are good reasons for thinking that dietary fat may play an important role in breast cancer incidence and mortality. Variations in the level of dietary fat that have been shown to have a significant effect on mammary tumorigenesis in animals are within the limits found in the diets of different human populations. Thus, in suggesting a reduction in dietary fat as a possible means of reducing the risk of breast cancer, it is not necessary to advocate an unnaturally low level. In fact, our recent studies in animals have indicated that reducing fat intake from 40 to 20% of calories inhibits mammary tumorigenesis as effectively as complete removal of fat from the diet (Kalamegham and Carroll, 1984).

It is important to continue with experiments in animals in order to obtain as much information as possible on effects of different types and amounts of dietary fat on mammary carcinogenesis and to increase our understanding of the mechanisms involved. It will be difficult, however, to establish whether or not dietary fat plays a significant role in human breast cancer without direct studies on human populations.

Although breast cancer is relatively common in North American women, it is probably impracticable to test the effects of lowering dietary fat in an unselected population. This would require monitoring a large population for a relatively long period of time to detect significant beneficial effects. A more useful approach is to study a population of women at increased risk of breast cancer. Examples of such populations include women with benign breast disease and women having close relatives with breast cancer.

It may also be possible to conduct trials on breast cancer patients themselves (Wynder and Cohen, 1982; de Waard, 1982). Recurrence is common in such patients and since the experimental data indicate that dietary fat acts by stimulating proliferation of cancer cells, it might be possible to delay or even prevent development of metastatic lesions.

There do not appear to be any serious risks associated with a reduction of dietary fat to as little as half the current level in North American diets.

Although dietary fat is the source of essential fatty acids, it seems unlikely that a deficiency would occur in a free-living population. Dietary fat also provides fat-soluble vitamins and enhances their absorption from the gut, but vitamin supplements could be provided if necessary.

In recent years there has been no indication of a downward trend in the death rate from breast cancer (Carroll et al., 1981). This suggests that any improvements in diagnosis and treatment are having little impact on the disease. A dietary approach may therefore be a worthwhile alternative to consider.

ACKNOWLEDGMENTS. The financial support of the National Cancer Institute of Canada is gratefully acknowledged. The author is a Career Investigator of the Medical Research Council of Canada.

REFERENCES

Abraham, S., and Hillyard, L. A., 1983, Lipids, lipogenesis, and the effects of dietary fat on growth in mammary tumor model systems, in: *Dietary Fats and Health* (E. G. Perkins and W. J. Visek, eds.), American Oil Chemists' Society, Champaign, Illinois, pp. 817–853.

Adelstein, A. M., Staszewski, J., and Muir, C. S., 1979, Cancer mortality in 1970–1972 among Polish-born migrants to England and Wales, *Br. J. Cancer* **40:**464–475.

Carroll, K. K., 1981, Neutral fats and cancer, *Cancer Res.* **41:**3695–3699.

Carroll, K. K., 1982, Dietary fat and its relationship to human cancer, in: *Carcinogens and Mutagens in the Environment,* Volume I, *Food Products* (H. F. Stich, ed.), CRC, Boca Raton, Florida, pp. 31–38.

Carroll, K. K., 1983, The role of dietary fat in carcinogenesis, in: *Dietary Fats and Health* (E. G. Perkins and W. J. Visek, eds.), American Oil Chemists' Society, Champaign, Illinois, pp. 710–720.

Carroll, K. K., and Khor, H. T., 1975, Dietary fat in relation to tumorigenesis, *Prog. Biochem. Pharmacol.* **10:**308–353.

Carroll, K. K., Hopkins, G. J., Kennedy, T. G., and Davidson, M. B., 1981, Essential fatty acids in relation to mammary carcinogenesis, *Prog. Lipid Res.* **20:**685–690.

Carter, C. A., Milholland, R. J., Shea, W., and Ip, M. M., 1983, Effect of the prostaglandin synthetase inhibitor indomethacin on 7,12-dimethylbenz(*a*)anthracene-induced mammary tumorigenesis in rats fed different levels of fat, *Cancer Res.* **43:**3559–3562.

Council for Agricultural Science and Technology, 1982, *Diet, Nutrition, and Cancer: A Critique,* Ames, Iowa.

Dao, T. L., and Chan, P. C., 1983, Hormones and dietary fat as promoters in mammary carcinogenesis, *Environ. Health Perspect.* **50:**219–225.

de Waard, F., 1969, The epidemiology of breast cancer: Review and prospects, *Int. J. Cancer* **4:**577–586.

de Waard, F., 1982, Nutritional etiology of breast cancer: Where are we now, and where are we going? *Nutr. Cancer* **4:**85–89.

El-Gazayerli, M. M., and Abdel-Aziz, A, S., 1963, On bilharziasis and male breast cancer in Egypt: A preliminary report and review of the literature, *Br. J. Cancer* **17:**566–571.

Gori, G. B., 1978, Diet and nutrition in cancer causation, *Nutr. Cancer* **1:**5–8.

Hems, G., 1980, Associations between breast-cancer mortality rates, childbearing and diet in the United Kingdom, *Br. J. Cancer* **41**:429–437.

Kalamegham, R., and Carroll, K. K., 1984, Reversal of the promotional effect of high-fat diet on mammary tumorigenesis by subsequent lowering of dietary fat, *Nutr. Cancer* **6**:22–31.

Kelsey, J. L., 1979, A review of the epidemiology of human breast cancer, *Epidemiol. Rev.* **1**:74–109.

Levine, L., 1981, Arachidonic acid transformation and tumor production, *Adv. Cancer Res.* **35**:49–79.

National Research Council, 1982, *Diet, Nutrition, and Cancer,* National Academy of Sciences, Washington, D.C.

Palmer, S., and Bakshi, K., 1983, Diet, nutrition, and cancer: Interim dietary guidelines, *J. Nat. Cancer Inst.* **70**:1153–1170.

Silverstone, H., and Tannenbaum, A., 1950, The effect of the proportion of dietary fat on the rate of formation of mammary carcinoma in mice, *Cancer Res.* **10**:448–453.

Tannenbaum, A., 1942, The genesis and growth of tumors III. Effects of a high-fat diet, *Cancer Res.* **2**:468–475.

Welsch, C. W., and Aylsworth, C. F., 1983, Enhancement of murine mammary tumorigenesis by feeding high levels of dietary fat: A hormonal mechanism? *J. Nat. Cancer Inst.* **70**: 215–221.

Wynder, E. L., and Cohen, L. A., 1982, A rationale for dietary intervention in the treatment of postmenopausal breast cancer patients, *Nutr. Cancer* **3**:195–199.

Wynder, E. L., McCoy, G. D., Reddy, B. S., Cohen, L., Hill, P., Spingarn, N. E., and Weisburger, J. H., 1981, Nutrition and metabolic epidemiology of cancers of the oral cavity, esophagus, colon, breast, prostate, and stomach, in: *Nutrition and Cancer: Etiology and Treatment* (G. R. Newell and N. M. Ellison, eds.), Raven, New York, pp. 11–48.

31

Calories and Chemical Carcinogenesis

DAVID M. KLURFELD, MAXINE M. WEBER, and DAVID KRITCHEVSKY

It is generally accepted that diet influences the development of cancer in humans and laboratory animals. The dietary component most thoroughly studied for effects on tumor development is fat (Kritchevsky and Klurfeld, 1981). High fat consumption by humans is correlated with cancers of the digestive system—colon, rectum, pancreas, and gall bladder—and of non-intestinal sites, such as breast, ovary, corpus uterus, and prostate (Modan *et al.*, 1975). In animal studies, both the amount and type of fat significantly affect chemically induced tumor growth. Carroll has summarized much of the work in this area of investigation and expressed the currently accepted working hypothesis that dietary fat provides conditions more favorable for tumor growth (Carroll, 1983). Those conditions may include alterations of target cell membranes, immunologic responses, hormone levels, fecal steroid concentrations, or prostaglandin production.

One aspect of dietary fat consumption relative to carcinogenesis that has not received much attention is its relative caloric density, which is more than twice that of carbohydrate or protein. Since polyunsaturated fat is significantly more effective in promoting tumor development than saturated fat, it is unlikely that caloric availability is completely responsible for the enhancing effects of fat. However, results of a series of experiments from our laboratory indicate that caloric availability may be a stronger determinant than fat content of the diet in susceptibility to chemical carcinogens (Kritchevsky *et al.*, 1984).

DAVID M. KLURFELD, MAXINE M. WEBER, and DAVID KRITCHEVSKY • The Wistar Institute of Anatomy and Biology, Philadelphia, Pennsylvania 19104.

In an experiment comparing fat content against caloric density for effects on mammary tumorigenesis in female Sprague-Dawley rats treated with 7,12-dimethylbenz(a)anthracene (DMBA), we used diets of low-fat, high-calorie (LF-HC, 3.73 kcal/g) and high-fat, low-calorie (HF-LC, 2.68 kcal/g) compositions (Table I). The diets were fed in a crossover design whose switch point was administration of DMBA. This yielded four treatment groups: (1) LF-HC → LF-HC; (2) LF-HC → HF-LC; (3) HF-LC → LF-HC; and (4) HF-LC → HF-LC. Diets were fed 1 month before and 4 months after DMBA; commercial ration was fed to all rats for 2 days before and after administration of carcinogen so diet would not influence its absorption. The results are presented in Table II. A significantly greater ($p < 0.01$) mammary tumor yield was found in the rats maintained on the low-fat, high-calorie diet throughout the study. Rats given low-calorie diets increased their food intake from 15 ± 1 to 23 ± 1 g/day ($p < 0.001$); these rats also consumed 3.4 ± 0.2 g/day of fat, while rats eating the low-fat, high-calorie diet ingested only 0.8 ± 0.02 g/day ($p < 0.001$). Despite this higher fat intake, tumor incidence was 33 and 40% compared to 50 and 67% in the rats given the low-fat, high-calorie diet during the promotion phase of tumor induction. These results suggest that caloric availability is a stronger determinant of tumor promotion than dietary fat content of DMBA-induced mammary cancer.

The previous study used cellulose as a nonnutritive filler to dilute the caloric density of the high-fat, low-calorie diet. While we had little reason to believe that dietary fiber would influence mammary tumorigenesis, it was decided to control for this variable. A subsequent experiment was performed in which pair-fed rats were subjected to 60% restriction of calorie consumption by rats allowed *ad libitum* access to food. Two groups of 24 rats each were housed individually and given 5 mg of DMBA dissolved in corn oil by gavage at 50 days of age. Ten days later, the rats were fed the diets described

TABLE I. Diet Composition

	Low fat, high calorie, %	High fat, low calorie, %
Sucrose	70.0	25.0
Casein	11.85	8.9
DL-Methionine	0.15	0.1
Coconut oil	4.0	14.0
Corn oil	1.0	1.0
Cellulose	8.0	46.0
Mineral mix	3.8	3.8
Vitamin mix	1.0	1.0
Choline dihydrogen citrate	0.2	0.2

TABLE II. Tumors in Rats Fed Diets of Different Fat and Calorie Contents

Group[a]	Tumor incidence		Tumor yield	Tumors/tumor-bearing rat
LF-HC→LF-HC	10/15	67%	29	2.9 ± 0.9
LF-HC→HF-LC	5/15	33%	13	2.6 ± 1.4
HF-LC→LF-HC	7/14	50%	13	1.9 ± 0.3
HF-LC→HF-LC	6/15	40%	12	2.0 ± 0.4

[a]LF-HC, Low-fat, high-calorie; HF-LC, high fat, low calorie.

under experiment 1 in Table III. Within 1 week, body weights of the food-restricted animals were significantly less than those of the rats allowed *ad libitum* access to their food. Final weights were 346 ± 13 and 234 ± 5 g in the *ad libitum* and restricted groups, respectively. Because of the different fat contents of the diets, rats in the group allowed free access to food consumed 0.8 g of fat per day, while the animals given restricted calories took in 1.7 g of fat per day. Fifty-eight percent of the rats in the *ad libitum* group developed mammary tumors by the end of 5 months, with a yield of 2.8 ± 0.5 tumors per tumor-bearing rat. No tumors were discovered in the group subjected to caloric restriction despite an intake of more than twice the fat of the *ad libitum* group.

In the previous study a relatively low yield of tumors may have been due to the fact that highly saturated coconut oil was the predominant fat or to reduced protein intake by the diet-restricted rats. Therefore, we conducted another experiment in DMBA-treated rats that were fed the two diets listed under experiment 2 of Table III. This study used corn oil as the only source of fat and altered the protein content of the diet fed to the rats restricted to 60% of calories so that the animals received the same amount of protein, as

TABLE III. Percent Composition of Pair-Fed Diets

	Experiment 1		Experiment 2	
	Ad lib	Restricted	*Ad lib*	Restricted
Sucrose	59.0	39.0	59.0	25.0
Casein	21.7	21.7	21.6	36.2
DL-Methionine	0.3	0.3	0.3	0.5
Coconut oil	2.9	13.0	--	--
Corn oil	1.0	1.0	4.0	13.1
Cellulose	10.1	16.8	10.1	16.8
Mineral mix	3.8	6.8	3.8	6.4
Vitamin mix	1.0	1.7	1.0	1.7
Choline dihydrogen citrate	0.2	0.2	0.2	0.3

well as cellulose, minerals, and vitamins as the animals allowed free access to food. Fat intake by the restricted rats was double that of the *ad libitum* group. Final body weights were 333 ± 11 and 208 ± 4 g in the *ad libitum* and restricted groups, respectively, at the end of 4 months on diet. The differences in body weights were reflected by differences in body fat. There was very little subcutaneous or other visible deposits of adipose tissue. Quantitation of renal fat pad weights showed 5.77 ± 0.99 g in the *ad libitum* rats and 0.74 ± 0.10 g in the restricted animals ($p < 0.001$). Tumor yields from this experiment are given in Table IV. All parameters that reflect tumor number, incidence, and size were significantly ($p < 0.001$) greater in the rats allowed the greater caloric intake.

The same diets described under experiment 2 in Table III were fed to male Fischer 344 rats for a study of colonic carcinogenesis. Rats were maintained on standard laboratory ration and given six weekly doses of 1,2-dimethylhydrazine (DMH) by gavage. Beginning 1 week after the last dose of DMH, the rats were fed the semipurified diets for 7 months. Tumor incidence in the *ad libitum* group was 100% and in the restricted group 53% ($p < 0.001$). The number of tumors per tumor-bearing rat was significantly lower in the rats given restricted calories, 3.5 ± 0.4 vs. 2.1 ± 0.6 tumors ($p < 0.02$). The incidence of extracolonic tumors (carcinomas of the duodenum and ear canal) was also significantly less in the restricted group, 32 vs. 11% ($p < 0.05$).

In an attempt to elucidate a mechanism by which restriction of caloric intake might be operative in inhibiting tumor development, we examined plasma lipoprotein levels. There is a substantial literature on the immunoregulatory activity of lipoproteins (reviewed in Klurfeld, 1983); alterations of the immune response may be significant for development of tumors, particularly during the promotion phase if the "immune surveillance" hypothesis is correct. Both lymphocyte and macrophage activities are depressed by exposure to lipoproteins primarily of the very low-density (VLDL) and intermediate-density (IDL) classes (Edgington and Curtiss, 1981; Morse *et al.*,

TABLE IV. Tumor Data from DMBA-Treated Rats Fed Diets Containing Corn Oil

	Ad libitum	Restricted
Tumor incidence	16/20 80%	4/20 20%
Tumors/tumor-bearing rat	4.0 ± 0.5	1.0 ± 0.0
Total tumor yield	62	4
Mean tumor weight, g	2.8 ± 1.1	0.2 ± 0.1
Mean tumor burden, g	11.1 ± 4.4	0.2 ± 0.1

1977; Klurfeld et al., 1979; Chapman and Hibbs, 1977; Takemura-Hattori et al., 1980).

All three pair-feeding studies showed similar results for plasma lipid levels as a function of caloric restriction (Table V). Both cholesterol and triglyceride concentrations were significantly reduced ($p < 0.001$) in rats restricted to 60% of calories in spite of provision of twice as much dietary fat as the unrestricted rats consumed. Decreases of plasma cholesterol ranged from 30 to 44% and decreases of triglycerides ranged from 38 to 65%. These alterations of plasma lipid concentrations suggested that significant changes in lipoprotein metabolism occurred during caloric restriction. Therefore, we analyzed lipoprotein concentrations by scanning densitometry of cellulose acetate electrophoretograms (Table VI). Significantly higher proportions of β-lipoproteins (corresponding to LDL) were found in the restricted rats treated with DMBA ($p < 0.05$) or DMH ($p < 0.001$). Pre-β-lipoproteins were significantly reduced ($p = 0.05$) in the DMBA-treated rats subjected to caloric restriction, but were unaffected in the DMH-treated rats. α-lipoproteins were unchanged in the DMBA-treated rats given reduced calories, but in the restricted DMH-treated rats a significant decrease ($p < 0.01$) was noted. The differences between these results of the two experiments may be a function of strain, sex, or carcinogen treatment of the rats. It should be noted that the absolute amounts of all the lipoproteins in the restricted rats were much lower than those of the unrestricted rats, as evidenced by the plasma lipid data (Table V). Therefore, differences in both quantity and quality of plasma lipoproteins are characteristic of restriction of caloric availability in rats. These differences may be responsible for some of the protective effects on tumor promotion exerted by caloric restriction.

TABLE V. Plasma Lipid Concentrations in Pair-Fed Rats (mg/dl)

	Ad libitum	Restricted
DMBA-treated female Sprague-Dawley rats fed saturated fat[a]		
Cholesterol	162 ± 10	114 ± 6
Triglycerides	185 ± 22	114 ± 4
DMBA-treated female Sprague-Dawley rats fed unsaturated fat[b]		
Cholesterol	83 ± 5	54 ± 3
Triglycerides	55 ± 10	19 ± 3
DMH-treated male F344 rats fed unsaturated fat[b]		
Cholesterol	81 ± 2	45 ±
Triglycerides	57 ± 3	29 ± 2

[a]Experiment 1, Table III.
[b]Experiment 2, Table III.

TABLE VI. Percent Composition of Plasma Lipoproteins in Pair-Fed Rats

	Ad libitum	Restricted
DMBA-treated female Sprague-Dawley rats		
fed unsaturated fat		
β-Lipoproteins	12.2±4.7	23.3±2.3
Pre-β-Lipoproteins	47.7±3.6	39.2±2.0
α-Lipoproteins	35.4±3.9	34.9±2.2
DMH-treated male F344 rats		
fed unsaturated fat		
β-Lipoproteins	3.8±1.5	18.8±2.8
Pre-β-Lipoproteins	31.2±2.2	28.4±3.3
α-Lipoproteins	55.7±1.6	47.2±2.4

The studies described above demonstrate that caloric availability is a stronger determinant than dietary fat content in the development of chemically induced mammary and colonic tumors. The protective effect of caloric restriction may be mediated through enhanced immunocompetence secondary to alterations in plasma lipoproteins. Forty years ago, Tannenbaum (1945), Lavik and Baumann (1943), and Boutwell et al. (1949) all reported that caloric restriction inhibited tumor development. Both fat and caloric intake affected the incidence of methylcholanthrene-induced skin tumors in mice; regardless of the amount of dietary fat, mice given high-calorie diets exhibited a greater tumor incidence than animals fed low-calorie diets (Lavik and Baumann, 1943). Benzpyrene-induced skin tumors and spontaneous mammary tumors in mice were inhibited proportionally to the degree of calorie restriction (Tannenbaum, 1945). Boutwell et al. (1949) concluded that the increased numbers of benzpyrene-induced skin tumors in mice fed a diet containing 27% fat vs. 2% fat could be explained by the greater net energy available from the high-fat diet.

A committee of the National Research Council (1982) reviewed the available evidence linking total caloric intake with cancer incidence epidemiologically and experimentally. The conclusions stated,

> Because the intake of all nutrients was simultaneously depressed in [the cited] studies, the observed reduction in tumor incidence or delayed onset of tumors might have been due to the reduction of other nutrients such as fat. It is also difficult to interpret experiments in which caloric intake has been modified by varying dietary fat or fiber, both of which may by themselves exert effects on tumorigenesis.

Our series of experiments addresses these uncertainties and demonstrates that caloric availability is more significant than dietary fat content in both mammary and colonic tumor formation in rats treated with chemical carcinogens.

ACKNOWLEDGMENTS. This work was supported in part by a grant-in-aid from the American Institute for Cancer Research, a Research Career Award (HL-00734) from the National Institutes of Health, and funds from the Commonwealth of Pennsylvania.

REFERENCES

Boutwell, R. K., Brush, M. K., and Rusch, H. P., 1949, The stimulating effect of dietary fat on carcinogenesis, *Cancer Res.* **9**:741–746.

Carroll, K. K., 1983, The role of dietary fat in carcinogenesis, in: *Dietary Fats and Health* (E.G. Perkins and W. J. Visek, eds.), American Oil Chemists Society, Champaign, Illinois, pp. 710–720.

Chapman, H. A., Jr., and Hibbs, J. B., Jr., 1977, Modulation of macrophage tumoricidal capability by components of normal serum: A central role for lipid, *Science* **197**:282–285.

Edgington, T. S., and Curtiss, L. K., 1981. Plasma lipoproteins with bioregulatory properties including the capacity to regulate lymphocyte function and the immune response, *Cancer Res.* **41**:3786–3788.

Klurfeld, D. M., 1983, Interactions of immune function with lipids and atherosclerosis, *CRC Crit. Rev. Toxicol.* **11**:333–365.

Klurfeld, D. M., Allison, M. J., Gerszten, E., and Dalton, H. P., 1979, Alterations of host defenses paralleling cholesterol-induced atherogenesis. II. Immunologic studies of rabbits, *J. Med.* **10**:49–64.

Kritchevsky, D., and Klurfeld, D. M., 1981, Fat and cancer, in: *Nutrition and Cancer: Etiology and Treatment* (G. R. Newell and N. M. Ellison, eds.), Raven, New York, pp. 173–188.

Kritchevsky, D., Weber, M. M., and Klurfeld, D. M., 1984, Dietary fat versus caloric content in initiation and promotion of 7,12-dimethylbenz(*a*)anthracene-induced mammary tumorigenesis in rats, *Cancer Res.* **44**:3174–3177.

Lavik, P. S., and Baumann, C. A., 1943, Further studies on the tumor-promoting action of fat, *Cancer Res.* **3**:749–756.

Modan, B., Barell, V., Lubin, F., Modan, M., Greenberg, R. A., and Graham, S., 1975, Low fiber intake as an etiologic factor in cancer of the colon, *J. Nat. Cancer Inst.* **55**:15–18.

Morse, J. H., Witte, L. D., and Goodman, D. S., 1977, Inhibition of lymphocyte proliferation stimulated by lectins and allogeneic cells by normal plasma lipoproteins, *J. Exp. Med.* **146**:1791–1803.

National Research Council, 1982, *Diet, Nutrition, and Cancer,* National Academy of Sciences, Washington, D. C., pp. 4-1-4-5.

Takemura-Hattori, R., Yamazaki, M., Kurisu, M., and Mizuno, D., 1980, Depression of macrophage function by lipoprotein from tumorous ascites, *Gann* **71**:206–212.

Tannenbaum, A., 1945, The dependence of tumor formation on the degree of caloric restriction, *Cancer Res.* **5**:609–615.

32

Enhancement of 7,12-Dimethylbenz(a)anthracene Mammary Carcinogenesis by a High Lard Diet

ADRIANNE E. ROGERS, BARBARA H. CONNER, CYNTHIA L. BOULANGER, SOON Y. LEE, F. ANN CARR, AND WILLIAM H. DUMOUCHEL

1. INTRODUCTION

Enhancement of 7,12-dimethylbenz(a)anthracene (DMBA)-induced mammary carcinogenesis in rats by diets containing 20–25% polyunsaturated vegetable oils or lard has been demonstrated in several laboratories (Carroll, 1980; Rogers *et al.*, 1982). In contrast to corn oil, which enhances tumorigenesis if fed after DMBA administration and has been considered to act only on promotion, lard enhanced tumorigenesis when it was fed before and after DMBA treatment but not when it was fed only after treatment (Rogers *et al.*, 1982; Wetsel *et al.*, 1981). Silverman *et al.* (1980) reported a similar timing of the enhancement of X-ray induced mammary tumorigenesis by lard. Dao and Chan (1983) reported that an effect of corn oil at initiation of tumorigenesis could be demonstrated by altering the standard protocols and that duration of feeding high-fat diets might be as important as timing.

ADRIANNE E. ROGERS • Department of Pathology, Boston University School of Medicine, Boston, Massachusetts 02118. BARBARA H. CONNER, CYNTHIA L. BOULANGER, SOON Y. LEE, F. ANN CARR and WILLIAM H. DUMOUCHEL • Department of Nutrition and Food Science and The Statistics Center, Massachusetts Institute of Technology, Cambridge, Massachusetts 02139.

2. MATERIALS AND METHODS*

Female Sprague-Dawley weanling rats, 40–45 g (Charles River Laboratories, Wilmington, Maryland, were fed either the control, 4% lard diet (C) or the same diet with 19% added lard substituted isocalorically for carbohydrate (Table I). Both diets contained 1% corn oil. DMBA (Sigma Chemical Co., St. Louis, Missouri) was given by gavage, 2.5 mg per rat in 0.2 ml sesame oil at 55 days of age.

Two experiments were performed. The first was designed to define the time period in which high-lard (HL) diet must be fed to increase mammary tumorigenesis by DMBA. The second experiment examined the possible contribution of increased caloric intake by rats fed the HL diet to enhancement of tumorigenesis.

Experiment 1. Rats were fed the HL diet or the C diet from weaning to age 53 days and then fed the C diet from age 53 to 57 days to eliminate a direct effect of diet on carcinogen absorption. They were given 2.5 mg DMBA in 0.2 ml sesame oil by gavage at 55 days. At 57 days the rats that had been fed the HL diet before DMBA treatment were divided into four groups (50 rats each) and fed: (1) the C diet to termination, (2) the HL diet for 3 weeks and then the C diet to termination, (3) the HL diet for 6 weeks and then the C diet to termination, or (4) the HL diet to termination. A fifth group fed the C diet from ∤he beginning of the experiment was fed that diet continously to termination.

Body weight, estrous cycles, day of vaginal opening, and appearance of palpable mammary tumors were monitored.

*The results of this work were reported in part elsewhere (Rogers, 1983).

TABLE I. Composition of Diets

Component	Percent in diet[a]	
	Control (C)	High lard (HL)
Casein (vitamin-free)	19.9	24.4
Sucrose, dextrose, dextrin	69.5	44.2
Lard[b]	4.0	23.3
Corn oil[c]	1.0	1.2
Minerals[d]	5.2	6.4
Vitamins[d]	0.4	0.5

[a] The diets were formulated to give equivalent nutrient intake on a caloric basis and incorporated into 5% aqueous agar.
[b] John Morrell Co.; fatty acid content, %: oleic (18:1), 40.4; palmitic (16:0), 24.2; stearic (18:0), 14.5; linoleic (18:2), 9.89; palmitoleic (16:1), 2.60; myristic (14:0), 1.41; eicosenoic (20:1), 0.901; linolenic (18:3), 0.660; all others 0.6% or less. BHA, 1.27 mg/kg, BHT, 6.26 mg/kg.
[c] Mazola
[d] Supplied in amounts recommended for rats (Rogers, 1979).

Experiment 2. Three groups, ten rats each, were fed throughout the experiment (1) the C diet *ad libitum* or (2) the HL diet *ad libitum,* or (3) were individually matched and pair-fed the HL diet by calories to rats fed the C diet. All rats were given 2.5 mg DMBA on day 55 and fed the C diet from day 53 to day 57.

In both experiments rats were necropsied when they bore a 2-cm tumor. Survivors were necropsied at 32 weeks. Location and size of all mammary tumors were recorded; all tumors were examined histologically.

Statistical analysis of the cumulative probability of bearing a palpable mammary tumor was performed using the product-limit (Kaplan–Meier) and the estimate of the survival distribution as programmed in BMDPIL (BMDP 79, 1979). The equality of the survival distribution between diet groups was tested with a nonparametric rank test developed by Breslow (1970). Relative risk for development of mammary tumors in experiment 1 was calculated as the ratio of tumor incidence in diet groups 1–4 to incidence in group 5. Associated *p* values were obtained by testing for a difference in proportion (incidence rate) between groups.

A logistic model was used to analyze the effects on tumor development of the duration of feeding the high-lard diet. Let P_{ti} be the probability of detecting a mammary tumor in a rat from diet group i ($i = 1-5$) during the examination t weeks after DMBA administration, conditional on that animal not having a detectable tumor preceding week t.

The statistical model used was

$$\log [P_{ti}/(1 - P_{ti})] = A_t + B_i$$

In this additive logistic model, the A's measure the way in which the odds of detecting a mammary tumor vary by week, while the B's measure the differences between the diet groups on the logit scale. Estimates and standard errors for the A's and B's were computed by maximum likelihood methods. For example, in comparing groups 4 and 5 (HL diet throughout vs. diet C), $B_4 - B_5 = 0.98$. Since $e^{0.98} = 2.67$, the odds of detecting a tumor in a rat in group 4 are 2.67 times greater than in a rat in group 5 at each week studied. A 95% confidence interval for this odds ratio is (1.6, 4.4).

3. RESULTS

Experiment 1. Mammary tumors were detected earlier in groups 1–4, all groups fed the HL diet, than in group 5, which was fed the C diet throughout the experiment. At 12 weeks after DMBA administration, the time after which rats with 2-cm tumors were killed, the differences from group 5 were statistically significant (Table II). Tumor latency and incidence and cumulative probability of bearing a palpable tumor were similar in groups 1, 3, and 4. Tumors appeared somewhat later in group 2 and last in

TABLE II. Incidence of Palpable Mammary Tumor 12 Weeks[a]
after DMBA Administration (Experiment 1)

Group	Period fed high-lard diet		Tumor incidence, %	p[b]
	Before DMBA	After DMBA		
1	+	0	32	<0.0001
2	+	3 weeks	18	0.015
3	+	6 weeks	34	0.0001
4	+	12 weeks	34	0.0001
5	0	0	8	—

[a] At a time before any rats were killed.
[b] Associated with testing for difference in proportion, compared to group 5.

group 5. Tumor number and weight were similar in all groups fed the HL diet and somewhat lower in group 5 (Table III).

The logistic model gave estimates for the B's as follows: group 1, -3.13; group 2, -3.48; group 3, -2.98; group 4, -2.84; group 5, -3.82. The standard error of each B_i is approximately 0.18, and they are approximately uncorrelated. Figure 1 depicts the estimates and the 95% confidence interval for the odds ratios for tumors, comparing each group to group 5. In order to test for a lard dose-related effect, we fitted a straight line to the points (likelihood ratio X^2 statistic for goodness of fit = 4.2, 2 df, $p = 0.12$). The test for trend has $p = 0.04$, one-sided, indicating that increasing duration of ingestion of the HL diet resulted in increasing odds of tumor development. There was an odds ratio of 1.64 in favor of occurrence of a palpable tumor in group 1, fed HL diet before DMBA only, compared to group 5.

The first and second mammary glands were approximately twice as likely to develop tumors as any of the lower glands. There was no difference

TABLE III. Period to First Palpable Tumor and Final Tumor
Incidence (Experiment 1)

Group	Time from DMBA to tumor, days	Final tumor incidence,[a] %	Per tumor-bearing rat	
			Number of tumors[b]	Weight of tumors, g
1	94	70	3.1 ± 0.3	4.5 ± 0.7
2	111	56	3.1 ± 0.4	4.7 ± 0.8
3	95	76	3.1 ± 0.3	4.4 ± 0.6
4	84	80	3.1 ± 0.4	4.4 ± 0.5
5	114	52	2.7 ± 0.3	3.5 ± 0.7

[a] At necropsy.
[b] Mean ± SEM.

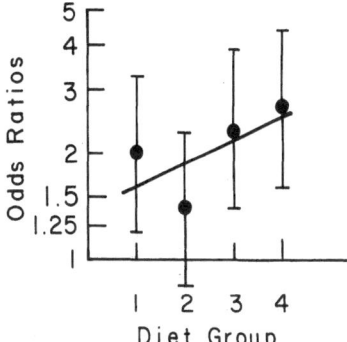

FIGURE 1. Estimated odds ratios with 95% confidence intervals comparing the age-adjusted proportions of rats with palpable mammary tumors in the groups fed the high-lard diet to the control group. Diet groups 1-4 had increasing exposure to the high-lard diet.

in distribution between the right and left sides; dietary treatment had no effect on tumor distribution (data not shown).

Diet had no significant effect on weight gain, age at vaginal opening, which was normally distributed and occurred at 33 ± 3 (SD) days, or on initiation, regularity, or duration of estrous cycles.

Experiment 2. Cumulative probability of bearing a palpable tumor was greater in both HL groups than in the C group (Fig. 2). Final tumor incidence was 90% in both HL groups and 60% in the C group (p = 0.002).

4. DISCUSSION

These experiments were performed to define more exactly the timing of the effect of lard on DMBA mammary tumorigenesis and to examine the specificity of the effect, i.e., whether it is due to lard itself or to increased caloric intake. We have found that the HL diet enhances tumorigenesis when it is fed only for the 5 weeks before DMBA treatment, and that further feeding increases the effect. Lard is therefore influencing events at the time of carcinogen exposure and tumor initiation, as well as later events in tumor development.

The mechanism by which lard acts on tumorigenesis is unknown; the demonstration that it is effective at initiation in the DMBA model directs attention to studies of carcinogen pharmacokinetics and metabolism and of cell division and differentiation in the mammary gland at the time of DMBA exposure. The similar result using X-irradiation to induce tumors (Silverman *et al.*, 1980) suggests that the condition of the mammary gland rather than carcinogen metabolism is an important factor.

Endocrine effects of high-fat diets have been reported (Chan *et al.*, 1977; Ip *et al.*, 1980). However, in a detailed study of plasma prolactin, progesterone, and estrogen in unanesthetized, unrestrained rats fed control or high-

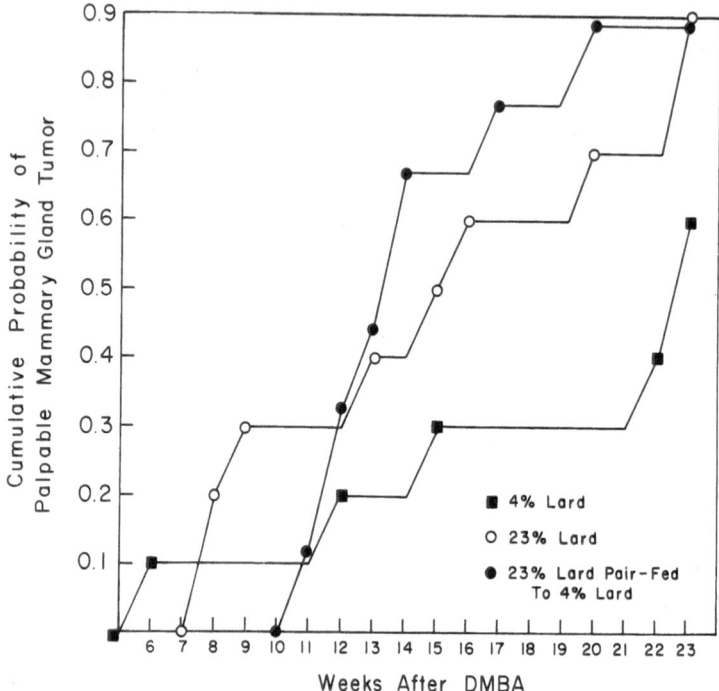

FIGURE 2. Cumulative probability of bearing a palpable mammary gland tumor in rats fed (O) the HL diet *ad libitum* or (●) pair-fed to rats fed (■) the C diet.

fat diets and bled serially over the estrous cycle, we have found that the hormone levels are identical in the two dietary groups at all stages in the cycle (Wetsel *et al.*, 1983). The different results reported by others may reflect a dietary inadequacy of essential fatty acids or may be related to the study of single rather than serial samples. Hepatic prolactin receptors also are not altered (Wetsel and Rogers, 1984).

The active components in lard are not known. We used food-grade lard, which gave consistent fatty acid analyses in different batches and contained very low levels of the antioxidants BHA and BHT. Although the fatty acid composition of lard may be expected to vary with the feed intake of the pigs from which it is derived, analyses of our samples gave results almost identical to the analysis reported by Carroll and Khor (1970) 12 years ago. BHT inhibits DMBA mammary carcinogenesis when fed at 0.3–0.7% of the diet (King *et al.*, 1979). The content in the HL diet was 0.00012% and was, of course, even lower in the C diet. Since the effect of BHT is inhibitory, the enhancing effect of the HL diet cannot be explained by its presence. Lard may contain a variety of trace substances derived from the animals or their feed that could influence tumorigenesis. Studies of lard fractions are indicated to identify the active components.

ACKNOWLEDGMENTS. This work was supported in part by U. S. Public Health Service grant R01 CA25538 from the National Cancer Institute, Department of Health and Human Services and by the MIT Undergraduate Research Opportunities Program.

REFERENCES

BMDP 79, 1979, in: *Biomedical Computer Programs P-Series* (W. J. Dixon and M. B. Brown, eds.), University of California Press, Berkeley.

Breslow, N., 1970, A generalized Kruskal–Wallis test for comparing *K* samples subject to unequal patterns of censorship, *Biometrika* **57**:579–594.

Carroll, K. K., 1980, Lipids and carcinogenesis, *J. Environ. Pathol. Toxicol.* **3**:253–271.

Carroll, K. D., and Khor, H. T., 1970, Effects of dietary fat and dose level of 7,12-dimethylbenz(*a*)anthracene on mammary tumor incidence in rats, *Cancer Res.* **30**:2260–2264.

Chan, P. C., Head, J. F., Cohen, L. A., and Wynder, E. L., 1977, Influence of dietary fat on the induction of mammary tumors by *N*-nitrosomethylurea: Associated hormone changes and differences between Sprague-Dawley and F344 rats, *J. Nat. Cancer Inst.* **59**:1279–1283.

Dao, T. L., and Chan. P.-C., 1983, Effect of duration of high fat intake on enhancement of mammary carcinogenesis in rats, *J. Nat. Cancer Inst.* **71**:201–205.

Ip, C., Yip, P., and Bernardis, L. L., 1980, Role of prolactin in the production of dimethylbenz-(*a*)anthracene-induced mammary tumors by dietary fat, *Cancer Res.* **40**:374–378.

King, M. M., Bailey, D. M., Gibson, D. D., Pitha, J. V., and McCay, P. B., 1979, Incidence and growth of mammary tumors induced by 7,12-dimethylbenz(*a*)anthracene as related to the dietary content of fat and antioxidant, *J. Nat. Cancer Inst.* **63**:657–663.

Rogers, A. E., 1979, Nutrition, in: *The Laboratory Rat*, Volume 1 (H. J. Baker, J. R. Lindsey, and S. H. Weisbroth, eds.), Academic, New York, pp. 123–152.

Rogers, A. E., 1983, Influence of dietary content of lipids and lipotropic nutrients on chemical carcinogenesis in rats, *Cancer Res.* **43**:2477s–2484s.

Rogers, A. E., Fernstrom, J. D., Ge, K., Wetsel, W. C., Yang, S. O., and Camelio, E. A., 1982, Endocrine interactions in the nutritional modulation of mammary carcinogenesis in rats, in: *Molecular Interrelations of Nutrition and Cancer* (M. S. Arnott, J. van Eys, and Y. M. Yang, eds.), Raven, New York pp. 381–399.

Silverman, J., Shellabarger, C. J., Holtzman, S., Stone, J. P., and Weisburger, J. H., 1980, Effect of dietary fat on x-ray-induced mammary cancer in Sprague-Dawley rats, *J. Nat. Cancer Inst.* **64**:631–634.

Wetsel, W. C., and Rogers, A. E., 1984, Hepatic prolactin binding in female Sprague-Dawley rats fed a diet high in corn oil, *J. Nat. Cancer Inst.* **73**:531–536.

Wetsel, W. C., Rogers, A. E., and Newberne, P. M., 1981, Dietary fat and DMBA mammary carcinogenesis in rats, *Cancer Detection Prevention* **4**:535–543.

Wetsel, W. C., Rutledge, A., and Rogers, A. E., 1983, Absence of an effect of dietary corn oil content on plasma prolactin, progesterone, and 17B-estradiol in female Sprague-Dawley rats, *Cancer Res.* **44**:1420–1425.

33

The Assessment of Individual Risk from Diet in Large Bowel Cancer Epidemiology

SHEILA A. BINGHAM

1. INTRODUCTION

The epidemiologic evidence for an etiologic role for diet in the causation of large bowel cancer is circumstantial. International correlation studies, using crude national statistics of food consumption, associate meat consumption with higher rates of colon cancer incidence (Armstrong and Doll, 1975). Studies using more direct indices of food consumption at the individual level suggest that nonstarch polysaccharide (dietary fiber) may have a protective role in populations that would otherwise be at high risk from high meat (and possibly fat) consumption (Jensen et al., 1982). However, case–control studies have yielded conflicting information. Out of ten "Westernized' population samples studied since 1966, one case–control study has supported a role for meat (Manousos et al., 1983), two a role for fat (Jain et al., 1980a; Potter et al., 1982), and none a clear role for dietary fiber. The situation is similar to that found in the study of diet and cardiovascular disease, where large-scale epidemiologic case–control and prospective studies have generally failed to confirm the predictions of experimental work and international comparative studies.

SHEILA A. BINGHAM • University of Cambridge and MRC Dunn Clinical Nutrition Centre, Cambridge, CB2 1QL, United Kingdom.

In large bowel cancer, however, the findings of case–control studies have to be viewed with caution because of the difficulties of assessing diet retrospectively, as detailed in Chapter 39 of this volume. This chapter discusses some nutritional factors pertinent to the prospective study of non-starch polysaccharide (NSP) intake in relation to large bowel cancer.

2. INDIVIDUAL VARIATION IN SUSCEPTIBILITY TO DIETARY STIMULI

In experimental studies of calcium absorption, fat and serum cholesterol, fiber and colonic function, and diet and thermogenesis, for example, it is consistently shown that individuals vary markedly in their physiological response to standard dietary stimuli (Keys *et al.*, 1959; Widdowson, 1962; Ahrens, 1979; Cummings and Stephen, 1980; Dallosso and James, 1984). This individual susceptibility will, of itself, tend to minimize any association between dietary intake and clinical or physiological effects.

In the case of NSP and colon function, individuals of the same age and sex on a standard intake of 20 g dietary fiber/day exhibit a threefold range in fecal weight (Cummings and Stephen, 1980). If high fecal weight is a protective factor in the development of colon cancer, via dilution, decreased transit, and microbial fermentation (Cummings and Branch, 1982), individuals at the right of the distribution will be at less risk from colon cancer than those to the left. Furthermore, on increasing the dietary fiber intake of all individuals, again by a standard amount, to a total of 40 g/day, the ranking of individual variation in fecal weight is maintained, although the distribution as a whole is shifted to the right. Even with a doubling of dietary fiber intake, individuals to the left of the fecal weight distribution may thus not have altered their risk profile appreciably (Cummings, 1984). In the absence of sufficient variation among individuals in dietary intake, observed differences in physiology and disease incidence within a single population are therefore a diffuse reflection of this individual susceptibility.

3. INDIVIDUAL VARIATION IN DIETARY INTAKE

3.1. Among Individuals

Within any one population, however, it is well known that individuals of the same age and sex vary substantially from one another in their intake of food and nutrients. This was first pointed out and emphasized by Widdowson and McCance in the 1930s and 1940s with their pioneering methods for measuring dietary intake in free-living individuals. Previously only average results from family food surveys were available. In summary, in 1945 they remarked that "One child was always found to be eating twice as much as another of the same age and sex, and exactly the same thing had previously been shown to be true of adults. All the separate dietary constituents varied just as much or more, and one boy of 2 years ate more than a boy of 17" (Widdowson and McCance, 1945). Hobson (1948) agreed that "This survey has shown a similar wide variation in the calorie intake of pregnant women, varying from 1600 to 3500 calories per day." Burke *et al.* (1959) remarked on the "enormous differences between individuals of the same age and sex.... At every age, among the boys as well as the girls, there was at least one child whose intake was approximately twice as high as that of one or more other children of the same age and sex." Wiehl (1944) also noticed that the "range in energy value of the diets is very great, 1120 to 3827 calories." More recent surveys have confirmed a minimum twofold variation in energy and nutrient intakes in adolescents, pregnant women, the elderly, and randomly selected adults (Darke *et al.*, 1980; Harries *et al.*, 1962; Bingham *et al.*, 1981).

This individual variation is also shown when NSP intake in individuals of the same age and sex is considered. Figure 1 shows the distribution of intakes of NSP in two randomly selected population groups of men aged 50–59 in rural Finland and Copenhagen. This readily demonstrates the marked effect of an apparently small difference in the average between two groups (5 g NSP in this case) on the distribution of intakes of individuals within any one group. Whereas half the population in rural Finland were consuming more than 18 g NSP/day, only 10% in Copenhagen did so. Colon cancer incidence rates in rural Finland are three times lower than in Copen-

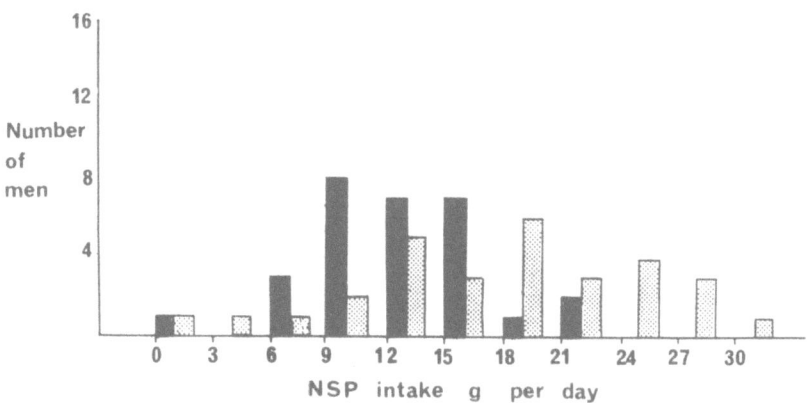

FIGURE 1. Distribution of NSP intake (g/day) in two randomly selected groups of men aged 50–59 in Scandinavia. Solid bars, Copenhagen; stippled bars, rural Finland.

hagen (Jensen *et al.*, 1982), whereas both populations consume high intakes of fat and meat.

However, populations also appear to differ in extent of individual variation. In Copenhagen, for example, the coefficient of variation in NSP intake between individuals was only 23%, whereas it was 33% in rural Finland (Table I). This is illustrated in Fig. 1; in Copenhagen the NSP intake of the majority of individuals is confined to a comparatively narrow range of 9–18 g/day. No other accurate data on individual variation on NSP intake are available, but if a similar narrow distribution of intakes occurs within populations at high risk for colon cancer, such as Australia, Canada, New Zealand, and the U. S., a failure of individual prospective studies within these "Westernized" populations to demonstrate a relationship between dietary fiber intake and colon cancer occurrence would not be surprising. Prospective studies within populations with higher intakes of NSP and a greater variation among individuals might prove more fruitful if they can also be assumed to be "at risk" from high meat and fat consumption, as in rural Finland.

3.2. Within Individuals

The epidemiology of diet and cardiovascular disease is analogous to studies relating NSP consumption to colon cancer incidence. Although the Seven Countries Heart Study (Keys, 1970) clearly demonstrates at the population level a relationship between two risk factors for coronary heart disease, saturated fat intake and serum cholesterol, this relationship has not been generally confirmed at the individual level by large-scale epidemiologic

TABLE I. Variation in NSP Intake in Relation to Fecal Weight among Individuals in Four Randomly Selected Groups of Men Aged 50–59 in Scandinavia

	Rural Finland	Rural Denmark	Helsinki	Copenhagen
Between-person coefficient of variation, B	33	30	30	23
Within-person coefficient of variation, W	27	21	30	28
Ratio B/W	1.19	1.42	1.02	0.82
Analyzed NSP intake vs. fecal weight				
r	0.59	0.51	0.41	−0.24
t	3.87	2.97	2.29	1.17
p	<0.001	<0.01	<0.05	>0.05

studies. Within any one population, however, Keys and Kimura (1970) point out that the errors associated with the measurement of blood cholesterol and saturated fat intake can be greater than the variation between individuals, and of sufficient magnitude to account for a lack of correlation between these two variables. When the ranges of both dietary intake and blood cholesterol were extended, by combining the individual studies in Japan, Greece, and the Netherlands, a significant association ($r = 0.6$) emerged. However, the objection to this international approach is the same as that often leveled at the findings of group comparisons: confounding variables that are not measured and which could account for the observed relationship are more likely to occur in these populations with very different lifestyles as well as diet. An alternative approach is to reduce the errors associated with the measurement of both blood cholesterol and dietary intake in individuals. Careful measurements in a small group of individuals have shown that fat intake (mostly saturated) is significantly associated with serum cholesterol ($r = 0.53$) (Easty, 1970).

Analysis of variance of 4-day records of dietary fiber consumption from all four randomly selected populations studied in Scandinavia (Jensen *et al.,* 1982; Englyst *et al.,* 1982) shows that, in addition to the variation in NSP intake among individuals, there is also substantial variation within individuals from day to day, as occurs with fat, foods, and other nutrients. Estimates of the within-person variation in dietary fiber intake in fact were almost as great as those among persons, from 21 to 30%/day when expressed as the coefficients of variation (Table I). With only a single day of dietary assessment, therefore, the individual values will be associated with a large component of random error.

In Copenhagen, this error actually exceeded the variation among individuals[ratio of among to within variations = 0.82 (Table I)]. In this area, two risk factors for colon cancer, NSP intake and fecal weight, were not significantly associated ($r = 0.24$, $t = 1.17$, n.s.). In all other three areas, however, where the variation among individuals exceeded the variation within individuals in NSP intake, NSP intake was significantly associated with fecal weight (Table I), particularly in rural Finland ($r = 0.59$, $t = 3.87$, $p < 0.001$). This is despite the fact that the daily variation in fecal output is as great as or greater than that in dietary intake.

Thus, in any population where the variation in dietary intake among individuals is small, large errors in assessing diet and other risk factors will obscure relationships between these factors and disease occurrence. Individual prospective studies must therefore be conducted in populations where the variance among individuals is maximal, in this case one where the risk for colon cancer is low. Alternatively, in homogeneous populations, in this case where colon cancer risks are high, it is crucial that the method chosen to assess diet prospectively is the most accurate available.

4. ERRORS IN THE ESTIMATION
OF DIETARY INTAKE

Variation in dietary intake from day to day is usually random, and the error can be substantially reduced by increasing the length of time each individual in a prospective study is observed, not necessarily over a period of consecutive days. The necessary length of time of observation can be predicted once the required degree of accuracy in a dietary survey is established, the nutrient or food of interest is clearly defined, and the extent of individual variation in that population known. For example, 7 days of observation would have been required to classify 80% of men living in Copenhagen into their correct third in the distribution of NSP intake, whereas 3–5 days would have been sufficient in the other areas (Englyst et al., 1982). This calculation, however, is based on the statistical assumption of an average (pooled) within-person variation, whereas in fact there is also a distribution in the extent to which people vary from day to day (Balogh et al., 1971). Longer periods of observation, depending on the degree of accuracy required, would be necessary to take account of variable dietary habits in some individuals.

Whereas the variance in nutrient intake among or between people is probably characteristic of the population under study, analysis of 15 population samples in America, Britain, Israel, Australia, and Hawaii shows that variability from day to day is closely related to the nutrient being studied. This is partly due to the use of food tables, but also to the foods ingested. In recent studies, pooled within-person coefficients of variation are usually 20–30% for energy, whereas those for fat are 20–40%. Calcium, iron, thiamin, and dietary fiber are within the range 30–50%, and riboflavin, vitamin C, cholesterol, and polyunsaturated fatty acids 40–70%. Daily variation is of greater magnitude than the variation in nutrient intake from week to week, which may be due to a lack of precision in the weekly means, from too short a period of observation. Daily variation in food consumption is even greater, and may require extended periods of observation (Bingham, 1984).

Because of this, alternatives to the weighed record method of assessing diet, which is the most accurate, have to be considered in epidemiology. However, the simpler methods, such as the daily (24 h) recall, diet history, questionnaire, or estimated record, are all associated with their own errors, which are far greater than generally assumed (Bingham, 1984). The diet history is said to be highly repeatable and in theory it offers a major advantage over daily methods of assessing diet if it is possible to obtain an estimate of the usual diet in a single interview. However, the method includes errors in the estimation of weights of food eaten and reporting error, as well as coding errors and those from food tables; in addition, the individual has to remember how often many different items of diet are eaten.

In only two instances, however, have the findings from the diet history been compared with records of food kept over a sufficient length of time to allow a comparison of these two estimates of usual diet. In the first (Huenemann and Turner, 1942), 21 adolescents and children kept weighed records of their food intake for 6 weeks, and the nutrient intakes obtained from these records were compared with the results from a diet history. The standard deviations of percentage differences between the two sets of results varied from 16% for protein and 40% for vitamin C, the slopes of the regression lines were not significant for energy, fat, and iron, and there was evidence of systematic bias in the results for energy, fat, thiamin, and calcium. In the study of Jain *et al.* (1980b), records with estimated weights over 30 days were obtained from 16 adult volunteers and the results again compared with those obtained from a diet history. Only 56, 50, and 63% of the subjects were classified into the same thirds of the distribution for energy, protein, and fat using either the diet history or the 30-day records, and the mean values for the group as a whole differed by 21% for fat, 28% for energy, and 52% for crude fiber, the higher values being obtained from the diet history. From these studies, it has to be concluded that the diet history does not measure actual food intake, as judged by comparisons with food records kept over a commensurate period of time.

Other published studies show that the errors associated with 24-h recalls of food intake and questionnaires, commonly used in cancer epidemiology, are even greater. Correlation coefficients show that questionnaires are rarely able to predict more than 4–20% of measured nutrient intake, and when expressed as a standard deviation of percentage differences between reported intakes and those actually measured, studies with children, students, and the elderly suggest that the total error over one day from the 24-h recall method ranges from 5 to 400% (Madden *et al.*, 1976; Todd *et al.*, 1983; Frank *et al.*, 1977). Several other studies with adults suggest that these large errors are routinely associated with one 24-h recall of food eaten (Linusson *et al.*, 1974; Pekkarinen, 1970; Morrison *et al.*, 1949; Young *et al.*, 1952). Errors of this magnitude would effectively obscure any association between diet and disease risk in a prospective study of NSP intake in relation to colorectal cancer.

5. SUMMARY

Within homogeneous population samples, a protective association between NSP intake and disease occurrence or other risk factors, such as fecal weight, is unlikely to be seen, given the inaccuracies of current methods of assessing these variables in large epidemiologic studies. In order to test the "fiber hypothesis" effectively, therefore, it is essential to confine studies to those populations with a demonstrable heterogeneity in NSP intake. On the limited evidence available, the variation in dietary NSP intake may be greater in populations at low or intermediate risk; this approach, however, would necessitate the prospective study of large cohorts. An alternative is to allocate far more resources to accurate methods of assessing the dietary intake of individuals than is customary in epidemiology at present.

REFERENCES

Ahrens, E. H., 1979, Dietary fats and coronary heart disease: Unfinished business, *Lancet* ii:1345.

Armstrong, B., and Doll, R., 1975, Environmental factors and cancer incidence in different countries, with special reference to dietary practices, *Int. J. Cancer* 15:617.

Balogh, M., Kahn, H. A., and Medalie, J. H., 1971, Random repeat 24-hour dietary recalls, *Am. J. Clin. Nutr.* 24:304.

Bingham, S., 1984, Surveillance of the dietary habit of the population with regard to cardiovascular disease: Premise and methods, in: *Euronut 2,* (G. G. de Backer and H. Tunstall-Pedoe, eds.), Wageningen, The Netherlands, pp. 21–42.

Bingham, S., McNeil, N. I., and Cummings, J. H., 1981, The diet of individuals: A study of a randomly chosen cross-section of British adults in a Cambridgeshire village, *Br. J. Nutr.* 45:23.

Burke, B. S., Reed, R. B., Van den Berg, A. S., and Stuart, H. C., 1959, Caloric and protein intakes of children between 1 and 18 years of age, *Pediatrics* 24:922.

Cummings, J. H., 1984, Constipation, dietary fiber and the control of large bowel function, *Postgrad. Med. J.* 60(3):98.

Cummings, J. H., and Branch, W. J., 1982, Postulated mechanisms whereby fiber may protect against large bowel cancer, in: *Dietary Fiber in Health and Disease* (G. V. Vahouny and D. Kritchevsky, eds.), Plenum, New York, p. 313.

Cummings, J. H., and Stephen, A. M., 1980, The role of dietary fiber in the human colon, *Can. Med. Assoc. J.* 123:1109.

Dallosso, H. M., and James, W. P. T., 1984, Whole body calorimetry studies in adult men. 1. The effect of fat overfeeding in 24 h energy expenditure, *Br. J. Nutr.* 52:49.

Darke, S. J., Disselduff, M. M., and Try, G. P., 1980, Frequency distribution of mean intakes of food energy and selected nutrients during nutrition surveys of different groups of people in Great Britain between 1968 and 1971, *Br. J. Nutr.* 44:243.

Easty, D. L., 1970, The relationship of diet to serum cholesterol levels in young men in Antarctica, *Br. J. Nutr.* 24:307.

Englyst, H. N., Bingham, S. A., Wiggins, H. S., Southgate, D. A. T., Seppanen, R., Helms, P., Anderson, V., Day, K. C., Choolun, R., Collinson, E., and Cummings, J. H., 1982, Non-starch polysaccharide consumption in four Scandinavian populations, *Nutr. Cancer* 4:50.

Frank, G. C., Berenson, G. S., Schilling, P. E., and Moore, M. C., 1977, Adapting the 24 hour recall for epidemiologic studies of school children, *J. Am. Diet. Assoc.* 71:26.

Harries, J. M., Hobson, E. A., and Hollingsworth, D. F., 1962, Individual variations in energy expenditure and intake, *Proc. Nutr. Soc.* 21:157.

Hobson, W., 1948, A dietary and clinical survey of pregnant women with particular reference to toxaemia of pregnancy, *J. Hyg.* 46:198.

Huenemann, R. L., and Turner, D., 1942, Methods of dietary investigation, *J. Am. Diet. Assoc.* 18:562.

Jain, M., Cook, G. M., Davis, F. G., Grace, M. G., Howe, G. R., and Miller, A. B., 1980a, A case control study of diet and colorectal cancer, *Int. J. Cancer* **26**:757.

Jain, M., Howe, G. R., Johnson, K. C., and Miller, A. B., 1980b, Evaluation of diet history questionnaire for epidemiologic studies, *Am. J. Epidemiol.* **111**:212.

Jensen, O. M., MacLennan, R., and Wahrendorf, J., 1982, Diet, bowel function, fecal characteristics and large bowel cancer in Denmark and Finland, *Nutr. Cancer* **4**:5.

Keys, A., 1970, Coronary heart disease in seven countries, *Circulation* **XLI** and **XLII** (Suppl. 1):162.

Keys, A., and Kimura, N., 1970, Diets of middle-aged farmers in Japan, *Am. J. Clin. Nutr.* **23**:212.

Keys, A., Anderson, J. T., and Grande, F., 1959, Serum cholesterol, *Circulation* **XIX**:207.

Linusson, E. E. I., Sanjur, D., and Erickson, E. C., 1974, Validating the 24 hour recall method as a dietary survey tool, *Arch. Latino Nutr.* **24**:277.

Madden, J. P., Goodman, S. J., and Guthrie, H. A., 1976, Validity of the 24 hr recall, *J. Am. Diet. Assoc.* **68**:143.

Manousos, O., Day, N. E., Trichopoulos, D., Gerovassilis, F., Tzonou, A., and Polychronopoulou, A., 1983, Diet and colorectal cancer: A case control study, *Int. J. Cancer* **32**:1.

Morrison, S. D., Russel, F. C., and Stevenson, J., 1949, Estimating food intake by questioning and weighing: A one day survey of eight subjects, *Proc. Nutr. Soc.* **3**:V.

Pekkarinen, M., 1970, Methodology in the collection of food consumption data, *World Rev. Nutr. Diet.* **12**:145.

Potter, J. D., McMichael, A. J., and Bonett, A. Z., 1982, Diet alcohol and large bowel cancer: A case control study, *Proc. Nutr. Soc. Aust.* **7**:123.

Todd, K. S., Hudes, M., and Calloway, D. H., 1983, Food intake measurement: Problems and approaches, *Am. J. Clin. Nutr.* **37**:139.

Widdowson, E. M., 1962, Nutritional individuality, *Proc. Nutr. Soc.* **21**:121.

Widdowson, E. M., and McCance, R. A., 1945, Individual dietary surveys, *Proc. Nutr. Soc.* **3**:110.

Wiehl, D. G., 1944, Medical evaluation of nutritional status, *Milbank Mem. Fund Q.* **22**:5-40.

Young, C. M., Chalmers, F. W., Church, H. N., Clayton, M. M., Hagan, G. C., Steele, B. F., Tucker, R. E., and Foster, W. D., 1952, Subjects' ability to estimate food portions, *Bull. Man. Agric. Exp. Stn.* **469**:63-77.

34

Dietary Studies of Cancer of the Large Bowel in the Animal Model

NORMAN D. NIGRO and ARTHUR W. BULL, Jr.

1. INTRODUCTION

Cancer of the large bowel is common in the U. S., Canada, and many countries of the Western world. About 125,000 Americans developed the disease in its clinically recognizable form in 1983. The 5-year survival rate is about 40%, virtually the same as it has been for some time. Curative treatment is surgical. Radiation and chemotherapy are sometimes given in conjunction with operation and often used to control symptoms in patients with advanced disease. Morbidity is excessive and the last 2 or 3 years of life are unusually difficult for most patients.

Improvements in early diagnosis and in therapy are being made, but progress is limited and slow. On the other hand, the prospects for prevention are brighter. Advances in our knowledge of some aspects of the etiology of the disease have been made from epidemiologic observations, clinical and laboratory studies, and animal experimentation. The purpose of this chapter is to describe the animal model as it is currently used and to review some information derived from it.

NORMAN D. NIGRO and ARTHUR W. BULL, Jr. • Department of Surgery, Wayne State University School of Medicine, Detroit, Michigan 48201.

2. CARCINOGENS

The induction of intestinal cancer in rodents by such chemicals as methylcholanthrene, aflatoxin, and certain biphenyls had been reported as early as 1941 (Lorenz and Stewart, 1941). However, these compounds induce a relatively low incidence of the disease, and some are difficult to administer. Consequently, the animal model was not widely used until Laqueur (1965) discovered that the plant product cycasin was a potent and organ-specific intestinal carcinogen. Cycasin was effective only when fed to conventional rats. The lack of effect in germ-free animals proved that the bacterial flora is essential for the activation of the compound. Cycasin was shown to contain methylazoxymethanol glucoside, which was hydrolyzed by bacterial β-glucosidases to release methylazoxymethanol (MAM), the proximate carcinogen (Laqueur, 1968). Druckrey (1970) and his associates discovered that the structurally related chemicals dimethylhydrazine (DMH) and azoxymethane (AOM) were also potent colon carcinogens in rodents.

When DMH is administered to animals, it is metabolized in azomethane, then to AOM, and finally to MAM (Fiala, 1977). Methylazoxymethylanol is either metabolized or decomposes spontaneously to the methyldiazonium ion, which is the ultimate carcinogen. Dimethylhydrazine, AOM, and MAM are all effective colon carcinogens when given to rodents by any of several routes. Their high degree of effectiveness and ease of administration are responsible for the marked increase in animal experimentation in colon cancer.

Of the three carcinogens, DMH is used most frequently, and has a greater effect when given subcutaneously. An average dose is 15 mg/kg injected at weekly intervals. Lower doses naturally are less effective, while higher doses increase tumor yield, although at some point high doses cause significant short-term toxicity (Deschner et al., 1979). Repeated injections at any dose level induce a rapidly cumulative tumor yield and a shorter latency period. The carcinogen is also given intragastrically, but is less effective compared to parenteral administration. DMH is obtained as the hydrochloride, which requires titration of pH each time it is prepared. Azoymethane is similar to DMH, but is slightly more potent and does not require titration after dilution. The average sc dose is 8 mg/kg. We have used AOM almost exclusively in our laboratory, and have developed the dose–response data shown in Table I. Initially we gave the carcinogen at weekly intervals for the duration of the experiment. We found that eight weekly injections of 8 mg/kg were as effective as 26 weekly injections at the same dose level. Methylazoxymethanol acetate is not as effective as DMH or AOM, so that higher doses are required to obtain the same effect. An average dose is 35 mg/kg per week. McConnell et al. (1980) published a study comparing

TABLE I. Azoxymethane Dose Responses for Intestinal Tumors in Rats[a]

Subcutaneous injections		Incidence, %	Number of intestinal tumors		
Dose, mg/kg	Number of weeks		Small	Large	Total
20	1	25	0.3	0.06	0.36
20	2	94	1.5	2.0	3.5
16	2	93	1.0	1.3	2.3
12	2	75	1.1	0.6	1.7
8	2	53	0.2	0.7	0.9
8	8	100	1.8	3.3	5.1
4	2	27	0.1	0.1	0.2

[a]Male Sprague-Dawley Rats from Charles River Breeding Laboratory, Portage, Michigan.

tumor yield of DMH and MAM. This report as well as others show that these intestinal carcinogens are slightly more effective in males. It is important to mention that one dose of any of these carcinogens will induce intestinal cancer in rodents. This fact is utilized in studies of the promotional stage of carcinogenesis.

Intestinal neoplasms can be induced with subcutaneous injections of 3,2'-dimethyl-4 aminobiphenyl (DMAB) (Spjut and Noall, 1970). The incidence rate for intestinal tumors, mostly benign, is about 33%. Tumors of other organs are far more frequent than with the hydrazine group of carcinogens.

Direct-acting colon carcinogens are also available, as first shown by Narisawa et al. (1971, 1976). Intrarectal instillation of N-methyl-N'-nitro-N-nitrosoquanidine (MNNG, 2 mg, twice a week) or methylnitrosourea (MNU, 2 mg/week) results in the formation of tumors in that portion of the colon exposed to these chemicals. These carcinogens are effective in several species of rodents, including guinea pigs, which are resistant to the hydrazine derivatives. A more comprehensive review of intestinal carcinogens has been published recently (Shamsuddin, 1983).

3. EXPERIMENTAL ANIMALS

Since spontaneous neoplasms of the intestinal tract are rare in most animals, especially rodents, and since we have good organ-specific carcinogens that are effective in the same animals, the model is particularly useful for the study of colon cancer. It is important to note that among rodents there are species and strain differences in the degree of susceptability to the carcinogens. Rats and mice are used most frequently, and several studies relating to strain differences are available (Diwan and Blackman, 1980; Pollard and Zedeck, 1978). In this country, the Sprague-Dawley rat is the most susceptible strain and therefore is used more often than any other variety.

A recent, rather exciting discovery is that spontaneously occurring cancer of the large bowel has been found to be very common in the cotton-top tamarin, a species of marmoset (Lushbaugh et al., 1978). This animal is a primate, and the disease occurs in both captured and laboratory-bred animals of both sexes. An interesting feature that is not present in the rodent model is that the cancers are associated with inflammatory bowel disease. This association makes the model useful for studying the relationship between colitis and cancer, a situation that occurs in humans.

Anatomic alterations of the intestinal tract can be used to develop useful information on the process of cancer formation in rats and mice. Examples of those that have been reported are: the resection of the distal part of the small intestine, which causes a compensatory hyperplasia of the mucosa of the large intestine (Oscarson et al., 1979). A segment of large intestine can be placed in the small intestinal circuit and vice versa (Gennaro et al., 1973). This, of course, exposes the large intestine to the small intestinal environment and the small intestine to the fecal stream of the large intestine, an alteration that evaluates the importance of luminal factors. Colostomies are done to defunctionalize the large intestine distal to the colostomy site (Campbell et al., 1975). This removes the fecal stream from the large bowel beyond that point. The same effect also can be achieved by isolating a loop of large bowel, attaching each end to the skin, and joining together what remains to reestablish intestinal continuity (Rubio and Nylander, 1981). The excluded loop has viable mucosa, which can be studied directly in several ways. The large intestine can be removed, or it can be bypassed but left in the animal (Celik et al., 1980). In one study, the latter operations suggested the need for colon mucosa to be present for the formation of tumors in the upper small intestine (Celik et al., 1980). Finally, the bile duct of the rat has been divided at its junction with the intestine near the outlet of the stomach, then joined to the small intestine at a more distal point (Chomchai et al., 1974). The effect of this is to increase the amount of bile that enters the large intestine. Naturally other operational procedures are possible.

The choice of a protocol for any particular study depends upon the objective of the experiment. While the spectrum of investigation is too great to establish guidelines for the choice of an animal model that would apply to any situation, some general guidance is possible. The principal variables are the carcinogen, the animal, and the dietary factors. Dimethylhydrazine and AOM are the most commonly used carcinogens. The most useful direct-acting carcinogens are N-methyl-N-nitrosourea (MNU) and N-methyl-N-

nitro-N'-nitrosoguanidine (MNNG). The dose, number of applications, route of administration, and timing of administration with respect to the experimental factors are all important. Rats and mice are used more often by far than other rodents. The strain of the animal is important because they have varying degrees of susceptibility to the carcinogens. For example, Sprague-Dawley rats are the most sensitive, while the Lobund-Wistar strain is least sensitive of the currently available strains of rats (Pollard and Zedeck, 1978). There are other strains with intermediate sensitivity. The composition of the diet is critical in all studies of intestinal carcinogenesis. This is a fact that needs emphasis because it is sometimes overlooked. For example, in assessing the effect of a single item of the diet, excessive amounts of some other component that may alter the effect of the experimental item must not be used. Semisynthetic (purified) diets should be used for obvious reasons. General nutrition and weight gain must be comparable in all animal groups in an experiment, at least until cancer develops to a degree that the disease causes loss of weight. Pair feeding theoretically would seem important enough to require widespread use, but has not been necessary because the diet in most experiments provides adequate levels of all essential dietary components. Dietary guidelines for experiments using rodents have been published (Bieri et al., 1977).

In designing a tumorigenesis study in animals, one must estimate as well as possible the degree of cancer challenge needed to show the effect of any single experimental factor. Cancer challenge can be moderated by the choice of carcinogen, its dosage, route of administration, and the number of applications. To some degree, it can be altered by dietary factors; for example, a high-fat diet increases the tumorigenic effect of most carcinogens. On the other hand, in studies of inhibition one must use an animal model that will develop a cancer incidence of about 50%, as Wattenberg (1978) has pointed out. A very high cancer challenge could bury the effect of inhibitors, at least those identified so far.

4. RELEVANCE OF THE RAT MODEL TO THE HUMAN DISEASE

While there necessarily must be differences between the disease in the animal and in the human, the similarities are rather striking (Table II). They are sufficient to make the model extremely useful for studying the disease. The genetic factors tend to have a less important role in the etiology of colon cancer than the environmental components in both animals and humans. The histopathology is strikingly similar between the two. Similarities extend to immunologic parameters and to cellular kinetics (Enker and Jacobitz,

TABLE II. Similarities between the Animal Cancer Model and Human Bowel Cancer

---

1. Pathology

2. Method of spread through intestinal wall to the regional lymph nodes

3. Sex differences

4. Cellular kinetics

5. Environmental factors

6. Tumor antigens

7. Genetic susceptibility

8. Elevation of ornithine decarboxylase levels in cancer tissue

---

1976). Enzyme levels, such as that of ornithine decarboxylase, are elevated in cancer tissue in both animals and humans (Rozhin *et al.*, 1984).

However, there are differences (Table III). An important one is that intestinal cancers in animals are almost always multiple, while this is uncommon in humans. Metastases to the lung and liver are not very common in the animal model, but are frequent in humans. All animals that develop the disease will die of it regardless of any treatment so far attempted (McCall *et al.*, 1977). This is not true of cancer in humans. Indeed, the evidence suggests that the cancer challenge in the animal model is far stronger than it is in humans.

5. ANIMAL STUDIES IMPLICATING FAT AND FIBER IN THE ETIOLOGY OF INTESTINAL CANCER

Burkitt (1969) published a paper implicating the lack of dietary fiber as the major environmental factor in the etiology of cancer of the large bowel.

TABLE III. Differences between the Animal Cancer Model and Human Cancer

	Animal	Human
Distant metastases	Rare	Common
Nature of carcinogens	Known	Unknown
Multiple cancers	Very common	Rare
Adenoma–carcinoma sequence	Slight evidence	Strong evidence
Cancer challenge	Very strong	Much weaker
Develops spontaneously	No[a]	Yes

[a]Exception: cotton-top tamaran (a primate).

At about the same time, Hill and his associates (Hill *et al.*, 1971) in London developed evidence to suggest that excessive dietary fat is important in the causation of large bowel cancer. They found a high concentration of fecal bile acids and an altered colonic bacterial flora in people who ate a high-fat, low-fiber diet, especially in patients with cancer of the large bowel. Hill proposed the hypothesis that high concentrations of bile acids interact with the bacterial flora to form substances that cause the development of cancer of the large bowel.

There are epidemiologic and other studies that support one or the other position, that is, either dietary fiber is the major environmental factor or excessive fat intake is. In 1978 Burkitt remarked, "that it is surely better to consider fat and fiber not as either/or but as both/and hypothesis" (Burkitt, 1978). Many studies have been done using the animal model in an attempt to answer questions such as this. Reddy (1982) recently reviewed this literature in considerable detail. Therefore, we limit our discussion to some evidence developed recently, using a few early studies for background material.

6. FAT EFFECT

Many experiments have shown that significant increases of fat in the diet of rats and mice strongly enhances intestinal cancer formation in animals treated with an appropriate carcinogen. For example, Reddy *et al.* (1974) fed rats semipurified diets with 0.5, 4, or 20% corn oil and used DMH as the carcinogen. Ninety percent of the animals on the high-fat diet developed colon tumors compared to 60% on the low-fat diet. In our laboratory (Nigro *et al.*, 1975), we fed rats either a 35 or a 5% beef fat diet and used azoxymethane as the carcinogen. Animals on the high-fat diet developed twice as many intestinal cancers as those on the low-fat regimen. The lesions in the rats fed the 35% fat were more anaplastic, and the animals had much more metastatic disease than those fed the low-fat diet. High-fat diet alone did not produce tumors.

As mentioned previously, high levels of bile acids that result from the ingestion of large quantities of fat were postulated to have an important role in the etiology of colorectal cancer by Aries *et al.* (1969). Consequently, the effect of excess bile acids in the colon has been studied extensively in the animal model. While the subject is discussed in chapters 36, 37, 39 and 41 in detail, it may be of interest to note that in the two studies just described, secondary bile acids were present in greater amounts in the feces of animals fed the high-fat diets compared to those on low-fat intakes.

In some cancer models, unsaturated fat appears to enhance carcinogenesis to a greater degree than saturated fat. For colon cancer, Reddy *et al.* (1976) found that at low levels of fat (5%) unsaturated fat potentiates tumor formation more than saturated fat, but this distinction vanished when rats were fed a high-fat (20%) diet. This effect was confirmed in a later study by the same group (Reddy and Maeura, 1984). However, the importance of the degree of saturation of fat in the etiology of colon cancer is not settled.

7. FIBER EFFECT

According to Kritchevsky (1982), the most widely accepted definition of fiber is that it is a substance of plant origin that cannot be digested by human endogenous enzymes. Investigations on the effect of various kinds of fiber have been done in the animal model rather extensively since Burkitt published his observations on the association of dietary fiber and intestinal diseases in humans. However, these studies have not yet clearly established the role of fiber in the development of cancer of the colon. The data developed from the animal studies are difficult to interpret, impossible to compare, and at times even contradictory. The confusion is due to the lack of uniformity in experimental protocols and to the complexity of fiber itself. As Eastwood and Passmore (1983) so aptly described, dietary fiber is "a biological unit not a chemical entity." Consequently, fiber activity is complex and variable, depending upon the type of fiber and even variations in fiber of the same kind, such as particle size.

Fiber products most frequently used in animal studies are wheat bran and cellulose. In studies reported by Bauer et al. (1979), Wilson et al. (1977), and Watanabe et al. (1979), the addition of wheat bran to the diet of rats had no inhibitory effect on colon carcinogenesis. On the other hand, experiments reported by Barbolt and Abraham (1978), Ward et al. (1973), and Freeman et al. (1978) demonstrated inhibition. The varied conclusions appear to be due to differences in the experimental protocols. Both type and amount of carcinogen varied, the rat strain differed, and, perhaps even more importantly, elements of the diet other than the fiber varied. Those that showed no inhibitory effect fed rats a high-fat diet, about four times normal for rats, while in those experiments that showed fiber to be inhibitory, the animals were fed a normal-fat diet.

Nigro et al. (1979) reported a study that confirmed the importance of the fat content of the diet in fiber experiments. Rats were fed diets containing 35% beef fat plus 10% fiber, either alfalfa, wheat bran, or cellulose. Other groups of animals were fed a 5% fat diet plus either 20% or 30% of one of three types of fiber. There were fiber-free groups and all rats were given weekly injections of AOM, 8 mg/kg. None of the fibers inhibited cancer formation in the rats fed the high-fat diet, whereas bran and cellulose did inhibit cancer in animals fed the normal-fat diet. While the fat and fiber levels were extreme in this study, the results show that in assessing the effect of fiber on colon cancer formation the amount of fat in the diet is important.

Fat in large amounts appears to be a stronger promoter of intestinal cancer than fiber is an inhibitor. More studies are needed to determine the level of fat in the diet that would permit an inhibitory response from a diet containing a reasonable amount of fiber.

Reddy *et al.* (1983) fed rats diets containing 15% corn bran or 7.5% lignin and gave a carcinogen. Corn bran was found to enhance colon cancer formation, whereas lignin reduced cancer incidence. Barnes *et al.* (1983) studied the effects of four dietary brans—wheat, rice, corn, and soybean—on DMH-induced colon tumors in rats. Colon tumors were inhibited in rats fed wheat, rice, and soybean bran, but increased sharply in those fed corn bran. They also found that wheat bran was inhibitory only if given no later than 4 weeks after carcinogen administration. Their conclusion was that inhibition was dependent upon both the source of bran and the time it was given in relation to carcinogen administration. Jacobs (1983) reported a study on the effect of feeding rats a 20% wheat bran-supplemented diet either during and/or after DMH administration. He found an increase in tumor yield in rats fed the fiber during carcinogen treatment, but in those animals fed the bran after carcinogen injections, tumor formation was inhibited compared to the fiber-free control group.

Pectin, a fiber present in fruit and vegetables, has been shown to inhibit colon cancer in animals in some studies but not others (Freeman *et al.*, 1980; Watanabe *et al.*, 1979). Again, experimental conditions varied significantly, so that the effect of pectin is unclear. Watanabe *et al.* (1978) found that carrageenan, a product of seaweed, fed at a 15% level in the diet of rats clearly increased colon cancer development.

Animal studies such as those just reviewed show that some types of fiber can inhibit colon cancer formation while others either have no effect on the process or stimulate it. We believe that the evidence from animal experimentation shows that wheat bran and cellulose can inhibit or reduce colon cancer formation. However, this effect appears to depend upon the proper mixture of many constituents of the diet, especially its fat content. Further studies are needed to learn more about the importance of the interaction between dietary factors that are suspected of having some influence on carcinogenesis. This information is needed to design an acceptable diet whose total effect would be inhibitory.

The multiple effects of fiber, both physical and metabolic, are discussed in detail elsewhere in this volume. However, it is appropriate here to mention the effects that may have an influence on carcinogenesis in the colon. These are increasing colon content, altering intestinal transit times, and changing the bacterial flora, as well as those arising from adsorptive properties of fiber. It appears that inhibition requires a combination of these effects. Naturally, this makes the elucidation of this mechanism difficult, to say the least.

The dilutional effect of fiber has some support from animal studies. In the study referred to above by Nigro *et al.* (1979), bran and cellulose, which inhibited carcinogenesis, increased the quantity of feces by two- to threefold. The concentration of fecal bile acids was also significantly reduced, although the total daily excretion was not. This dilutional effect could have been part of the mechanism by which fiber inhibited carcinogenesis. The experiments mentioned above by Watanabe *et al.* (1979), Barbolt and Abraham (1978), and Freeman *et al.* (1978) also showed that wheat bran increased fecal bulk considerably in animals. Fecal bile acid concentration presumably was also diminished. Interestingly, Reddy *et al.* (1983) found that corn bran, which enhances carcinogenesis, increases the concentration of fecal bile acids as well as the total output. Fecal bulk was increased but to a lesser degree than that caused by wheat bran or cellulose.

The effect of fiber on intestinal mucosal growth has been studied recently by Jacobs and White (1983). They found that in rats, 20% wheat bran stimulated cell replication in the colon, with some variation among different segments of the colon. Alterations in the structure of the intestinal mucosa with loss of microvilli and cell injury have also been found by Cassidy *et al.* (1982) in animals fed a high-fiber diet. On the other hand, Shiau and Chang (1983) found that rats fed a high-fiber diet had reduced mucinase and β-glucuronidase levels in the lower intestine. High levels of these enzymes enable bacteria to degrade mucins, which protect the mucosal cells. These results suggest that the dilutional effect of some fibers may be of greater importance than their irritative properties, so that the net effect is still inhibitory.

8. ROLE OF MINOR DIETARY CONSTITUENTS

Wattenberg (1971) was the first to emphasize that among the normal defenses against carcinogens are a number of minor items in the diet. These include phenols, indoles, plant sterols, selenium, protease inhibitors, ascorbic acid, tocopherols, retinol, and carotenes (Wattenberg, 1983). He suggests that there are no doubt many more compounds not yet identified. Most of these substances occur in the diet of practically everyone, but the amount of each varies. Animal studies designed to improve the inhibitory effect of diet for many types of cancer by the addition of increased amounts of one or more of these compounds are in progress. Some of these inhibitory components are present in high-fiber diets either bound to the fiber itself or present in the fruits and vegetables taken to yield the high fiber content of the diet.

9. CONCLUSIONS

The animal model for the study of intestinal carcinogenesis is simple to use and it has striking similarities to the human disease. This relatively new tool has sharply increased the tempo of investigation of all aspects of colon cancer, including the role of dietary factors in its etiology. Not unexpectedly, current studies clearly demonstrate the difficulty of determining the influence of any single item of the diet on cancer formation and even more importantly the increased complexity that arises due to the interaction of many items taken simultaneously. Nevertheless, a reduction in the incidence of colorectal cancer in humans is possible through dietary alteration. However, it appears that it will require several changes together to convert a diet whose total effect is enhancement of cancer to one that is inhibitory (Nigro, 1981).

REFERENCES

Aries, V., Crowther, J. S., Drasar, B. S., Hill, M. J., and Williams, R. E. O., 1969, Bacteria and etiology of cancer of the large bowel, *Gut* **10**:334-335.

Barbolt, T. A., and Abraham, R., 1978, The effect of bran on dimethylhydrazine-induced colon carcinogenesis in the rat, *Proc. Soc. Exp. Biol. Med.* **157**:656-659.

Barnes, D. S., Clapp, N. K., Scott, D. A., Oberst, D. L., and Berry, S. G., 1983, Effects of wheat, rice, corn, and soybean bran on 1,2-dimethylhydrazine-induced large bowel tumorigenesis in F344 rats, *Nutr. Cancer* **5**:1-9.

Bauer, H. G., Asp, R., Oste, A., Dahlquist, A., and Fredlund, P. E., 1979, Effect of dietary fiber on the induction of colorectal tumors and fecal B-glucuronidase activity in the rat, *Cancer Res.* **39**:3752-3756.

Bieri, J. G., Stoewsand, G. S., Briggs, G. M., Phillips, R. W., Woodard, J. C., and Knapka, J. J., 1977, Report of the American Institute of Nutrition *ad hoc* committee on standards for nutritional studies, *J. Nutr.* **107**:1340-1348.

Burkitt, D. P., 1969, Related disease—Related cause?, *Lancet* **i**:1229-1231.

Burkitt, D. P., 1978, Colonic-rectal cancer: Fiber and other dietary factors, *Am. J. Clin. Nutr.* **31**:558-564.

Campbell, R. L., Singh, D. V., and Nigro, N. D., 1975, Importance of the fecal stream on the induction of colon tumors by azohymethanc in rats, *Cancer Res.* **35**:1369-1371.

Cassidy, M. M., Lightfoot, F. G., and Vahouny, G. V., 1982, Dietary fiber, bile acids, and intestinal morphology, in: *Dietary Fiber in Health and Disease* (G. V. Vahouny, and D. Kritchevsky, eds.), Plenum, New York, pp. 239-264.

Celik, C., Mittleman, A., Lewis, D., Paolini, N. S., and Holyoke, E. D., 1980, Effect of colectomy on carcinogenicity of symmetrical dimethylhydrazine in rats, *Surg. Forum* **31**:415-417.

Chomchai, C., Bhadrachori, N., and Nigro, N. D., 1974, The effect of bile on the induction of experimental intestinal tumors in rats, *Dis. Colon Rectum* **17**:310-312.

Deschner, E. E., Long, F. C., and Maskens, A. P., 1979, Relationship between dose, time, and tumor yield in mouse dimethylhydrazine-induced colon tumorigenesis, *Cancer Lett.* **8**:23-28.

Diwan, B. A., and Blackman, K. E., 1980, Differential susceptibility of 3 sublines of C57BL/6 mice to the induction of colorectal tumors by 1,2-dimethylhydrazine, *Cancer Lett.* **9**:111-115.

Druckrey, H., 1970, Production of colonic carcinoma by 1,2-dialkylhydrazines and azohyalkanes, in: *Carcinoma of the Colon and Antecedent Epithelium* (W. J. Burdette, ed.), C. C. Thomas, Springfield, Illinois, pp. 267-279.

Eastwood, M. A., and Passmore, R., 1983, Dietary fibre, *Lancet* **ii**:202-206.

Enker, W. E., and Jacobitz, J. L., 1976, Experimental carcinoma of the colon induced by 1,2-dimethylhydrazine-di HCl: Value as a model of human disease, *J. Surg. Res.* **21**:291-299.

Fiala, E. S., 1977, Investigations into the metabolism and mode of action of the colon carcinogens 1,2-dimethylhydrazine and azomethan, *Cancer* **40**:2436–2445.

Freeman, H. J., Spiller, G. A., and Kim, Y. S., 1978, A double-blind study on the effect of purified cellulose dietary fiber on 1,2-dimethylhydrazine-induced rat colon neoplasia, *Cancer Res.* **38**:2912–2917.

Freeman, H. J., Spiller, G. A., and Kim, Y. S., 1980, A double-blind study on the effects of differing purified cellulose and pectin fiber diets on 1,2-dimethylhydrazine-induced rat colonic neoplasia, *Cancer Res.* **40**:2661–2665.

Gennaro, A. R., Villanueva, R., Sukonthaman, Y., Vathanophos, V., and Rosemond, G. P., 1973, Chemical carcinogenesis in transposed intestinal segments, *Cancer Res.* **33**:536–541.

Hill, M. J., Drasar, B. S., Aries, V., Crowther, J. S., Hawksworth, G., and Williams, R. E. O., 1971, Bacteria and aetiology of cancer of large bowel, *Lancet* **i**:95–100.

Jacobs, L. R., 1983, Enhancement of rat colon carcinogenesis by wheat bran consumption during the stage of 1,2-dimethylhydrazine administration, *Cancer Res.* **43**:4057–4061.

Jacobs, L. R., and White, F. A., 1983, Modulation of mucosal cell proliferation in the intestine of rats fed a wheat bran diet, *Am. J. Clin. Nutr.* **37**:945–953.

Kritchevsky, D., 1982, Dietary fiber and disease, *Bull. N. Y. Acad. Med.* **58**:230–241.

Laqueur, C. L., 1965, The induction of intestinal neoplasms in rats with the glycoside cycasin and its aglycone, *Virchows Arch. Pathol. Anat. Physiol.* **340**:151–163.

Laqueur, G. L., and Spatz, M., 1968, Toxicology of Cycasin, *Cancer Res.* **28**:2262–2267.

Lorenz, E., and Stewart, H. L., 1940, Intestinal carcinoma and other lesions in mice following oral administration of 1,2,5,6-dibenzanthracene and 20-methylcholanthrene, *J. Nat. Cancer Inst.* **1**:17–40.

Lushbaugh, C. C., Humason, G. L., Swartzendruber, D. C., Richter, C. B., and Gengozian, N., 1978, Spontaneous colonic adenocarcinoma in marmosets, in: *Primates in Medicine,* Volume 10 (E. I. Goldsmith and J. Moor-Jankowski, eds.), S. Karger, Basel, pp. 119–134.

McCall, D. C., Lawrence, R., and Goldenberg, I. S., 1977, The effect of surgical resection of experimental "primary" adenocarcinoma of the colon on survival and incidence of metastases, *Cancer* **40**:1492–1496.

McConnell, E. E., Wilson, R. E., Moore, J. A., and Haseman, J. R., 1980, Dose response of 1,2-dimethylhydrazine and methylazoxymethanol acetate in the F344 rat, *Cancer Lett.* **8**:271–278.

Narisawa, T., Sato, T., Hayakawa, M., Sakuma, A., and Nakano, H., 1971, Carcinoma of the colon and rectum of rats by rectal infusion of *N*-methyl-*N'*-nitro-*N*-nitrosoguanidine, *Gann* **63**:231–234.

Narisawa, T., Wong, C. Q., Maronpot, R. R., and Weisburger, J. H., 1976, Large bowel carcinogenesis in mice and rats by several intrarectal doses of methylnitrosourea and negative effect of nitrite plus methylurea, *Cancer Res.* **36**:505–510.

Nigro, N. D., 1981, Fat, fiber, and other modifiers on intestinal carcinogenesis: A strategy for prevention, in: *Banbury Report 7, Gastrointestinal Cancer: Endogenous Factors* (W. R. Bruce, P. Correa, M. Lipkin, S. R. Tannenbaum, and T. D. Wilkins, eds.), Cold Spring Harbor Laboratory, Cold Spring Harbor, New York, pp. 83–93.

Nigro, N. D., Bull, A. W., Klopfer, B. A., Pak, M. S., and Campbell, R. L., 1979, Effect of dietary fiber on azoxymethane-induced intestinal carcinogenesis in rats, *J. Nat. Cancer Inst.* **62**:1097–1102.

Nigro, N. D., Singh, D. V., Campbell, R. L., and Pak, M. S., 1975, Effect of dietary beef fat on intestinal tumor formation by azoxymethane in rats, *J. Nat. Cancer Inst.* **54**:439–442.

Oscarson, J. E. A., Veen, H. F., Ross, J. S., and Malt, R. A., 1979, Ileal resection potentiates 1,2-dimethylhydrazine induced colonic carcinogenesis, *Ann. Surg.* **189**:503–508.

Pollard, M., and Zedeck, M. S., 1978, Induction of colon tumors in 1,2-dimethylhydrazine-resistant Lobund-Wistar rats by methylazoxymethanol acetate, *J. Nat. Cancer Inst.* **61**:493–494.

Reddy, B. S., 1982, Dietary fiber and colon carcinogenesis, A critical review, in: *Dietary Fiber in Health and Disease* (G. V. Vahouny and D. Kritchevsky, eds.), Plenum, New York, pp. 265–285.

Reddy, B. S., and Maeura, Y., 1984, Promoting effect of amount and source of dietary fat on azoxymethane-induced colon carcinogenesis in female F344 rats, *J. Nat. Cancer Inst.* **75**:745–750.

Reddy, B. S., Maeura, Y., and Wayman, M., 1983, Effect of dietary corn bran and autohydrolyzed lignin on 3,2-dimethyl-4-aminobiphenyl-induced intestinal carcinogenesis in male F344 rats, *J. Nat. Cancer Inst.* **71**:419–423.

Reddy, B. S., Narisawa, T., Vukusich, D., Weisburger, J. H., and Wynder, E. L., 1976, Effect of quality and quantity of dietary fat and dimethylhydrazine in colon carcinogenesis in rats, *Proc. Soc. Exp. Biol. Med.* **151**:237–239.

Reddy, B. S., Weisburger, J. H., and Wynder, E. L., 1974, Effects of dietary fat level and dimethylhydrazine on fecal acid and neutral sterol excretion and colon carcinogenesis in rats, *J. Nat. Cancer Inst.* **52**:507–511.

Rozhin, J. R., Wilson, P. S., Bull, A. W., and Nigro, N. D., 1984, Studies on ornithine decarboxylase activity in the rat and human colon, *Cancer Res.,* **44**:3326–3230.

Rubio, C. A., and Nylander, G., 1981, Further studies on the carcinogenesis of the colon of the rat with special reference to the absence of intestinal contents, *Cancer* **48**:951–953.

Shamsuddin, A. K. M., 1983, *In vivo* induction of colon cancer, Dose and animal species, in: *Experimental Colon Carcinogenesis* (. Autrup and G. M. Williams, eds.), CRC, Boca Raton, Florida, pp. 51–62.

Shiau, S. Y., and Chang, G. W., 1983, Effects of dietary fiber on fecal mucinase and β-glucuronidase activity in rats, *J. Nutr.* **113**:138–144.

Spjut, H. J., and Noall, M. W., 1970, Colonic neoplasms induced by 3,2'-dimethyl-4-aminobiphenyl, in: *Carcinoma of the Colon and Antecedent Epithelium* (W. J. Burdette, ed.), C. C. Thomas, Springfield, Illinois, pp. 280–288.

Ward, J. M., Yamamoto, R. S., and Weisburger, J. H., 1973, Cellulose dietary bulk and azoxymethane-induced intestinal cancer, *J. Nat. Cancer Inst.* **51**:713–715.

Watanabe, K., Reddy, B. S., Wong, C. Q., and Weisburger, J. H., 1978, Effect of dietary undegraded carrageenan on colon carcinogenesis in F344 rats treated with azoxymethane of methylnitrosourea, *Cancer Res.* **38**:4427–4430.

Watanabe, K., Reddy, B. S., Weisburger, J. H., and Kritchevsky, D., 1979, Effect of dietary alfalfa, pectin, and wheat bran on azoxymethane- or methylnitrosourea-induced colon carcinogenesis in F344 rats, *J. Nat. Cancer Inst.* **63**:141–145.

Wattenberg, L. W., 1971, Studies of polycyclic hydrocarbon hydroxylases of the intestine possibly related to cancer: Effect of diet on benzpyrene hydroxylase activity, *Cancer* **28**:99–102.

Wattenberg, L. W., 1978, Inhibitors of chemical carcinogens, *Adv. Cancer Res.* **26**:197–226.

Wattenberg, L. W., 1983, Inhibition of neoplasia by minor dietary constituents, *Cancer Res.* **43**:24485–24535.

Wilson, R. B., Hutcheson, D. P., and Wideman, L., 1977, Dimethylhydrazine-induced colon tumors in rats fed diets containing beef fat or corn oil with and without wheat bran, *Am. J. Clin. Nutr.* **30**:176–181.

35

Animal Experimentation and Prevention of Colorectal Cancer

NORMAN D. NIGRO

1. INTRODUCTION

Epidemiologic studies indicate that dietary factors play an important role in the etiology of colorectal cancer (Wynder and Reddy, 1974). This suggests that its incidence can be reduced by dietary alterations in countries like the U.S. where the incidence is high. The questions that need an answer are: What changes in the diet are required to reduce the risk of developing cancer? Second, can such a diet be nutritionally adequate and at the same time acceptable to the general public?

At present, there is considerable controversy regarding the desirability of suggesting dietary changes to prevent cancer (Pariza, 1984). Nevertheless, the majority favor offering some general guidelines relating to the intake of fat, fiber, fruit, and vegetables for the purpose of reducing cancer risk. These suggestions deal with substantial changes of the major items of the diet. Another approach is to add supplements of one or more of the minor dietary constituents that would add enough inhibitory strength to make the total effect of the entire diet inhibitory. This should permit less drastic changes in the fat and fiber content, making the change more acceptable to the public.

The objective of this chapter is to present evidence obtained from animal studies on the reduction of bowel cancer by the addition of chemicals to the diet that inhibit neoplasia, as suggested by Wattenberg (1983), who

NORMAN D. NIGRO • Department of Surgery, Wayne State University School of Medicine, Detroit, Michigan 48201.

calls such substances minor dietary constituents. Conclusions arrived at from animal studies certainly are speculative when applied to humans. However, evidence from human studies correlate fairly well with those from animal experiments. Therefore, such speculations are worth considering.

2. FAT-FIBER RELATIONSHIP

We did a study that adds support to the importance of the fat–fiber relationship in intestinal carcinogenesis in the animal model (Nigro *et al.*, 1979). The experiment consisted of two parts. In the first, rats were fed a semisynthetic diet containing 35% beef fat and 10% fiber. The fiber was either alfalfa, bran, or cellulose. In the second part, the animals were fed about 5% beef fat and either 20 or 30% of one of the fibers. Each study had a fiber-free group, and all rats were given weekly, subcutaneous injections of azoxymethane (AOM), 8 mg/kg. The entire experiment was terminated at the end of 23 weeks. All animals injected with the carcinogen developed intestinal cancers.

The results confirmed the fact that excessive dietary fat is a strong positive modifier of intestinal carcinogenesis in this animal model, whereas the inhibitor effect of fiber is relatively small. The rats fed the high-fat, fiber-free diet developed an average of 8.4 intestinal cancers per animal. The addition of 10% of any one of the three fibers had no significant inhibitory effect; the lowest rate was 7.6 per rat in the group fed wheat bran. On the other hand, the animals fed the low-fat, fiber-free diet developed an average of 4 intestinal tumors per rat. The addition of 20 or 30% of any one of the three fibers reduced the average number of tumors significantly in all groups except the 20% alfalfa group. Greatest inhibition occurred in the 30% cellulose group, where the average number of tumors was 1.9. In this group, nutritional deprivation due to the insignificant digestibility of cellulose may have been partially responsible for the inhibition of carcinogenesis.

The inhibition of cancers by fiber may be due, in part, to the dilution of fecal biliary steroids. The concentration of fecal biliary steroids was lowered significantly in the rats with reduced tumor frequencies, whereas the total daily excretion did not show a similar correlation. All rats fed diets containing fiber excreted more feces than those fed a fiber-free diet, and the greatest increases occurred in the 30% fiber group.

Further studies are needed to determine the optimum proportion of these two major dietary components for the effective inhibition of colorectal cancer. However, it is clear that the necessary alterations of fat and fiber in the diet would have to be substantial in order to reduce cancer incidence. As we suggested earlier, another strategy that should be considered is the addition of supplements to the diet that would interrupt or delay the carcinogenic process. These include chemicals that would effectively modify the carcinogen, thereby reducing the initiation effect, or would inhibit the promotional phase of the process or even increase the latency period sufficiently so that, for all practical purposes, it would constitute prevention.

3. INHIBITION BY MINOR DIETARY CONSTITUENTS

Known inhibitors of carcinogenesis include vitamins, trace metals, plant sterols, indoles, and phenols, all of which are present to some degree in our diets. Others not included in our food are disulfiram, cyanates, α-difluoro-methylornithine (DFMO), and some others (Wattenberg, 1983).

We have investigated the use of a combination of selenium, 13-*cis*-retinoic acid, and β-sitosterol (Nigro *et al.*, 1982). We gave rats one basic 5% fat diet, to which was added one, two, or all three inhibitors in various combinations. The amount of each of these three supplements in our study was far less than that generally used when one compound is given alone. At the end of 26 weeks, the animals were sacrificed, and we found that there was a significant reduction in the average number of intestinal tumors in only two of the seven experimental groups. One was the group that received the combination 13-*cis*-retinoic acid and selenium. These animals developed 3.7 tumors per animal, compared with 5.07 tumors in the controls. This was a small but significant reduction. On the other hand, when all three compounds were used together, the animals developed 2.75 tumors per animal, nearly a 50% reduction when compared with the control group.

The result of the study adds support to the concept that the use of small amounts of several agents that inhibit cancer offers an additional opportunity for the development of a chemoprevention program for humans. It is apparent, however, that we need to identify other nontoxic inhibitors that would function in this manner. Currently, we are investigating the effect of such compounds as β-carotene, calcium, and DFMO.

4. SHORT-TERM ASSAYS TO IDENTIFY INHIBITORS

One approach for the identification of tumor inhibitors is the use of short-term assays to screen a large number of compounds. This would permit a better selection of agents to use for tumorigenesis studies, which are time-consuming and expensive.

Studies of tumor promoters in the mouse skin demonstrate that several biological responses occur shortly after the application of promoters. One of these is an increase in DNA synthesis. While this response is not specific for tumor promoters, it is present when agents that cause hyperplasia are used.

Of course, not all hyperplastic agents are tumor promoters, so this assay alone is not sufficient to use as a screening mechanism for tumorigenesis studies.

The effect of various agents on colonic [³H] thymidine incorporation is shown in Table I. The results of this investigation demonstrate that bile salts and a variety of other compounds to which the colonic mucosa is commonly exposed induced an increase in the incorporation of [³H] into colonic DNA. This is analogous to the effect of phorbol ester tumor promoters in the well-characterized mouse skin system. While the stimulation is probably not specific for tumor promoters, it is significant that compounds that possess tumor-enhancing properties elicit this response. It also suggests that numerous compounds in the intestinal lumen can exert a mitogenic influence on the mucosa, which under the proper conditions could influence the enhancement of tumorigenesis (Bull *et al.*, 1983). This assay identifies agents that promote carcinogenesis more accurately than those that inhibit the process.

The induction of ornithine decarboxylase (ODC) activity plays an important part in tumor promotion, which was demonstrated initially in the mouse skin (O'Brien, 1976). We found that a high level of dietary fat caused an increase in ODC activity in the rat colon, as did the rectal instillation of bile salts. The study showed that DFMO given in the drinking water inhibited ODC activity and also intestinal tumor frequency in rats (Table II). In assaying ODC activity in cancer tissue, it was found to be higher than in normal colonic mucosa in both rats and humans (Rozhin *et al.*, 1984).

5. CONCLUSIONS

Animal studies suggest that the incidence of colorectal cancer can be reduced by supplementing the diet with chemicals that inhibit intestinal

TABLE I. Effect of various Agents on Colonic [³H]Thymidine Incorporation

Agent[a]	Percent increase over control ± SD
Deoxycholate	383±137
Lithocholate (25 mM in saline)	33±12
Lithocholate (in mineral oil)	179±34
Cholate	178±64
Beef fat[b]	217±83
Mineral oil[b]	14±13

[a]All at 50 mM in saline unless otherwise noted.
[b]Neat.

TABLE II. Effect of DFMO on AOM-Induced Intestinal Cancer in Rats

Treatment	Intestinal cancer frequency[a]		
	Small	Large	Total
Control	2.36±2.0	2.28±2.2	4.6±2.8
0.01% DFMO	2.24±1.4	1.80±1.5	4.04±2.4
0.1% DFMO	1.21±1.3***	0.54±0.8**	1.75±1.5*
1.0% DFMO	0.09±0.29*	0.26±0.5*	0.35±0.5*

[a]Mean number of cancers/rat ± SD; 26th week of experiment; significance compared to controls:* $p < 0.005$, ** $p < 0.005$, *** $p < 0.025$.

carcinogenesis. At present, there is no single substance that will accomplish this effectively without toxicity. However, small amounts of several chemicals given at low, nontoxic doses may have an additive or even a synergistic effect that may be sufficient to convert a diet to one whose total effect is inhibitory. The evidence suggests that the strategy is appropriate (Nigro, 1982). We now need to identify substances that will act effectively to accomplish this purpose.

REFERENCES

Bull, A. W., Marnett, L. J., Dawe, E. J., and Nigro, N. D., 1983, Stimulation of deoxythymidine incorporation in the colon of rats treated intrarectally with bile acids and fats, *Carcinogenesis* **4**:207–210.

Nigro, N. D., 1982, A strategy for prevention of cancer of the large bowel, *Dis. Colon Rectum* **25**:755–758.

Nigro, N. D., Bull, A. W., Klopfer, B. A., Pak, M. S., and Campbell, R. L., 1979, Effect of dietary fiber on azoxymethane-induced intestinal carcinogenesis in rats, **62**:1097–1102.

Nigro, N. D., Bull, A. W., Wilson, P. S., Soullier, B. K., and Alousi, M. A., 1982, Combined inhibitors of carcinogenesis: Effect of azoxymethane-induced intestinal cancer in rats, *J. Nat. Cancer Inst.* **69**:103–107.

O'Brien, T. G., 1976, The induction of ornithine decarboxylase as an early, possibly obligatory, event in mouse skin carcinogenesis, *Cancer Res.* **36**:2644–2653.

Pariza, M. W., 1984, A perspective on diet, nutrition, and cancer, *J. Am. Med. Assoc.* **251**:1455–1458.

Rozhin, J., Wilson, P., Bull, A., and Nigro, N., 1984, Studies on ornithine decarboxylase activity in the rat and human colon, *Cancer Res.* **44**:3326–3230.

Wattenberg, L. W., 1983, Inhibition of neoplasia by minor dietary constituents, *Cancer Res.* (*Suppl.*) **43**:2448s–2453s.

Wynder, E. L., and Reddy, B. S., 1974, Metabolic epidemiology of colorectal cancer, *Cancer* **34**:801–806.

36

The Role of Bile Acids in Colon Cancer

BERTRAM I. COHEN and ERWIN H. MOSBACH

1. BACKGROUND

Cancer of the large bowel has been a topic of intensive investigation for many years. Several epidemiologic studies suggested that colorectal cancer varies with geographic areas and socioeconomic levels. Incidence is high in Northwestern Europe and North America and low in Central and South America, Africa, and Asia. Apparently, environmental factors rather than genetic and social factors are important (Doll, 1969; Armstrong and Doll, 1975; Burkitt, 1975; Jain et al., 1980).

The role of diet on cancer of the large bowel has been studied by various laboratories (Reddy, 1975; Reddy et al., 1975a,b; Wynder and Reddy, 1975; Cohen et al., 1980; Kay, 1981; Zaridge, 1981). Populations consuming diets high in protein and fat (mainly meat-rich diets) have an increased risk of developing colon cancer compared to populations consuming diets low in fat and protein (mainly vegetarian diets) (Carroll and Khor, 1975; Phillips, 1975; Enig et al., 1978; Reddy, 1981; McCay, 1983). Dietary fiber although widely discussed, has not been positively correlated with the incidence of colon cancer (Burkitt, 1980). Metabolic epidemiologic studies have shown that high-risk populations have increased concentrations of bile acids and cholesterol (or its metabolites) in the feces (Reddy et al., 1976a, 1977a, 1980; Reddy and Wynder, 1977). In addition, these populations have increased concentrations of intestinal anaerobic bacteria and an enhanced metabolic

BERTRAM I. COHEN and ERWIN H. MOSBACH • Departments of Surgery, Beth Israel Medical Center and Mount Sinai School of Medicine of the City University of New York, New York, New York 10003.

activity of these bacteria (Hill *et al.*, 1971; Hill, 1974, 1983; van der Werf *et al.*, 1983). Thus, in groups of individuals consuming diets rich in meat (and consequently high in fat), the bacterial metabolism of the primary bile acids [cholic acid (I, Fig. 1) and chenodeoxycholic acid (II, Fig. 1)] was greater than in individuals on a low-meat, low-protein diet (Reddy *et al.*, 1975b, 1976a). Patients with colorectal cancer and subjects with adenomatous polyps both have higher concentrations of fecal bile acids than controls (Reddy and Wynder, 1977). The amounts of secondary bile acids [deoxycholic acid (III, Fig. 1) and lithocholic acid (IV, Fig. 1)] were higher in the colon cancer patients than controls (Reddy *et al.*, 1977b). Among the hypotheses offered for the increased incidence of large bowel cancer in the American population were that diet can affect (1) the type and amounts of bile acids and neutral sterols in the feces, (2) the concentration and metabolic activities of certain bacteria that can alter the structure of bile acids, or (3)

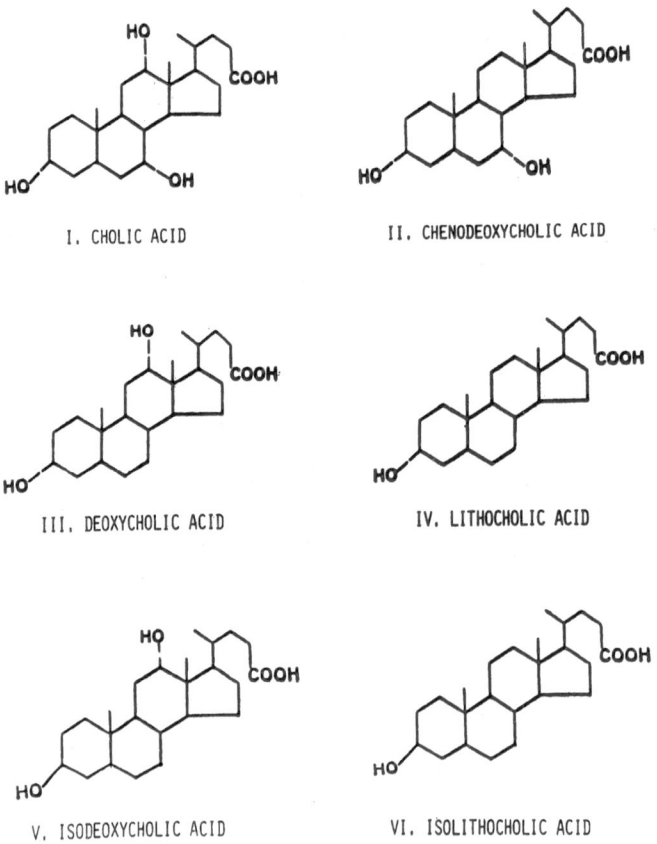

I. CHOLIC ACID

II. CHENODEOXYCHOLIC ACID

III. DEOXYCHOLIC ACID

IV. LITHOCHOLIC ACID

V. ISODEOXYCHOLIC ACID

VI. ISOLITHOCHOLIC ACID

FIGURE 1. Structures of primary and secondary bile acids in man.

the nature of the intestinal flora, causing an increased incidence of colon cancer in an unknown manner. This review will deal with the bile acids as potential tumor promoters.

2. BILE ACIDS: STRUCTURE AND FUNCTION

Bile acids are formed in the biodegradative metabolism of cholesterol. The primary bile acids of higher vertebrates possess 24 carbon atoms. Structurally, these carbon atoms are present as a cyclopentanoperhydrophenanthrene nucleus and are derivatives of 5β-cholanoic acid. The major primary bile acids are cholic acid (I) ($3\alpha,7\alpha,12\alpha$-trihydroxy-5β-cholanoic acid) and chenodeoxycholic acid (II) ($3\alpha,7\alpha$-dihydroxy-5β-cholanoic acid). These bile acids undergo bacterial modification (7α-dehydroxylation) in the gut to form deoxycholic acid (III) ($3\alpha,12\alpha$-dihydroxy-5β-cholanoic acid) and lithocholic acid (IV) (3α-hydroxy-5β-cholanoic acid), respectively. Several epimers of the secondary bile acids have been detected (Danielsson *et al.*, 1963; Norman and Palmer, 1964). These compounds include isodeoxycholic acid (V) ($3\beta,12\alpha$-dihydroxy-5β-cholanoic acid) and isolithocholic acid (VI) (3β-hydroxy-5β-cholanoic acid).

The possible role of bile acids as colon tumor promoters has been studied in animal models treated with carcinogens (Reddy *et al.*, 1977b; Cohen *et al.*, 1980). Lithocholic acid and taurodeoxycholic acid instilled intrarectally acted as colon tumor promoters in rats given the carcinogen *N*-methyl-*N'*-nitro-*N*-nitrosoguanidine (MNNG) (Reddy *et al.*, 1976b). In addition, intrarectal instillation of sodium cholate and sodium chenodeoxycholate increased tumors in germ-free rats given MNNG (Reddy *et al.*, 1977b). In conventional rats these bile acids further elevated the number of colon tumors. Our laboratory has studied the role of dietary bile acids on colon cancer (Sarwal *et al.*, 1979; Cohen *et al.*, 1980). These studies likewise implicated bile acids as colon tumor promoters in a system where tumors were chemically induced.

3. BILE ACIDS AND COLON CANCER

3.1. Cholic Acid and *N*-Methyl-*N*-nitrosourea (MNU)

Carcinogenesis studies in our laboratory were designed to study colon tumor promotion or inhibition in a rat model using the carcinogen *N*-methyl-*N*-nitrosourea (MNU). Intrarectal administration of MNU was chosen since (1) tumors were produced only in the colon and histopathologically resemble colon cancer in man, and (2) MNU is direct-acting, so that any changes would be independent of the metabolism of the carcinogen.

The tumor-promoting effects of cholic acid feeding were examined in Caesarean-derived F344 rats treated with intrarectally administered MNU. The animals were divided into four treatment groups. Group 1 received control chow; group 2 received control chow and bile acid (0.2%); group 3 received control chow and 8 mg MNU; and group 4 received control chow and bile acid (0.2%) plus MNU (8 mg). After 28 weeks the animals were sacrificed. Rats in groups 1 and 2 had no tumors (experiment 1, Table I). MNU-treated animals had a tumor incidence of 49% (1.00 tumors/animal). Significantly, more tumors (62%) were seen in the cholic acid–MNU group than with MNU alone (group 3) (χ^2, $p < 0.05$). Tumors were primarily adenomas, but invasive adenocarcinomas were also detected. The tumors increased in average size from adenomas (0.38 cm) to adenocarcinomas (0.79 cm) ($p < 0.025$). As expected, in the cholic acid-fed rats fecal total bile acid output was elevated compared to their controls. The major fecal bile acid in the bile acid-fed groups 2 and 4 was deoxycholic acid. The latter is presumed to be the primary tumor promoter. Cell kinetics was measured at week 5. The cumulative effect of MNU and cholic acid feeding increased the numbers of epithelial cells that underwent DNA synthesis (Deschner et al., 1981). The heightened cell turnover allowed tumors to occur with greater frequency in the cholic acid/MNU-treated group (Deschner et al., 1981).

3.2. Chenodeoxycholic Acid and MNU
(Experiment 2, Table I; Sarwal et al., 1979)

We examined the effects of chenodeoxycholic acid feeding on tumor incidence in rats treated with MNU (Table I). After 28 weeks, pathological

TABLE I. Tumor Incidence at Week 28: Bile Acid Feeding[a]

Group	Diet (number of animals)		Carcinogen	Animals with tumors Number	Percent	Tumors/ animal	Tumors/ tumor-bearing animal
Experiment 1. Cholic acid							
1	Control (Purina chow)	(30)	−	0	0	0	0
2	Cholic acid (0.2%)	(10)	−	0	0	0	0
3	Control (Purina chow)	(91)	+	45	49	1.00	2.11
4	Cholic acid (0.2%)	(42)	+	26	62*	1.80*	2.92*
Experiment 2. Chenodeoxycholic acid							
5	Control (Purina chow)	(30)	−	0	0	0	0
6	Chenic acid (0.2%)	(9)	−	0	0	0	0
7	Control (Purina chow)	(91)	+	45	49	1.00	2.11
8	Chenic acid (0.2%)	(42)	+	26	62*	1.11	1.79

[a]Asterisk indicates significant difference from control, $p < 0.05$.

and histological examination revealed no tumors in groups 1 and 2. The MNU group (group 3) had a tumor incidence of 49%, compared to the MNU plus chenodeoxycholic acid group (group 4) in which 62% of the animals had tumors (1.1 tumors/animal). The tumors were primarily adenomas, but three carcinomas were also detected. Fecal total bile acids were higher in chenodeoxycholic acid-fed rats compared to control chow-fed rats. Major fecal bile acids in the chenodeoxycholic acid-fed rats were chenodeoxycholic acid, lithocholic acid, α-muricholic acid, β-muricholic acid, and ω-muricholic acid. The ability of rats to 6-hydroxylate bile acids may protect them from the increased number of tumors observed in other carcinogen—bile acid experiments.

The important findings of the carcinogen—bile acid experiments are: (1) In animals treated with a carcinogen, bile acids delivered in physiological amounts and in a physiological manner (admixed with feces) promote colon cancer formation, and (2) different bile acids are not equally potent in this regard.

3.3 Iso-Bile Acids

3.3.1 Detection in Feces

An improved method for the isolation, quantitation, and identification of fecal secondary bile acids was developed in our laboratory (Takahashi *et al.*, 1978). This method employed silica gel TLC to separate 3α-hydroxycholanoic acids from 3β-hydroxycholanoic acids, and GLC-MS to confirm the identity of the compounds. Using this method, we analyzed the fecal samples obtained from the animals in the cholic acid—MNU and chenodeoxycholic acid—MNU studies (Table II). In the cholic acid study, the concentration of isodeoxycholic acid in feces increased significantly in the cholic acid-fed animals compared to their controls. Interestingly, animals treated with MNU alone (group 3) had higher amounts of isodeoxycholic acid in the feces than the control animals. In the animals treated with chenodeoxycholic acid, increased amounts of isolithocholic acid were present in the feces. The mechanism of iso-bile acid formation as well as the significance of its presence in the feces is not yet determined.

3.3.2. Iso-Bile Acids and Colon Cancer

Our laboratory examined the effects of isolithocholic acid and lithocholic acid in an animal model for cancer. Rats were treated intrarectally with the chemical carcinogen MNU. The experimental design involved dividing the animals as follows: group 1, control; group 2, intrarectal lithocholic acid, 6 mg/week, no MNU; group 3, intrarectal isolithocholic acid 6

TABLE II. Iso-Bile Acids in Bile Acid–Carcinogen Rats

Group	Diet	Carcinogen	Isolithocholic acid		Isodeoxycholic acid	
			μg/g	Percent[a]	μg/g	Percent[b]
Experiment 1. Cholic acid						
1	Control chow	–	–	–	26	3
2	Control chow + cholic acid (0.2%)	–	–	–	1100[c]	18
3	Control chow	+	–	–	119	18
4	Control chow + cholic acid (0.2%)	+	–	–	512[c]	14
Experiment 2. Chenodeoxycholic acid						
5	Control chow	–	97	39	–	–
6	Control chow + chenic acid (0.2%)	–	372[d]	21	–	–
7	Control chow	+	136	38	–	–
8	Control chow + chenic acid (0.2%)	+	298[d]	21	–	–

[a]Isolithocholic acid/isolithocholic acid + lithocholic acid.   [c]Differs from groups 1 and 3 $p<0.01$.
[b]Isodeoxycholic acid/isodeoxycholic acid + deoxycholic acid.   [d]Differs from groups 5 and 7, $p<0.01$.

mg/week, no MNU; group 4, intrarectal MNU, no bile acid; group 5, intrarectal lithocholic acid plus intrarectal MNU; group 6, intrarectal isolithocholic acid plus intrarectal MNU. The carcinogen (total dose 8 mg/animal) was administered in divided 2-mg doses on days 1, 4, 7, and 10 of the experiment. The bile acids were sonicated into peanut oil and administered three times a week for 28 weeks (2 mg/instillation). All animals were fed rat chow for 28 weeks. After 28 weeks, pathological and histological examinations were performed on all the animals. No tumors were present in groups

TABLE III. Effect of Iso-Bile Acids on Incidence of Colon Tumors in Rats[a]

Group	Treatment	Number of animals	Carcinogen	Animals with tumors		Tumors/ animal	Tumors/ tumor-bearing animal
				Number	Percent		
1	Control	10	–	–	–	–	–
2	Lithocholic acid	6	–	–	–	–	–
3	Isolithocholic acid	6	–	–	–	–	–
4	Control	59	+	28	47	0.93	1.96
5	Lithocholic acid	23	+	15	65	1.39	2.13
6	Isolithocholic acid	24	+	12	50	0.92	1.83

[a]Animals were given MNU in four divided doses (2 mg/dose) on days 1, 4, 7, and 10. The bile acids (2 mg/dose) were given three times per week for 28 weeks. Histopathology was carried out at sacrifice.

1, 2, and 3 (Table III). The MNU group (group 4) had a tumor incidence of 47% (0.93 tumor/animal; 1.96 tumors/tumor-bearing animal). In the group given MNU and intrarectal lithocholic acid (group 5), 65% of the animals had tumors and there were 1.39 tumors/animal (2.13 tumors/tumor-bearing animal). Interestingly, the group given MNU and intrarectal isolithocholic acid had fewer animals with tumors (50%) and fewer tumors/animal (0.92) compared with group 5. This is suggestive of a real difference between lithocholic acid and isolithocholic acid in promoting colon tumors with MNU. Others have already shown that secondary bile acids are more effective colon tumor promoters than primary bile acids, although the mechanism of action of iso-bile acids remains to be elucidated.

3.4. Deoxycholic Acid, Semi-synthetic Diets, and Colon Cancer in Rats

The results of carcinogenesis experiments of the type described above have not always been consistent from laboratory to laboratory. These phenomena were attributed to variations in the composition of the commercial diets fed to the animals (Newberne, 1975; Greenman et al., 1980). The need for defined diets was eventually established and investigators have gradually changed from the standard commercial diets to ones of defined composition, for example, AIN-76 (Clarke et al., 1977). Our laboratory has investigated the effects of increasing doses of MNU in animals on a defined diet (AIN-76 rodent diet). Dose response with respect to tumor formation and the effects of a secondary bile acid on tumor promotion were studied in this model.

3.4.1. MNU Dose Response to Tumor Formation

These studies were carried out to examine the effect of different amounts of carcinogen (MNU) in Fisher rats fed a semisynthetic diet (AIN-76). MNU was administered according to the protocol shown in Table IV. The animals

TABLE IV. Dose Response of MNU on Colon Cancer in Rats Fed a Semisynthetic diet[a]

Treatment group	Diet	MNU dose, mg	Incidence of large bowel neoplasms	
			Percent	Tumors/animal
1	Semisynthetic diet (AIN-76)	2	18	0.24
2	Semisynthetic diet	4	60	0.73
3	Semisynthetic diet	8	84	2.00
4	Purina chow	8	47	1.00

[a] Animals were given MNU dissolved in sterile saline (2 mg/dose) or sterile saline alone on days 1, 4, 7, and 10 of the experiment. Animals were sacrificed at week 28.

were given the carcinogen and fed the semisynthetic diet for 28 weeks. Pathological evaluation showed that tumors were produced in a dose-responsive manner. Interestingly, the same dose of MNU in rats fed a chow diet gave a significantly lower number of animals with tumors as well as tumors/animal. This is suggestive of an inhibitor(s) being present in chow diets, but not in the defined diet. In contrast, rats given MNNG have more tumors when fed a chow diet (88%) vs. a semipurified diet (65%) (Reddy, 1975). Therefore, the type and dose of carcinogen and the nature of the diet must be carefully controlled in animal studies of chemical carcinogenesis.

3.4.2. Deoxycholic Acid and Colon Cancer

The secondary bile acids have been shown to be more potent tumor promoters than the primary bile acids (Reddy et al., 1977b; Cohen et al., 1980). These studies had used only the chow diet. In an attempt to control dietary variability, our laboratory examined the effects of deoxycholic acid (0.2%) in rats fed a semisynthetic diet and given MNU in a dose-responsive manner. These studies resulted in several interesting findings. First, we were able to detect the effects of different doses of MNU (and 0.2% deoxycholic acid) on the number of animals with tumors (%) as well as tumors/animal. The tumors increased in a dose-responsive manner when increasing amounts of MNU were given to the animals. Second, we were unable to show that deoxycholic acid promoted tumors in the animals. For example, animals treated with 8 mg MNU had a similar tumor incidence (84%, 2 tumors/animal; (Table IV) as rats receiving 8 mg MNU plus 0.2% dietary deoxycholic acid (76% tumor incidence, 1.75 tumors/animal; Table V). Similarly,

TABLE V. Dose Response of MNU and Deoxycholic Acid on Colon Carcinogenesis in Rats[a]

Treatment group	Diet	MNU dose, mg	Incidence of neoplasms		Number of neoplasms	
			Percent	Tumors/animal	Adenoma	Adenocarcinoma
1	Semisynthetic diet (SSD) +0.2% deoxycholic acid (DA)	0	0	0	0	0
2	SSD + 0.2% DA	2	12	0.12	2	0
3	SSD + 0.2% DA	4	53	0.80	11	1
4	SSD + 0.2% DA	8	76	1.75	145	2

[a]Animals were fed the semisynthetic diet (AIN-76) with deoxycholic acid (0.2%) simultaneously with the first dose of MNU (2 mg/dose). Animals in group 3 received two doses (4 mg total) and animals in group 4 received four doses (8 mg total dose).

tumor promotion by deoxycholic acid feeding in MNU-treated animals was not observed even when lower doses of MNU were given to the animals. This suggests that the entire colonic milieu (colonic epithelium, colonic contents, etc.) may be an important determinant in the tumor promotion capability of bile acids. To date, the mechanism of action of bile acids in colon carcinogenesis has not been determined.

4. CONCLUSIONS AND FUTURE DIRECTIONS

The studies presented are suggestive that some bile acids act at the promotional stage of tumor development. By themselves, bile acids have not been found to be either tumor initiators or tumor promoters. However, in animal models where colon cancer is initiated via a chemical carcinogen, bile acids appear to promote carcinogenesis. Definitive studies on the role of bile acids in this regard must await further experimentation in animal models.

ACKNOWLEDGMENTS. This work was supported in part by grant CA-27438 from the National Cancer Institute as part of the National Large Bowel Cancer Project, and by grant HL-24061 from the National Heart, Lung and Blood Institute.

REFERENCES

Armstrong, B., and Doll, R., 1975, Environmental factors and cancer incidence and mortality in different countries with special reference to dietary factors, *Int. J. Cancer* **15**:617.

Burkitt, D. P., 1975, Large bowel carcinogenesis—An epidemiological jigsaw puzzle, *J. Nat. Cancer Inst.* **54**:3.

Burkitt, D. P., 1980, Fiber and etiology of colorectal cancer, in: *Colorectal Cancer: Prevention, Epidemiology and Screening* (S. J. Winower, D. Schottenfeld, and P. Sherlock, eds.), Raven, New York, pp. 13–19.

Carroll, K. K., and Khor, H. T., 1975, Dietary fat in relation to tumorigenesis, *Prog. Biochem. Pharmacol.* **10**:308.

Clarke, H. E., Coates, M. E., Eva, J. K., Ford, D. J., Milner, C. K., O'Donoghue, P. N., Scott, P. P., and Ward, R. J., 1977, Dietary standards for laboratory animals: Report for the Laboratory Animal Centre Diets Advisory Committee, *Lab. Anim.* **11**:1.

Cohen, B. I., Raicht, R. F., Deschner, E. E., Takahashi, M., Sarwal, A. N., and Fazzini, E., 1980, Effect of cholic acid feeding on N-methyl-N-nitrosourea-induced colon tumors and cell kinetics in rats, *J. Nat. Cancer Inst.* **64**:573.

Danielsson, H., Eneroth, P., Hellstrom, K., Lindstedt, S., and Sjövall, J., 1963, Synthesis of some 3β-hydroxylated bile acids and the isolation of 3β,12α-dihydroxy-5β-cholanic acid from feces, *J. Biol. Chem.* **238**:331.

Deschner, E. E., Cohen, B. I., and Raicht, R. F., 1981, The acute and chronic effect of dietary cholic acid on colon epithelial cell proliferation, *Digestion* **21**:290.

Doll, R., 1969, The geographical distribution of cancer, *Br. J. Cancer* **23**:1.

Enig, M. G., Mann, R. J., and Kerney, M., 1978, Dietary fat and cancer trends–A critique, *Fed. Proc. Fed. Am. Soc. Exp. Biol.* **37**:2215.

Greenman, D. L., Oller, W. L., Littlefield, N. A., and Nelson, C. J., 1980, Commercial laboratory animal diets: Toxicant and nutrient variability, *J. Toxicol. Environ. Health* **6**:235.

Hill, M. J., 1974, Bacteria and the etiology of colonic cancer, *Cancer* **34**:815.

Hill, M. J., 1983, Bile, bacteria and bowel cancer, *Gut* **24**:871.

Hill, M. J., Drasar, B. S., Aries, V. C., Crowther, J. S., Hawksworth, G. B., and Williams, R. E. Q., 1971, Bacteria and the etiology of cancer of the large bowel, *Lancet* **1**:95.

Jain, M., Cook, G. M., Davis, F. G., Grace, M. G., Howe, G. R., and Miller, A. B., 1980, A case control study of diet and colorectal cancer, *Int. J. Cancer* **26**:757.

Kay, R. M., 1981, Effects of diet on the fecal excretion and bacterial modification of acidic and neutral steroids, and implications for colon carcinogenesis, *Cancer Res.* **41**:3774.

McCay, P. B., 1983, Dietary fat and cancer, An overview, in: *Diet, Nutrition and Cancer: From Basic Research to Policy Implications* (D. Roe, ed.), Alan R. Liss, New York, pp 7–17.

Newberne, P. M., 1975, Diet: The neglected experimental variable, *Lab. Anim.* **4**:20.

Norman, A., and Palmer R. H., 1964, Metabolites of lithocholic acid-24-C^{14} in human bile and feces, *J. Lab. Clin. Med.* **63**:986.

Phillips, R. L., 1975, Role of life style and dietary habits in risk of cancer among Seventh-Day Adventists, *Cancer Res.* **35**:3513.

Reddy, B. S., 1975, Role of bile metabolites in colon cancer, Animal models, *Cancer* **36**:2401.

Reddy, B. S., 1981, Dietary fat and its relationship to large bowel cancer, *Cancer Res.* **41**:3700.

Reddy, B. S., and Wynder, E. L., 1977, Metabolic epidemiology of colon cancer: Fecal bile acids and neutral sterols in colon cancer patients with adenomatous polyps, *Cancer* **39**:2533.

Reddy, B. S., Narisawa, T., Maronpot, R., and Wynder, E. L., 1975a, Animal models for the study of dietary factors and cancer of the large bowel, *Cancer Res.* **35**:3421.

Reddy, B. S., Weisburger, J. H., and Wynder, E. L., 1975b, Effects of high risk and low risk diets for colon carcinogenesis on fecal microflora and steroids in man, *J. Nutr.* **105**:878.

Reddy, B. S., Mastromarino, A., Gustafson, C., Lipkin, M., and Wynder, E. L., 1976a, Fecal bile acids and neutral sterols in patients with familial polyposis, *Cancer* **38**:1694.

Reddy, B. S., Narisawa, T., Weisburger, J. H., and Wynder, E. L., 1976b, Promoting effect of sodium deoxycholate on colon adenocarcinomas in germfree rats, *J. Nat. Cancer Inst.* **56**:441.

Reddy, B. S., Martin, C. W., and Wynder, E. L., 1977a, Fecal bile acids and cholesterol metabolites of patients with ulcerative colitis, a high risk group for development of colon cancer, *Cancer Res.* **37**:1697.

Reddy, B. S., Watanabe, K., Weisburger, J. H., and Wynder, E. L., 1977b, Promoting effect of bile acids in colon carcinogenesis in germfree and conventional F344 rats, *Cancer Res.* **37**:3238.

Reddy, B. S., Sharma, C., Darby, L., Laakso, K., and Wynder, E. L., 1980, Metabolic epidemiology of large bowel cancer: Fecal mutagens in high- and low-risk populations for colon cancer, A preliminary report, *Mutat. Res.* **72**:511.

Sarwal, A. N., Cohen, B. I., Raicht, R. F., Takahashi, M., and Fazzini, E., 1979, Effects of dietary administration of chenodeoxycholic acid on N-methyl-N-nitrosourea-induced colon cancer in rats, *Biochem. Biophys. Acta* **574**:423.

Takahashi, M., Raicht, R. F., Sarwal, A. N., Mosbach, E. H., and Cohen, B. I., 1978, An improved method for the identification and quantitation of secondary bile acids in biological samples, *Anal. Biochem.* **87**:594.

Van der Werf, S. D., Nagengast, F. M., van Berge-Henegouwen, G. P., Huijbregts, A. W., and van Tongeren, J. H., 1983, Intracolonic environment and the presence of colonic adenomas in man, *Gut* **24**:876.

Wynder, E. L., and Reddy, B. S., 1975, Dietary fat and colon cancer, *J. Nat. Cancer Inst.* **53**:7.

Zaridge, D. G., 1981, Diet and cancer of the large bowel, *Nutr. Cancer* **2**:241.

37

Bile Acids and Colorectal Cancer in Humans

MICHAEL J. HILL

1. BACKGROUND

The relation between diet and the causation of large bowel cancer is widely accepted, although there is still little agreement regarding the component of the diet that is of most importance (Table I). In an attempt to provide a mechanism for this link with diet, Aries *et al.* (1969) postulated that diet provided substrates for metabolism by bacteria to yield products that either cause or promote colorectal cancer. The original substrate postulated was the bile acids, and there have been many studies relating the fecal bile acid (FBA) concentrations in populations to the risk of large bowel cancer (LBC) in those populations (Table II); this correlation must now be accepted as established.

The attempts to establish a similar correlation in case–control studies have been less successful (Table III), but in only one of these studies (that by Hill *et al.*, 1975) was a suitable patient control group chosen; the others all used healthy persons as controls, thereby adding the confounding factor of loss of appetite associated with bowel disease. In addition, only one study (Hill *et al.*, 1975) contained a low proportion of patients with liver metastases; this has been shown by Moskovitz *et al.* (1979) to be extremely important and we have confirmed this (Table IV). Our study indicates that the FBA concentration is a factor in carcinogenesis of the rectosigmoid but not of the right colon, and that liver metastases interfere with FBA loss. Never-

MICHAEL J. HILL ● PHLS Centre for Applied Microbiology and Research, Salisbury, Wiltshire SP4 0JG, United Kingdom.

TABLE I. The Relation between Diet and Colorectal Cancer
in Epidemiologic Studies

Dietary component	Role[a]	Type of study
Total fat	Causal	Population studies[b]
		Case-control studies
Animal fat	Causal	Population studies
Unsaturated fatty acid	Causal	Population studies
Cholesterol	Causal	Population studies
Animal protein	Causal	Population studies
Meat	Causal	Population studies
	Protective	Prospective study
Beef	Causal	Population study
Dietary fiber	Causal	Population studies
Crude	Protective	Case-control studies
Pentosan	Protective	Population studies
Vitamins A, C, E	Protective	Population studies
	Protective	Case-control studies
Beer	Causal	Population studies
	Causal	Case-control studies
Milk	Protective	Population study
	Protective	Prospective study

[a]"Causal" means that the dietary item has been correlated with colorectal cancer incidence, while "protective"
factors have been inversely correlated.
[b]In almost all cases there have been a number of studies failing to show the correlation described.

TABLE II. Relation between Mean Fecal Bile Acid (FBA) Concentration and
Incidence of Large Bowel Cancer (LBC)

Type of Study	Observation	Reference
Comparison of populations in six countries	FBA correlated with LBC	Hill et al. (1971)
Comparison of populations in New York	FBA correlated with LBC	Wynder and Reddy (1974)
Comparison of three income groups in Hong Kong	FBA correlated with LBC	Crowther et al. (1976)
Comparison of populations in Scandinavia	FBA correlated with LBC	Wynder and Reddy (1978), Hill et al. (1982)
Comparison of religious groups in California	FBA correlated with LBC	Turjman et al. (1982)

TABLE III. Case–Control Studies Relating Fecal Bile Acids (FBA) and Colorectal Carcinogenesis

Cases	Controls	Observation	Reference
Colorectal cancer (44)	Patients with no malignant/gastrointestinal disease (99)	FBA higher in cases	Hill et al. (1975)
Colorectal cancer (84)	Healthy control persons (100)	FBA higher in Dukes A and B cases in the sigmoid and rectum, not in the right colon or in metastatic cancer	Hill (1981)
Colon cancer	Healthy controls	FBA higher in cases	Reddy and Wynder (1978)
Colorectal cancer	Healthy controls	No difference	Blackwood et al. (1978)
Colorectal cancer	Healthy controls	No difference	Mudd et al. (1978)
Colorectal cancer	Healthy controls	No difference	Moskovitz et al. (1978)
Colorectal cancer (15)	Healthy controls	No difference	Kaibara et al. (1983)

TABLE IV. Relation between Fecal Bile Acids (FBA) and Colorectal
Carcinogenesis by Histological Stage and by Subsite

	Number assayed	FBA, mg/g dry weight	Percent carrying NDC
All colorectal cancers			
Dukes A	17	10.6	88
Dukes B	36	10.7	72
Dukes C	28	9.6	80
Dukes C2	10	7.0	0
All colon cancers	30	10.6	80
Cecum + transverse	10	9.0	80
Descending + sigmoid	20	11.4	80
All rectal cancers	38	10.3	79
Upper third	13	10.3	85
Mid third	12	10.8	67
Lower third	13	10.0	85
Normal healthy persons	100	7.9	38

theless, there is an overlap between the cases and controls in FBA concentration, indicating that a more refined approach is necessary. Some suggestions for this are made later.

The conclusions of the histopathologists are that there is a histopathological sequence in colorectal carcinogenesis (Morson et al., 1983). The evidence for this dysplasia–carcinoma sequence has been summarized by Morson and Konishi (1980) and a schematic formulation (Fig. 1) has been proposed by Hill et al. (1978). In general, dysplasia is manifest as discrete raised adenomas, although in ulcerative colitis and occasionally in the uninflamed colon dysplasia may be in the plane of the mucosa (and therefore difficult to detect except by random biopsy). In determining the etiology of colorectal cancer it is necessary to determine the factors causing (1) initiation of dysplasia, (2) increase in the area of dysplasia, (3) increase of severity of dysplasia, and (4) the progression from severe dysplasia to carcinoma. The role of bile acids in these four stages has been investigated in adenoma patients and in patients with chronic ulcerative colitis.

In the original hypothesis by Aries et al. the role of diet in determining the FBA concentration was regarded as crucial. However, it is now clear that many factors other than diet are important in determining the FBA concentration, and indeed diet may not be the most important factor. This will be discussed later. Bacterial metabolism was also of importance in the original hypothesis, and two enzymic reactions have been found to be of importance. Mastromarino *et al.* (1976) showed that the activity of 7α-dehydroxylase was greater in colorectal cancer cases than in controls; since this enzyme produces the two secondary bile acids shown to be tumor promoters (deoxycholic acid and lithocholic acid) from the primary bile acids, this observation is likely to be of importance. A number of groups have demonstrated that those clostridia able to produce unsaturated bile acids, referred to as NDC (Hill *et al.*, 1975), are carried by a high proportion of colorectal cancer cases compared with controls (Table V). A number of groups have claimed to have failed to demonstrate the increased carriage rate of NDC (Moskovitz *et al.*, 1979; Moore and Holdman, 1975; Finegold *et al.*, 1975); however, none of these groups actually attempted to assay carriage of the enzyme, but merely looked for marker species. The role of NDC will also be discussed in this review.

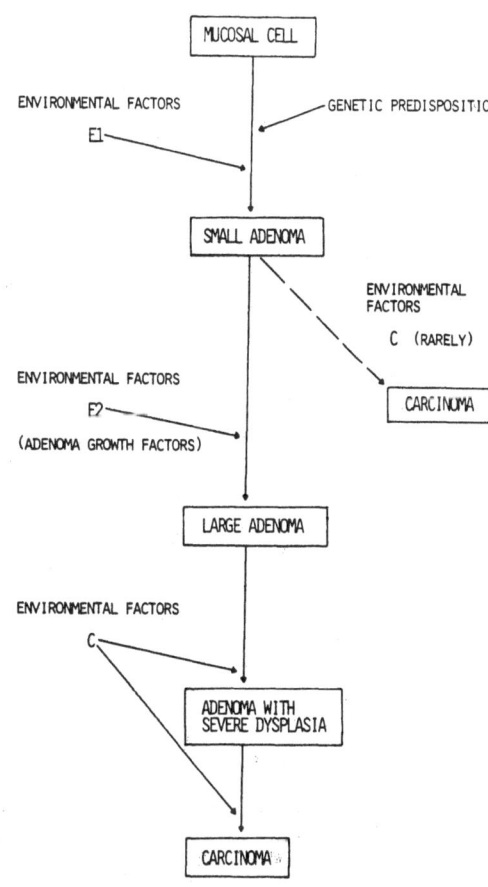

FIGURE 1. The postulated mechanism of the adenoma/carcinoma sequence.

TABLE V. The Carriage of NDC in Colorectal Cancer
Cases and Controls in Two Studies

	Carriage rate of NDC, %	
	Colorectal cancer	Controls
Hill et al. (1975)	86	43
Blackwood et al. (1978)	83	58

2. BACTERIAL ENZYMES AND COLORECTAL CANCER

There have been a few studies attempting to relate bacterial enzymes to
large bowel cancer risk. In some studies enzymes that might have a causal
role have been examined, while in others enzymes are used as markers of
bacterial activity. The results of these are summarized in Table VI. The first
enzyme to be examined was cholanoyl 7-dehydroxylase; this followed early
evidence that the concentration of deoxycholic acid, the product of 7-
dehydroxylation of cholic acid was highly correlated with bowel cancer risk
(Hill et al., 1971). Narisawa et al. (1974) then demonstrated that bile acids
are more cocarcinogenic in conventional than in germ-free rats (implicating
a role for bacterial metabolites) and that the products of 7-dehydroxylation,
deoxycholic acid and lithocholic acid, are tumor promoters, while the primary bile acids are not. Mastromarino et al. (1976) showed that the activity
of 7-dehydroxylase in the feces of colorectal cancer cases was higher than
in controls; we have confirmed this (Jivraj and Hill, unpublished results).

TABLE VI. Bacterial Enzymes Related to Colorectal Carcinogenesis

Enzyme	Evidence	Reference
Cholanoyl 7-dehydroxylase	Strong correlation between deoxycholic acid concentration and LBC	Hill et al. (1971)
	Higher activity of 7-dehydroxylase in LBC cases than in controls	Mastromarino et al. (1976)
β-Glucuronidase	Higher activity in New York populations with higher LBC risk	Wynder and Reddy (1974)
Cholanoyl 4-5 dehydrogenase	Relation between organisms producing the enzyme and LBC in populations and in case–control studies (in three countries)	Hill et al. (1975); Blackwood et al. (1978)

The second enzyme to be studied was β-glucuronidase, which might release carcinogens from the conjugates produced as detoxification products of hepatic enzymes. After initial studies relating fecal β-glucuronidase to the intake of dietary fat (Reddy et al., 1974) interest waned. In our studies the day-to-day variation in β-glucuronidase activity was very wide, as was the variation in activity among persons; these variations made it impossible to detect effects of diet, etc., or differences between groups of bowel cancer patients and controls. Cholanoyl 4-5 dehydrogenase is an enzyme produced by certain clostridia referred to as NDC (bile acid nuclear dehydrogenating clostridia). NDC do not belong to a single species of the genus *Clostridium*. Although a high proportion of strains of *C. paraputrificum, C. tertium,* and *C. butyricum* produce the enzyme together with a small proportion of *C. indolis* and representatives of a large number of other species of lecithinase-negative clostridia, representatives of the "high-risk" species from feces of Japanese and Hong Kong persons did not produce the enzyme. Thus it is clearly useless to identify species and infer their NDC status, and only assay of the enzyme can be used to determine whether a person carries NDC. The three groups who have assayed 4-5 dehydrogenase activity have shown that a higher proportion of colorectal cancer cases than controls carry NDC (Hill et al., 1975; Blackwood et al., 1978; Haralambie and Linzemeier, 1981). A range of "sentinel enzymes" (including β-glucosidase, azoreductase, nitro-reductase, and β-glucuronidase has been used to monitor changes in the bacterial flora produced by dietary manipulation (e.g., Goldin et al., 1978, 1981), but these have not been directly implicated in colorectal carcinogenesis.

The effects of diet on the various bacterial enzymes described above are summarized in Table VII. We have not seen any major effects of diet on NDC carriage, and most of the evidence concerns the sentinel enzymes.

TABLE VII. The Relation between Diet and Fecal Bacterial Enzymes

	Diet difference	Change in enzyme activity
Reddy et al. (1974)	High meat vs. no meat	Higher β-glucuronidase on high meat
Drasar et al. (1976)	High bran vs. low bran	No difference in β-glucuronidase
Goldin et al. (1978)	Including dietary bran	No effect on a range of enzymes
Bauer et al. (1979)	Pectin supplements in rats	Tenfold increase in β-glucuronidase
Shiau and Chang (1983)	No fiber vs. 15% fiber	β-glucuronidase and mucinase higher on fiber-free diet

3. FBA AND NDC IN THE DYSPLASIA-CARCINOMA SEQUENCE

We have carried out two studies of the role of FBA and NDC in the dysplasia-carcinoma sequence; in one, patients with colorectal adenomas were compared with control persons (Hill et al. 1983), while in the other, patients with ulcerative colitis with total colonic involvement were investigated.

3.1 Adenoma Patients

In a study of 133 patients with colorectal adenomas and 22 patients with nonadenomatous polyps (e.g., fibromas, hamartomatous polyps, metaplastic polyps), all attending the outpatient clinic at St. Mark's Hospital, London, fecal analyses were no different from those of healthy control persons (Table VIII). Further, there was no relation between the number of colorectal adenomas detected during the period of study (1974–1981) and the fecal analyses (Table IX). This suggests that the FBA/NDC discriminant is not involved in the initial causation of epithelial dysplasia in the colon (factor E1 in Fig. 1).

When the adenoma patients were subdivided on the basis of adenoma size (Table X) there was a good correlation between the mean diameter of the adenoma and both FBA concentration ($p < 0.01$) and carriage rate of NDC ($p < 0.05$), suggesting that the FBA/NDC discriminant may be important in adenoma growth or in increasing the rate of proliferation of dysplastic mucosal cells (factor E2 in Fig. 1).

When the adenoma patients were segregated into those with only mild dysplasia and those with moderate or severe dysplasia (Table XI) there was again a correlation between the severity of epithelial dysplasia and the FBA concentration ($p < 0.01$) and the carriage rate NDC, suggesting that, as well as causing an increase in the rate of proliferation of dysplastic tissues, the FBA/NDC factor may also be responsible for the increase in severity of epithelial dysplasia (factor C in Fig. 1).

TABLE VIII. Fecal Analysis in Patients with Adenomas or Nonadenomatous Polyps and Healthy Control Persons

	Number of patients	FBA, mg/g dry weight	Percent carrying NDC
Control persons	100	8.7 ± 2.5	37
Patients with adenomas	133	8.8 ± 2.2	42
Patients with other polyps	22	6.9 ± 1.2	38

TABLE IX. Relation between Number of Adenomas Carried
and Fecal Analysis

Number of adenomas	Number of patients	Fecal analysis	
		FBA, mg/g dry weight	Percent carrying NDC
0	100	8.7±2.5	37
1	57	8.3±2.2	33
2	32	9.4±2.5	42
3 or 4	21	8.8±2.0	38
>4	20	9.4±3.4	65

3.2 Patients with Ulcerative Colitis

Patients with chronic ulcerative colitis involving the whole of the large bowel whose history of symptoms covers more than 10 years are at above average risk of developing colorectal cancer and so are usually advised to have a prophylatic colectomy. A number of such patients elect not to have surgery and instead have a regular colorectal examination for signs of precancer, which is detected histologically. (Morson and Pang, 1967). We have followed a group of 110 such patients since 1974; during that time seven have had a serious relapse in their colitis prompting a colectomy, seven have died, and 43 have developed epithelial dysplasia (Table XII). Those who needed a colectomy because of the severity of their colitis tended to have below average FBA concentration and an average carriage rate of NDC. Those who died had, as expected, average fecal analyses.

In patients in whom dysplasia of any grade was detected the fecal analyses were similar to those of the whole group, indicating (as with the adenoma patients) no role for the FBA/NDC factor in the causation of dysplasia *per se*. When this small group was segregated into those with

TABLE X. Relation between Fecal Analysis and
Size of Adenoma Carried by the Patient

Mean diameter of the largest adenoma, mm	Number of patients	Fecal Analysis	
		FBA, mg/g dry weight	Percent carrying NDC
< 5	26	6.7±1.2	7
5–10	30	7.9±1.5	37
10–20	45	8.0±2.6	45
> 20	32	11.4±2.4	70

TABLE XI. Relation between Severity of Epithelial Dysplasia in an Adenoma and Fecal Analysis

Severity of epithelial dysplasia	Number of patients	Fecal analysis	
		FBA, mg/g dry weight	Percent carrying NDC
Mild	84	8.3 ± 2.4	38
Moderate or severe	39	10.0 ± 2.1	49

moderate or severe dysplasia compared with those with only mild dysplasia there was a clear difference in the mean FBA concentration and the carriage rate of NDC between the two groups. These results support the conclusion that the role of bile acid metabolites in the causation of colorectal cancer is not in the initiation of the precursor benign lesion but in its progression to malignancy.

4. FACTORS DETERMINING BILE ACID METABOLISM

We have carried out a number of types of experiment to determine the factors controlling bile acid metabolism in the gut. These include investigations of the site of metabolism, the mechanism by which diet affects FBA loss, and the reasons for the between-person variations in FBA loss.

TABLE XII. Relation between Fecal Analysis and Severity of Epithelial Dysplasia in 110 Patients with Ulcerative Colitis

Grade of dysplasia	Number of patients	Fecal analysis	
		FBA, mg/g dry weight	Percent carrying NDC
Severe	13	10.5	46
Moderate	8	9.5	13
Mild	22	7.4	25
None	67	7.2	27
Still alive	53	7.2	32
Colectomy	7	7.0	—
Died	7	7.4	—
Total group	110	7.8	28
All dysplasia	43	8.7	27

4.1 Site of Steroid Metabolism in the Body

Because of the relative simplicity of neutral steroid analysis (compared with that of bile acids) we have studied the subsite of metabolism of cholesterol in the gut at autopsy and in patients with partial colonic resection. In a study of persons at autopsy (Boyer *et al.,* 1984) there were three patterns of cholesterol metabolism (Fig. 2); in only 21% was metabolism continuous throughout the colon, and in the remaining 79% it had reached completion (i.e., the level attained by the sigmoid colon) before reaching the transverse colon, suggesting that the main site of metabolism was the cecum. This conclusion was supported in a study of patients who had partial colonic resection; where the resected specimen was from the left colon the extent of cholesterol metabolism and of metabolism of tyrosine to urinary volatile phenols was similar to that in persons with a complete colon (Table XIII). Interestingly, when part of the right colon (cecum of ascending colon) was resected this was accompanied by a big decrease in microbial degradation of cholesterol (Table XIII), although there was clear evidence of adaptation with time (Fig. 3). There was no relation between the length of the resected specimen and the effect on metabolism of cholesterol, and the difference in effect or removal of part of the left compared with part of the right colon

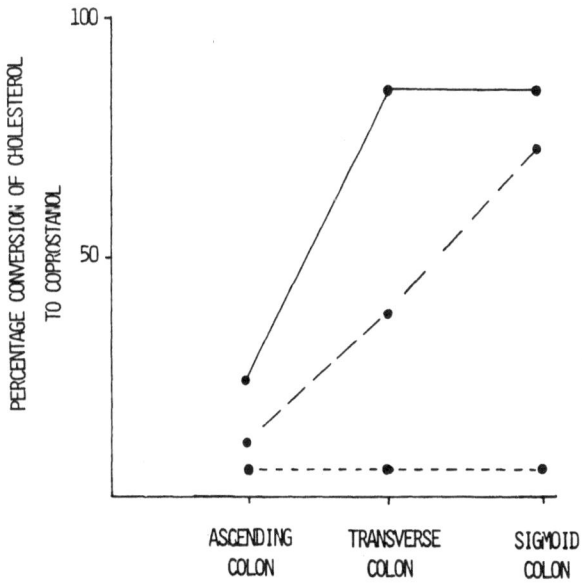

FIGURE 2. Patterns of cholesterol metabolism. (A) Metabolism complete by the mid-colon (61% of persons); (B) no metabolism of cholesterol (18% of persons); (C) metabolism continuous throughout the colon (21% of persons).

TABLE XIII. Metabolism of Cholesterol and of Tyrosine in the Colon of Persons Who Had Undergone Colonic Resection

	Site of the initial tumor			Normal persons
	Right colon	Left colon	Rectum	
Number of patients	10	20	14	—
Length of resection	39 ± 21	29 ± 14	21 ± 12	—
Percent of undegraded cholesterol	47 ± 21	29 ± 16	25 ± 13	—
Number of patients	—	3	—	10
Total urinary volatile phenols	—	62	—	62
Ratio p-cresol/phenol	—	11.8	—	5.3

ᵃResults shown are mean±standard deviation.

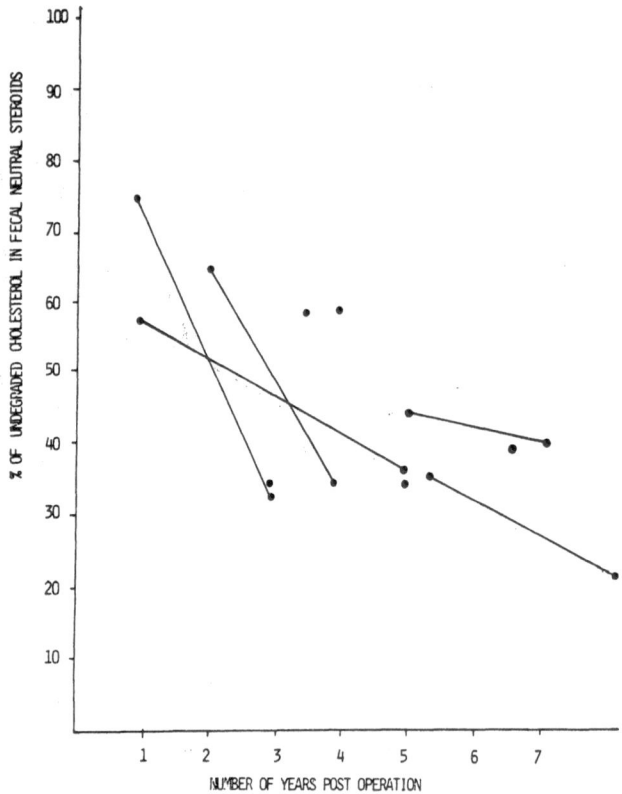

FIGURE 3. The variation in the extent of cholesterol metabolism with time after resection of part of the right colon.

must be sought in the different functions and types of propulsive movements between the two subsites.

It is clear from these studies that events in the right colon, before the gut contents have become dehydrated and viscous, are the main determinants of bacterial metabolism in the large bowel.

4.2 The Mechanism by Which Diet Affects Gut Bacterial Metabolism

It is clear from previous studies (Cummings, *et al.,* 1976, 1978, 1979) that diet has a profound affect on the amounts of bacterial metabolites producted in the colon, and this could be due to affects on substrate concentration, on cecal physiology, on colorectal transit time, or on the composition of the cecal bacterial flora. Studies of ileostomy patients by Hori *et al.* (1983) and Fernandez *et al.* (1983, 1984) have indicated clearly that dietary changes result in differences in the amounts of nutrients and substrates delivered to the cecum, and also profoundly affect the composition of the flora of the terminal ileum. This work has been dealt with in more detail elsewhere (Fadden, this volume, Chapter 8).

4.3 Between-Person Variations

In studies conducted in collaboration with various groups (e.g. Cummings *et al.*, 1976, 1978, 1979; Walters *et al.*, 1975) we have noted very large variations among persons eating similar diets in the fecal loss of bile acids (Fig. 4). Clearly, although diet is an important factor in determining fecal bile acid loss, it is not the only factor (and may not even be the most important factor). Bile acids are very efficiently absorbed by active transport from the terminal ileum and only 1–4% is lost into the large bowel with each of the 6–10 cycles of the enterohepatic circulation per day. The number of enterohepatic circulations per day is dependent in part on diet and in addition on host factors; the amount lost with each cycle will depend on events in the terminal ileum, which again appear to be determined by host factors. Since similar variations are found in all other measures of bacterial metabolism (e.g., cholesterol metabolites, amino acid metabolites, undegraded dietary fiber), it is clear that, if bacterial metabolites are implicated in the causation of large bowel cancer, host factors may be among the most important determinants of risk and are certainly important modulators of the effects of environmental factors.

5. Characteristics of High-Risk Populations

Comparisons of populations in epidemiologic studies have revealed a number of risk factors in colorectal carcinogenesis, the most important of

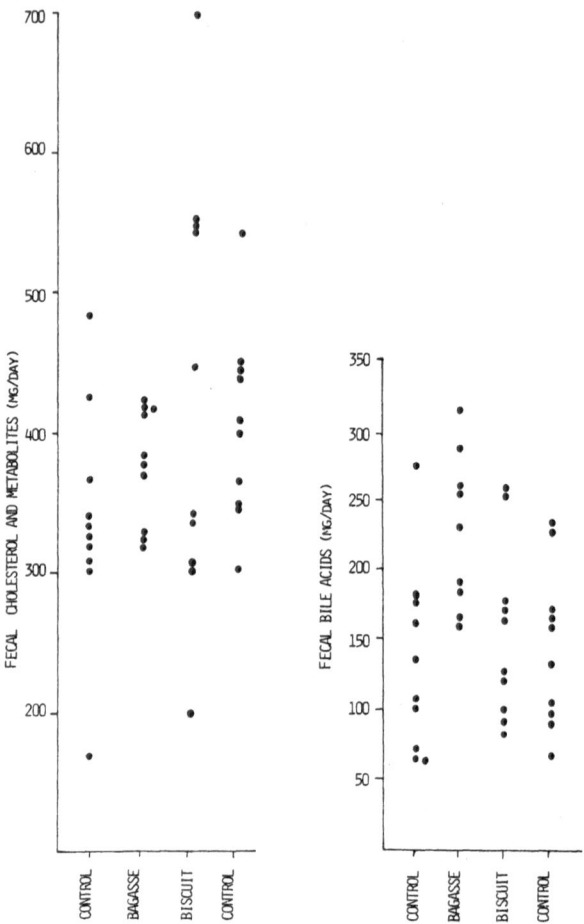

FIGURE 4. The variation in daily fecal neutral steroid and bile acid loss in persons eating identical diets. (For details of the diets see Walters *et al.*, 1975.)

which is diet (Wynder and Shigematsu, 1967; Drasar and Irving, 1973; Armstrong and Doll, 1975), particularly dietary meat or fat. Metabolic epidemiology of colorectal cancer in populations reveals a strong correlation with FBA concentration (Table II). These correlations that are very strong in comparisons of populations seem to disappear when case–control studies are carried out, and this is almost certainly because of the strength of modulating factors characteristic of the individual. These modulating factors include "adenoma-proneness," variations among individuals in digestive processes, and particularly the ecology of the terminal ileum and cecum.

There is a well-documented variation in sensitivity of different strains of rodents to the action of a variety of carcinogens and it would be surprising if there were not a similar genetically determined variation in sensitivity among humans. It has been postulated that this is manifest in humans as a variation in risk of developing the precurser adenoma ["adenoma-proneness" (Veale, 1965)] and this has been discussed at length by Morson *et al.* (1983). Thus, within a population at high risk because of their diet there is a subpopulation at higher risk (because they are adenoma-prone), with the remainder being at little risk (because they are not sensitive to the adenogenic properties of the "high-risk" diet). This is certain to confound any case–control study unless it is taken into account.

Although certain diets are associated with a high risk of colorectal cancer in populations, Aries *et al.* (1969) postulated that this was because they contained components that were metabolized by bacteria to factors implicated in carcinogenesis. It has already been noted that the production of bacterial metabolites is determined by events in the terminal ileum and cecum and that host factors are important determinants of these events. Thus, in the production of metabolites important in colorectal carcinogenesis the important determinants are diet (which supplies the substrates), the efficiency with which the host metabolizes that diet, the nature of the flora, and the physiology of the cecum (where the metabolism is to take place). In addition to the amount of metabolites, the sensitivity of the host mucosa to the adenogenic properties of the metabolite will also be important in determining cancer risk. In the light of this, it is important to reiterate that case–control studies are unlikely to provide a good test of hypotheses of colorectal carcinogenesis unless the confounding factors are taken into account in the study design.

ACKNOWLEDGMENTS. This work is financially supported by the Cancer Research Campaign.

REFERENCES

Aries, V. C., Crowther, J. S., Drasar, B. S., Hill, M. J., and Williams, R. E. O., 1969, Bacteria and the etiology of cancer of the large bowel, *Gut* **10**:334–335.

Armstrong, B., and Doll, R., 1975, Environmental factors and the incidence and mortality from cancer in different countries with special reference to dietary practice, *Int. J. Cancer.* **15**:617–631.

Bauer, H. G., Asp, N., Oste, R., Dahlqvist, A., and Fredlund, P., 1979, Effect of dietary fibre on the induction of colorectal tumours and fecal β-glucuronidase activity in the rat, *Cancer Res.* **39**:3752–3756.

Blackwood, A., Murray, W. R., Mackay, C., and Calman, K., 1978, Faecal bile acids and clostridia in the aetiology of colorectal cancer and breast cancer, *B. J. Cancer* **38**:175.

Boyer, J. A., Day, D. W., and Hill, M. J., 1984, Site of cholesterol degradation in the human gut, *Biochem. Soc. Trans.* **12**:1104–1105.

Crowther, J. S., Drasar, B. S., Hill, M. J., MaClennan, R., Magnin, D., Peach, S., and Teoh-

Chan, C. H., 1976, Faecal steroids and bacteria and large bowel cancer in Hong Kong by socio-economic groups, *Br. J. Cancer* **34**:191–198.

Cummings, J. H., Hill, M. J., Bone, E. S., Branch, W. J., and Jenkins, D. J., 1979, The effect of meat protein with and without dietary fibre on colonic function and metabolism II: Bacterial Metabolites in faeces and urine, *Am. J. Clin. Nutr.* **32**:2094–2107.

Cummings, J. H., Hill, M. J., Jenkins, D. J., Pearson, J. R., and Wiggins, H. S., 1976, Changes in fecal composition and colonic function due to cereal fiber *Am. J. Clin. Nutr.* **29**: 1468–1473.

Cummings, J. H., Wiggins, H. S., Jenkins, D. J. A., Houston, H., Jivraj, T., Drasar, B. S., and Hill, M. J., 1978, Influence of diets high and low in animal fat on bowel habit, gastro-intestinal transit time, fecal microflora, bile acid and fat excretion, *J. Clin. Invest.* **61**: 953–963.

Drasar, B. S., and Irvine, D., 1973, Environmental factors and cancer of the colon and breast, *Br. J., Cancer* **27**:167–172.

Drasar, B. S., Jenkins, D. J. A., and Cummings, J. H., 1976, The influence of a diet rich in wheat fibre on the human faecal flora, *J. Med. Microbiol.* **9**: 423–431.

Fernandez, F., Kennedy, H., Truelove, S., and Hill, M. J., 1983, The effect of changes in the amount of dietary protein on the composition of ileostomy fluid, *Proc. Nutr. Soc.* **42**:109A.

Fernandez, F., Kennedy, H., Todd, E., Truelove, S., and Hill, M., 1984, Diet and the steroid composition of ileostomy fluid, *Biochem. Soc. Trans.* **12**:1103–1104.

Finegold, S. M., Flora, D., Attebury, H., and Sutter, V., 1975, Fecal bacteriology of colonic polyp patients and control patients, *Cancer Res.* **35**:3407–3417.

Goldin, B., Dwyer, J., Gorbach, S. L., Gordon, W., and Swenson, L., 1978, Influence of diet and age on fecal bacterial enzymes, *Am. J. Clin. Nutr.* **31**:5136–5140.

Haralambie, E., and Linzenmeier, G., 1981, Clostridia of the human gut, in: *Recent Advances in Germfree Research,* Tokai University Press, pp. 207–211.

Hill, M. J., 1981, Metabolic epidemiology of large bowel cancer, in: *Gastrointestinal Cancer* (J. De Cosse and P. Sherlock, eds.), Martinus Nijhoff, New York, pp. 187–226.

Hill, M. J., Drasar, B. S., Aries, V. C., Crowther, J. S., Hawksworth, G., and Williams, R. E. O., 1971, Bacteria and etiology of cancer of large bowel, *Lancet* **i**:95–100.

Hill, M. J., Drasar, B. S., Williams, R. E. O., Meade, T., Simpson, J., and Morson, B. C., 1975, Fecal bile acids, clostridia and the etiology of cancer of the large bowel, *Lancet* **i**:535–539.

Hill, M. J., Morson, B. C., and Bussey, H. J. R., 1978, Aetiology of adenoma–carcinoma sequence in bowel, *Lancet* **i**:245–247.

Hill, M. J., Morson, B. C., and Thomson, M. H., 1983, The role of faecal bile acids in large bowel carcinogenesis, *Br. J. Cancer* **48**:143.

Hill, M. J., Taylor, A., Thompson, M., and Wait, R., 1982, Fecal steroids and urinary volatile phenols in four Scandinavian populations, *Nutr. Cancer* **4**:67–73.

Hori, S., Berghouse, L., Hill, M., Hudson, M., Rogers, E., and Lennard-Jones, J., 1983, The effect of dietary fibre on the bacterial flora of ileostomy fluid, *J. Med. Microbiol.* **16**:viii.

Kaibara, N., Sasaki, T., Ikeguchi, M., Kog, A. S., and Ikawa, S., 1983, Fecal bile acids and neutral sterols in Japanese with large bowel carcinoma, *Oncology* **40**:255–258.

Mastromarino, A., Reddy, B. S., and Wynder, E. L., 1976, Metabolic epidemiology of colon cancer: Enzymic activities of fecal flora, *Am. J. Clin. Nutr.* **29**:1455–1460.

Moore, W. E. C., and Holdman, L. V., 1975, Discussion of recent bacteriological investigations of the relationships between intestinal flora, diet and colon cancer, *Cancer Res.* **35**: 3418–3420.

Morson, B. C., and Konishi, F., 1980, Dysplasia of the colorectum, in: *Recent Advances in Gastrointestinal Pathology* (R. Wright, ed.), W. B. Saunders, London, pp. 331–343.

Morson, B. C., and Pang, L. S. G., 1967, Rectal biopsy as an aid to cancer control in ulcerative colitis, *Gut* **8**:423–434.

Morson, B. C., Bussey, H. J. R., Day, D. W., and Hill, M. J., 1983, Adenomas of the large bowel, *Cancer Surv.* **2**:451–477.

Moskovitz, M., White, C., Barnett, R. N., Stevens, S., Russell, E., Vargo, D., and Floch, M. H., 1979, Diet, faecal bile acids and neutral sterols in carcinoma of the colon, *Dig. Dis. Sci.* **24**:746–751.

Mudd, D. G., McKelvey, S. T., Sloan, J. M., and Elmore, D. T., 1978, Faecal bile acid concentrations in patients at increased risk of large bowel cancer, *Acta Gastroenterol. Belg.* **41**:241–244.

Narisawa, T., Magadia, N. E., and Wynder, E. L., 1974, Promoting effect of bile acids on colon carcinogenesis after intrarectal instillation of N-methyl-N-nitroso-N-nitroguanidine in rats, *Cancer Res.* **53**:1093–1097.

Reddy, B. S., Weisburger, J. H., and Wynder, E. L., 1974, Fecal bacterial β-glucuronidases control by diet, *Science* **183**:416–417.

Reddy, B. S., and Wynder, E. L., 1977, Metabolic epidemiology of colon cancer: Fecal bile acids and neutral steroids in colon cancer patients and patients with adenomatous polyps, *Cancer* **39**:2533–2539.

Shiau, S., and Chang, G. W., 1983, Effects of dietary fibre on faecal mucinase and β-glucuronidase activity in rats, *J. Nutr.* **113**:138–144.

Turjman, N., Guidry, C., Jaeger, B., Mendeloff, A. I., Calkins, B., Phillips, R. L., and Nair, P. P., 1982, Faecal bile acids and neutral sterols in Seventh Day Adventists and the general population of California, in: *Colon and Nutrition* (H. Kaspar and H. Geobell, eds.), MTP, Lancaster, England, pp. 291–298.

Veale, A. M. O., 1965, Intestinal Polyposis, in: *Eugenics Lab. Memoirs Series, 40,* Cambridge University Press, London.

Walters, R. L., Baird, I. M., Hill, M. J., Drasar, B. S., Southgate, D. A. T., Green, J., and Morgan, B., 1975, Effects of two types of dietary fibre on faecal steroid and lipid excretion, *Br. Med. J.* **2**:536–538.

Wynder, E. L., and Reddy, B. S., 1974, Metabolic epidemiology of colorectal cancer, *Cancer* **34**:801–806.

Wynder, E. L., and Reddy, B. S., 1978, Etiology of cancer of the colon, in: *Colon Cancer* (H. Grundmann, ed.), Gustav Fischer, Stuttgart, pp. 1–14.

Wynder, E. L., and Shigematsu, T., 1967, Environmental factors in cancer of the colon and rectum, *Cancer* **20**:1520–1561.

38

Cancer Patterns in Different Ethnic Groups in South Africa

A. R. P. WALKER, M. I. ODENDAAL, and I. SEGAL

1. INTRODUCTION

Early and some later workers (Higginson and Oettlé, 1960; Robertson *et al.*, 1971; Schonland and Bradshaw, 1968; Rose and Fellingham, 1981; Isaacson *et al.*, 1978) noted pronounced differences in the incidence rates of cancers in South African interethnic populations. These currently include blacks (about 19 million), whites (4½ million), coloreds (Eur-African-Malays) (2½ million), and Indians (3/4 million). The pattern of differences from the incidence studies was in substantial agreement with the pattern based on mortality rates (Bradshaw and Harington, 1982; Bradshaw *et al.*, 1982, 1983). Understandably, while there are some limitations to the validity of death certificates even in developed populations (Percy *et al.*, 1981), there are much greater uncertainties in certification in the cases of less privileged or less developed populations.

The previously acquired information indicated the following:

Blacks: Total mortality rate from cancer was much lower than that in whites. In urban black men, by far the commonest cancer was esophageal cancer, followed, with much lower mortality rates, by lung and liver cancers. In women, apart from a very high mortality from invasive cervix cancer, and much less commonly, esophageal cancer, tumors in other sites were relatively rare.

A.R.P. WALKER ● School of Pathology, South African Institute for Medical Research, and University of the Witwatersrand, Johannesburg, South Africa. M. I. ODENDAAL ● Department of Physiology, University of Potchefstroom, Potchefstroom, South Africa. I. SEGAL ● Department of Gastroenterology, Baragwanath Hospital, Johannesburg, South Africa.

Indians: Cancer mortality rate was lower than that for whites. In men, stomach and lung cancers, and in women, breast and stomach cancers, predominated.

Coloreds: Total cancer mortality rate exceeded that in whites. In men there were very high rates for lung, stomach, and esophageal cancers. In women highest rates were for cervix and breast cancers.

Whites: The total mortality from cancer was somewhat low, and little different from that in Canada and the U. S. (Anonymous, 1974). The rates were much lower, for example, than that in Scotland (Anonymous, 1974; World Health Organization, 1982). In South African white men, the most frequent cancer sites were lung, stomach, and colon–rectum. In women, breast cancer was by far the commonest.

2. PRESENT STUDIES

The above information concerns situations that were obtained one or two decades or more ago. More recent data on mortality rates have therefore been secured, for the year 1979. The figures to be given relate to total ethnic populations, save in the case of blacks; their data refer to that moiety of the population living in urban areas (the proportion is about 40%). The requisite information was derived from publications by the Central Statistical Services (Central Statistical Services, 1982). As already noted, there are limitations to the accuracy of the figures, particularly on the blacks; among urban dwellers, excluding deaths from violence, almost 40% of deaths were certified as from "unknown" or "natural causes." Among Indian, colored, and white populations, corresponding proportions in these categories were approximately 20, 15, and 5%, respectively. The mortality rates per 100,000 are standardized to world population (Doll and Peto, 1982).

Table I relates to data on black, Indian, colored, and white populations. For comparison, data for 1980 for England and Wales are also given. Table II provides further comparative data, mainly for 1980, on a number of European populations, as recently reported by the World Health Organization (World Health Organization, 1982).

The cancer mortality rates depicted indicate that the present general situation has scarcely altered compared with that prevailing in the past.

3. DISCUSSION

Blacks: In urban dwellers, bearing in mind the changes that have occurred in lifestyle, higher rates would have been expected than those depicted. Yet the low rates, at least in the big cities, may well be valid, for intensive studies by social and other workers indicate that the huge majority of urban patients with cancer do ultimately seek medical attention.

TABLE I. Cancer Mortality Rates in South African Populations and in U. K. Population per 100,000[a]

Site	Blacks		Indians		Coloreds		Whites		U. K. population[b]	
	M	F	M	F	M	F	M	F	M	F
Esophagus	30	8	7	4	29	5	6	2	9	6
Stomach	6	3	21	11	35	11	16	7	27	18
Colon, rectum	3	2	9	6	8	8	13	12	32	35
Liver	14	4	7	4	13	7	6	4	2	1
Lung	17	3	20	6	66	11	44	14	112	33
Breast	—	5	—	12	—	20	—	24	—	48
Cervix	—	14	—	8	—	26	—	5	—	8
Prostate	7	—	4	—	12	—	16	—	21	—
Other	30	14	27	32	50	36	54	40	84	89
All sites	107	53	95	83	213	124	155	108	287	238

[a] Standardized to world population.
[b] World Health Organization (1982).

TABLE II. Death Rates from Cancer in 1980 (per 100,000)[a]

Country	Males	Females
Austria	274.7	241.0
Bulgaria	162.2	115.3
Germany	266.1	244.2
Greece	214.8	132.7
Hungary	292.7	223.9
Netherlands	259.4	174.8
Poland	191.4	145.4
Romania	149.5	114.4
England and Wales	287.2	238.9
Yugoslavia	145.6	106.6
South Africa (Whites)	155.1	108.7

[a]World Health Organization (1982).

Regarding the high rates from *esophageal cancer,* these have been attributed to consumption of a predominantly maize diet with associated deficiencies of micronutrients (van Rensburg, 1981), as well as to particular smoking and drinking practices (Bradshaw and Schonland, 1974). The precise etiology remains obscure. Survival is very short, with 50% mortality occurs in 3–4 months (Walker *et al.*, 1984b), half of the period with white patients (Cancer Statistics Group, 1982).

The high rates for *liver cancer,* especially in certain parts of the country, are believed to be linked with the consumption of mouldy food (especially cereals and legumes), with consequent exposure to aflotoxin (van Rensburg, 1977). The high prevalence of chronic hepatitis B virus infection is also believed to be strongly influential (Kew, 1982; Kew *et al.*, 1983). The frequency of this cancer is falling in both rural and urban populations.

The low frequency of *breast cancer* is undoubted, as is the rarity of colon–rectum cancers. Many rural hospitals that serve huge populations have never had a càse of the latter cancers. Breast cancer patients experience 50% mortality in 1.4 years (Walker *et al.*, 1984c), about a quarter of the time obtaining with white patients (Cancer Statistics Group, 1982), partly because three-quarters of patients present late, at stages III and IV.

As to incidence rates, no recent studies have been published. In unpublished studies an examination for 1981 and 1982 of the pattern of admissions of blacks with cancer to Baragwanath Hospital, Soweto, has revealed substantially the same picture as that indicated by Isaacson (1978) regarding the cancer situation at this hospital a decade ago. Among black men, cancer of the esophagus remains by far the commonest, 31% of the total. Among black women, invasive cancer of the cervix continues to be by far the most frequent, constituting 54% of total cancers; the situation depicted resembles that in some rural South American populations (Walker *et al.*, 1984a).

Among *rural* blacks, limited studies indicate little change from the situation described two decades ago (Robertson *et al.*, 1971; Rose and Fellingham, 1981). From enquiries at hospitals where satisfactory records are kept, it appears that the frequency of total cancer is low, that its occurrence is not significantly increasing, and that cancers of the esophagus and liver in men, and of cervix in women, head admissions to hospital for cancer (Walker *et al.*, 1984a).

Indians: Frequency of cancer among this population undoubtedly is low, as it is in the population of India (Jussawalla *et al.*, 1971). The validity of the low frequency is supported by unpublished studies on the number and type of cancer seen in patients admitted to hospitals and nursing homes in Durban, where there is the biggest concentration of Indians. The low frequency prevailing is remarkable, given the excessively high frequency in Indians of other disease burdens of Westernization, namely, diabetes and coronary heart disease (Walker, 1980).

Coloreds: This population has much higher rates for certain cancers than can be readily explained [as is the case with the population in Scotland (Anonymous, 1974)]. While the high frequencies of smoking (van der Burgh, 1979) and of alcohol consumption are powerfully contributory, these factors alone cannot account for the excessive occurrences described.

Whites: Their *pattern* of cancers is similar to that of most Western populations. Yet the somewhat low rates depicted, which are just over half the rates published for Scotland (Anonymous, 1974), are not explicable, given, e.g., the very high frequency of coronary heart disease (Walker, 1980), an index of high prosperity.

4. SUMMARY

Among South African populations, mortality rates from cancer are relatively high in colored (Eur-African-Malay) and white populations (although their rates are lower than those of many Western populations); rates are much lower in black and Indian populations. The main sites affected are, in blacks, esophagus, lung, and liver in men, and cervix in women; in Indians, stomach and lung in men, and breast and stomach in women; in coloreds, lung, stomach, and esophagus in men, and cervix and breast in women; in whites, lung, stomach, prostate, and colon–rectum in men, and breast and colon–rectum in women. With progressive rises in socioeconomic state and associated Westernization of diet and manner of life in the less privileged populations, their cancer patterns are likely to approach the pattern exhibited by whites. Thus, there will be falls in cancers at some sites (esophagus, liver), yet rises in others (lung, breast, colon–rectum). Rural blacks, especially in some areas, are at an exceptionally low risk to colon–rectum, stomach, prostate, and breast cancers; hence, such populations are worthy of intensive characterization.

ACKNOWLEDGMENTS. Investigations are supported by grants from the National Cancer Association of South Africa and the Anglo-American and De Beers Chairman's Fund.

REFERENCES

Anonymous, 1974, Annual global data on mortality (1970-1972), *World Health Stat. Rep.* **27**:196-197.

Bradshaw, E., and Harington, J. S., 1982, A comparison of the cancer mortality rates in South Africa with those in other countries, *S. Afr. Med. J.* **61**:943-946.

Bradshaw, E., and Schonland, M., 1974, Smoking, drinking and oesophageal cancer in African males in Johannesburg, South Africa, *Br. J. Cancer* **30**:157-163.

Bradshaw, E., McGlashan, N. D., Fitzgerald, D., and Harington, J. S., 1982, Analysis of cancer incidence in Black gold miners from Southern Africa (1964-79), *Br. J. Cancer* **46**:737-748.

Bradshaw, E., Harington, J. S., and McGlashan, N. D., 1983, Geographical distribution of lung and stomach cancers in South Africa (1968-1972), *S. Afr. Med. J.* **64**:655-663.

Cancer Statistics Group, 1982, *Trends in Cancer Survival in Great Britain*, Cancer Research Campaign, London, pp. 35-41.

Central Statistical Services, 1982, *Deaths of Blacks*, Report no. 07-05-02 (1979), Government Printer, Pretoria, South Africa.

Doll, R., and Peto, R., 1982, Morbidity versus mortality, *J. Nat. Cancer Inst.* **69**:549-550.

Henson, D. E., 1983, Meeting highlights: Conference and workshop on cancer in Latin America, *J. Nat. Cancer Inst.* **70**:979-984.

Higginson, J., and Oettlé, A. G., 1960, Cancer incidence in the Bantu and "Cape Coloured" races of South Africa: Report of a cancer survey in the Transvaal (1953-55), *J. Nat. Cancer Inst.* **24**:589-671.

Isaacson, C., Selzer, G., Kaye, V., Greenberg, M., Woodruff, D., Davies, J., Ninin, D., Vetten, D., and Andrew, M., 1978, Cancer in the urban blacks of South Africa, *S. Afr. Cancer Bull.* **22**:49-84.

Jussawalla, D. J., Deshpande, V. A., and Standfast, S. J., 1971, Assessment of risk patterns in cancer of the cervix: A comparison between Greater Bombay and Western countries, *Int. J. Cancer* **7**:259-268.

Kew, M. C., 1982, Tumours of the liver, in: *Hepatology* (D. Zakim and T. D. Boyer, eds.), W. B. Saunders, Philadelphia, pp. 1048-1083.

Kew, M. C., Rossouw, E., Paterson, A., Hodkinson, J., Dusheiko, G. M., and Whitcutt, M., 1983, Hepatitis-B virus status of Black women with hepatocellular carcinoma, *Gastroenterology* **84**:693-696.

Percy, C., Stanck, E., and Gloeckler, I., 1981, Accuracy of death certificates and its effect on cancer mortality statistics, *Am. J. Public Health* **71**:242-250.

Robertson, M. A., Harington, J. S., and Bradshaw, E., 1971, The cancer pattern in Africans of the Transvaal Lowveld, *Br. J. Cancer* **25**:377-384.

Rose, E. F., and Fellingham, S. A., 1981, Cancer patterns in the Transkei, *S. Afr. J. Sci.* **77**:555-561.

Schonland, M., and Bradshaw, E., 1968, Cancer in the Natal African and Indian (1964-66), *Int. J. Cancer* **3**:304-316.

Van der Burgh, C., 1979, Smoking behaviour of white, black, coloured and Indian South Africans: Some statistical data on a major public health hazard, *S. Afr. Med. J.* **55**:975-978.

Van Rensburg, S. J., 1977, Mycotoxoses in the tropics, in: *Medicine in a Tropical Environment* (J. S. Gear, ed.), South African Medical Research Council, Cape Town, South Africa.

Van Rensburg, S. J., 1981, Epidemiological and dietary evidence for a specific nutritional predisposition to esophageal cancer, *J. Nat. Cancer Inst.* **67:**243–251.

Walker, A. R. P., 1980, Epidemiology of ischaemic heart disease in the different populations in Johannesburg, *S. Afr. Med. J.* **57:**748–752.

Walker, A. R. P., Gilpin, J., Evans, J., and Walker, B. F., 1984a, Disease patterns of admissions of blacks to Murchison Hospital, Kwa-Zulu, *S. Afr. Med. J.* (in press).

Walker, A. R. P., Walker, B. F., Isaacson, C., Segal, I., and Pryor, S., 1984b, Low survival of blacks with oesophageal cancer in Johannesburg, South Africa, *S. Afr. Med. J.* **66:**877–878.

Walker, A. R. P., Walker, B. F., Tshabalala, E. N., Isaacson, C., and Segal, I., 1984c, Low survival of South African urban Black women with breast cancer, *Br. J. Cancer* **49:**241–245.

World Health Organization, 1982, Vital statistics and causes of death, in: *World Health Annual Statistics,* World Health Organization, Geneva, p. 46.

39

Epidemiology of Dietary Fiber and Colorectal Cancer: Current Status of the Hypothesis

SHEILA A. BINGHAM

1. INTRODUCTION

Much of the evidence supporting a role for fiber in large bowel cancer rests on epidemiologic observations. The causative agent in human large bowel cancer, or the mechanisms by which fiber may protect against it, have never been firmly established. Current views on the promoting effects of fat are discussed in Chapters 34, 35, 36, and 37 of this volume, and Cummings has postulated mechanisms by which dietary fiber may protect against large bowel cancer (Cummings and Branch, 1982). The purpose of this chapter is to concentrate on the question of whether or not a reduced intake of dietary fiber, or "deficiency" of it, is associated with a higher risk of large bowel cancer, both in populations and individuals.

2. DETERMINATION OF DIETARY FIBER INTAKE

In seeking associations between dietary fiber intake and large bowel cancer risk, it is readily apparent that the dietary fiber content of the majority of the world's foods is unknown. Elsewhere (Bingham and Cummings, 1980) we have reported that the intake of dietary fiber for the

SHEILA A. BINGHAM • University of Cambridge and MRC, Dunn Clinical Nutrition Centre, Cambridge CB2 1QL, United Kingdom.

majority of the world's population is unmapped. Some time ago we were fortunate in having David Southgate's analyses for the fiber content of some foods available to us and were able, using a variety of new and older studies in the literature, to make some limited observations on the amount of fiber eaten in Britain, Europe, America, and parts of rural Africa. There have been some more recent data available for New Zealand and Australia, based on the British Food Tables, which also show the fiber intakes of these other "Westernized" countries to be similar to those found in U. S. and Britain, about 20 g/day. These studies have shown that it is quite true to say that fiber intakes are higher in some parts of rural Africa than in Western populations (Burkitt, 1969). However, this is not the only difference between the diet of rural Africans and that eaten in the U. S. The rural African eats minimal fat and meat, which have also been associated epidemiologically with large bowel cancer (Gregor et al., 1969).

The most recent and interesting data we have is from Japan (Minowa et al., 1983). Rates for colon cancer and diverticular disease in Japan are still, despite recent postwar changes, some of the lowest in the world (Narasaka et al., 1975; Sato et al., 1976; Inoue, 1980) and these rates for cancer in migrants change to those of the host country within one or two generations (Haenszel and Kurihara, 1968). However, fiber cannot be the reason for these low rates. Intakes in Japan are 20 g/day, that is, no greater than in countries such as Britain, U. S., and New Zealand, with the highest colon cancer rates in the world.

The reason for this is that the fiber content of rice is low, whatever method of analysis is used (Table I) and as a consequence, despite the recent trends toward Westernization of the Japanese diet, there have been no major changes in the Japanese fiber intake over the past 50 years (Minowa et al., 1983). However, intakes of fat and animal protein are low, and, despite recent changes, the Japanese still only eat 70 g meat, compared with about 160 g in Britain, and half the fat. It is therefore necessary to look at the role

TABLE I. Total Dietary Fiber (g/100 g fresh weight)

Method	White rice	White bread	Cabbage
Hellendoorn et al. (1975)	1.4	2.4	2.1
Southgate et al. (1978)	2.4	2.7	3.4
Holloway et al. (1977)	—	2.4	2.1
NDF (Van Soest 1978)	—	1.5	1.1
Angus et al. (1981)	1.7	2.0	1.0
Englyst et al. (1983)	0.7	1.6	—

of dietary fiber in countries that can otherwise be supposed to be at high risk of colon cancer from a "Westernized" type of diet or lifestyle.

Even this, however, is no easy matter. As can be seen from Table I, different methods of chemical analysis give different results for the dietary fiber content of important staple foods such as white bread, potato, and rice. Critical to this confusion are differences of opinion of the definition of dietary fiber. Some order has been imposed by the suggestion that analytical methods should confine themselves to measuring chemically defined nonstarch polysaccharides (NSP) (Cummings, 1980). Food table values, based on well-researched methods, capable of measuring nonstarch polysaccharides, uncontaminated with starch, and the cellulose, pentose, hexose, and uronic acid fractions are prerequisite conditions for definitive epidemiologic studies. To date, however, values for dietary fiber are published in only one widely available set of food tables (Paul and Southgate, 1978) and the method on which these are based has itself been criticized (Selvendran et al., 1981). As discussed in Chapters 1 and 2 of this volume, results from even the two probable official methods of fiber analysis in Britain and the U. S. are systematically different. This error will introduce bias, which will make worldwide comparisons impossible. The second problem that will become evident in this chapter concerns the difficulties associated with the measurement of food consumption. Unless these two sources of potential systematic errors are eliminated, it will not be possible to establish, for example, a recommended intake for dietary fiber on the basis of reduced risk from colon cancer.

3. TIME TRENDS

A cornerstone of the hypothesis relating fiber intake to the etiology of colon cancer was the suggested decline in intakes following the introduction of roller milling of wheat in Britain, Europe, and the U. S. around 1880. This allowed cheap white flour to be produced and distributed, whereas previously it had been more expensive than brown. However, while it is clear that all types of bread were eaten throughout the 19th century, exactly how much was eaten by which social class is difficult to determine. In Britain, interest in the food supply of the general population and its nutritional value was only aroused at the beginning of the 20th century following the discovery of widespread and hitherto unrecognized malnutrition (Drummond and Wilbraham, 1958). Limited data on the supply of wheat and potatoes in farm laborers' diets, however, suggest that total fiber intakes may have been between 37 and 47 g/day in 1860. This compares with present-day intakes in Britain of 20 g/day (Bingham and Cummings, 1980).

In countries with stable and well-documented population bases, per capita national statistics of food produced and imported with corrections for exported food are probably valid indicators of trends. In Britain, these statistics are available for selected years from 1909, and continuously from 1940. They have been reinterpreted to examine trends in crude fiber consumption (Robertson, 1972) and, more recently, dietary fiber consumption (Southgate *et al.*, 1978). Similar data are available for crude fiber trends in consumption for the U. S. (Heller and Hackler, 1978) and for total dietary fiber (Bingham and Cummings, 1980), and for total dietary fiber consumption from 1950 to 1976 in the Netherlands (Van Staveren *et al.*, 1982). The general trend emerging from these statistics is the decline in cereal fiber consumption, which has been offset somewhat in Britain and the Netherlands in the 20th century by an increase in vegetable dietary fiber consumption.

The most striking feature in Britain over the 20th century was a probable doubling of total dietary fiber intake due to an increase in the extraction rate of flour and increases in consumption of bread to conserve population food supplies during World War II. McMichael *et al.* (1979) noted that time trends in colon cancer mortality rates could be associated in Britain and the U. S. with changes in crude fiber intakes, particularly in Britain, where there was a marked postwar fall in mortality. This analysis has recently been extended by Powles and Williams (1984), using more accurate analyses for nonstarch polysaccharide (NSP) consumption, based on the data of Englyst *et al.* (1983), to include four other countries. The estimated war-time increases in NSP from flour were 15 g in Ireland, 12 g in England and Wales, 10 g in Switzerland, and 4 g in New Zealand, with virtually no change in Australia and the U. S. In these two latter countries the ratio of observed to expected mortality 11–15 years after the increase, extrapolating from prewar trends, was about 0.8, but only 0.6 in Ireland, the population that experienced the greatest increase in NSP consumption. Over the six populations studied, the correlation coefficient between these two variables was −0.88 (Powles and Williams, 1984). The most obvious problem with this type of analysis, however, is that changes in dietary habits rarely occur in isolation; in Britain, for example, fat consumption fell from 39% of total energy in the 1930s to 33% of total energy in 1947 (Greaves and Hollingsworth, 1966).

4. CORRELATION STUDIES

4.1. Food Balance Sheets

FAO food balance sheets, which are equivalent to the national statistics of food available to populations mentioned above (Section 3), are available for the majority of countries in the world. Numerous comparisons between data from these statistics and disease occurrence have been published, and, over the past 10 years, seven have attempted to relate large bowel, usually colon, cancer mortality or incidence to indicators of dietary fiber consumption (Table II). Protective associations have usually been found. However, the relationship became nonsignificant when controlling for meat consumption in the study of Armstrong and Doll (1975). Since all these studies used the same data bases, this would have been the probable fate of the correlation coefficients for fiber indicators noted by other workers. The overriding factor emerging from these studies, therefore, is the positive association between colon cancer occurrence and meat consumption (Armstrong and Doll, 1975).

However, there are several difficulties with this type of analysis. Per capita indicators of food consumption rely on accurate population estimates, and the proportion of men, women, and children eating different amounts of food within any one population may vary markedly from one population to another. In addition, regional differences in food intake and disease incidence are obscured. Rates for large bowel cancer incidence differ between rural

TABLE II. Correlation Studies

Reference	Number of countries	Colon cancer occurrence[a]	Item	Correlation coefficient	Partial correlation Controlled for	Partial coefficient[b]
Drasar and Irving (1972)	37	I,m	Crude fiber	0	—	ND
Irving and Drasar (1973)	37	I,m	Cereals	−0.30	—	ND
Howell (1975)	33	I,m	Vegetable calories	−0.18	—	ND
Armstrong and Doll (1975)	23	I,m	Cereals	−0.52	Meat	NS
Schrauzer (1976)	17	M,m	Cereals	−0.69	Meat	NS[c]
Liu et al. (1979)	20	M,m,f	Vegetable calories	−0.71	Cholesterol	NS
McKeown-Eyssen and Bright-See (1983)	48	M,m	Dietary fiber	−0.66	Fat Meat	"Significant" ND

[a]M, mortality; I, incidence; m, male; f, female.
[b]ND, not determined; NS, not significant.
[c]Meat vs. cereals, $r = -0.70$; meat vs. colon cancer mortality, males, $r = 0.95$.

and urban Denmark and Finland, for example, and between Scotland and England/Wales. A third problem is that national statistics do not measure food actually consumed by the population; waste occurring within the system or in the home, for example, is not measured.

Table III shows the nutrients contained in the U. K. diet as measured by three different methods: first those calculated from the national statistics which in Britain are called *Foods Moving into Consumption;* next, the results from the *National Food Survey,* which is a household survey of about 6500 households every year (Ministry of Agriculture, Fisheries and Food, 1953–1983); and finally, the results from a randomly selected population group of adults aged 20–80 years who weighed everything they ate for 1 week (Bingham *et al.,* 1979a). As can be seen, the amount of food available per head calculated from the national statistics is some 25% greater than that actually consumed by representative individuals, mainly because there is an overestimation of the amount of fat consumed. There is no guarantee that error operates to the same extent and in the same direction in all countries of the world, particularly in developing countries.

4.2. Household Surveys

Food intakes assessed from household survey techniques on a national basis can provide information on regional dietary differences. Recent changes in the Japanese diet have been most marked in the urban areas, for example. In the ten largest cities in 1979, 57.5 g/day of fat was eaten and 52% of protein derived from animal foods. Carbohydrate and dietary fiber intakes were

TABLE III. The U. K. Diet

	National statistics (1980)	National household survey (1980)	Individual survey (1977)
Energy, MJ	12.7[a]	9.4	9.1[a]
Protein,g	81.7	72.7	72.3
Fat,g	128	106	97.1
Polyunsaturated:saturated fat ratio	—	0.20	—
Sucrose,g	121	—	72.9
Starch,g	—	—	148
Dietary fiber,g	23[b]	20[c]	20
Percent fat	37	43	40
Percent sucrose	15	—	13
Percent starch	—	—	26

[a] Including alcohol.
[b] 1970.
[c] 1976.

also lower, 296 and 17.7 g, in these areas. This compares with less fat, 50.6 g, less protein from animal sources, 48.2%, more carbohydrate, 332 g, and more dietary fiber, 20.2 g, in towns and villages. There is a clear trend between these extremes, depending on the size of the city (Minowa *et al.*, 1983). Mortality rates for colon cancer are greater in urban versus rural areas, but no formal studies have yet been published.

Two studies in the literature have compared food intakes, calculated from household surveys, with regional differences in standardized colon cancer mortality rates in France (Meyer, 1977) and with age-adjusted colorectal cancer mortality rates by income group in Hong Kong (Hill *et al.*, 1979). Both showed positive associations between the consumption of all fiber-containing foods, although the correlation coefficient was not significant in the French study. Consumption of fruit was negatively associated with mortality ($r = -0.84$), but all items of diet were interrelated and partial correlation was not conducted. In neither of these household studies was total dietary fiber consumption measured.

Analyses for the dietary fiber content of British foods are available, however (Southgate *et al.*, 1976, 1978). In addition, regional intakes of foodstuffs have been documented every year since 1940 by the British National Food Survey, under the auspices of the Ministry of Agriculture, Fisheries and Food (1953–1983). The housewife is asked to keep a record of her purchases for 1 week and from this the average quantity of food eaten per person per day in the household is calculated. Between 300 and 2400 households in nine standard regions of the U. K. take part every year. Intakes of dietary fiber and its components have been calculated from these data and compared with 5-year age and sex-standardized truncated colon and rectal cancer mortality rates in the same standard regions. Rectal and colon cancer were considered separately, recognizing the difficulties incurred in classifying tumors at the rectosigmoid junction. However, in a small study of normal subjects without diarrhea the rectum was usually empty (McNeil and Rampton, 1981), which suggests that colon and rectal cancer may have different etiologies. Due to boundary reorganizations, it was not possible to compare mortality data with dietary data collected some time previously and the two variables were therefore compared over the same period of time, 1969–1973. Regional variations in alcohol and tobacco consumption, together with regional variations in social class, were also considered.

In summary, intakes of fat and animal protein were high in all regions. Total dietary fiber intake was not significantly associated with either colon or rectal cancer mortality and there were no significant associations with nutrients, apart from vitamin C ($r = -0.842$). However, a protective association ($r = -0.960$) was found between the consumption of one of the components of dietary fiber, the pentosan fraction, and mortality from colon cancer. Total vegetable consumption, excluding potatoes, and fresh green vegetable consumption were also inversely correlated ($r = -0.940$ and $r = -0.861$). Partial correlation, controlling for pentosan intake, reduced all other significant associations, for vegetables, fresh green vegetables, vitamin C, substances analyzing as lignin, and tobacco expenditure, to insignificance.

Although the pentosan fraction of dietary fiber has been shown to be the most effective component of dietary fiber in increasing fecal weight (Cummings *et al.*, 1978), thereby diluting putative carcinogens in contact with the colonic mucosa, associations do not prove causation and a number of potential confounding variables could not be assessed. The regional pattern of colon cancer death rates is similar to that of many diseases in Britain, with higher rates in the north and west than in the south and east. To discount the possibility that regional associations were reflecting a coincidence of geography in both diet and disease, 5-year death rates for bronchitis, a disease not associated with diet, were also compared with the dietary variables. No significant association with the intake of dietary fiber or its components was found.

However, as with all studies of this type, actual food consumption by individuals is not measured, and there are too few cancer registries in Britain to have allowed a regional comparison with colon cancer incidence. Regional survival rates from colon cancer, for example, are known to differ (Silman and Evans, 1981). More important, improved methods of analysis of non-starch polysaccharides and component sugars have since become available (Englyst *et al.*, 1983) and the regional variations in NSP intake require confirmation by these improved methods.

4.3. Studies of Representative Groups of Individuals

Established cancer registries in Scandinavia show a three- to fourfold range in colon cancer incidence within an area with a fairly homogeneous population. Age-standardized truncated colon cancer incidence rates per 100,000 men are lowest in rural Finland (6.7) and highest in Copenhagen (22.8). Rates in rural Denmark and Helsinki are intermediate (12.9 and 17.0). In collaboration with the International Agency for Research on Cancer, a study was undertaken to characterize the diets eaten by representative population samples in each area, with particular reference to the consumption of NSP using the method of Englyst (Jensen *et al.*, 1982; Bingham *et al.*, 1982; Englyst *et al.*, 1982). Thirty men aged 50–59 were randomly selected from population registers in each of the four areas: Parikkala in the Kymi region of southeast Finland; Them, in Jutland; Helsinki; and Copenhagen. Response rates among those approached were: Parikkala, 83.3%; Helsinki, 74.4%; Copenhagen, 75%; and Them, 62.5%.

Each of the 120 men was asked to keep a weighed food record for 4 days, in order to assess nutrient intake from local food tables. Because analyses for dietary fiber are generally not available in food tables, the amounts of NSP eaten in each of the four areas had to be established from direct chemical analysis of duplicate diets in Cambridge. However, it is notoriously difficult to collect complete duplicates of food eaten from free-living individuals, and a number of methodological checks were built into the protocol. On the final day of the survey, the men were asked to make a complete weighed duplicate of all food eaten, a 24-h urine collection, and a 24-h fecal collection. The weights of the food collected were compared with that recorded to have been eaten, and the chemically analyzed content of fat, carbohydrate, and nitrogen (N) in the duplicate collections compared with calculated intakes for the same day, using food tables and the food records. In summary, as judged by the evidence available from weighing and analysis, the food samples were virtually complete duplicates. The overall correlation coefficient between protein intake calculated from food tables and that in the duplicates, for example, was 0.86, slope 0.99, intercept 2.3 g protein. The standard deviations of individual percentage differences between analyzed and calculated intakes of protein ranged from 8 to 16% in the four areas, and those for fat from 7 to 21%.

Fourteen of the 119 24-h urine samples collected during the survey were excluded from the analysis because they were reported to be incomplete or contained less than 10 mmol (1.1 g) creatinine per 24 h. Nitrogen was not determined for an additional two samples. The average N excretion from the remaining 103 samples and fecal N excretion from pooled collections was 14.5 g, and the average N intake from all 119 diets was 14.3 g. Between areas the average values for 24-h urine N excretion corresponded with the average N intake, with the highest values in Parikkala and lowest in Copenhagen. Overall, therefore, average dietary intake was equal to or related to average fecal and urine N excretion, with no evidence of systematic bias incurred as a consequence of attempting to obtain duplicate day's diets. In addition there was no evidence of a change in dietary habits during the survey, since a comparison of constituents of 24-h urines collected on the day of the survey with those collected 3–6 weeks after the study showed no significant differences (Bingham et al., 1982).

As in the British study, average intakes of fat and animal protein were high, fat ranging from 102 to 146 g/day, and meat consumption from 148 to 214 g/day. There were no significant associations with fat, cholesterol, or meat consumption and large bowel cancer incidence. The simple correlation coefficient between nonstarch polysaccharide consumption and large bowel cancer incidence was −0.776, although more sophisticated statistical techniques demonstrated a significant relationship (Jensen et al., 1982). The simple correlation coefficient between pentosan consumption and large bowel cancer was −0.904 (not significant) and that between pentose consumption and colon cancer was −0.992, $p < 0.01$ (Fig. 1).

Two other studies were carried out in Finland, Sweden, and New York (Reddy *et al.*, 1978; Domellof, 1982). In the first, fiber intake was not measured, but fecal fiber excretion of volunteers living in rural Finland was higher than that of volunteers living in New York. In the second, the food intake of 21 male and female volunteers living in Umea, Sweden, was assessed by diet history and calculated from food tables. Again, a protective association was shown, fiber intakes being greater in the lower cancer area of Sweden compared with the intakes of 22 men and 18 women volunteers in New York.

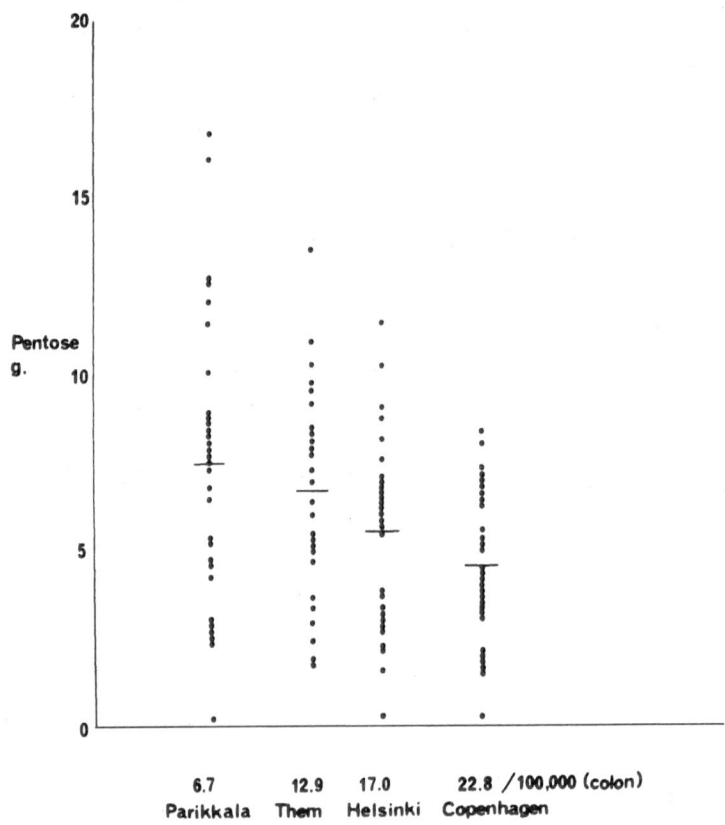

FIGURE 1. Individual and average intakes of fiber pentose from chemical analysis of a complete, duplicate day's diets in four Scandanavian populations in relation to regional truncated age-standardized colon cancer incidence.

A further study in Edinburgh, Scotland also assessed dietary fiber intake, as part of a cross-country collaborative study of heart disease in Stockholm and Edinburgh (Thompson *et al.*, 1982). In a randomly selected population sample of 97 males, who weighed and recorded their food intake for 7 days, fat intakes were again high, 120 g/day, and fiber intakes assessed from the British food tables (Paul and Southgate, 1978) were substantially lower than the national average for Britain, 17 g/day. Dietary fiber intakes of two other randomly selected population samples of men, in Westray in the Orkney Islands of Scotland and in Cambridge, were 16.5 and 20 g/day (Bull *et al.*, 1982; Bingham *et al.*, 1979a).

Unfortunately, all of these data cannot be directly compared, due to methodological differences. The British, Danish, and Finnish data were obtained from randomly selected population groups of men who kept records of food consumption, whereas those for New York and Sweden were obtained by interview of volunteer men and women to obtain a diet history. Dietary intakes of volunteers may be different from those of randomly selected population groups and comparative studies in the literature show that different methods of assessing dietary intake are associated with systematic differences when compared with each other (Bingham, 1984). There are also sex differences in fiber intake (Bingham and Cummings, 1980).

If only the seven representative populations are considered, there are also differences in the methods of analysis on which the "fiber" values are based. With this proviso in mind, however, the protective association between fiber intake and colon cancer incidence noted in the Scandinavian studies described above remains ($r = -0.90$; Fig. 2). Intakes of fat and protein were high in all seven areas studied and not associated with colon cancer incidence ($r = +0.38$ fat, $+0.39$ protein).

5. CASE-CONTROL STUDIES

The epidemiologist looks for evidence of exposure from risk factors in relation to disease at the individual level, since in the group approach the data on exposure and outcome may relate to different groups in the population (National Research Council, 1982). This calls for accurate assessment of the habitual diet of free-living individuals, which is no easy undertaking.

Twelve case–control studies that specifically looked at intakes of fiber or fiber-containing foods in large bowel cancer have been reported (Table IV). Four controlled studies might be considered to lend definite support for a protective role for fiber in large bowel cancer, since in these the cases were reported to eat vegetables or fiber-containing foods less frequently (Bjelke, 1970; Modan *et al.*, 1975; Graham *et al.*, 1978; Manousos *et al.*, 1983).

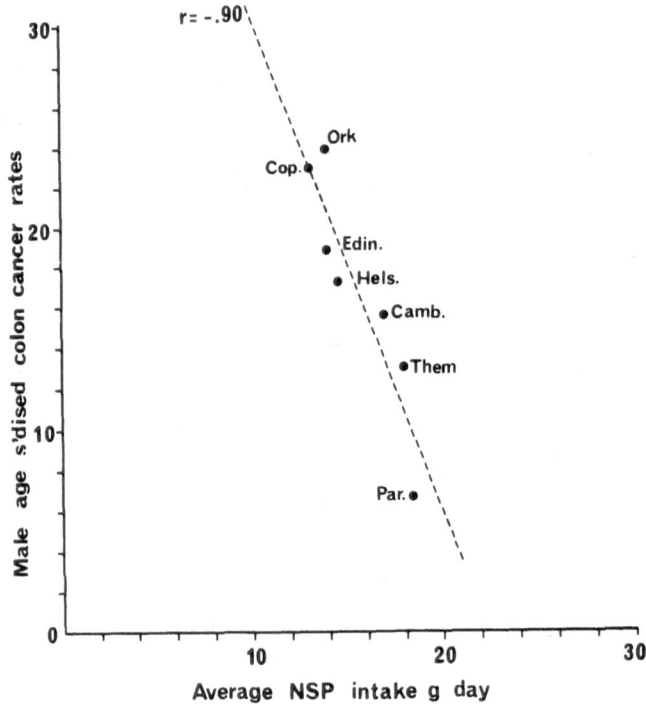

FIGURE 2. Nonstarch polysaccharide intake (as polysaccharides and excluding "lignin") in seven randomly selected male population samples in relation to colon cancer incidence. [Waterhouse *et al.* (1982).]

However, colorectal cancer patients are likely to alter their food intake at the onset of symptoms such as altered bowel habit and abdominal pain (Cummings, 1981). Authors have attempted to control for this by asking all subjects to give information only concerning food intake by up to 3 years previously, but this in fact is probably not possible.

Jain *et al.* (1980b), for example, obtained diet histories from 26 pairs of patients with large bowel cancer and their healthy controls, covering the time immediately before the interview (time 1) and 6 months earlier (time 2). This was repeated 6 months later, so that time 2 of the second diet history coincided with time 1 of the first. For cases this meant the period immediately before surgery. Since the same time period was being asked about, the results should have been identical. For controls, the correlation coefficients were, for example, 0.79 for protein and 0.67 for fat, and there were no significant differences in the mean results. However, the agreement was much worse for the patients' two diet histories (for example, 0.28 for protein and 0.48 for fat). The authors interpret this to mean that the cases had altered their diet since surgery and that the reported retrospective diet history of 6 months ago was actually a current diet history of recent food habits.

Jensen *et al.* (1984) reinvestigated individuals who had taken part in a dietary survey 15–25 years before, by asking the subjects to recall their dietary habits at that time, using a diet history. In addition, present-day dietary habits were assessed, also by diet history. For food intake there was greater agreement between the two diet histories (correlation coefficients ranging from 0.32 to 0.69) than between the two estimates of past diets (correlation coefficients 0.15–0.41). The authors concluded that "recall of past diets is strongly influenced by present dietary habits." Garland and Ibrahim [quoted in National Research Council (1982)] also found that there was greater similarity between usual (present) diet histories and usual diet of 20 years ago and reassessed recently than there was between past diet assessed recently and actual diet histories taken at the time. When subjects were asked in 1964 about their use of certain food items before World War II and the questions were repeated after an interval of 3–6 months, the answers were "too variable to be of any scientific value" (Acheson and Doll, 1964). On the basis of these findings, studies in which colorectal cancer cases have apparently eaten less vegetables or fiber-containing foods must be treated with caution.

Two well-controlled studies in Toronto and Adelaide (Miller *et al.*, 1983; Potter *et al.*, 1982) have recently been reported in which a quantitative estimate of fiber consumption was made using the British food tables. In both, the cases consumed more fat, but a protective effect of fiber was not seen, apart from slight weakening of the risk for males only consuming high-fat diets in Adelaide. In Toronto, however, when cases and controls were subdivided into extremes of fiber consumption, there was no lessening of risk either when controlled or uncontrolled for fat consumption. This is despite the fact that individuals in the high extreme were eating more than 28 g of fiber per day, an amount greater than the average consumed by men in rural Finland, where the colon cancer risk is one of the lowest. However, numerical comparisons are difficult, because of the problems with systematic bias in methods of assessing food consumption and the analysis of dietary fiber. The particular method used in Toronto, for example, may overestimate crude fiber consumption by 56%, at least when compared with records of actual food eaten (Jain *et al.*, 1980b). Table I shows that the British food tables (Southgate analysis) may overestimate the NSP for common foods such as white bread by 50%.

In addition, methods for assessing the dietary intake of individuals are prone to random errors leading to misclassification when an attempt is made of divide the distribution into, for example, thirds for characterization of

TABLE IV. Case–control Studies[a]

Reference	Area or subjects	Number[a]	Dietary[a] method	Cancer[a]	Item	p
Higginson (1966)	Kansas	340 ca 1020 co	Q (R 2 years)	CR	Fruit, vegetables	NS
Haenszel et al .(1973)	Hawaiian Japanese	179 ca 357 co	Q	CR	Starches, legumes	(Increased risk)
Bjelke (1970)	Norway	278 ca 1394 co	Q (R 1 year)	CR	Vegetables	<0.05
Modan et al. (1975)	Israel	198 ca 396 co	Q (R 1 year)	C	Fiber-containing foods	<0.001
Phillips (1975)	California Seventh-Day Adventists	41 ca 123 co	Q	C	Green vegetables	NS

Dales (1978)	San Francisco	99 ca 280 co	Q (R 3 year)	CR	Fiber-containing foods	NS
Graham et al. (1978)	Buffalo	453 ca 1136 co	Q (R)	C	Vegetables	<0.002
Hunter et al. (1980)	Miami	25 ca 25 co	DH (R)	C	Fiber-containing foods	NS
Calder et al. (1980)	Kenya	12 ca 91 co	DH	C	Food items	NS
Potter (1982)	Adelaide	400 ca 800 co	Q	CR	Dietary fiber	NS
Jain (1980), Miller et al. (1983)	Toronto	542 ca 1619 co	DH (R 6 months)	CR	Dietary fiber	NS
Manousos et al. (1983)	Greece	100 ca 100 co	Q (R)	CR	Vegetables	<0.05

[a] ca, cases; co, controls; Q, questionnaire; R, retrospective; DH, diet history; C, colon; CR, colorectal; NS, not significant.

extremes of risk. The questionnaire used by Potter *et al.* (1982), for example, was tested for its ability to produce the same result when used to assess the intake of a group of controls initially and 6 months later. The *r* value between fiber intake assessed initially and 6 months later was only 0.57, so that less than half of individuals would have been classified into the same third of intake at each occasion. In the Toronto study, the correlation coefficient between crude fiber intake assessed by diet history and by records of food consumption was 0.24.

6. PROSPECTIVE STUDIES

The findings of a large prospective study in Japan contrast markedly with those of case–control studies. In 1965, 265,118 adults aged 40 years and above were interviewed throughout Japan. By 1978 there were 368 male and 357 female deaths from colorectal cancer. SMRs for colorectal cancer were 33 for subjects who had eaten less than 180 cm³ of rice and wheat per day, and only 20 in those who had eaten more than 720 cm³/day. No effect of vegetables was seen, and subjects who died from colorectal cancer had eaten less meat than others. Dietary fiber intakes have not yet been assessed (Hirayama, 1981). Kromhout *et al.* (1982) also report that dietary fiber intake was significantly lower in 44 cases of cancer within a population of 871 men followed for 10 years. However, the data were not controlled for smoking habit, and the majority of deaths were from lung cancer (17), with only five deaths from colon cancer recorded.

7. CONCLUSIONS

Support for a protective role for dietary fiber in the etiology of large bowel cancer, particularly colon cancer, is apparent in some types of epidemiologic study. However, results are highly method-dependent. Worldwide comparisons using gross national statistics of food consumption are of questionable value, due partly to the interrelationship of staple starch-containing foods with meat consumption in particular. Studies of a limited number of population samples using accurate methods in Britain and Scandinavia suggest that dietary fiber may be protective in populations that would otherwise be at risk from an excess of meat and fat, but to date the majority of case–control studies at the individual level have failed to confirm this. Possible reasons for this conflict are further discussed in Chapter 33 of this volume.

REFERENCES

Acheson, E. D., and Doll, R., 1964, Dietary factors in carcinoma of the stomach: A study of 100 cases and 200 controls, *Gut* **5:**126.

Angus, R., Sutherland, T. M., and Farrell, D. J., 1981, Insoluble dietary fibre content of some local foods, *Proc. Nutr. Soc. Aust.* **6:**161.

Armstrong, B., and Doll, R., 1975, Environmental factors and cancer incidence in different countries, with special reference to dietary practices, *Int. J. Cancer* **15:**617.

Bingham, S., 1984, Surveillance of the dietary habits of the population with regard to cardiovascular disease: Premise and methods, in: *Euronut 2* (G. G. de Backer, H. Tunstall-Pedoe, and P. Ducimetiere, eds.), Wageningen, The Netherlands, pp. 21–42.

Bingham, S., and Cummings, J. H., 1980, Intakes and sources of dietary fibre in man, in: *Medical Aspects of Dietary Fiber* (G. A. Spiller and R. M., Amen, eds.), Plenum, New York, p. 261.

Bingham, S., Cummings, J. H., and McNeil, N. I., 1979a, Intakes and sources of dietary fiber in the British population, *Am. J. Clin. Nutr.* **32:**1313.

Bingham, S. A., Williams, D. R. R., Cole, T. J., and James, W. P. T., 1979b, Dietary fibre consumption and regional large bowel cancer mortality in Britain, *Br. J. Cancer* **40:**456.

Bingham, S., Wiggins, H. S., Englyst, H., Seppanen, R., Helms, P., Strand, R., Burton, R., Jorgensen, I. M., Poulsen, L., Paerregaard, A., Bjerrum, L., and James, W. P. T., 1982, Methods and validity of the dietary assessments in four Scandinavian populations, *Nutr. Cancer* **4:**23.

Bjelke, E., 1970, Case control study of cancer of the stomach, colon and rectum, in: *Oncology 1970: Being the Proceedings of the Tenth International Cancer Congress, Volume V* (R. L. Clark, R. W. Cumley, J. E. McCay, and M. M. Copeland, eds.), Yearbook Medical, Chicago, p. 320.

Bull, N. L., Smart, G. A., and Judson, H., 1982, Food and nutrient intakes on Westray in the Orkney Islands, *Ecol. Food Nutr.* **12:**97.

Burkitt, D. P., 1969, Related disease—Related cause, *Lancet* **2:**1229.

Calder, J. F., Wachira, M. W., Van Sant, T., Malik, M. J., and Bowry, R. N., 1980, Diverticular disease, carcinoma of the colon and diet in urban and rural Kenyan Africans, *Diagn. Imag.* **49:**23.

Cummings, J. H., 1980, Some aspects of dietary fibre metabolism in the human gut, in: *Food and Health Science and Technology* (G. G. Birch and K. J. Parker, eds.), Applied Science, London, p. 441.

Cummings, J. H., 1981, Dietary fibre and large bowel cancer, *Proc. Nutr. Soc.* **40:**7.

Cummings, J. H., and Branch, W. J., 1982, Postulated mechanisms whereby fiber may protect against large bowel cancer, in: *Dietary Fibre in Health and Disease* (G. Vahouny and D. Kritchevsky, eds.), Plenum, New York, p. 313.

Cummings, J. H., Southgate, D. A. T., Branch, W., Houston, H., Jenkins, D. J. A., and James, W. P. T., 1978, Colonic response to dietary fibre from carrot, cabbage, apple, bran and guar gum, *Lancet* **1:**5.

Dales, L. G., Friedman, G. D., Ury, H. K., Grossman, S., and Williams, S., 1978, A case control study of relationships of diet and other traits to colorectal cancer in American blacks, *Am. J. Epid.* **109:**132–144.

Domellof, L., Darby, L., Hanson, D., Mathews, L., Simi, B., and Reddy, B. S., 1982, Fecal sterols and bacterial β-glucuronidase activity: A preliminary metabolic study of healthy volunteers from Umea, Sweden and Metropolitan New York, *Nutr. Cancer* **4:**120.

Drasar, B. S., and Irving, D., 1972, Environmental factors and cancer of the colon and breast, *Br. J. Cancer* **27:**167.

Drummond, J.C., Wilbraham, A., 1958, The Englishman's Food, Jonathan Cape, London.

Englyst, H. N., Anderson, V., and Cummings, J. H., 1983, Starch and non-starch polysaccharides in some cereal foods, *J. Sci. Food Agric.* **34:**1434.

Englyst, H. N., Bingham, S. A., Wiggins, H. S., Southgate, D. A. T., Seppanen, R., Helms, P., Anderson, V., Day, K. C., Choolun, R., Collinson, E., and Cummings, J. H., 1982, Nonstarch polysaccharide consumption in four Scandinavian populations, *Nutr. Cancer* **4:**50.

Graham, S., Dayal, H., Swanson, M., Mittelman, A., and Wilkinson, G., 1978, Diet in the epidemiology of cancer of the colon and rectum, *J. Nat. Cancer Inst.* **61:**709.

Greaves, J. P., and Hollingsworth, D. F., 1966, Trends in food consumption in the United Kingdom, *World Rev. Nutr. Diet* **6:**34.

Gregor, O., Toman, R., and Prusova, F., 1969, Gastrointestinal cancer and nutrition, *Gut* **10:**1031.

Haenszel, W., Berg, J. W., Segi, M., Kurihara, M., and Locke, F. B., 1973, Bowel cancer in Hawaiian Japanese, *J. Nat. Cancer Inst.* **51:**1765.

Haenszel, W., and Kurihara, M., 1968, Studies of Japanese migrants: Mortality from cancer and other diseases among Japanese in the United States, *J. Nat. Cancer Inst.* **40:**43.

Hellendoorn, E. W., Noordhoff, M. G., and Slagman, J., 1975, Enzymatic determination of the indigestible residue content of human food, *J. Sci. Food Agric.* **26:**1461.

Heller, S. N., and Hackler, L. R., 1978, Changes in the crude fiber content of the American diet, *Am. J. Clin. Nutr.* **31:**1510.

Higginson, J., 1966, Etiological factors in gastrointestinal cancer in man, *J. Nat. Cancer Inst.* **37:**527.

Hill, M., MacLennan, R., and Newcombe, R., 1979, Diet and large bowel cancer in three socioeconomic groups in Hong Kong, *Lancet* **1:**436.

Hirayama, T., 1981, A large scale cohort study on the relationship between diet and selected cancers of digestive organs, in: *Banbury Report 7, Gastrointestinal Cancer: Endogenous Factors* (W. R. Bruce, P. Correa, M. Lipkin, S. R. Tannenbaum, and T. D. Wilkins, eds.), Cold Spring Harbor Laboratory, Cold Spring Harbor, New York, p. 409.

Holloway, W. D., Tasman-Jones, C., and Maher, D., 1977, Towards an accurate measurement of dietary fibre, *N. Z. Med. J.* **85:**420.

Howell, M. A., 1975, Diet as an etiological factor in development of cancer of the colon and rectum, *J. Chronic Dis.* **28:**67.

Hunter, K., Linn, M. W., and Harris, R., 1980, Dietary pattern and cancer of the digestive tract in older patients, *J. Am. Geriatr. Soc.* **28:**405.

Inoue, M., 1980, Diverticular disease of the colon in Japan, *Stomach Intestine* **15:**807.

Irving, D., and Drasar, B. S., 1973, Fibre and cancer of the colon, *Br. J. Cancer* **28:**462.

Jain, M., Cook, G. M., Davis, F. G., Grace, M. G., Howe, G. R., and Miller, A. B., 1980a, A case control study of diet and colo-rectal cancer, *Int. J. Cancer* **26:**757.

Jain, M., Howe, G. R., Johnson, K. C., and Miller, A. B., 1980b, Evaluation of a diet history questionnaire for epidemiologic studies, *Am. J. Epidemiol.* **111:**212.

Jensen, O. M., MacLennan, R., and Wahrendorf, J., 1982, Diet, bowel function fecal characteristics and large bowel cancer in Denmark and Finland, *Nutr. Cancer* **4:**5.

Jensen, O. M., Wahrendorf, J., Rosenquist, A., and Geser, A., 1984, The reliability of questionnaire-derived historic dietary information and temporal stability of food habits in individuals, *Am. J. Epidemiol.,* **120:**281.

Kromhout, D., Bosschieter, E. B., and Coulander, C. de L., 1982, Dietary fibre and 10 y mortality for CHD, cancer and all causes, *Lancet,* **2:**518.

Liu, K., Stamler, J., Moss, D., Garside, D., Persky, U., and Soltero, I., 1979, Dietary cholesterol, fat and fibre and colon-cancer mortality, *Lancet* **2:**782.

Malhotra, S. L., 1977, Dietary factors in a study of cancer colon, *Med. Hypoth.* **3:**122.

Manousos, O., Day, N. E., Trichopoulos, D., Gerovassilis, F., Tzonou, A., and Polychrono-poulou, A., 1983, Diet and colorectal cancer: A case control study, *Int. J. Cancer* **32**:1.

McKeown-Eyssen, G., and Bright-See, E., 1983, Colon cancer mortality and fibre consumption: An international study, in: *Fibre in Human and Animal Nutrition,* Royal Society of New Zealand, Bulletin 20, Abstract, p. 35.

McMichael, A. J., Potter, J. D., and Hetzel, B. S., 1979, Time trends in colorectal cancer mortality in relation to food and alcohol consumption, *Int. J. Epidemiol.* **8**:295.

McNeil, N. I., and Rampton, D. S., 1981, Is the rectum usually empty? A quantitative study in subjects with and without diarrhea, *Dis. Colon Rectum* **24**:596.

Meyer, F., 1977, Relations alimentatation-cancer en France, *Gastroenterol. Clin. Biol.* **1**:971.

Miller, A. B., Howe, G. R., Jain, M., Craib, K. J. P., and Harrison, L., 1983, Food items and food groups as risk factors in a case control study of diet and colorectal cancer, *Int. J. Cancer* **32**:155.

Ministry of Agriculture, Fisheries and Food (1953–1983), Household Food Consumption and Expenditure 1950–1981, Annual Reports of the National Food Survey Committee, Her Majesty's Stationery Office, London.

Minowa, M., Bingham, S., and Cummings, J. H., 1983, Dietary fibre intake in Japan, *Hum. Nutr.* **37A**:113.

Modan, B., Barell, V., Lubin, F., Modan, M., Greenberg, R., and Graham, S., 1975, Low-fiber intake as an etiologic factor in cancer of the colon, *J. Nat. Cancer Inst.* **55**:15.

Narasaka, T., Watanabe, H., Yamagata, S., Munakata, A., Tajima, T., and Matsunaga, F., 1975, Statistical analysis of diverticulosis of the colon, *Tohoku J. Exp. Med.* **115**:271.

National Research Council, 1982, *Diet, Nutrition and Cancer,* National Research Council, National Academy of Sciences, Washington, D. C.

Paul, A. A., and Southgate, D. A. T., 1978, *McCance and Widdowson's The Composition of Foods,* 4th ed., Her Majesty's Stationery Office, London.

Phillips, R. L., 1975, Role of life style and dietary habits in risk of cancer among Seventh Day Adventists, *Cancer Res.* **35**:3513.

Potter, J. D., McMichael, A. J., and Bonett, A. Z., 1982, Diet, alcohol and large bowel cancer: A case control study. *Proc. Nutr. Soc. Aust.* **7**:123.

Powles, J., and Williams, D. R. R., 1984, Trends in bowel cancer in selected countries in relation to war-time changes in flour-milling, *Nutr. Cancer* **6**:40.

Reddy, B. S., Hedges, A. R., Laakso, K., and Wynder, E., 1978, Metabolic epidemiology of large bowel cancer, *Cancer* **42**:2832.

Robertson, J., 1972, Changes in the fibre content of the British diet, *Nature* **238**:290.

Sato, E., Ouchi, A., Sasano, N., and Ishidate, T., 1976, Polyps and diverticulosis of the large bowel in autopsy, *Cancer* **37**:1316.

Schrauzer, G. H., 1976, Cancer mortality correlation studies, *Med. Hypoth.* **2**:39.

Selvendran, R. R., Ring, S. G., and Du Pont, M. S., 1981, Determination of the dietary fiber content of EEC samples and a discussion of the various methods of analysis, in: *The Analysis of Dietary Fiber in Foods* (W. P. T. James and O. Theander, eds.), Marcel Dekker, New York, p. 95.

Silman, A. J., and Evans, S. J. W., 1981, Regional differences in survival from cancer, *Comm. Med.* **3**:291.

Southgate, D. A. T., Bailey, B., Collinson, E., and Walker, A. F., 1976, A guide to calculating intakes of dietary fibre, *J. Hum. Nutr.* **30**:303.

Southgate, D. A. T., 1978, Dietary fibre: analysis and food sources. *Am. J. Clin. Nutr. (Supp.)* **31**:S107.

Southgate, D. A. T., Bingham, S., and Robertson, J., 1978, Dietary fibre in British diet, *Nature* **274**:51.

Thompson, M., Logan, R. L., Sharman, M., Lockerbie, L., Riemersma, R. A., and Oliver, M.

F., 1982, Dietary survey in 40 year old Edinburgh men, *Hum. Nutr. Appl. Nutr.* **36A**:272.

Van Soest, P. J., 1978, Fibre analysis tables, *Am. J. Clin. Nutr. (Suppl.)* **31**:S284.

Van Staveren, W. A., Hautvast, J. G. A. J., Katan, M. B., van Montfort, M. A., and Van Oosten-van der Goes, H. G. C., 1982, Dietary fiber consumption in an adult Dutch population, *J. Am. Dietet. Assoc.* **80**:324.

Waterhouse, J., Muir, C., Shanmugaratnam, K., and Powell, J., 1982, *Cancer Incidence in 5 Continents,* Volume IV, IARC Scientific Publications 42, International Agency for Research on Cancer, Lyon.

40

Colon Cancer: Future Directions

BANDARU S. REDDY

1. INTRODUCTION

During the past two decades, epidemiologic studies have investigated the role of dietary factors on the incidence and mortality of colon cancer and suggested not only that the diets particularly high in total fat and low in certain dietary fibers, cruciferous vegetables, and selenium are generally associated with an increased risk of colon cancer in man, but high dietary fiber may be a protective factor in populations consuming diets high in total fat (Wynder, 1975; Burkitt, 1971, 1975; Reddy et al., 1980; Reddy, 1983a,b). Although the major strength of epidemiologic studies is their focus on human populations, the conduct and interpretation of these studies is complicated by inherent problems in testing the dietary practices for their reliability, validity, and sensitivity to reveal narrow but biologically significant differences, and to achieve some degree of dose stratification (Schottenfled, 1983). However, when another line of evidence, based on experimental studies, support human epidemiologic studies and suggest that dietary fat and certain micronutrients play an important role in the etiology of colon cancer, the relationship between diet and colon cancer deserves attention (Palmer, 1983). The biological plausibility of the role of dietary factors in the etiology of colon cancer is reflected in a number of hypotheses for a mechanism of action (Hill, 1982; Reddy, 1983a,b). The concept that dietary fat and certain fibers and micronutrients distinct from chemical contaminants of diet and other environmental and genetic factors are important determinants

BANDARU S. REDDY • Naylor Dana Institute for Disease Prevention, American Health Foundation, Valhalla, New York 10595.

of colon cancer risk is reinforced by metabolic epidemiologic and laboratory animal studies that have been used to test various hypotheses for a mechanism of action (Wynder and Reddy, 1983).

The purpose of this chapter is to evaluate scientific evidence for a dietary etiology of colon cancer and to propose additional studies in this area.

2. HUMAN STUDIES

The strength of the evidence that diet and nutrition play a role in colon cancer came from epidemiologic and metabolic epidemiologic studies, which have been reviewed extensively (Burkitt, 1975; Correa and Haenszel, 1978; Doll and Peto, 1981; Graham et al., 1978; Reddy, 1982; Wynder, 1975). Briefly, these studies suggest that diets high in total fat and low in fiber are associated with an increased risk of colon cancer in man. In several populations consuming diets high in total fat and saturated fat, certain dietary fibers and cruciferous vegetables are associated with a reduced risk for colon cancer.

Case-control studies in Canada and in Utah Mormons indicated an elevated risk for those with an increased intake of total fat and saturated fat (Miller et al., 1983; West et al., 1983). It was also found in Athens, Greece that colon cancer patients reported significantly more frequent consumption of meat (notably beef and lamb) and less consumption of vegetables, such as beets, spinach, lettuce, and cabbage, compared to controls (Manousos et al., 1983). There was no significant difference in the consumption of olive oil between cases and controls. A recent Hawaiian study indicated no association within countries of regional or ethnic colon cancer rates in relation to meat (Kolonel et al., 1981). These conflicting results could be explained on the basis that several of these studies neglected to take into consideration possible confounding factors, such as consumption of cruciferous vegetables, dietary fiber, and other food items and micronutrients that have been shown to reduce the risk of colon cancer. For example, the Finnish population consumes high amounts of fat, mainly saturated fat; but the low incidence of colon cancer in that country may be explained in part by the fact that the Finns consume diets high in cereal fiber (Jensen et al., 1982; Reddy et al., 1978). In addition, several studies have combined cases of colon and rectal cancer, despite the evidence that these conditions do not have an identical etiology. Finally, some of these studies may have been hampered by the possibility that diets within communities have been too uniform to permit associations between diet and disease to be detected (McKewon-Eyssen, 1983). However, the majority of case-control studies support a role of dietary fat and fiber in the incidence of colon cancer.

When one visualizes the overall relationship between diet and colon cancer, one very large unexplored area is the interaction of micronutrients, dietary fiber, and dietary fat. Since most of these macro- and micronutrients interact with each other to elicit maximum biological effects, it is likely that the aggregate effect of groups of nutrients, rather than a single nutrient, will be the critical parameter in determining whether a protective or enhancing effect is exerted in carcinogenesis. Therefore, additional studies are needed to gain new insights into the interaction of macro- and micronutrients and dietary fibers in colon cancer.

The search for genotoxic carcinogens associated with the etiology of colon cancer has been initiated by several laboratories, using Ames' *Salmonella typhimurium*/mammalian microsomal assay system to determine the mutagenic (or presumptive carcinogenic) activity in the feces in an attempt to understand the nature of these compounds and their relevance to colon cancer (Ehrich *et al.*, 1979; Reddy *et al.*, 1980b; Mower *et al.*, 1982; Kuhnlein *et al.*, 1981; Bruce *et al.*, 1977). These studies demonstrate that populations that are at high risk for colon cancer and consuming either a high-fat and/or nonvegetarian diet excrete increased levels of fecal mutagens compared to low-risk populations who are consuming either a low-fat, high-fiber diet, a high-fat, high-fiber diet, or a vegetarian diet. Although mutagenicity assays of fecal extracts have yet to provide detailed information on the presence of biologically active species in the feces, an important finding was that of Hirai and Kingston (1982), who noted that the mutagenicity of feces of certain donors appears to be due to a type of compound, namely (*S*)-3-(1,3,5,7,9-dodecapentaenoyloxy)-1,2-propanediol, produced by anaerobic bacteria. Other studies demonstrated the presence of different types of mutagenic compounds in the feces that probably play a role in human colon cancer (Mower *et al.*, 1982; Reddy *et al.*, 1984). Identification of these mutagens is of great importance.

In addition, a distinct and direct means of determining the presence and effect of such compounds (mutagens), the culture of intact fragments of colon in organ culture and the DNA repair system offers realistic test systems in which the action of these mutagens or agents on isolated mammalian tissue can be studied under rigidly controlled conditions and also facilitates the examination of critical events in the genotoxic actions of these substances at the molecular and cellular levels in the putative target organ. This novel approach to the detection of these substances should aid in the effort to isolate the compounds that seemingly play a role in colon cancer. An area that also requires immediate attention is the determination of carcinogenic activity of these mutagens in animal models.

Another area that requires attention is diet intervention studies in high-risk patients. Since the same factors that affect colon cancer incidence in various population groups also influence the recurrence of benign adenomatous polyps after polypectomy, transformation of adenomas into carcinomas of the colon, and recurrence of colon carcinomas after surgical intervention in cancer patients, dietary intervention in these patients should result in an objective increase in their disease-free survival and overall survival. The same holds for symptomatic and asymptomatic patients affected with autosomal, dominantly inherited nonpolyposis colorectal cancer syndrome, which may account for as much as 5–7% of all colorectal cancer. The overall goal is to reduce the incidence of colon cancer in these high-risk groups. Randomized prospective clinical trials should be performed in patients at high risk for colon cancer with the aim of reducing the incidence of new polyps or carcinomas.

3. LABORATORY ANIMAL MODEL STUDIES

The possible role of dietary fat and certain dietary fibers on colon carcinogenesis has received support from studies in animal models (Freeman, 1983; Nigro and Bull, 1983; Reddy, 1983a; Wargovich and Felkner, 1983). In several earlier studies on dietary fat and colon cancer, interpretation of results between high- and low-fat diets was complicated by the use of diets of varying caloric density and confounded by different intakes of other nutrients. In addition, a recent study in which all experimental diets were made in a 5% agar solution and contained slightly higher levels of minerals and vitamins over recommended levels suggests that high dietary fat had no measurable effect in colon carcinogenesis (Nauss et al., 1983). It has been shown that dietary agar and the related sulfated polysaccharide carrageenan enhance colon carcinogenesis in animal models (Glauert et al., 1981; Watanabe et al., 1979). Therefore, it is difficult to interpret the results generated with this type of experimental design.

Studies carried out in our laboratory to determine the effect of high dietary fat on colon tumor induction by a variety of carcinogens, 1,2-dimethylhydrazine (DMH), methylazoxymethanol (MAM acetate), 3,2′-dimethyl-4-aminobiphenyl (DMAB), or methylnitrosourea (MNU), which not only differ in metabolic activation, but also represent a broad spectrum of exogenous carcinogens, indicate that, irrespective of the colon carcinogens, animals fed a diet containing 20% beef fat, corn oil, or lard had a greater incidence of colon tumors than did rats fed a diet containing 5% fat.

A recent study from our laboratory, in which the intake of all nutrients and calories except fat calories were controlled, provided evidence for the effect of types and amount of fat on colon carcinogenesis (Reddy and Maeura, 1984). AOM-induced colon tumor incidence was increased in F344 rats fed 23.5% corn oil or 23.5% safflower oil diet compared to those fed 5%

corn oil or safflower oil diets (Table I). However, diets containing 23.5% olive oil or coconut oil had no enhancing effect on colon tumor promotion. In another study, Sprague-Dawley rats fed a diet containing 10% corn oil had more DMH-induced colon tumors than did those fed a diet containing 5% corn oil or 9% coconut oil + 1% linoleic acid (Wargovich and Felkner, 1983). Another study suggested that dietary unsaturated fats have colon tumor-promoting activity (Sakaguchi et al., 1984). These results suggest that not only the amount, but also the types of fat (differing in fatty acid composition) are important factors in colon tumor promotion.

Although the concept of dietary fiber involvement in colon carcino-genesis is of great importance, studies examining the possible role of various types of dietary fiber in animal models appear to have provided conflicting results (Reddy, 1982). This discrepancy might have been due in part to the nature of the carcinogen used, to differences in the susceptibility of different rat strains to carcinogen treatment, to variation in the composition of diets, to qualitative and quantitative differences in administered intact fibers and their components, to relative differences in food intake by the animals, and/or to differences in experimental design and duration of the experiment. In recent studies, when diets containing 20% wheat bran were fed to rats only during, but not after, carcinogen treatment, there was an increase in colon tumor incidence (Jacobs, 1983; Barnes et al., 1983). It is possible that in these studies, a switch from a high-fiber experimental diet to a standard or a fiber-free diet during the post-carcinogen treatment period failed to show any protective effect of wheat bran. It is also possible that a high-wheat bran (20%) diet, when fed during the period of carcinogen administration, caused unavailability of certain essential trace elements that are involved in carcino-gen metabolism and detoxification, thereby enhancing colon tumorigenesis.

TABLE I. Effect of Types and Amount of Fat on Azoxymethane-Induced Colon Carcinogenesis in Rats

	Percent animals with colon tumors		
Diet group	Total with tumors	Adenoma	Adenocarcinoma
5% Corn oil	17	10	7
23.5% Corn oil	46[a]	14	32
5% Safflower oil	13	7	6
23.5% Safflower oil	36[a]	14	22
5% Olive oil	10	7	3
23.5% Olive oil	13	10	3
23.5% Coconut oil	13	10	3

[a]Significantly different from their respective 5% fat diet at $p < 0.05$.

Our recent studies on the relationship between dietary fiber and colon cancer indicate that animals fed diets containing 15% wheat bran or citrus fiber had a lower incidence of AOM- or DMAB-induced colon tumors, whereas a diet containing 15% corn bran enhanced DMAB-induced colon tumors (Reddy, 1983). The relationship between the components of dietary fiber has been studied in our laboratory (Reddy, 1983; Watanabe et al., 1979). Animals fed diets containing 15% pectin or 7.5% lignin had a lower colon tumor incidence compared to those fed control diets (Table II). These studies thus indicate that protection against colon cancer in animal models depends on the types or components of fiber taken.

Studies thus far conducted in various laboratories have used two levels of dietary fat and of dietary fiber to demonstrate the effect of fat or fiber on colon carcinogenesis. In addition, the modulating effects of most nutrients are often studied individually, with little regard for interacting effects with other nutrients. However, people are constantly exposed to multiple nutritional insults, so that the justification for multifactorial studies is apparent. The interrelationship and synergistic effects of various micronutrients such as trace minerals and vitamins and saturated and unsaturated fats have been well recognized in nutrition. Further, there are reports of decreased mineral balances when the level of fiber in the diet is increased (Judd et al., 1983). Decreased absorption of minerals due to binding by fiber is not so important if mineral intakes are sufficiently high to maintain near-zero or positive balances. As discussed earlier, since most of these macro- and micronutrients and dietary fiber interact with each other to produce biological effects, it is likely that synergistic and aggregate effects of groups of nutrients, rather than a single nutrient, will be the critical factors in yielding a protective or enhancing effect in carcinogenesis.

Therefore, additional studies are needed to: (1) determine threshhold levels, if any, of saturated and unsaturated fats, and of various dietary fibers that exhibit measurable enhancing or protective effects, respectively, on colon carcinogenesis; (2) determine the role of dietary excess, adequacy, or deficiency of certain trace minerals and vitamins individually or in combination in colon carcinogenesis; and (3) determine the interaction among trace

TABLE II. Effect of Dietary Lignin on DMAB-Induced Colon Carcinogenesis in Rats

Diet group	Percent animals with colon tumors	Tumors/tumor-bearing animal	
		Adenoma	Adenocarcinoma
Control diet	30	0.78±0.20	0.56±0.11[a]
7.5% Lignin diet	26	0.82±0.12	0.18±0.10

[a]Significantly different at $p < 0.05$.

minerals, vitamins, saturated and unsaturated fats, and various types of dietary fiber on colon carcinogenesis.

4. MECHANISMS OF NUTRITIONAL FACTORS IN COLON CANCER

Currently, much of our knowledge on the mechanism of dietary fat in colon carcinogenesis is based on experiments conducted in humans (metabolic epidemiology) and in animal models (Reddy, 1983a). The major significance of these studies is that the primary effect of dietary fat appears to be during the promotional phase of carcinogenesis rather than during the initiation phase (Nigro and Bull, 1983). The amount of dietary fat modulates the concentration of intestinal bile acids as well as the metabolic activity of gut microflora, which, in turn, metabolize these sterols and other substances into tumorigenic compounds in the colon. These studies have demonstrated that high-fat diets increase the excretion of bile acids into the gut. These bile acids have been shown to act as colon tumor promoters, but do not have the properties of genotoxic carcinogens. This is important, since the current views on properties of promoters note that the effect of such agents is highly dependent on dose and on length of exposure, and this provides an opportunity of reducing the risk of colon cancer development by lowering the concentration of bile acids by dietary means.

The mechanism by which a protective effect might be exerted by dietary fiber, which comprises a heterogeneous group of carbohydrates, including cellulose, hemicellulose, and pectin, and a noncarbohydrate substance, lignin, has been the subject of a recent workshop (Vahouny and Kritchevsky, 1982). The protective effect of dietary fiber in colon carcinogenesis depends on the nature and source of fiber in the diet. The protective effect of dietary fiber may be due to adsorption, dilution, and/or metabolism of cocarcinogens, promoters, and yet to be identified carcinogens by the components of the fiber. Different types of nonnutritive fiber could bind the tumorigenic compounds and affect the enterohepatic circulation of tumorigenic compounds, as well as dilute potential carcinogens and cocarcinogens by their bulking effect.

Additional studies are needed not only to determine the effect of dietary fat or dietary fiber on colon carcinogenesis during the stage of initiation, but also the mode of action of dietary fat and fiber during initiation.

5. CONCLUSIONS

During the last decade, a substantial amount of progress has been made in understanding the relationship between dietary constituents and the development of colon cancer. Although the information base on the effects of fat and fiber on colon cancer is sufficiently convincing, further studies may eventually define the exact mechanism for the effect exerted by various dietary fats, fibers, and other dietary components and delineate the precise diets capable of counteracting some of these effects.

The general recommendations for additional studies are summarized as follows.

Epidemiologic studies:

1. Better nutritional data-gathering methods should be developed to monitor and quantify dietary intake of various nutrients in human populations, to establish more clearly the relationship of dietary pattern and occurrence of colon cancer.

2. Case-control studies should be conducted to assess the interaction of various micro- and macronutrients and dietary fiber in colon carcinogenesis.

3. Intervention studies should be conducted using foods or food components believed to be associated with a lower colon cancer risk.

Animal model studies:

1. The relative roles of the level and types of fat in both initiation and postinitiation stages of carcinogenesis as well as the threshold levels at which dietary fat begins to exert measurable effects on carcinogenesis should be studied.

2. The relative roles of the levels and types of dietary fiber in all phases of tumor formation should be investigated.

3. The interaction of the levels and types of fat with micronutrients (vitamins and minerals) and dietary fibers as it relates to the incidence of colon tumors should be studied.

4. The interaction of the amount and type of fiber with micronutrients should be explored.

ACKNOWLEDGMENTS. This work was supported in part by grants CA-17613, CA-29602, CA-36892, CA-37663, and CA-32617 and contract CP-85659 from the National Cancer Institute. The author acknowledges the assistance of Arlene Banow in preparation of the manuscript.

REFERENCES

Barnes, D. S., Clapp, N. K., Scott, D. A., Oberst, D. L., and Berry, S. G., 1983, Effects of wheat, rice, corn, and soybean bran on 1,2-dimethylhydrazine-induced large bowel tumorigenesis in F344 rats, *Nutr. Cancer* **5**:1–9.

Bruce, W. R., Varghese, A. J., Furrer, R., and Land, P. C., 1977. A mutagen in the feces of normal humans, in: *Origins of Human Cancer* (H. H. Hiatt, J. D. Watson, and J. A. Winsten, eds.), Cold Spring Harbor Laboratory, Cold Spring Harbor, New York, pp. 1641–1646.

Burkitt, D. P., 1971, Epidemiology of cancer of the colon and rectum, *Cancer* **28**:3–13.

Burkitt, D. P., 1975, Large bowel carcinogenesis. An epidemiologic jigsaw puzzle, *J. Nat. Cancer Inst.* **54**:3–6.

Clayson, D. B., 1975, Nutritional and experimental carcinogenesis, *Cancer Res.* **35**:3292–3300.

Correa, P., and Haenszel, W., 1978, Epidemiology of large bowel cancer, in: *Advances in Cancer Research*, Volume 26 (G. Klein and S. Weinhouse, eds.), Academic, New York, pp. 1–141.

Doll, R., and Peto, R., 1981, The causes of cancer: Quantitative estimates of avoidable risks of cancer in the United States today, *J. Nat. Cancer Inst.* **66**:1191–1308.

Ehrich, M., Ashell, J. E., van Tassell, R. L., Wilkins, T. D., Walker, A. R. P., and Richardson, N. J., 1979 Mutations in the feces of 3 South African populations at different levels of risk for colon cancer, *Mutat. Res.* **64**:231–240.

Freeman, H. J., 1983, Dietary fibers and colon cancer, in: *Experimental Colon Carcinogenesis* (H. Autrup and G. M. Williams, eds.), CRC, Boca Raton, Florida, pp. 267–279.

Glauert, H. P., Bennink, M. R., and Sander, C. H., 1981, Enhancement of 1,2-dimethylhydrazine-induced colon carcinogenesis in mice by dietary agar, *Food Cosmet. Toxicol.* **19**: 281–286.

Graham, S., Dayal, H., Swanson, M., Mittelman, A., and Wilkinson, G., 1978, Diet in the epidemiology of cancer of the colon and rectum, *J. Nat. Cancer Inst.* **61**:709–714.

Hill, M. J., 1982, Bile acids and human colorectal cancer, in: *Dietary Fiber in Health and Disease* (G. V. Vahouny and D. Kritchevsky, eds.), Plenum, New York, pp. 299–312.

Hirai, N., and Kingston, D. G. I., 1982, Structure elucidation of a potent mutagen from human feces, *J. Am. Chem. Soc.* **104**:6149.

Jacobs, L. R., 1983, Enhancement of rat colon carcinogenesis by wheat bran consumption during the stage of 1,2-dimethylhydrazine administration, *Cancer Res.* **43**:4059–4061.

Jensen, O. M., MacLennan, R., and Wahrendorf, J., 1982, Diet, bowel function, fecal characteristics and large bowel cancer in Denmark and Finland, *Nutr. Cancer* **4**:5–19.

Judd, J. T., Kelsay, J. L., and Mertz, W., 1983, Potential risks from low-fat diets, *Semin. Oncol.* **10**:273–280.

Kolonel, L. N., Hankin, J. H., Lee, J., Chu, S. Y., Nomura, A. M. Y., and Ward, H. M., 1981, Nutrient intakes in relation to cancer incidence in Hawaii, *Br. J. Cancer* **44**:332.

Kuhnlein, U., Bergstrom, D., and Kuhnlein, H., 1981, Mutations in feces from vegetarians and non-vegetarians, *Mutat. Res.* **45**:1–12.

Manousos, O., Day, N. E., Trichopoulos, D., Gerovassilis, F., and Tzonou, A., 1983, Diet and colorectal cancer: A case control study, *Int. J. Cancer* **32**:1–5.

McKeown-Eyssen, G., 1983, A diet to prevent colon cancer: How do we get there from here, in: *Diet, Nutrition and Cancer: From Basic Research to Policy Implications* (D. A. Roe, ed.), Alan R. Liss, New York, pp. 243–256.

Miller, A. B., Howe, G. R., Jain, M., Craib, K. J. P., and Harrison, L. 1983, Food items and food groups as risk factors in a case–control study of diet and colorectal cancer, *Int. J. Cancer* **32**:155–161.

Mower, H. F., Ichinotsubo, D., Wang, L. W., Mandel, M., Stemmerman, G., Nomura, A., Heilbrun, L., Kamiya, S. and Shimada, A. 1982, Fecal mutagens in two Japanese populations with different colon cancer risks, *Cancer Res.* **42**:1164–1169.

Nauss, K. M., Locniskoor, M., and Newberne, P. M., 1983, Effect of alterations in the quality and quantity of dietary fat on 1,2-dimethylhydrazine-induced colon tumorigenesis in rats, *Cancer Res.* **43**:4083–4090.

Nigro, N. D., and Bull, A. W., 1983, The two-step concept of intestinal carcinogenesis, in: *Experimental Colon Carcinogenesis* (H. Autrup and G. M. Williams, eds.), CRC, Boca Raton, Florida, pp. 215–224.

Palmer, S., 1983, Diet, nutrition and cancer: The future of dietary policy, *Cancer Res.* **43**: 2059S–2514S.

Reddy, B. S., 1982, Dietary fiber and colon carcinogenesis: A critical review, in: *Dietary Fiber in Health and Disease* (G. V. Vahouny and D. Kritchevsky, eds.), Plenum, New York, pp. 265–285.

Reddy, B. S., 1983a, Dietary lipids and their relationship to colon cancer, in: *Diet, Nutrition and Cancer: From Basic Research to Policy Implications* (D. A. Roe, ed.), Alan R. Liss, New York, pp. 17–31.

Reddy, B. S., 1983b, Dietary fat and colon cancer, in: *Experimental Colon Carcinogenesis* (H. Autrup and G. M. Williams, eds.), CRC, Boca Raton, Florida, pp. 225–239.

Reddy, B. S., Cohen, L., McCoy, G. D., Hill, P., Weisburger, J. H., and Wynder, E. L., 1980, Nutrition and its relationship to cancer, in: *Advances in Cancer Research,* Volume 32 (G. Klein and S. Weinhouse, eds.), Academic, New York, pp. 237–345.

Reddy, B. S., Hedges, A. T., Laakso, K., and Wynder, E. L., 1978, Metabolic epidemiology of large bowel cancer: Fecal bulk and constituents of high-risk North American and low-risk Finnish population, *Cancer* **42:**2832–2838.

Reddy, B. S., and Maeura, Y., 1984, Tumor promotion by dietary fat in azoxymethane-induced colon carcinogenesis in female F344 rats: Influence of amount and source of dietary fat, *J. Nat. Cancer Inst.* **72:**745–750.

Reddy, B. S., Maeura, Y., and Wayman, M., 1983, Effect of dietary corn bran and auto-hydrolyzed lignin on 3,2′-dimethyl-4-aminobiphenyl-induced intestinal carcinogenesis in male F344 rats, *J. Nat. Cancer Inst.* **71:**419–423.

Reddy, B. S., Sharma, C., Darby, L., Laakso, K., and Wynder, E. L., 1980b, Metabolic epidemiology of large bowel cancer: Fecal mutagens in high- and low-risk population for colon cancer, A preliminary report, *Mutat. Res.* **72:**511–522.

Reddy, B. S., Sharma, C., Mathews, L., and Engle, A., 1984, Fecal mutagens from subjects consuming a mixed-Western diet, *Mutat. Res.* **135:**11–19.

Sakaguchi, M., Hiramatsu, Y., Takada, H., Yamamura, M., Hioki, K., Saito, K., and Yamamoto, M., 1984, Effect of dietary unsaturated and saturated fats on azoxymethane-induced colon carcinogenesis in rats, *Cancer Res.* **44:**1472–1477.

Schottenfeld, D., 1983, Overview, in: *Diet, Nutrition and Cancer: From Basic Research to Policy Implications* (D. A. Roe, ed.), Alan R. Liss, New York, pp. 197–201.

Vahouny, G. V., and Kritchevsky, D. (eds.), 1982, *Dietary Fiber in Health and Disease,* Plenum, New York.

Wargovich, M. J., and Felkner, I. C., 1983, Metabolic activation of DMH by colonic microsomes: A process influenced by type of dietary fat, *Nutr. Cancer* **4:**146–153.

Watanabe, K., Reddy, B. S., Weisburger, J. H., and Kritchevsky, D., 1979, Effect of dietary alfalfa, pectin and wheat bran on azoxymethane or methylnitrosourea-induced colon carcinogenesis in F344 rats, *J. Nat. Cancer Inst.* **63:**141–145.

West, D. W., Lyon, J. L., Gardner, J. W., Schuman, K., Stanish, W., Mahoney, A., Sorenson, A., and Avlon, E. 1983, Epidemiology of Colon Cancer in Utah, 1983 Workshop: A Decade of Achievements and Challenges in Large Bowel Carcinogenesis, National Large Bowel Cancer Project, Houston, Texas, pp. 3–5.

Wynder, E. L., 1975, The epidemiology of large bowel cancer, *Cancer Res.* **35:**3388–3394.

Wynder, E. L., and Reddy, B. S., 1983, Dietary fat and fiber and colon cancer, *Semin. Oncol.* **10:**264–272.

41

Bile Acids and Colon Cancer: Future Prospectives

MICHAEL J. HILL

1. INTRODUCTION

At St. Mark's Hospital, London, we believe that colorectal carcino-genesis is a multistage process (Morson, 1974; Hill *et al.*, 1978) and that prevention of the disease might be achieved by interfering with any of those stages. Thus, our approach has been to try to identify high-risk patient groups and to monitor those persons as intensively as resources allow in order to prevent or to diagnose the disease at an early stage; the alternative of mass screening is expensive in time and resources and is highly invasive in the vast majority of the population, who are probably at very low risk of the disease. The first priority must therefore be to identify the persons at greatest risk.

In the future, it is likely that the high-risk groups will be studied not only clinically, but also biochemically. Clinical prevention of colorectal cancer can be achieved by polpectomy or, in some conditions, by prophylactic colectomy. We also hope in the future to be able to achieve prevention of the disease by dietary change.

Persons are thought to be at increased risk of colorectal carcinogenesis if they are closely related to a colorectal cancer case, if they have a history of colorectal adenomas, if they have adenomatosis coli, or if they belong to "cancer families." In all of these situations there is a genetic predisposition to

MICHAEL J. HILL • PHLS Centre for Applied Microbiology and Research, Salisbury, Wiltshire SP4 0JG, United Kingdom.

colorectal carcinogenesis, which is thought to be expressed as a result of environmental factors, especially in the colonic environment. This expression may be inhibited by decreasing the rate of adenoma formation or by decreasing the rate of progression from adenoma to carcinoma.

Dietary changes that might decrease the risk of colorectal cancer could at the same time increase the risk of other diseases; for example, Kinlen has shown that vegetarians (i.e., those eating a high-fiber diet), although having a slightly below average risk of colorectal cancer, have an above average risk of gastric cancer (Kinlen *et al.*, 1983), a disease with a much poorer prognosis. It would therefore be extremely unwise in view of this risk to recommend dietary changes for the whole population, and this provides a further reason for concentrating on those at high risk of colorectal cancer.

2. IDENTIFYING HIGH RISK GROUPS

It has been postulated that there is an autosomal recessive gene that confers adenoma-proneness on an individual (Veale, 1965), that is, increased sensitivity of the colonic mucosa to environmental factors. The evidence for this is largely based on studies of the risk of colorectal cancer in relatives of index cases with the disease. It is essential that an attempt be made soon to test this hypothesis in an autopsy series of patients. It could only be tested in a country where there is a very high proportion of autopsies and where the colon is routinely examined; in addition, it could only be done in a country where record linkage allows the identification of close relatives. The risks to be measured would be (1) that of colorectal adenomas in the brothers and sisters of an index case compared with that in the normal population; (2) that of colorectal adenomas in children of a parent with colorectal adenomas and in children both of whose parents had colorectal adenomas compared with that in the normal population. If the Veale hypothesis is correct, then close relatives of persons with colorectal adenomas are at increased risk of developing adenomas and therefore of developing colorectal cancer. The hypothesis is, however, very difficult to test.

It is easier to identify colorectal cancer cases, since these are registered. It has been demonstrated by many groups that the risk of colorectal cancer is increased in relatives of index cases (Table I). This should be taken further; the risk of the disease in the normal population should be compared with that in persons where one parent or both parents had colorectal cancer. Again, if the Veale hypothesis is correct, the risk of carcinogenesis in a person both of whose parents had the disease ought to be high and such persons should be given special attention in any screening program.

Bile acids have been implicated as risk factors in the causation of

TABLE I. Large Bowel Cancer Incidence in Relatives of Index Cases,
Relative to That Expected from the Normal Populations

| | Incidence of large bowel cancer | | | |
| | Parents | | Siblings | |
Reference	Expected	Observed	Expected	Observed
Woolf (1958)	1	10	7	16
Macklin (1960)	5.2	17	45	14
Burdette (1971)	64	435	—	—
Lovett (1976)	8.3	23	3.4	18
Duncan and Kyle (1982)	—	—	1	8
Woolf et al. (1955)	—	—	2.6[a]	25[a]

[a] Adenomas.

colorectal cancer and a number of studies have shown a higher prevalence of bile acid receptors in the colon of cancer cases than in controls. For example, Summerton et al. (1983) found bile acid receptors in the colonic mucosa of 31% of colorectal cancer cases and only 2.6% of controls; it would be of great interest to carry out a prospective study of the fate of persons with colonic mucosal bile acid receptors, because this might be a useful marker in identifying high risk patient groups.

3. PREVENTION OF ADENOGENESIS

The environmental factors causing the formation of adenomas in adenoma-prone persons can only be investigated in persons identified as adenoma-prone. This can be achieved by studying the rate of recurrence of adenomas in persons who have already been diagnosed with an adenoma. In a pilot study of patients at St. Mark's Hospital the rate of recurrence was 3.3% per year in men under 55 years of age, nearly 4% per year in men over 55 years of age, 1.5% per year in women under 55 years of age, and 2.5% per year in women over 55 years of age. Over a 10-year followup period, following removal of an adenoma, the cumulative risk of a second adenoma was 35% in men and 20% in women, but some patients developed no further adenomas, while others developed one each year. Populations exist, therefore, for the study of the factors causing adenoma formation. Determination of such factors would then provide another means of cancer prevention.

At present we have no clues to the identity of any of the factors causing adenoma formation.

4. FACTORS CAUSING THE PROGRESSION OF ADENOMAS TO CARCINOMAS

There is a growing body of evidence implicating bile acids in this stage of colorectal carcinogenesis. This includes (Table II):

1. The detection of bile acid-binding sites in the colonic mucosa of colorectal cancer cases but not of controls (e.g., Summerton *et al.*, 1983).
2. The demonstration that bile acids cause dysplastic changes in the colonic mucosa (Wargovich *et al.*, 1983).
3. The demonstration that bile acids are more readily taken up by the mucosa of adenoma patients than of control persons (Van der Werf *et al.*, 1983).
4. The correlation between FBA concentration and adenoma size (Hill *et al.*, 1983).
5. The demonstration that bile acids are comutagenic (Wilpart *et al.*, 1983) as well as cocarcinogenic (Narisawa *et al.*, 1974).

Recently the role of bile acids has been refined as a result of *in vivo* and *in vitro* studies. Wilpart *et al.* (1983) showed that certain secondary bile acids are comutagenic (Table III); structure–activity studies showed that the co-mutagenic activity was decreased by the presence of a 7-hydroxyl group, that 3β-hydroxy steroids were less active than their 3α-hydroxy analogues, and that 5α-steroids were more active then their 5β isomers. They also showed that although deoxycholic and lithocholic acids were both comutagenic, they were antagonistic; in mixtures of the two, the ratio was a better indicator of activity than the sum or the difference. A similar *in vivo* observation was made by Owen *et al.* (1983), who showed that the ratio of lithocholic to deoxycholic acid (L/D) was much higher in colorectal cancer cases than in controls, and in adenoma patients was related to adenoma size.

TABLE II. Evidence Relating Bile Acids to Colorectal Carcinogenesis

Study	Observation
Comparison of populations	Fecal bile acid (FBA) concentration correlated with colorectal cancer (CRC) incidence
Animal studies	Diet or surgical changes that increase FBA increase CRC incidence
Studies with pure bile acids	Secondary bile acids are comutagenic and cocarcinogenic, and cause dysplasia in the colonic mucosa
Bile acid receptors	Bile acid receptors are found in the mucosa of CRC patients, not controls

TABLE III. Structure–Activity Relationships to Comutagenicity
of Bile Acids[a]

Structural change	Effect on comutagencity
Loss of 7α-hydroxyl group	Increase
Inversion of 3α-hydroxyl group to 3β	Decrease
Inversion of 5β carbon to 5α	Increase

[a] Data from Wilpart *et al.* (1983).

Bile acids with a 5α configuration are readily detected in human feces (Wait *et al.*, 1984), and their higher comutagenic activity might provide the explanation for the association between clostridia with cholanoyl 4-5 dehydrogenase activity (the first stage in inversion at the 5 position) and colorectal cancer.

Further studies are necessary to see whether the L/D ratio has any value in predicting the risk of colorectal carcinogenesis; in addition, the factors determining the L/D ratio still have to be elucidated. Any action that increases the proportion of chenodeoxycholic acid in bile will increase the L/D ratio; cholecystectomy both increases the proportion of chenodeoxycholic acid (Van der Linden *et al.*, 1983) and increases the risk of bowel cancer.

5. CONCLUSIONS

Colorectal cancer is most likely to be conquered by concentrating resources on those at highest risk of the disease. The first priority is therefore to improve the identification of those at high risk.

In such patients, colorectal cancer may be prevented by preventing adenoma formation or by preventing the progression from adenoma to carcinoma.

ACKNOWLEDGMENT. This work is financially supported by the Cancer Research Campaign, to whom I express my sincere thanks.

REFERENCES

Burdette, W. J., 1971, Identification of antecedents of colorectal cancer, *Cancer* **28**:51–56

Duncan, J. L., and Kyle, J., 1982, Family incidence of carcinoma of the colon and rectum in north-east Scotland, *Gut* **23**:169–171.

Hill, M. J., Morson, B. C., and Bussey, H. J. R., 1978, Aetiology of the adenoma–carcinoma sequence in large bowel, *Lancet* **ii**:535–538.

Hill, M. J., Morson, B. C., and Thompson, M. H., 1983, The role of faecal bile acids in large bowel carcinogenesis, *Br. J. Cancer* **48**:143.

Kinlen, L. J., Hermon, C., and Smith, P. G., 1983, A proportionate study of cancer mortality among members of a vegetarian society, *Br. J. Cancer* **48**:355–361.

Lovett, E., 1976, Family studies in cancer of the colon and rectum, *Br. J. Surg.* **63**:13–18.

Macklin, M. T., 1960, Inheritance of cancer of the stomach and large intestine in man, *J. Nat. Cancer Inst.* **24**:551–571.

Morson, B. C., 1974, The polyp–cancer sequence in the large bowel, *Proc. R. Soc. Med.* **67**: 451–457.

Narisawa, T., Magadia, N. E., and Wynder, E. L., 1974, Promoting effect of bile acids on colon carcinogenesis after intrarectal instillation of N-methyl-N-nitroso-N-nitroguanidine in rats, *Cancer Res.* **53**:1093–1097.

Owen, R. W., Dodo, M., Thompson, M. H., and Hill, M. J., 1983, The faecal ratio of lithocholic acid to deoxycholic acid may be an important aetiological factor in colorectal cancer, *Eur. J. Cancer. Clin. Oncol.* **19**:307.

Summerton, J., Flynn, M., Cooke, T., and Taylor, I., 1983, Bile acid receptors in colorectal cancer, *Br. J. Surg.* **70**:549–551.

Van der Linden, W., Katzenstein, B., and Nakayama, F., 1983, The possible carcinogenic effect of cholecystectomy. No post operative increase in the proportion of secondary bile acids, *Cancer* **52**:1265–1268.

Van der Werf, S. D., Nagengast, F. M., Henegouwen, G. P., Huijbregts, A. W., and Van Tongeren, J., 1983, Intracolonic environment and the presence of colonic adenomas in man, *Gut* **24**:876–880.

Veale, A. M. O., 1965, *Intestinal Polyposes*, Eugenics Laboratory Memoirs, Series 40, Cambridge University Press, London.

Wait, R., and Thompson, M. H., 1984, Minor faecal bile acids and large bowel cancer, *Biochem. Soc. Trans.* **12**:1134–1135.

Wargovich, M. J., Eng, V. W., Newmark, H. L., and Bruce, W. R., 1983, Calcium amelioriates the toxic effect of deocycholic acid on colonic epithlium, *Carcinogenesis* **4**:1205–1207.

Wilpart, M., Mainguet, P., Maskens, A., and Roberfroid, M., 1983, Structure–activity relationship amongst biliary acids showing co-mutagenic activity towards dimethylhydrazine, *Carcinogenesis* **4**:1239–1241.

Woolf, C. M., 1958, A genetic study of carcinoma of the large intestine, *Am. J. Hum. Genet.* **10**:42–47.

Woolf, C. M., Richards, B. C., and Gardner, E. J., 1955, Occasional discrete polyps of the colon and rectum showing an inherited tendency in a kindred, *Cancer* **8**:403–408.

42

Dietary Fiber and Cancer: Future Research Directions

WILLIAM D. DEWYS, RITVA R. BUTRUM, and PETER GREENWALD

An increasing body of knowledge supports the hypothesis that dietary fiber has a protective role against carcinogenesis. The evidence includes results from studies in experimental animal models and epidemiologic studies in human populations. In general we feel that leads from laboratory and epidemiologic research should be considered for further testing in clinical trials and/or translated into recommendations for the public. We therefore raise two questions: Which leads from our fund of information should now be subjected to further study in human clinical trials, and what recommendations should we be proposing for the public?

Related questions are: What is the role of scientists in making recommendations as to public policy, and how much evidence is needed in order to reach conclusions and/or make recommendations? Different scientists will answer the question on the role of scientists differently. These answers in general can be classified into three categories:

1. Nonrecommenders: the role of scientists is to discover facts, not to make recommendations of public policy.
2. Hesitant recommenders: we are not sure that changes in diet will reduce the risk of cancer, and are concerned that changes in diet might have unexpected, unfavorable effects.

WILLIAM D. DEWYS, RITVA R. BUTRUM, and PETER GREENWALD • National Cancer Institute, Bethesda, Maryland 20205.

3. Recommenders: scientists should periodically review the available data and recommend guidelines for the public even if these recommendations are of an interim nature and subject to later revision and refinement.

The question as to how much additional evidence is needed in order to make recommendations on dietary fiber requires continuing attention.

Regarding results from animal models, we should view these from the perspective of uncertainties as to the relevance of a particular model for the human situation. The animal models usually involve the administration of a large single dose of carcinogen, whereas humans more likely are exposed to low doses of carcinogens on a chronic basis. Also, we are not sure which carcinogens humans are exposed to, except in rare industrial exposures, and therefore we must raise a question as to the relevance of the carcinogen used in the animal models. Furthermore, the physiological effects of dietary fiber and the intestinal microflora of the animal model may differ appreciably from those in humans. Thus, we would urge a healthy skepticism regarding the translation of animal model results into human recommendations.

Which foods should we be recommending for clinical trials or for incorporation into dietary guidelines? This question can be resolved into two subquestions; namely, which forms of dietary fiber are protective against carcinogenesis, and which foods contain these fibers in significant quantities? To resolve these questions, we need to expand the data base of comparative studies comparing a variety of different fiber types. We need more studies in animal models comparing the protective effects of different dietary fibers studied either as purified preparations or in foods that contain a predominance of a specific fiber component. We also require comparative studies in humans using a variety of fiber types in which the endpoint of the study is measurement of physiological or physiochemical effects thought to be relevant to carcinogenesis. As these studies clarify which fiber types are most relevant and most important, we will increasingly need to know which foods supply these fiber types. Accordingly, we need to expand our capabilities to analyze the fiber content of food and to perform systematic analyses of the major food sources of specific dietary fibers.

Which physiological and physiochemical effects of fiber are most relevant to carcinogenesis and to the prevention of carcinogenesis? Many mechanisms have been proposed and have been studied in both animals and humans, but the relative contribution of each of these effects or mechanisms is not well understood. Since these physiological and physicochemical effects may differ with different fiber types, resolution of this question has more than academic interest. If dilution of carcinogens or promoters is viewed as the predominant mechanism, then we should focus on fibers having the greatest effect on retaining fluid within the fecal contents and thus diluting any harmful chemicals. Alternatively, if adsorption of carcinogens or pro-moters to the fiber is an important mechanism, then one would wish to select dietary fibers having the greatest adsorptive capacity. Another possibility is that changes in fecal pH may be important either for metabolism of carcino-gens or for the metabolism of fecal bacteria and the production of fecal mutagens. If acidification is the major protective mechanism, then one could speculate that dietay fiber is not the only means of achieving acidification of the fecal contents. Administration of other chemicals, such as lactulose or sorbital, could also result in acidification of the fecal contents. Another possible mechanism is that byproducts of fermentation of fiber may have protective or chemopreventive effects either locally or systemically. An example is butyrate, which diffuses from the fecal contents into the colonic mucosal cells. In some cell systems butyrate has been found *in vitro* to cause differentiation of undifferentiated cells. In addition, we need to question whether the relevant effect is different for different carcinogens and/or different promoters. Perhaps we should aim for a spectrum of physiological changes rather than focusing on any one mechanism.

We also need more information of the dose–response relationships both for physiological effects and for protection against carcinogenesis. For ex-ample, if the protective effect increases with dose up to a threshold, then we need only assure an intake reaching this threshold level (Fig. 1). In contrast, the protective effect may continue to increase progressively with increasing dose (Fig. 2). In this case, if there are no unfavorable effects from the specific substance, one would recommend a maximum intake within the limits of a balanced diet. If there were unfavorable effects, the dose–response relation of these unfavorable effects should be clarified (Fig. 3). Risk/benefit ratios would then need to be considered in recommending a level of intake. Possible unfavorable effects from fiber, such as interference with absorption of minerals, require further quantitative study. As an example, in human studies one would not wish to increase the incidence of osteoporosis due to interference with absorption of calcium.

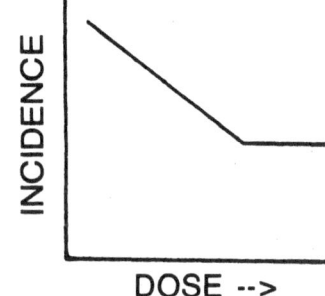

FIGURE 1. Dose-response relation with a thres-hold. Dietary intake above the threshold assures maximum protection.

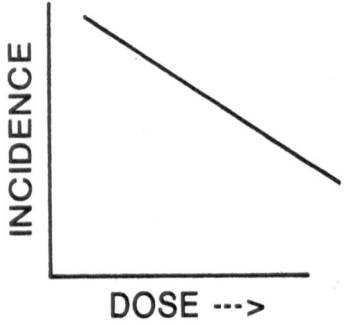

FIGURE 2. Linear dose-response relation without toxicity. Recommendation on intake is determined by the constraints of achieving a balanced diet.

Finally, we should raise a question regarding associated and/or reciprocal changes in the diet that may confound the effects of dietary fiber. By associated effects we have in mind that food sources of dietary fiber contain many important micronutrients that may themselves be protective against carcinogenesis. Thus it will be important to compare the effects of fiber in food versus the effects of that same fiber in pure form to dissect the contribution from the associated micronutrients in the food. Similarly, a diet high in fiber often has reciprocal changes in the dietary fat content and some of the observed effects may be attributed to these changes. This is particularly of concern in epidemiologic studies. Theoretically at least, in animal studies, one can control for this by administering diets of similar fat content but differing in their fiber content. While this is theoretically attractive, one must record appropriate indices of dietary intake to indeed document that comparable fat intake was achieved, since the other components of the diet, such as the dietary fiber, may influence the volume of food consumed and/or the amount of nutrients absorbed.

In this brief overview we have attempted to raise some of the questions requiring further attention and discussion. It is hoped that volumes such as the present one will begin to provide some clarification as to where there has been most progress, as opposed to areas where greater attention and resources are required.

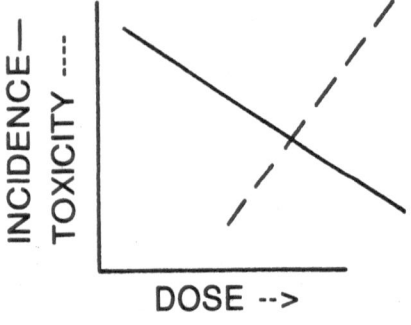

FIGURE 3. Linear dose-response relations for a protective effect and for an unfavorable effect. Recommendation on intake is based on a benefit/risk ratio.

Index